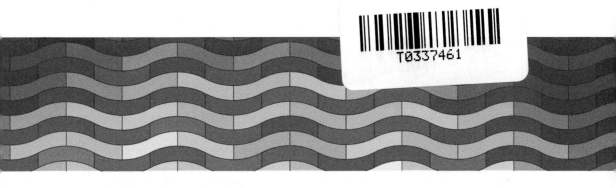

GREEN'S CHILD & ADOLESCENT CLINICAL PSYCHOPHARMACOLOGY

6TH EDITION

RICK T. BOWERS, MD
Clinical Professor
Division of Child and Adolescent Psychiatry
Wright State University Boonshoft School of
   Medicine
Dayton, Ohio

CHRISTINA G. WESTON, MD
Associate Clinical Professor
Division of Child and Adolescent Psychiatry
Wright State University Boonshoft School of
   Medicine
Dayton, Ohio

RYAN C. MAST, DO, MBA
Assistant Professor
Training Director of CAP Fellowship
Division of Child and Adolescent Psychiatry
Wright State University Boonshoft School of
   Medicine
Dayton, Ohio

SUZIE C. NELSON, MD
Assistant Professor
Associate Training Director
Division of Child and Adolescent Psychiatry
Wright State University Boonshoft School of
   Medicine
Dayton, Ohio

JULIA C. JACKSON, MD
Adult, Child, and Adolescent Psychiatrist
United States Air Force

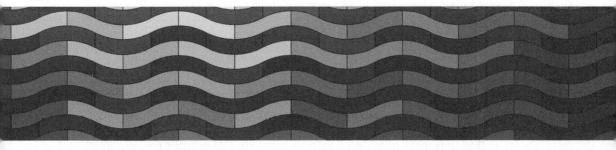

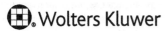
. Wolters Kluwer

Philadelphia • Baltimore • New York • London
Buenos Aires • Hong Kong • Sydney • Tokyo

Acquisitions Editor: Chris Teja
Editorial Coordinator: Tim Rinehart
Editorial Assistant: Brian Convery
Marketing Manager: Rachel Mante Leung
Production Project Manager: Linda Van Pelt
Design Coordinator: Holly McLaughlin
Manufacturing Coordinator: Beth Welsh
Prepress Vendor: S4Carlisle Publishing Services

Sixth edition

9 8 7

Printed in the United States of America

Library of Congress Cataloging-in-Publication Data

Names: Bowers, Rick (Physician), author. | Weston, Christina, author. | Mast,
    Ryan C., author. | Nelson, Suzie C., author. | Jackson, Julia, author. |
    Preceded by (work): Klykylo, William M. Green's child and adolescent
    clinical psychopharmacology.
Title: Green's child and adolescent clinical psychopharmacology / Rick T.
    Bowers, Christina G. Weston, Ryan C. Mast, Suzie C. Nelson, Julia C. Jackson.
Other titles: Child and adolescent clinical psychopharmacology
Description: 6th edition. | Philadelhia, PA: Wolters Kluwer, [2019] |
    Preceded by Green's child and adolescent clinical psychopharmacology /
    William M. Klykylo. Fifth edition. [2014]. | Includes bibliographical
    references and index.
Identifiers: LCCN 2018027356 | ISBN 9781975105600 (paperback : alk. paper)
Subjects: | MESH: Mental Disorders—drug therapy | Child |
    Psychopharmacology—methods | Psychotropic Drugs—therapeutic use |
    Adolescent
Classification: LCC RJ504.7 | NLM WS 350.2 | DDC 616.89/18—dc23 LC record available at
    https://lccn.loc.gov/2018027356

To our teachers, our students, our patients, and our families for their contributions and support, to editor Wayne Hugo Green for providing the foundation for our efforts, and, of course, to our personal mentor William Klykylo for his inspiration and guidance.

Contributors

Matthew J. Baker, DO
Assistant Professor
Division of Child and Adolescent
    Psychiatry
Wright State University Boonshoft
    School of Medicine
Dayton, Ohio

Rick T. Bowers, MD
Clinical Professor
Division of Child and Adolescent
    Psychiatry
Wright State University Boonshoft
    School of Medicine
Dayton, Ohio

Robert P. Cusser, DO
Clinical Instructor
Division of Child and Adolescent
    Psychiatry
Wright State University Boonshoft
    School of Medicine
Dayton, Ohio

Bethany L. Harper, MD
Assistant Professor
Director of Medical Student Education
    in Psychiatry
Division of Child and Adolescent
    Psychiatry
Wright State University Boonshoft
    School of Medicine
Dayton, Ohio

Kari S. Harper, MD
Clinical Instructor
Division of Child and Adolescent
    Psychiatry
Wright State University Boonshoft
    School of Medicine
Dayton, Ohio

Julia C. Jackson, MD
Adult, Child, and Adolescent
    Psychiatrist
United States Air Force

Ryan C. Mast, DO, MBA
Assistant Professor
Training Director of CAP Fellowship
Division of Child and Adolescent
    Psychiatry
Wright State University Boonshoft
    School of Medicine
Dayton, Ohio

Suzie C. Nelson, MD, DFAACAP
Assistant Professor
Associate Training Director
Division of Child and Adolescent
    Psychiatry
Wright State University Boonshoft
    School of Medicine
Dayton, Ohio

Natosha S. Osansanya, MD, MPH
Assistant Professor
Division of Child and Adolescent
    Psychiatry
Wright State University Boonshoft
    School of Medicine
Dayton, Ohio

Kaitlyn T. Pollock, DO
Clinical Instructor
Division of Child and Adolescent
    Psychiatry
Wright State University Boonshoft
    School of Medicine
Dayton, Ohio

Ronne J. Proch, DO, MA
Clinical Instructor
Department of Psychiatry
Wright State University Boonshoft
    School of Medicine
Dayton, Ohio

Ravinder S. Sandhu, MD
Clinical Instructor
Division of Child and Adolescent
    Psychiatry
Wright State University Boonshoft
    School of Medicine
Dayton, Ohio

Jamie L. Snyder, MD
Associate Professor
Training Director—Child and
    Adolescent Psychiatry and PPPP
Vice-Chair for Psychiatry Education
Creighton University
Omaha, Nebraska

Christina G. Weston, MD
Associate Clinical Professor
Division of Child and Adolescent
    Psychiatry
Wright State University Boonshoft
    School of Medicine
Dayton, Ohio

Preface

In the fifth edition's preface, Dr. William Klykylo paid warranted homage to the founding editor, Dr. Hugo Green, who was responsible for the early acclaim that his book series garnered, before the editorial duties were later assumed by chief editor Dr. Klykylo in the last edition. In kind, Dr. Klykylo has now passed the torch to the current editors to not just continue, but also evolve the important discussion of psychopharmacology in children and adolescents. Dr. Klykylo trained the current editors, and his influence continues to permeate the Child Psychiatry Department at Wright State University, which he headed for over two decades. He has been an invaluable mentor to us in our professional careers as child and adolescent psychiatrists, as well as a "life mentor" in so many areas outside our immediate vocations. His generosity of time and guidance can never be sufficiently repaid.

While this series has always highlighted the potential risks of medications for this age group, it is promising that researchers are now reporting that the appropriate implementation of select medicines early in treatment may result in observable neuroprotective effects on neurons in the brain. It is hoped that these neuroprotective effects will alter the pernicious course of brain degradation and disease progression that is the archetypal life experience for so many individuals with serious mental illnesses. This finding is immensely important in the risk/benefit analysis whenever medications are employed but is especially pertinent given that the neurodegenerative brain processes occurring in many mental health conditions seem to have their onset in childhood for a significant number of patients. Chronic depression, bipolar disorder, and schizophrenia are all now appreciated as neurodegenerative diseases that benefit from early medication interventions and various other forms of therapy, such as cognitive-behavioral therapy, when delivered in a prescribed fashion.

One cannot overstate the importance of assessing and addressing the entire psycho-social-cultural experience of this young population of patients. Even the most knowledgeable psychopharmacologist is often humbled when he or she realizes that his or her well-thought-out medication regimen is likely to be of minor benefit when juxtaposed with the continual onslaught of trauma and other social stressors that impede recovery and normal development. Although medication treatment alone is inappropriate for most patients, it is noteworthy that in treatment studies for conditions such as attention-deficit/hyperactivity disorder (ADHD), major depressive disorder (MDD), bipolar disorder, and schizophrenia, the single largest treatment effects are the result of medication interventions, not counseling therapy interventions. However, as one might expect, the best overall outcomes and remission rates are achieved when the treatment plan utilizes combined therapy. The modest overall effect sizes in MDD with counseling alone speak to the need for identifying those patients who will best respond to counseling and then initiating specialized talk therapy such as cognitive-behavioral therapy for these patient groups. Just as the counseling services that our youth receive need to be enhanced, so do the medical treatments currently used to treat conditions such as depression or schizophrenia via the development of new medications with novel mechanisms of action.

Despite the clear limitations of our current therapies, it is still amazing to note that when the first edition of this book was published, there were few pediatric mental health conditions other than ADHD for which any medication was Food and Drug Administration (FDA) approved to treat. Even by the fourth edition, the only FDA-approved pediatric medications were the selective serotonin reuptake inhibitors (SSRIs) of fluoxetine (MDD and obsessive-compulsive disorder [OCD]), sertraline (OCD), and fluvoxamine (OCD). At that time, there were no pediatric indications for second-generation antipsychotics (SGAs). The fifth edition saw the addition of several SGAs approved for schizophrenia and bipolar disorder, such as risperidone, olanzapine, quetiapine, aripiprazole, and paliperidone. However, progress remains slow in the FDA approval of agents to be utilized in the treatment of pediatric depression and anxiety; currently only the SSRI escitalopram (MDD) and, more recently in 2015, the serotonin and norepinephrine reuptake inhibitor (SNRI) duloxetine (generalized anxiety disorder) were added to the list of FDA-approved agents for the adolescent age group. Other new significant approved medications for this edition include the SGA asenapine (schizophrenia) and lurasidone (schizophrenia and bipolar disorder). Today, for all the major mental health conditions, such as anxiety, depression, schizophrenia, and bipolar disorder, there are medications that are FDA-approved for pediatric use. There are many other agents whose usage in these conditions is supported by numerous pediatric clinical studies that attest to their effectiveness.

While the availability of seemingly safer and more effective medications led to an increase in utilization of these various agents in the pediatric population, a treatment dilemma developed. When several agents belonging to the atypical antipsychotic class received new FDA indications for their usage as effective mood stabilizers in adults, this led to their subsequent application for treatment in suspected pediatric bipolar disorder. Indeed, mood stabilization is by far the primary reason these atypical agents are prescribed in the United States, so much so that now there is a realization that these medications are overprescribed, and efforts are under way, supported by academia and insurance, to reduce their usage for safety and monetary reasons given their side effects and extreme costs to the healthcare system. This edition contains a new chapter, "Deprescribing: The Prescription for Polypharmacy in the Child and Adolescent Psychiatric Population," addressing this concerning practice in our field. Drs. Proch and Weston, in their chapter on deprescribing, discuss the appropriate push to reduce polypharmacy in children and adolescents, especially with the high side-effect burden from medications such as second-generation antipsychotic/mood stabilizers, whenever possible.

Although there are many other timely additions to this edition of the book series, the general format was carried on from previous editions, but with some modifications to condense clinical management materials and highlight clinical "pearls."

In Section One, the "General Principles" chapter was restructured with the addition of very useful tables that summarize the most widely used and accredited rating scales for depression, anxiety, OCD, substance abuse, and ADHD. As a benefit to the reader, all scales available in the public domain are placed in the appendix. Because of the ongoing recognition of the ethical as well as legal challenges related to the use of psychotropic medication in minors, we continue to advocate reviewing the section on the ethics of psychopharmacology.

We have updated the "Sympathomimetic Amines, Central Nervous System Stimulants, and Executive Function Agents" chapter to include various new medications that enhance attentional function. In the past few years, a large number of long-acting stimulants were approved for use in the treatment of ADHD. These new medicines can be taken in various forms, such as liquids and dissolvable tablets, that utilize basically the same methylphenidate or amphetamine chemical compounds but differ in their D- and L-isomer ratios.

The "Antidepressant Medications" chapter incorporates new tables to consolidate information about FDA indications that are current for this edition as well as dosing guidelines, for ease of use in practice. Additional reviews of the evidence base for this broad medication class in the treatment of a multitude of conditions are included, and the discussion of clinical use of duloxetine and commentary on emerging antidepressants provide important updates on current practice. The "Antiepileptic Mood Stabilizers and Lithium Carbonate" and "Non-SSRI/SNRI Anxiety Medication" chapters are updated and reformatted to better allow the quick assimilation of the results of multiple studies and for ease of reading.

The "Second- and Third-Generation Antipsychotic/Mood Stabilizer Medications" chapter is now updated to include third-generation antipsychotics with a greater emphasis on clinical treatment, which acknowledges that over 90% of the time these medications are used in child and adolescent psychiatry for their mood-stabilizing effects, not for their antipsychotic properties. The fact that clinicians and news reports often reference the medications as being solely "antipsychotics" can be harmful to the profession as well as to the mission of improving the lives of a vulnerable population. This terminology continues to confuse and scare parents. When used in articles and news reports, the term *antipsychotics* supports the misinformed opinion that prescribers choose to "drug kids" with inappropriate medication interventions. The term *mood stabilizer* more correctly represents their FDA-approval status as to why they are used. The term *mood stabilizer* also has less of a negative connotation while making more pragmatic sense to patients and caregivers. A section in this chapter also introduces the new long-acting injectable antipsychotic/mood-stabilizing agents that are improving outcomes in many of the select pediatric patients who utilize them, albeit in an off-label manner.

It is a sad commentary on our society that we felt compelled to add a new chapter, "Medications Used to Treat Substance Use Disorders in Adolescents," which addresses the all-too-common finding that many of our youth have succumbed to the addiction of prescription opiate pain pills and even heroin. The use of medication-assisted treatment (although not a specific class of medications) has become standard in treating opioid and alcohol use disorders in adults, and studies of medication-assisted treatment of substance use disorders in adolescents are reviewed in this much-needed chapter. Across the country, medication overdoses are the leading cause of death for Americans under the age of 50, claiming more lives than car crashes, gun deaths, and the AIDS virus did at their peaks. The treatments in this chapter can truly be life saving but take a concerted effort by the entire community to be effective in this true modern-day epidemic.

Finally, the "Other Useful Medications for Specific Conditions of Interest" chapter expands the discussion of the scope of medications that may be prescribed in the pursuit of stabilizing weight or to evoke actual weight loss as one combats the unwanted side effect of weight gain that occurs with many medication classes, but especially the second-generation antipsychotics/mood stabilizers. Also new in the chapter is the section on the treatment of the new *DSM-5* diagnosis of disruptive mood dysregulation disorder, for which currently there are no FDA-approved medications, nor even an expert panel list of recommendations.

Inevitably, indications (and possible contraindications) will continue to appear after any book goes to print, and the reader is strongly encouraged to maintain currency with www.fda.gov and related sources.

We hope that this edition will continue the book's tradition of authority and utility. Whatever its merits, preparing it required the help of many others. Dr. Klykylo has been personally supportive as always, and we would not have undertaken this project without his kind encouragement. The staff of Wolters Kluwer, most notably Acquisitions Editor Chris Teja and Editorial Coordinator Tim Rinehart, have made our work pleasurable through their encouragement, advice, and patience. Bette S. Sydelko, Medical and Education Librarian, Wright State University, and University Libraries assisted with literature research. No such work as this could ever come about without the assistance of our colleagues and the tolerance of our families, to whom we are forever in debt.

Rick T. Bowers, MD

Contents

General Principles

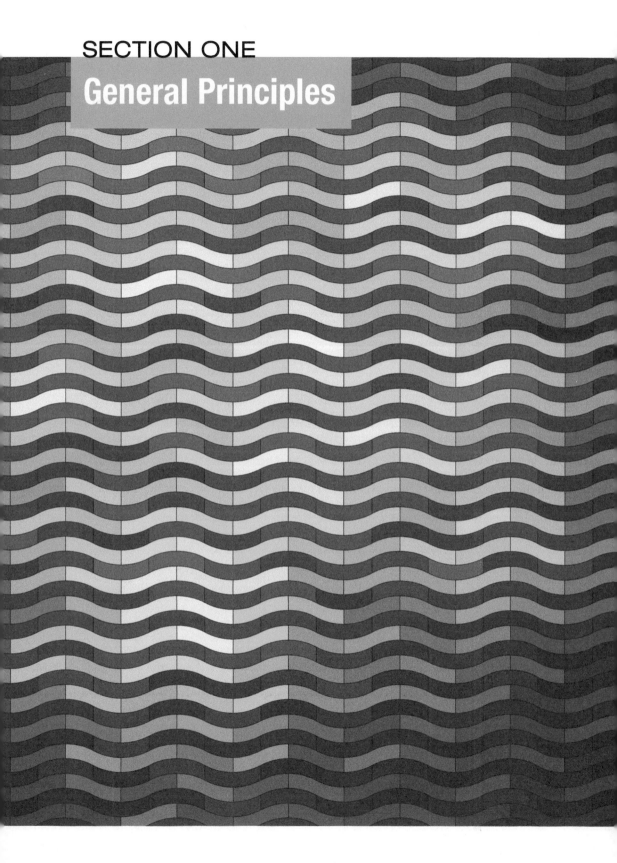

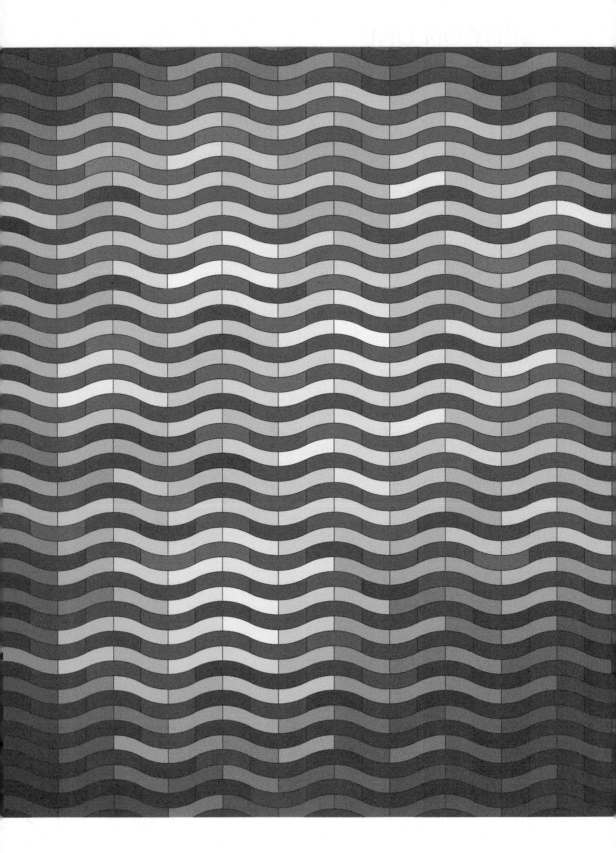

CHAPTER 1

Introduction

RICK T. BOWERS

INTRODUCTION

The sixth edition of *Child and Adolescent Clinical Psychopharmacology* attempts to synthesize and summarize, in a clinically useful manner, the ever-expanding pool of data regarding the medical treatment options that are now available to those clinicians attempting to improve the lives of children with mental health conditions. In the fifth edition of Wayne H. Green's series, Dr. William Klykylo, as editor, put forth in his eloquent and cogent prose a masterful summary of the process of assessment, and, if indicated, the cautious initiation and maintenance of medication therapies that in many instances were not U.S. Food and Drug Administration (FDA) approved for that condition. Since that time, the pendulum has swung to a point that, for most major pediatric mental health conditions, there are now approved medicines. Dr. Klykylo's approach to rational and safe prescribing remains as relevant as ever; so with his approval, the current editors chose to build upon his literary framework in the last edition and highlight the advances in the field as well as new challenges the field must address.

As in the previous editions, this book reviews selected topics and medications used in child and adolescent psychopharmacology from a practical, clinically oriented perspective. It is intended primarily for clinicians actively engaged in treating children and adolescents with psychoactive medications. These include child psychiatrists, pediatricians, family physicians, residents in child and adolescent psychiatry, residents in general psychiatry, pediatric residents, and other health care professionals such as advanced clinical nurse practitioners or physician assistants who may prescribe medications to patients in this age group. In addition, other clinicians and mental health personnel who work with children on psychoactive medication may wish to review the medications their patients are taking, as may some parents/caregivers of such children.

The first part of this book focuses rather intensively on the general principles of psychopharmacotherapy for children and adolescents. This section, although updated by the current editors, is unabashedly derivative of Dr. Green's work, restating his enduring standards. The reader is presented with a clinically useful way of thinking about psychopharmacotherapy, beginning with the initial clinical contact and continuing through the psychiatric evaluation, psychodynamic formulation, diagnosis and development of the treatment plan. For those cases in which psychoactive medication is recommended as a part of the treatment plan, the necessary medicolegal responsibilities of the clinician in introducing and explaining the purpose of medication to the relevant caretakers and the patient, steps to obtain parental informed consent and patient assent to administer medication, ways of maximizing the chances of the legal guardian's and patient's acceptance of a trial of the medication, and the necessary documentation of these facts in the clinical record are reviewed. Following this, the entire process of administering medication is discussed. This begins with a consideration of which medication to choose for the initial trial of medication and subsequent medications, should the first choice(s) not result in adequate clinical improvement. Examples of algorithms, which are often helpful in medicating complicated clinical cases, are also included. The necessary documentation of target symptoms, any baseline behavioral ratings that will be useful in assessing clinical response, or the development of untoward effects and the baseline physical and laboratory assessments to be selected are then discussed. This part of the book ends with a detailed presentation of the principles of administering psychoactive medication from the initial dose, through titration and determining the optimal dose, to maintenance therapy, duration of treatment, and issues in terminating medication. These principles are generalizable and provide clinical guidelines for selecting and administering any psychoactive medication to children and adolescents.

The second portion of this book begins with a short chapter discussing the history of child psychopharmacology and some issues concerning psychopharmacologic research in children and adolescents. The purpose of this review is to remind the reader where the information that follows is placed in the history of child psychopharmacology and of the importance of research and a critical assessment of the presented data for informed clinical practice.

After these brief introductory comments, the remainder of Section Two focuses on specific psychopharmacologic agents that are presently the most important in the clinical practice of child and adolescent psychiatry. This section is, necessarily, more extensively modified than the first. The medications are presented by their class. Many specific psychoactive medications are presently used to treat diverse psychiatric disorders or symptoms across psychiatric diagnoses (e.g., second-generation antipsychotics [SGAs]/mood stabilizers and third-generation antipsychotics [TGAs]/ mood stabilizers or lithium for their anti-aggressive effects), and this method of organization avoids repeating similar information under several diagnoses. There are exceptions to this rule, for example, with metformin and topiramate, which are covered twice, because of two particularly divergent uses for these agents.

As we learn more about the etiopathogenesis of psychiatric disorders, it becomes increasingly useful and important, both scientifically and clinically, to think about how medications affect basic neurotransmitter and psychoneuroendocrine functioning across diagnoses. Most medicines affect more than one neurotransmitter system. For example, the atypical antipsychotics or SGAs and TGAs have a very complex mixture of pharmacologic properties. They influence not only the serotonin and dopamine systems as antagonists, and even agonists in the case of TGAs, but also the noradrenergic and cholinergic systems, and have antihistaminic and other properties (Stahl, 2000). Likewise, a specific neurotransmitter system may be important in one or more diagnostic categories. For example, there appears to be a relationship between the serotonergic system's functioning and aggressive or violent behavior and self-destructive behavior, among various diagnostic groups (Linnoila et al., 1989; Mann et al., 1989).

As might be expected in a clinically oriented book, the standard, often older psychopharmacologic treatments established by investigational and clinical studies as both efficacious and safe for use in children and adolescents and approved by the

FDA for advertising as such, are still included. The literature reviews determining the efficacy of these treatments, however, are kept to a minimum, and usually only referenced if they contain information related to the off-label treatment of specialized populations, such as individuals with a low intelligence quotient or autism or in younger children below the age for which the agent is approved. In some cases, such as infrequently used first-generation antipsychotics, these agents are now placed in appendices, because comprehensive reviews are readily available elsewhere.

For the first time in child and adolescent psychiatry, it can now be stated that most of the first-line medicines prescribed to treat psychiatric disorders in children and adolescents are FDA approved and on-label for the age (except for young children) or indication, or both. The current first-line agents are the newer selective serotonin reuptake inhibitors (SSRIs), serotonin–norepinephrine reuptake inhibitors as well as the SGA and TGA medications. These medications are generally deemed to be more effective, to have fewer or less serious untoward/adverse effects, or both, compared to older FDA-approved medications. From a historical perspective, it is interesting to note that in actuality, even before their respective official FDA approvals in youth, the SSRIs and SGAs were more frequently prescribed for non–FDA-approved indications in children and adolescents than were the FDA-approved medications at the time. In a historical perspective, it is also interesting to note that the prior first-line tricyclic antidepressant agents, which were surpassed by the SSRIs in the total number of prescriptions written many years ago, were never approved for use in treating depression in children below age 12, even after the SSRI fluoxetine received approval for use in children aged 7 years and older. In addition, substantial data from long-term adult studies have accumulated pertaining to the side effects of these FDA-approved medications in adults, which can be valuable in selecting which agents to initiate treatment with and how to monitor them in ongoing treatment.

Medications that appear to be likely candidates for eventual FDA approval (if the necessary studies are funded and carried out) or which are beginning to be used in standard practice are thoroughly addressed as well. Because reviews of these medications are usually less readily available and some studies are very recent, only summaries of relevant studies are included. Although in those warranted cases where there is discussion of the current literature on medications used for non–FDA-approved or off-label indications over FDA-approved medications may seem paradoxical, it is deliberate and reflects current clinical practice. This is because there is significant difficulty when patients do not respond with sufficient amelioration of symptoms to FDA-approved pharmacologic treatments currently available, or, even more importantly, no FDA-approved medication is approved for the treatment indication, or untoward effects prevent the medication's use in efficacious doses. When the patient's symptoms prevent him or her from functioning in a psychosocial environment that will facilitate normal growth, maturation, and development, many clinicians use FDA-approved medications for non–FDA-approved indications to treat their patients. Although this book does not proselytize for the use of medication for non–FDA-approved uses, it does present the clinician with possible alternative treatments for patients who are resistant to standard pharmacologic treatments. In fact, the use of many of these medications for off-label indications is medically accepted in standard clinical practice, for example, the use of methylphenidate formulations in children younger than 6 years. As with FDA-approved treatments, the physician must consider, perhaps even more carefully, the risks versus the potential benefits of using any medication for non–FDA-approved indications. Medicolegal, ethical, and some practical issues of using medications for non–FDA-approved indications are considered in appropriate sections of the book.

We emphasize that no book can substitute a careful reading of the FDA-approved labeling (manufacturer's labeling/package insert) which contains additional information on all FDA-approved medications discussed in this book. To address this issue in a focused manner, only the most clinically salient labeling information is summarized in the discussions of these various agents. No medication should be prescribed without the physician having read and become familiar with its labeling information; to do so is a disservice to one's patient and renders one vulnerable to professional liability. This information, however, focuses on the medication's use for indications approved by the FDA and for many psychotropic medications, there is often little controlled data about the medication's use for non–FDA-approved indications in children and adolescents.

The staff have made great efforts to include and explicate the most current pharmacologic findings and treatment practices in the field of child and adolescent psychiatry. However, the knowledge base of medicine is ever expanding at such an astounding rate that it creates obstacles to print textbooks detailing the most cutting edge material once in print. To address this clinical issue, it is planned that yearly electronic updates on select topics will be made available to the reader to ensure this latest edition remains a valuable quick reference for clinicians treating mental health conditions in children and adolescents.

General Principles of Psychopharmacotherapy with Children and Adolescents

SUZIE C. NELSON

PSYCHIATRIC DIAGNOSIS AND PSYCHOPHARMACOTHERAPY

Psychopharmacotherapy should always be part of a comprehensive treatment plan arrived at after a thorough psychiatric evaluation results in a diagnosis, or at least a working diagnosis. It is indefensible to initiate treatment without first attempting to formulate as clear an understanding of the clinical picture as possible. This will enable clinicians to institute the most appropriate and rational treatment(s) available in their therapeutic armamentaria for the situation at hand.

Current Psychiatric Diagnostic Nomenclature

A challenge with the official American Psychiatric Association (APA) nomenclature, the *Diagnostic and Statistical Manual of Mental Disorders*, Fifth Edition (DSM-5) (APA, 2013), and, indeed, with current psychiatric nomenclatures is that etiology is not always taken into account when formulating a diagnosis. One reason for this is that we do not know the etiologies of many conditions. Autistic disorder, as an example, is not etiologically homogeneous. Hence, at times we are left treating specific constellations of behavioral symptoms without fully understanding their biologic and genetic underpinnings, or how they interact with psychosocial and physical environments.

Theoretically, for a given psychiatric disorder, treatments may be effective by correcting the condition(s) leading to it (or them) or by influencing events somewhere along the usually complex pathways between the hypothesized abnormality(ies) and its subsequent psychological and/or behavioral consequences. Therefore, specific psychoactive medications may be effective in dissimilar disorders because they influence or modify neurotransmitters and psychoneuroendocrine events in the brain along or near the end of these interacting, partially confluent, or final common pathways. Current research suggests that there are genetic bases for these phenomena (Cross-Disorder Group, 2013).

Other psychoactive medications appear to exert their therapeutic effects through entirely different mechanisms in different diagnostic entities—for example, imipramine in depression, attention-deficit/hyperactivity disorder (ADHD), and enuresis.

Some patients with a specific diagnosis (e.g., ADHD, autistic disorder, or schizophrenia) will not have a satisfactory clinical response or will be refractory to a specific medication—even one known to be highly effective in statistically significant double-blind studies—or will even have a worsening of symptoms. This may reflect differences in genetic makeup or other biologically determined conditions, psychosocial environments, and/or internalized conflicts and the contributions each makes to the etiopathogenesis of each patient's psychiatric disorder.

Although diagnostic issues are not discussed specifically in this book, it is emphasized that an accurate diagnosis is of critical importance in choosing the correct medication. At times, the lack of expected clinical response to a medication should suggest to the clinician the possibility of an incorrect diagnosis and that a careful diagnostic reconsideration should be undertaken.

Other unfortunate clinical consequences may result from incorrect diagnoses. For example, antidepressants may precipitate an acute psychotic reaction when given to some individuals with schizophrenic disorder. Stimulant medications, too, may precipitate psychosis when given in sufficient doses to some children or adolescents with borderline personalities or unrecognized schizophrenia.

Wender (1988) noted that clinical experience suggested that some children diagnosed with ADHD were treated with stimulants and rapidly developed tolerance to them but were actually suffering from a major depressive disorder, and that they responded to treatment with tricyclic antidepressants (TCAs) with remarkable improvement.

Changing diagnostic criteria may also complicate matters. For example, some of the controversy regarding the efficacy of stimulants in patients with development disabilities may have resulted from diagnostic issues. Until the publication of DSM-II (APA, 1968), there was no specific APA diagnosis for what was commonly known as the hyperactive child. There were various labels for this condition, including *hyperactive child, hyperkinetic syndrome, minimal brain dysfunction (MBD)*, and *minimal cerebral dysfunction*. Intellectual disability was considered evidence of more than "minimal" dysfunction, and the various etiologies were thought to be biologic. Because of this concept, children with intellectual disabilities were excluded from the possibility of receiving a codiagnosis of MBD, hyperactive child, or an equivalent diagnosis, and some clinicians may not have tried stimulant medication in their patients who had even mild disabilities.

The situation changed with the publication of DSM-II, which noted that "in children, mild brain damage often manifests itself by hyperactivity, short attention span, easy distractibility, and impulsiveness" (APA, 1968, p. 31). It also suggested that unless there are significant interactional factors (e.g., between child and parents) that appear to be responsible for these behaviors, the disorder should be classified as a nonpsychotic, organic brain syndrome and not as a behavior disorder.

In DSM-III (APA, 1980a), the diagnosis of attention-deficit disorder with hyperactivity (ADDH) was based on the presence of a specific constellation of symptoms, and no etiology was hypothesized. Hence, children of any intelligence could exhibit such features. DSM-III additionally notes that mild or moderate mental retardation may predispose one to the development of ADDH and that the addition of this diagnosis to the severely and profoundly retarded child is not clinically useful because these symptoms are often an inherent part of the condition.

DSM-III-R redefined ADDH somewhat, renamed it (ADHD), and refined its relation with mental retardation. It noted that many features of ADHD may be present in mentally retarded people because of the generalized delays in intellectual development. DSM-III-R (APA, 1987), DSM-IV (APA, 1994), DSM-IV-TR (APA, 2000), and DSM-5 (APA, 2013) note that a child or an adolescent with an intellectual disability should be additionally diagnosed with ADHD only if the relevant symptoms significantly exceed those that are compatible with the child's or adolescent's mental age. These changes in diagnostic criteria, although directed toward greater precision in identification and classification of disorders, have often complicated the process of treatment planning for clinicians.

DIAGNOSIS AND TARGET SYMPTOMS

In making the decision about which psychoactive medication to select initially, two major issues should be addressed: diagnosis and target symptoms. Both are important and are often interrelated. It is important to make the most accurate diagnosis possible using the available data and to identify and quantify target symptoms to choose an efficacious medication and to assess the results of medication. The target symptoms must be of sufficient severity and must interfere so significantly with the child's or adolescent's current functioning and future maturation and development that the potential benefits of the medication will justify the risks concomitant with its administration.

The initial medication may be chosen with respect to either diagnosis or target symptoms, or both. Sometimes the decision is not difficult because the same medication is appropriate for both the target symptoms and the diagnosis. For example, antipsychotics are the medications of first choice for treating schizophrenia and are appropriate for most of the significant target symptoms (e.g., hallucinations, thought disorder, and delusions). The symptom "hyperactivity," however, is present in numerous childhood psychiatric disorders, but all hyperactivity is not the same (Fish, 1971). The clinician should be fully aware of the diagnosis in treating this symptom. Hyperactivity in a youngster with ADHD would be expected to respond favorably to the administration of a stimulant, whereas a schizophrenic youngster who is in relative remission but exhibits marked hyperactivity would have a risk of having his or her psychotic symptoms reexacerbated if stimulant medication were used. Stimulant drugs, the medications of choice in ADHD, are sometimes considered to be relatively contraindicated in schizophrenia and may cause worsening of psychotic symptoms. More recently, however, clinicians have prescribed stimulants to psychotic children who are maintained on antipsychotic medication but have residual symptoms of hyperactivity, distractibility, and inattention, with resulting clinical improvement.

Medication can also be prescribed to treat specific diagnoses. Lithium, for example, has a certain specificity for treatment of mania in patients diagnosed with bipolar disorder, manic, but also appears to have an antiaggressive action that cuts across various diagnoses. Lithium has been used effectively to treat aggression directed against others or self-injurious behavior in children and adolescents diagnosed with conduct disorder, mental retardation with disturbance of behavior, and autistic disorder.

SPECIAL ASPECTS OF CHILD PSYCHOPHARMACOTHERAPY

Maturational/Developmental Issues

Physiologic Factors

The relation between biologic developmental issues and psychopharmacotherapy has been long recognized and emphasized by Popper (1987b), Geller (1991), and many other authors. Children and adolescents may require larger doses of psychoactive medication per unit of body weight compared with adults to attain similar blood levels and therapeutic efficacy. It is usually assumed that two factors explain this situation: more rapid metabolism by the liver and an increased glomerular filtration rate in children compared with that in adults.

Teicher and Baldessarini (1987) pointed out that children may respond to medications differently compared with adults because of pharmacodynamic factors (medication-effector mechanisms) that are caused by developmental changes in neural pathways or their functions (e.g., Geller et al. (1992) reported that prepubescent subjects treated with the TCA nortriptyline reported almost no anticholinergic adverse effects; especially noteworthy was the lack of any prominent dry mouth frequently reported by adults) or because of pharmacokinetic factors caused by developmental changes in the distribution, metabolism, or excretion of a medication.

Jatlow (1987) noted that, although the rapid rate of medication disposition may decrease gradually throughout childhood, there may be an abrupt decline around puberty. Medication disposition usually reaches adult levels by middle to late adolescence. Clinically, this would indicate that the clinician should be especially alert to possible changes in pharmacokinetics during the period around puberty and be ready to adjust dose levels if necessary. When they are available, it may be useful to obtain plasma concentration levels if there appears to be a change in the clinical efficacy of a medication as a child matures into an adolescent.

Puig-Antich (1987) summarized some of the evidence that catecholamine (norepinephrine, epinephrine, and dopamine) systems are not fully anatomically developed and operationally functional until adulthood. The fact that younger children may respond to stimulant medication differently than do older adolescents and adults may be explained by the immaturity of the catecholamine systems (Puig-Antich, 1987); it could also be considered to result from developmental pharmacodynamic factors.

The pharmacokinetics of many medications have been observed to change over the course of life. For example, children and adolescents below 15 years of age treated with clomipramine had significantly lower steady-state plasma concentrations for a given dose than did adults (*Physicians' Desk Reference [PDR]*, 1990). Similarly, Rivera-Calimlim et al. (1979) reported that children and adolescents 8 to 15 years of age required larger doses of chlorpromazine than those required by adults to attain similar plasma concentrations.

There may also be differences between acute and chronic pharmacokinetics. For example, Rivera-Calimlim et al. (1979) reported a decline in plasma chlorpromazine levels in most child and adolescent patients who were on a fixed dose, and suggested it might be due to autoinduction of metabolic enzymes during long-term treatment, as was reported in adults. The consequences of autoinduction and its cellular basis have been extensively reported (Bonate & Howard, 2005).

A clear relationship between plasma concentrations and clinical response to imipramine was noted for prepubescent subjects and older adults with endogenous depression, but not for adolescents and young adults (Burke & Puig-Antich, 1990). The authors hypothesized that the relatively poor clinical efficacy of TCAs in post-pubescent adolescents and young adults compared with the clinical response of prepubescent children and older adults is secondary to a negative effect of increased sex hormone levels on the antidepressant action of imipramine.

Herskowitz (1987) reviewed the developmental neurotoxicity of pharmacoactive drugs. Developmental neurotoxicity concerns stage-specific, medication-induced biochemical or physiologic changes, morphologic manifestations, and behavioral symptoms. For example, stimulant medication may adversely affect normal increases in height and growth, at least temporarily, in some actively growing children and adolescents. Similarly, some psychoactive medications taken during early pregnancy have significant potential for damaging the fetus (e.g., lithium may cause cardiac malformations).

Cognitive/Psychological/Experiential Factors

The maturation and development of the central nervous system as well as the life experiences accumulating since infancy determine much of the specific level of functioning of a given child or adolescent. Although detailed knowledge of these factors is essential to evaluate any child or adolescent psychiatrically, this book addresses only their specific relevance to psychopharmacotherapy.

In general, the younger the patient, the less the verbal facility available to convey information to the clinician and, reciprocally, the less the cognitive ability available to understand information the clinician wishes to impart. Part of the psychiatric evaluation leading to a decision that psychotropic medication is indicated will provide the clinician with an assessment of the level of the patient's ability to communicate his or her emotional status and of his or her cognitive/linguistic ability to understand the proposed treatment and reliably report the effect of the treatment.

In the very young child or the child with no communicative language, the clinician can only observe behavioral effects of medication directly or learn of them as reported by others. The younger the child, the fewer the compliments or complaints about the beneficial or adverse effects. Also, the young child has less-differentiated emotions and more limited experience with feelings and emotions and with communicating them to others than do older children. In addition, some chronically depressed or anxious children may not have had a sufficiently recent normal emotional baseline with which they can compare their present mood. Such children may experience a depressed mood as their normal, usual state of being and, therefore, do not have a normal baseline frame of reference upon which to draw in describing how they feel.

The younger the child, the less accurate his or her time estimates. Until approximately 10 years of age, concepts of long periods of time are often not easily understood. It can be very useful and at times essential to use concrete markers of time in discussing time concepts and chronology of events with children. For example, the clinician may enquire whether something occurred before or after the last birthday, specific holidays (e.g., Christmas, Thanksgiving, or Halloween), specific events (e.g., separation or divorce of parents, when the family moved to another home, an operation, a relative's death, or the birth of a sibling), the seasons or weather (e.g., winter, snow, cold, or summer, hot), or the school year (e.g., specific teacher's name or grade, or Christmas, spring or Easter, or summer vacation).

Concepts such as concentration, distractibility, and impulsivity may be beyond the understanding of some early latency-age children. Different children may use different words or expressions to mean the same concept. It is important to be certain that a child knows the meaning of a specific word and not assume an understanding because the child responds to a question. If there is any doubt, ask what something means or explain it in another way. It can be very useful to ask the same thing in several different ways.

In the final analysis, once the patient's psychopathology and his or her developmental experiential factors are taken into account, it is the quality of the relationship between the clinician and the child or adolescent that becomes paramount in determining the usefulness of information shared.

Relationship to the Patient's Family or Caregivers

Diagnosis, Formulation, and Development of the Treatment Plan

A complete psychiatric assessment, including appropriate psychological tests, resulting in a working diagnosis and comprehensive treatment plan; appropriate physical and laboratory examinations; and baseline behavioral measurements should be completed as minimum prerequisites before the initiation of psychopharmacotherapy. The treatment plan should be developed in conjunction with either the parent(s) or the primary caretaker and should include participation of the child or adolescent as appropriate to his or her understanding. Treatment with psychoactive medications should always be part of a more comprehensive treatment regimen and is rarely appropriate as the sole treatment modality for a child or an adolescent.

At variance with this traditional wisdom, however, are the results of several studies comparing the treatment of hyperactive children with stimulant medication alone versus stimulant medication combined with other interventions, such as cognitive training, attention control, social reinforcement, and parent training. A review of these studies concluded that "the additional use of various forms of psychotherapies (behavioral treatment, parent training, cognitive therapy) with stimulants has not resulted in superior outcomes than medication alone" (Klein, 1987, p. 1223). One possible factor contributing to this result is that in several studies children who were treated with methylphenidate alone showed improvement in social behavior. Following this course of treatment, adults—both parents and teachers—related to the children more positively (Klein, 1987). The Multimodal Treatment Study Group of Children with Attention-Deficit/Hyperactivity Disorder (MTA) Cooperative Group also found that stimulant medication was the most important factor in improving ADHD symptoms. This is further discussed in Chapter 5 (MTA Cooperative Group, 1999a, 1999b).

It seems clinically unlikely, however, that all the difficulties of ADHD children are secondary to the target symptoms that improve with psychostimulants. Those difficulties that result from other psychosocial problems, including psychopathologic familial interactions and long-standing maladaptive behavioral patterns, would be expected to benefit from additional interventions; until it is possible to differentiate those children whose difficulties arise from their attention deficit per se from children whose symptoms are of multidetermined origin, a comprehensive treatment program is recommended for all children. Obviously, this same principle applies to all psychiatric disorders, regardless of their responsiveness to medications.

The legal guardian/caregiver and the child or adolescent patient, to the degree appropriate for the patient's age and psychopathology, should participate in formulating the treatment plan. The use of medication, including expected benefits and possible short- and long-term adverse effects, should be reviewed with the caregivers/parents and patient in understandable terminology. It is essential to carefully assess the attitude and reliability of the persons who will be responsible for administering the medication. Unless there is a positive or at least an honestly neutral attitude toward medication and some therapeutic alliance with the parents, it will be difficult or infeasible to make a reliable assessment of drug efficacy and adherence. Likewise, to store and administer medication safely on an outpatient basis requires a responsible adult, especially if there are young children in the home or if the patient is at risk of suicide.

It should be explained to parents that, even if medication helps some biologically determined symptoms (e.g., in some cases of ADHD), the disorder's presence may have caused psychological difficulties in the child or adolescent as well as disturbances in familial and social relationships. Controlling or ameliorating the biologic difficulty does not usually correct the long-standing internalized psychological or interpersonal problems and long-standing maladaptive patterns of behavior immediately. Resolving these difficulties will take time and may often require concomitant individual, group, family, or other therapeutic intervention.

Adherence

Treatment adherence is an issue of particular importance in child and adolescent psychiatry. Because the parents or other caretakers are usually interposed between the physician and patient, adherence is somewhat more complex than in adult psychiatry, in which the patient usually relates directly to the physician.

Obviously, for psychopharmacotherapy to be effective in the disorder for which it is prescribed, the medication should be taken following the prescribed directions. Erratic adherence or running out of medication may cause the patient to undergo what is in effect an abrupt withdrawal of medication. Withdrawal syndromes may sometimes be confused with adverse effects, worsening of the clinical condition, or inadequate medication levels. In some cases, such as when an antipsychotic is used, the patient is at increased risk for an acute dystonic reaction if the physician restarts the medication at the optimal dose after the medication was discontinued for several days or more. In addition, when medication is stopped, it may sometimes require a higher dose of medication to regain the same degree of symptom control. For example, Sleator et al. (1974) found that 7 of 28 hyperactive children who showed clinical worsening during a month-long placebo period after having received methylphenidate for 1 to 2 years required an increase in dose to regain their original clinical improvement. Hence, it is very important to emphasize to parents that running out of medication is to be avoided.

Many factors may interfere with adherence. Some parents will withhold medication if their child appears to be doing well, or, conversely, increase the medication without the physician's approval if behavior worsens, or even administer the medication to the child as a punishment.

When parents or legal guardians seek treatment for their children primarily because of pressure from others such as a school, a child welfare agency, or a court, there may be considerable resistance to both treatment and medication. Some of these parents may delay filling the prescription, lose it, or simply not fill it. Other parents consider it something to be done when convenient, especially if they have to travel any distance to get the prescription filled. If money is involved, even the amount necessary for travel to the pharmacy or to pay for the medication, limitations may delay some families from purchasing the medication for legitimate financial reasons. These issues may come into play each time the prescription is renewed; in addition, it is common in many clinics for parents to miss appointments, including those when medication is to be renewed.

At times, some children and adolescents, both outpatients and inpatients, actively try to avoid ingesting medication. Their techniques may include pretending to place the pill in their mouths and later discarding it, or placing the pill under the tongue or between teeth and the cheek when swallowing and later spitting it out. Adherence in these cases may improve if the person administering the medication observes it in the mouth and watches the patient swallow it. Crushing the medication may be helpful in some cases, but one must be certain that absorption rates will not be so significantly altered as to cause decreased clinical efficacy or adverse or toxic effects. If available, switching to a liquid form of the medication may be indicated for some patients.

Adverse effects are another factor that influences adherence, particularly in older children and adolescents. For example, if they feel "funny" or different, or if they develop a stomachache, they may be more reluctant to take medication. Adolescents may be especially sensitive to adverse effects affecting sexual functioning. When a child or an adolescent is primarily responsible for administering his or her own medication, unpleasant or adverse effects are generally more likely to interfere with adherence. Richardson et al. (1991) reported that children and adolescents who developed parkinsonism while receiving neuroleptics were very aware of the symptoms and described them as "zombie-like" and a reason for nonadherence with outpatient treatment. These and other adverse effects can have similar influences on children and adolescents.

Nonadherence may be lessened sometimes if an adequate, understandable explanation of the simple pharmacokinetics of the medication is given to parents and patients when initially discussing medication. For example, the importance of keeping blood levels fairly constant by taking the medication as prescribed can be emphasized and reviewed again if lack of adherence becomes important. Conversely, when parents continue to sabotage treatment consciously, or unconsciously, because of their own psychopathology, or for other reasons, and this behavior seriously interferes with the psychiatric treatment of a child or an adolescent, it may be necessary to report the patient to a government agency as a case of medical neglect, and request legal intervention. Likewise, it may be necessary to discontinue medication if adherence is very poor or so unacceptably erratic as to be potentially dangerous.

Explaining Medication to the Child or Adolescent

The clinician should discuss the medication with the child or adolescent as appropriate to the patient's psychopathology and ability to understand. Giving the patient an opportunity to participate in his or her treatment is helpful for many reasons.

The patient can feel like an active partner in the treatment. This can alleviate feelings of passivity (i.e., that treatment is something over which the patient has no control). Letting the patient know that he or she should pay attention to the effects of the medication to report them to the therapist, that the patient will be listened to, and that the information the patient conveys will be considered seriously in regulating the medicine also helps the therapeutic relationship. The patient can also be informed that although medication may provide some relief or help, it cannot do everything, and he or she must still contribute effort toward reaching the treatment goals. This can be particularly important during adolescence, when issues of autonomy and control over one's own body are normal developmental concerns.

Because the patient is experiencing firsthand the disorder being treated, in many cases valuable information necessary for regulating the medication can be obtained directly. Some fairly young children can express whether the medicine makes them feel better, more calm, or quiet; less mad or less like fighting; happier or sadder; less afraid, upset, nervous, or anxious; or worse, sleepy, tired, more bored, "madder," or harder to get along with; and so on. Although parents or caretakers can provide much useful information, they may be unaware of some information that the patient can provide if time is taken to learn the words or expressions that the child uses to communicate feelings and experiences.

Adverse effects should be explained so that the child or adolescent understands them. The patient's awareness that adverse effects may be transient (e.g., that tolerance for sedation may develop) or reversible with dose reduction may be helpful in gaining cooperation during the titration period. Foreknowledge also increases the sense of control and can decrease fear of some adverse effects. For example, if an acute dystonic reaction is a possibility, it is important to realize how frightening this can be to some patients (and their parents). Explaining beforehand that if this reaction occurs, medicine will help, and the condition will go away can make the experience less frightening. Also, if a rapidly effective oral medication such as diphenhydramine, an antihistamine with anticholinergic properties, is made available and patients and parents are aware of what is happening, the medication may be administered earlier in the process, frequently aborting a potentially more severe reaction.

Children who ride bicycles and adolescents who drive a car, motor bike, or motorcycle, or operate potentially dangerous machinery should be cautioned if a medication may cause sedation or other impairment. They should be told to wait until they are sure how they are reacting to the medication before engaging in these activities. Similarly, if an adolescent is likely to use alcohol or other psychoactive drugs, he or she should be warned of possible additive or other adverse effects. Medications such as monoamine oxidase inhibitors are too risky to recommend except in very cooperative patients who are able to follow the necessary strict dietary restrictions to avoid a potential hypertensive crisis.

Medicolegal Aspects of Medicating Children and Adolescents

Medicolegal issues usually involve concerns about the clinician's clinical competence or performance. These issues arise primarily when something goes wrong. Incidentally, that "wrong something" may have nothing to do with the clinician's specific treatment or competence, but may, for example, be an outcome that displeases the patient or guardian. Even then, for a medicolegal issue to arise, someone who has become aware of it must decide to pursue the matter legally.

The importance of these issues is that the clinician's relationship with the patient and his or her family or caretakers can either increase or decrease the likelihood of legal proceedings. As a general rule, the better the quality of the relationship and rapport between the physician and the patient and his or her family, the less the likelihood for legal proceedings to occur. Parents, who are angry at their child's physician or who feel neglected or not cared about, are more likely to institute legal proceedings. Taking time to explain what the medicine may or may not do is important; no medication can be guaranteed to be clinically effective and safe for every patient.

If there is a risk that a depressed patient may attempt suicide and yet the patient is not hospitalized, this should be discussed with all concerned parties. Public perception of the association of suicidal ideation with a number of psychotropic agents has intensified the importance of these concerns. The patient may be asked to commit verbally or in writing to a contract to contact the clinician before any attempt to take his or her own life. Legal guardians should be informed of and concur with the decision that their child or ward will not be hospitalized and that, although there is a risk, the degree of risk is acceptable to avoid hospitalization. The guardians should be asked to provide more formal supervision until the depression improves sufficiently. If such measures are carried out and documented and a working rapport established, the risk of legal action and/or liability will be lessened should a suicide attempt, successful or otherwise, occur.

The clinician should make a genuine effort to establish a working rapport with parents who have consented under duress to the treatment of their child or adolescent (e.g., if their child has been removed from their care by a governmental agency because of abuse or neglect or where medication may be a prerequisite for remaining in a particular educational program), although this is frequently difficult.

Holzer (1989) noted that most, if not all, malpractice claims occur in cases with either an unexpected clinical outcome or an event that is perceived by the patient (or parents) as avoidable or preventable. The aspects of psychopharmacotherapy that have potential for medicolegal implications parallel this book's entire section on general principles of psychopharmacotherapy. Lawsuits are most frequently brought if something is omitted or if something that could reasonably have been prevented goes wrong. It should be emphasized that proper documentation in the clinical record is essential. If this is not done, the clinician's position is precarious in case legal difficulties arise. Although the ascendancy of electronic health records (EHRs) made it possible for physicians to document their assessments and interventions more fully, EHRs also make every aspect of patient care easily discoverable. Particular areas of concern are discussed later.

For a comprehensive overview of malpractice issues in child psychiatric practice, see Benedek et al. (2010).

Ethical Issues in Child and Adolescent Psychopharmacology

Ethical concerns are paramount in the practice of psychiatry, and especially with children because of their inherent vulnerability and their special reliance upon others and their environment. Contemporary medical ethics rests upon a set of major principles (Veatch, 1991): beneficence, maleficence, autonomy, veracity, fidelity, and avoidance of killing. These principles are often designated consequentialist (beneficence and nonmaleficence—having to do with good outcome) and nonconsequentialist (having to do with inherent morality—autonomy, fidelity, veracity, avoidance of killing, and justice). Although many today assign a higher lexical ranking to the nonconsequentialist principles, this stance may be questioned in view of the vulnerability of children and their inherent lack of autonomy. In any case, it is the duty of the practitioner to recognize and appropriately balance the application of these principles.

The consequentialist principles of beneficence and nonbeneficence are usually the instinctive first consideration of clinicians. All medications that we use have both desirable and adverse effects, and each prescription represents an attempt to balance these effects for an individual patient. The history of psychopharmacology is replete with misapprehensions of these. The neuromuscular and metabolic effects of neuroleptics compared with their limited effectiveness in many off-label uses are a prime example.

Another such example would be the use of a psychostimulant in a child whose inattentive behavior in school results not from an attention-deficit disorder but from a language-based learning disability. The child would demonstrate less activity when receiving the medication to the possible satisfaction of adults; however, this child would not be adequately educated, and the occurrence of dysphoria or other adverse effects might hurt the child.

It is an intrinsic duty (based on the principle of fidelity) for a physician to pursue beneficence and avoid maleficence. It is obvious that a physician can do so only with a comprehensive biopsychosocial diagnostic understanding of the child patient. The physician must also have as full a familiarity as possible with the effects of any agents to be considered. Ignorance is unethical.

The nonconsequentialist principles present a more nuanced challenge. Avoiding killing is a clearly defined and almost universally accepted principle among physicians, despite concerns about euthanasia. Fidelity, the adherence to behavioral and professional standards, in the context of a doctor–patient relationship depending on a social contract, is universally accepted. Justice in the context of medical ethics refers to the allocation of resources among a larger population; its application involves a range of political and cultural issues that are constantly debated.

Veracity in today's context requires not only the avoidance of falsehoods but the telling of the "whole truth." Two complications arise here. First of all, doctors and patients considering pharmacologic treatment face an intimidating volume of information. The pages of fine print in the *PDR* are intimidating to many patients and families and contain information of varying relevance to physicians. The full possibility of adverse effects from any agent can never be absolutely known. In this situation, physicians should offer as much information as they judge families can digest at a given time, with the added proviso that other information is available, that it can be acquired from the physician and other sources, and that no other information can be absolutely complete. At times, physicians fear that information may be daunting to families and will discourage the acceptance of beneficial agents. Parents almost always have the autonomous right to refuse to give psychotropic agents to their children, despite the concerns of physicians. Coercion is usually unethical and seldom successful. These issues can be resolved only through communication, and the ability to communicate with authority, empathy, and clarity is as essential a skill in psychopharmacology as is scientific knowledge (Krener & Mancina, 1994).

The second complication of veracity is the cognitive level of the child patient. One must provide a clear and developmentally appropriate explanation of risks, benefits, and possible adverse effects of medication; this is important not only from an ethical standpoint but also to assure that the child can recognize positive and/or adverse effects and report them.

Autonomy is the most complicated ethical issue in child psychopharmacology. In general, parents have absolute authority in decisions related to the treatment of minor children. Concurrently, however, children, despite their intrinsically limited autonomy, are seen as having the right to assent or refuse treatment. Assent is "agreement obtained from those who are unable to enter a legal contract" (Ford et al., 2007). Dockett and Perry (2011) describe assent as "a relational process whereby children's actions and adult's responses taken together reflect children's participation in decisions"; this is an interactive process. In their masterful review, Krener and Mancina (1994) describe various models for decision making and demonstrate that autonomy in child patients, as well as adherence, is engendered by a communicative rather than an authoritative or prescriptive stance.

This same principle is obtained in addressing the autonomy of parents or guardians. In rare cases, this autonomy may be superseded by legal interventions as in overt abuse or neglect; however, this almost never occurs regarding issues of psychopharmacology. Consequently, for both ethical and pragmatic reasons, the clinician must respect the nearly total autonomy of parents. Krener and Mancina provide models and examples for decision making. In all of these cases, there is a framework of communication that is respectful, empathetic, and complete.

The most specific application of autonomy arises in informed consent. Today, most physicians are aware of the absolute necessity for documentation of informed consent to all treatments, for legal as well as ethical reasons. Informed consent involves information and voluntariness. Patients and families are provided with a diagnosis, the nature and purpose of an intervention, and the risks and benefits of all options, including no treatment (American Medical Association [AMA], 2016). These principles are accepted throughout much of the world (Malhotra & Subodh, 2009).

A special problem that involves all principles of ethics arises from the use of psychotropic agents in the face of inadequate or inappropriate psychosocial services or environmental settings. This most often occurs with the intent of managing or attenuating aggressive behavior. Massive public attention was recently directed toward the alleged misuse or overuse of psychotropic agents, notably neuroleptics among children in foster care (Kutz, 2011). Similar concerns were raised for children in other treatment settings (MMDLN, 2011). It is charged that these medications were given involuntarily (autonomy) and without full information (veracity) to children. Adverse effects arose (nonmaleficence) with few if any concurrent benefits (beneficence). Implicit and explicit accusations are made that these agents are used for behavioral control in the absence of appropriate environments and psychosocial treatments (justice). Clinicians involved in these issues may be overwhelmed by massive numbers of needy children and very sparse treatment resources. In certain circumstances, clinicians may opine that medications given in a resource-starved setting constitute a more beneficent alternative than placement in restrictive settings, multiple brief foster or residential placements, incarceration, or abandonment. The obvious answer to this ethical dilemma is the development of comprehensive environmental and treatment resources. In the absence of that blessed circumstance, clinicians must approach these questions with a broad awareness of all ethical principles involved, applying them with both rationality and sensitivity; this approach to ethics facilitates all medical practice. The Codes of Ethics and the Ethics Committees of the American Psychiatric Association and the American Academy of Child and Adolescent Psychiatry provide assistance in assessing these dilemmas (Sondheimer & Klykylo, 2008).

Treatment Planning

Issues Concerning Diagnosis and Implications for Medication Choice and Premedication Work-Up

Areas of primary importance include making a correct psychiatric diagnosis and being aware of coexisting medical conditions. Obtaining accurate medical and psychiatric histories, including previous medications and the patient's response to them, as well as adverse effects and allergic reactions, is essential. Nurcombe (1991) notes that the physician may be held liable if adverse reactions or medication interactions that could have been prevented by taking an accurate and adequate history occur. History taking must be followed by a proper premedication work-up; if the patient has a medical condition, the physician must consider how the psychotropic medication may affect that condition. Physicians must also determine whether interactions with other medications the patient is taking may occur. Examples to avoid include (a) making an incorrect diagnosis and prescribing the wrong medication, or failing to detect or recognize coexisting conditions that would contraindicate the chosen medication; (b) prescribing a medication that will interact adversely with another medication the patient is taking or a medication to which the patient has previously been allergic; or (c) failing to perform a baseline and serial electrocardiograms (ECGs) or to monitor serum levels when tricyclics are used because of possible cardiotoxicity.

Issues Concerning Informed Consent

The treatment plan should be discussed and agreed upon by the legal guardian and the patient as appropriate for his or her age and understanding. The diagnosis and the risks and benefits of the proposed treatment and alternative treatment possibilities should be reviewed. To give informed consent, a patient (or legal guardian) must be mentally competent, have sufficient information available, and not be coerced. Adolescents 12 years of age and older should participate formally in developing their treatment plans and in giving informed "assent." If this is not possible, it should be so stated in the clinical record. It is wise to have both the legal guardian and, when appropriate, the patient sign the treatment plan and/or an informed consent ("assent" for underage individuals) for medication. If this is not done, at a minimum the clinician must document the discussion of the treatment plan and the response of the patient and legal guardian in the clinical record.

Nurcombe (1991) recommends that the following be discussed:

1. The nature of the condition that requires treatment.
2. The nature and purpose of the proposed treatment and the probability that it will succeed.
3. The risks and consequences of the proposed treatment. (It should be noted, e.g., if the proposed medication is an off-label use and that possible rare or long-term treatment-emergent adverse events or unknown interactions may occur, especially for newer medications where there is relatively little clinical experience. Also newer, postinitial medication marketing adverse events must be explained clearly and not minimized which could be interpreted as misleading in order to obtain consent, e.g., the recent warning for all antidepressants that they increased suicidal thinking and behavior in short-term studies in children and adolescents with major depressive and other psychiatric disorders should not be downplayed. Another example would be to discuss possible prolactin increase, weight gain, and onset of type 2 diabetes with risperidone.)
4. Alternatives to the proposed treatment and their attendant risks and consequences.
5. Prognosis with and without the proposed treatment (p. 1132).

Popper (1987a) adds that it should be explicitly stated that there may be unknown risks in taking the medication, especially when using novel psychopharmacologic treatments or treatments in which risks versus benefits are uncertain.

Involuntary medication of patients occurs primarily in emergency rooms and inpatient wards. This is usually permissible in a true emergency, but Nurcombe (1991) cautions that even involuntary commitment to a hospital for psychiatric treatment permits involuntary medication only in narrowly defined circumstances. Administering medication forcibly without judicial approval in a nonemergency situation may be considered battery. Physicians should become thoroughly familiar with their state laws and local hospital policies governing these matters.

Issues Concerning the Administration of Medication

Issues that concern the administration of medication include justification for the decision to use medication in treating the psychiatric condition (risks vs. benefits), rationale for the initial agent chosen, and administration of the medication by the appropriate route, usually orally, and in a clinically efficacious dose. If a patient is suicidal, the prescribing physician should ascertain to the best of his or her ability and document that only sublethal amounts of medication are accessible to the patient. It is best to have a responsible adult, usually a parent, have control of the medication—keeping it where the patient does not have access to it and dispensing it to the patient as directed. The medication should be completely or nearly finished before more is prescribed. The clinician must monitor the medication adequately for the duration of the therapy and should either discontinue the medication or attempt to do so at appropriate intervals, or document in the clinical record the reasons for the decision not to follow this protocol. Responsible deprescribing guidelines and considerations are discussed in Chapter 4.

Examples of behavior that may increase medicolegal risk include failing to prescribe medication for a condition for which most practitioners would, prescribing a medication without personally evaluating the patient (e.g., based on another physician's report), prescribing an inappropriate medication for the diagnosis (e.g., amphetamines to a drug abuser), using an unsatisfactory rationale to justify the choice of medication, administering an inappropriate dosage for the disorder (e.g., subtherapeutic levels), or administering medication by an inappropriate route (e.g., continuing to give medication intramuscularly when it is no longer indicated or necessary). A patient's use of a prescribed medication to attempt or successfully complete a suicide may also result in legal action.

■ *Off-label Prescribing/Deviating from a Manufacturer's Labeling of a Medication*

This book discusses many uses of psychoactive medications that are different from those formally recommended by the manufacturer or approved by the U.S. Food and Drug Administration (FDA) for advertising as safe and effective. Many of these off-label uses are medically accepted, but others are not yet common medical practice. Deviating from the usual clinical practice may increase the risk of legal action. Although legally permissible, using FDA-approved medications for non–FDA-approved indications and using FDA-approved medications for approved indications in children below the age limit for which they are approved may increase the potential for liability. Similarly, not adhering to the recommendations of the manufacturer (in the package insert or as reprinted in the *PDR*)—for example, exceeding recommended dosages—should alert the clinician to carefully document the rationale for doing so. In general, however, clinicians are on solid ground if they have assessed the risk–benefit ratio for prescribing a medication for a non–FDA-approved indication and have documented a scientifically reasonable rationale for choosing a particular medication over other possible treatments in the medical record.

It should be clear that the preceding discussion of off-label use applies primarily to situations where data were lacking at the time of application for approval by the FDA and subsequent research and clinical practice support a rationale for their use. Most frequently, there were insufficient data to determine efficacy and safety in the pediatric age group or the medication was being used for a diagnosis not initially studied. It should be clear that ignoring specific safety recommendations contained in the package insert that are based on verifiable data is an entirely different situation and is not condoned.

In clinical practice, standard treatments and off-label (non–FDA-approved) but clinically accepted treatments that may be efficacious with less risk should almost always be tried before less clinically accepted or riskier medications. Concurrence of a consultant and appropriate psychopharmacologic references supporting such use may be helpful when the off-label use is not commonly accepted (Nurcombe, 1991). As a general principle, the more novel the treatment or uncertain the risk–benefit ratio, the more severely disabling the condition should be for which it is used.

■ *Issues Concerned with Documenting Ongoing Appropriate Attention to Medication and Related Matters in the Clinical Record*

The patient's clinical record should reflect continued appropriate monitoring of the medication's efficacy; monitoring for the presence or absence of adverse effects, including tardive dyskinesia; results of laboratory tests or other procedures (e.g., ECG) performed at appropriate intervals to monitor adverse effects; justifications for increases or decreases in dosage or changes in times of administration; decisions to employ a medication holiday or discontinue medication; and consequences of discontinuing the medication, including any change in symptomatology, reexacerbation of symptoms, rebound effects, or withdrawal syndromes such as a withdrawal dyskinesia.

When patients are hospitalized, it is important for the clinician to address in the medical record not only his or her own observations of the patient but also those of other professionals who have reported or recorded behaviors or symptoms that may indicate adverse effects of medication (e.g., unsteadiness of gait reported by a nurse or falling asleep in class reported by a teacher).

The reviews of Nurcombe (1991), Nurcombe and Partlett (1994), and Benedek et al. (2010) of medicolegal aspects of the entire practice of child and adolescent psychiatry, including specific court cases and decisions, are recommended to the interested reader. Popper (1987a) has written a chapter that remains relevant on ethical considerations of the relationship between obtaining consent for the use of medication from parents and children and adolescents and incomplete or unknown medical knowledge of the risks and long-term effects of psychoactive medication used during childhood and adolescence.

BASELINE ASSESSMENTS BEFORE INITIATION OF MEDICATION

All patients should have a complete medical history and physical and neurologic examinations. These examinations are essential to identify any organic factors contributing to the psychiatric symptomatology and any coexisting medical abnormalities. In addition, all medications may cause adverse physical and psychological effects; hence, a baseline examination before the initiation of psychopharmacotherapy should be mandatory.

Although there is considerable information available for stimulant medications, relatively little information is available concerning the long-term adverse effects of psychoactive medications on the growth and development of children and adolescents. Because of this fact as well as the potential medicolegal ramifications, particularly when medications are used for non–FDA-approved indications, it is recommended that the premedication work-up be reasonably comprehensive. The reader who wishes a more detailed review of laboratory tests and diagnostic procedures applicable to general psychiatry than that provided in the subsequent text is referred to the review of Realmuto (2012).

Physical Examination

The physical examination should include recording baseline temperature, pulse and respiration rates, and blood pressure. Height and weight should be entered on standardized growth charts, such as the Centers for Disease Control National Center for Health Statistics Growth Charts (CDC, 2000), so that serial measurements and percentiles may be plotted over time. Effects of medications on both stature and weight are discussed in detail in respective medication chapters.

Laboratory Tests and Diagnostic Procedures

The following are frequently recommended premedication laboratory tests and diagnostic procedures. Some of these tests may have already been done as a part of the pediatric/medical evaluation that should be a part of any comprehensive psychiatric evaluation. These tests are addressed more specifically under each class of medications or, if appropriate, for specific medications when they are discussed. Obviously, the premedication work-up will be influenced by and should be modified to accommodate any particular abnormal findings in the medical history or examination, such as renal, thyroid, and cardiac abnormalities, or by any initial abnormal laboratory results themselves.

Laboratory tests routinely or frequently recommended as part of a comprehensive, complete, pediatric examination, and/or premedication work-up include the following:

1. Complete blood cell count, differential, and hematocrit
2. Urinalysis
3. Blood urea nitrogen level
4. Serum electrolyte levels for sodium (Na^+), potassium (K^+), chloride (Cl^-), calcium (Ca^{2+}), phosphate (PO_4^{3-}), and carbon dioxide (CO_2) content
5. Liver function tests: aspartate aminotransferase or serum glutamic oxaloacetic transaminase, alanine aminotransferase or serum glutamic pyruvic transaminase, alkaline phosphatase, lactic dehydrogenase, and bilirubin (total and indirect)
6. Blood glucose, especially when second-generation antipsychotics will be prescribed, because they can cause metabolic syndrome and cause or exacerbate type 2 diabetes. The American Diabetes Association published, in collaboration with the APA, a protocol for monitoring adult patients treated with second-generation antipsychotics. Fasting plasma glucose and a fasting lipid profile are recommended (American Diabetes Association & American Psychiatric Association, 2004).
7. Lipid profile: hyperlipidemia with elevated triglyceride and cholesterol serum levels have been reported as an adverse effect of some second-generation antipsychotics. Sheitman et al. (1999) reported an increase of almost 40% in serum triglycerides in adults taking olanzapine.
8. Serum lead level determination in children below 7 years of age and in older children when indicated
9. If substance abuse (alcohol or drugs) is suspected, screening of urine and/or blood is usually indicated.

Other laboratory tests may be recommended before using specific psychoactive medications.

Pregnancy/Pregnancy Test

Because medications may have known or unknown adverse effects on the developing fetus, a serum beta human chorionic gonadotropin test for pregnancy should be considered for any adolescent capable of becoming pregnant, at a time as close to beginning the medication as convenient and reasonable. A related issue is that, if an adolescent is considered to be at significant risk for becoming pregnant despite birth control counseling, certain medications (e.g., lithium) should not be prescribed if at all possible, because the embryo would usually be exposed to the medication before pregnancy was detected.

Risk versus benefit must be carefully considered for both the patient and the (potential) embryo/fetus if a woman is on medication and has unprotected sexual intercourse or attempts to become pregnant. As is also well known, pregnancies occur at times even with "protected" sex. Once pregnancy is verified, serious concerns about teratogenic risk to the embryo/fetus arise. "A pregnant woman should not take any drug unless it is necessary for her own health or that of her fetus" (Friedman & Polifka, 1998, p. ix). Additional concerns occur when mothers who are taking medication wish to breastfeed their infants, as some agents and/or their metabolites are secreted in breast milk. Overall consideration of the health of a pregnant or nursing mother includes adequate maintenance of mental health, both to support healthy pregnancy as well as to support appropriate attachment in the infancy period while caring for the child. An example review of the importance of appropriate management of depression during pregnancy is available (Yonkers et al., 2009).

Discussion of these very important issues on a medication-by-medication basis is beyond the scope of this book.

Thyroid Function Tests

There is a strong association between clinical thyroid disease and psychiatric disorders, particularly mood disorders (Esposito et al., 1997). Thyroid function tests (thyroxine [T_4], triiodothyronine resin uptake [T_3RU], and thyroid-stimulating hormone or thyrotropin) are recommended before the use of TCAs and lithium. Abnormal thyroid function can aggravate cardiac arrhythmias that may occur as an adverse effect of TCAs (*PDR*, 1995). Lithium has been reported to cause hypothyroidism with lower T_3 and T_4 levels and elevated ^{131}I uptake.

Kidney Function Tests

Many medications are excreted at least partially through the kidney and in the urine. Because of reported adverse effects of lithium carbonate on the kidney, baseline evaluation of kidney function should be determined. Jefferson et al. (1987) suggest that a baseline serum creatinine and urinalysis are usually adequate and that more extensive testing (e.g., creatinine clearance, 24-hour urine volume, and maximal urine osmolality) is not practical or necessary for most patients.

Prolactin Levels

Prolactin is a polypeptide protein hormone synthesized and secreted by lactotrophs of the anterior pituitary gland. Prolactin stimulates breast tissue development and production of milk and lactation. Prolactin secretion is controlled by the tuberoinfundibular dopamine pathway and the inhibitory action of dopamine on D_2 receptors located on the surface of pituitary lactotrophs (Ayd, 1995; Stahl, 2000). Medications that antagonize dopamine D_2 receptors, that is, with D_2 blocking action such as antipsychotics and cocaine, as well as medications that may indirectly influence dopaminergic function such as fluoxetine, therefore have the capability of causing elevated prolactin levels (hyperprolactinemia) that have been associated with inhibition of gonadotropin secretion, with galactorrhea and amenorrhea in women, and with gynecomastia, decreased testosterone level, and impotence in men (Kane & Lieberman, 1992). In their seminal review, Correll and Carlson (2006) indicated that the relative potency of antipsychotics in inducing hyperprolactinemia is approximately: risperidone > haloperidol > olanzapine > ziprasidone > quetiapine > clozapine > aripiprazole.

The long-term clinical implications/effects of hyperprolactinemia on the general maturation and development of children and adolescents, and, in particular, on their endocrine and central nervous systems, are uncertain. However, the review of Correll (2008) suggests that there may be multiple adverse consequences associated with this condition, including pituitary tumors. Because of this, a baseline prolactin level may be useful before initiating treatment with an agent known to affect prolactin secretion. Baseline and continued monitoring should take into consideration variations in prolactin levels, such as typical variation over a 24-hour period and that activities such as nipple stimulation result in moderate increases in levels. Medications such as estrogens, TCAs, opiates, amphetamines, cimetidine, and some antihypertensives can also cause elevated levels. Ideally, specimen collection to monitor prolactin levels would be taken about 3 to 4 hours after awakening, because prolactin levels rise during sleep and peak in the early morning.

Wudarsky et al. (1999) reported prolactin levels in 35 subjects (22 males, 13 females; mean age 14.1 ± 2.3 years, age range 9.1 to 19 years) diagnosed with schizophrenia ($N = 32$) or psychotic disorder not otherwise specified (NOS) ($N = 3$)

before age 13 who were treated with haloperidol, olanzapine, and/or clozapine for 6 weeks. Reference normal plasma prolactin values used for this study were as follows: adult range (combined male and female), 1.39 to 24.2 ng/mL; mean for adult males, 5.6 ng/mL (range, 1.61 to 18.77 ng/mL), and for adult females, 7.97 (range, 1.39 to 24.2). Conventional normal reference values for prepubescent males are 4.0 ± 0.5 ng/mL and for prepubescent females, 4.5 ± 0.6 ng/mL.

Mean baseline prolactin levels were measured after a mean washout period of 3 weeks and were below normal limits. Prolactin levels during the sixth week were significantly elevated from baseline for all three medications (haloperidol, 9.0 ± 4.2 ng/mL vs. 47.8 ± 30.6 ng/mL [$P < .001$]; clozapine, 9.0 ± 3.4 ng/mL vs. 11.2 ± 4.0 ng/mL [$P < .007$]; olanzapine, 10.0 ± 4.7 ng/mL vs. 23.7 ± 7.7 ng/mL [$P < .003$]). The mean plasma prolactin level for the 10 subjects on haloperidol was above the upper limit of normal (ULN), and nine subjects had levels above the ULN. The mean plasma prolactin value for the 15 subjects on clozapine, although significantly elevated from baseline, remained within the ULN, and plasma prolactin levels remained within the normal range for all 15 subjects. The mean plasma prolactin level for the 10 subjects on olanzapine was above the ULN, and 7 of the subjects had plasma prolactin levels above the ULN. The authors noted that plasma prolactin levels usually returned to baseline values within a few days of the medication being discontinued, but persisted for up to 3 weeks in a few cases. When compared with adults, these younger subjects had more robust increases in plasma prolactin levels on haloperidol and olanzapine but not clozapine, perhaps because of a greater number or sensitivity of dopamine receptors in the tuberoinfundibular systems of children and adolescents. The authors called for additional studies of prolactin response to various medications in this age group and the effects of hyperprolactinemia on their development and maturation (Wudarsky et al., 1999).

Saito et al. (2004) conducted a prospective study of 40 subjects (22 males, 18 females; mean age, 13.4 years, age range 5 to 18 years) that examined the change in prolactin levels from baseline to a mean of 11.2 weeks of treatment with risperidone ($N = 21$), olanzapine ($N = 13$), or quetiapine ($N = 6$). Primary diagnoses were schizophrenia/psychosis ($N = 14$); mood disorder ($N = 14$); disruptive behavior disorder ($N = 9$); intermittent explosive disorder ($N = 1$); pervasive developmental disorder NOS ($N = 1$); and eating disorder NOS ($N = 1$); 80% of the subjects were taking two or more psychotropic medications. The authors hypothesized that, because of risperidone's relatively high affinity for D_2 receptors in the pituitary, children and adolescents receiving risperidone would develop hyperprolactinemia to a greater extent than those subjects receiving olanzapine and quetiapine. Baseline prolactin levels were drawn before beginning the atypical antipsychotic in 17 (43%) subjects and within 1 week of beginning treatment in 23 (57%). The reference range for normal was 3.9 to 25.4 ng/mL for all children, 4.1 to 18.4 ng/mL for males, and 3.4 to 24.1 ng/mL for females. Baseline prolactin levels, pubertal status, and gender were not significantly different among the three groups. Hyperprolactinemia was present in 53% of the subjects at end point. A greater percentage of subjects receiving risperidone (15/21 or 71%) had elevated prolactin levels (group mean end-point level 46.8 ± 33.3 mg/mL) than subjects receiving olanzapine (5/13 or 38%) with a group mean end-point level of 24.5 ± 17.8 ng/mL or subjects receiving quetiapine (1/6 or 17%) with a group mean end-point level of 16.7 ± 10.1 ng/mL. The end-point level of risperidone was significantly higher than that of olanzapine ($P = .008$) and that of quetiapine ($P = .027$). Prolactin levels in the olanzapine and quetiapine groups were not significantly different from each other. Regarding end-point prolactin levels, there were no significant gender differences, and postpubertal females did not have significantly different levels from the entire group. In addition, end-point prolactin levels were not associated with changes in weight. Interestingly, 25% (seven women and three men) of the entire group reported sexual adverse effects: breast tenderness ($N = 4$), irregular menses ($N = 3$), decreased libido ($N = 3$), erectile dysfunction ($N = 3$), galactor-rhea, and amenorrhea ($N = 1$); the authors suggested that this rather high level resulted from their asking specific questions rather than recording only spontane-ous reports. There was no association between the medication taken and sexual side effects; five of these subjects were on risperidone; three were on olanzapine; and two were on quetiapine. The authors also noted that the lower incidence of hyperprolactinemia in their study compared with that of Alfaro et al. (2002) is likely because the doses they employed were only approximately one half those used in the Alfaro et al. study. This study also suggested that children and adolescents may be more likely than adults to develop hyperprolactinemia at a specific dose of atypical antipsychotic.

Pappagallo and Silva (2004) reviewed the literature through 2003 on the effect of atypical antipsychotic medications in children and adolescents. They identified 14 studies with a total of 276 subjects. The authors concluded that, of the atypical antipsychotics, risperidone was more frequently associated with hyperprolactinemia than clozaril, the least; however, they noted that aripiprazole has partial D_2 agonist properties and may result in smaller increases in prolactin levels; to date, studies in adults have shown no significant prolactin elevations; values in children and ado-lescents had not been reported. The authors note that there is some evidence that prolactin levels may decrease over time without dose reduction. When prolactinemia is present, the authors suggest that other possible causes, including oral birth con-trol pills, opiates, and pregnancy, be considered. If the increase in prolactin is mild and adverse effects associated with prolactin are not troublesome, one can elect to continue to administer the medication with close monitoring of clinical effects and periodic prolactin levels. It is noted that data elucidating the long-term effects of hyperprolactinemia on the physical and emotional development of such children and adolescents are not yet available.

Croonenberghs et al. (2005) conducted an international multisite 1-year open-label trial of risperidone with 504 patients (419 males, 85 females; mean age 9.7 ± 2.5 years, range 4 to 14 years). Mean serum prolactin levels at baseline were 7.7 ± 7.1 ng/mL for boys (ULN 18 ng/mL) and 10.1 ± 8.1 ng/mL for girls (ULN 25 ng/mL). Prolactin levels rose rather sharply and peak average prolactin levels occurred at week 4 in both boys and girls and were above normal limits for both (boys, 28.2 ± 14.2 ng/mL and girls, 35.4 ± 19.1 ng/mL). Prolactin levels then gradually decreased until, by the ninth month of treatment, they were again within normal limits for both; and remained there for the duration of the study, although they remained higher than baseline. The following adverse effects, which could possibly be related to hyperprolactinemia, were noted: mild to moderate gynecomastia in 25 subjects (22 men and 3 women); menstrual disturbances in 6 subjects; galactorrhea in 1 patient; and moderately severe menorrhagia in 1 patient. However, as these symptoms can occur in normal populations, it is impossible to assess the added risk attributed by risperidone without a control group.

Electrocardiogram

Many psychiatric medications may have adverse effects on the cardiovascular sys-tem, both on the electroconductivity of the heart, as evidenced by the ECG, and on hemodynamics (e.g., blood pressure). Before prescribing psychoactive medication, a careful cardiac history should be done. A personal history of palpitations, syncope, or near-syncope, or a family history of long-QT syndrome, cardiac conduction defects, or sudden, unexplained death warrant further work-up (Gutgesell et al., 1999). The physical examination should include baseline heart rate and blood pressure. Some experts recommend baseline ECG as part of the complete physical examination of every child before prescribing psychoactive medication; it should be mandatory in any person with a history of, or clinical findings suggestive of, cardiovascular disease. ECGs are noninvasive and relatively inexpensive.

The American Heart Association (AHA) issued guidelines regarding cardiovascular monitoring of children and adolescents receiving psychotropic medications (Gutgesell et al., 1999); this particular review addressed cardiac monitoring in children for a multitude of psychotropic medication classes. A review of the literature reveals that in the years since those guidelines were initially issued, there has been continued and at times contentious discussion regarding necessity for routine pretreatment ECGs, particularly for children with ADHD. Concerns about potential associations between stimulant treatment and sudden cardiac death led to a series of FDA advisory statements about these possible cardiac risks (Stevens et al., 2014). However, a lack of evidence base to support routine pretreatment ECGs has rendered current guidelines that echo some of those original AHA recommendations. Thus, monitoring recommendations do not include routine pretreatment ECG, but do include routine pretreatment review of personal and family cardiovascular risk factors and assessment of heart rate and blood pressure as well as reassessing these same risk factors and vital signs during treatment (Hammerness et al., 2011).

A baseline ECG should be recorded before the administration of TCAs to determine any preexisting conduction or other cardiac abnormality because clinically important cardiotoxicity may occur, especially at higher serum levels. The ECG should be monitored with dose increases and periodically thereafter if tricyclics are used (this is discussed in detail in Chapter 8 under "Tricyclic Antidepressants and Cardiotoxicity").

Most of the antipsychotics, both standard and atypical, may cause ECG changes, including prolongation of the QTc interval. Lithium may also cause cardiac abnormalities, and an ECG is recommended before initiating therapy. Carbamazepine may also prolong the QTc interval.

It also frequently occurs that if the response to a particular medication is not clinically satisfactory, it is discontinued and another is prescribed or another agent may be added to the initial medication. In some such cases, the new medication or combination of medications would make an ECG necessary for optimal clinical practice.

Polypharmacy may also cause drug–drug interactions; of particular importance are interactions where one medication may affect the metabolism of a second agent (e.g., by inhibiting metabolism by the cytochrome P450 enzyme system). For example, two sudden deaths were reported when clarithromycin, which inhibits the cytochrome P450 enzyme system, and pimozide, which is metabolized by the P450 enzyme system, were administered simultaneously, giving rise to the possibility that their interaction was a contributing or causal factor.

Electroencephalogram

An electroencephalogram (EEG) may be considered for patients who have a history of seizure disorder, who are on an antiepileptic agent for a seizure disorder, or who may be at risk for seizures (e.g., following brain surgery or head injury), as antipsychotics, TCAs, or lithium have all have been associated with either lowered threshold for seizures or other EEG changes.

Blanz and Schmidt (1993) reported a significant increase in pathologic EEG findings (short biphasic waves) in child and adolescent patients receiving clozapine. Similarly, Remschmidt et al. (1994) reported EEG changes in 16 (44%) of 36 adolescents being treated with clozapine. Baseline EEG and periodic monitoring of EEG while on clozapine should be mandatory.

Baseline Behavioral Assessment

Clinical Observations

Baseline observations and careful characterizations of both behavior and target symptoms must be recorded in the clinical record. These should include direct observations by the clinician in the waiting room, office, playroom, and/or ward, as well as those reported by other reliable observers in locations such as the home and school. It is important to include usual eating and sleeping patterns, because these may be altered by medications. These observations should be described both qualitatively and quantitatively (amplitude and frequency), and the circumstances in which they occur should be noted in the clinical record.

It is also essential to record an accurate baseline rating in the clinical record before beginning psychopharmacotherapy in children or adolescents who have existing abnormal movements or who are at risk of developing them (e.g., patients diagnosed with autistic disorder or severe intellectual disability and/or patients who will be treated with antipsychotics). This documentation is necessary both to follow the patient's clinical course and to be able to differentiate among recrudescence of preexisting involuntary movements, stereotypies, and mannerisms and any subsequent withdrawal dyskinesias or new stereotypies that may occur when medication, particularly an antipsychotic, is discontinued. The availability of these longitudinal data becomes even more critical if the treating physician changes. Although the baseline data can be documented in the clinician's records, the use of a rating scale such as the Abnormal Involuntary Movement Scale (AIMS) (Rating Scales, 1985) or the Extrapyramidal Symptom Rating Scale (ESRS) (Gharabawi et al., 2005) that assesses abnormal movements is strongly recommended.

To be able to assess the efficacy of a specific medication, a baseline observation period, with reasonably stable or worsening target symptoms, is necessary. For inpatients, this will permit assessment of the combined effects of hospitalization and a therapeutic milieu and the removal of the identified patient from his or her living situation on the patient's psychopathology and symptoms. For outpatients, this observation period will give the clinician an opportunity to see the effect of the clinical contact and assessment on the symptom expression of the patient and the psychodynamic equilibrium of the family. During this observation period, some children and adolescents, both inpatients and outpatients, will improve enough such that psychopharmacotherapy will no longer be indicated. Unfortunately, because of the high cost of inpatient hospitalization and pressure by various managed care organizations, patients are often medicated before there is time to assess their responses to the inpatient environment.

Rating Scales

Rating scales are an essential component of psychopharmacologic research. They provide a means of recording serial qualitative and quantitative measurements of behaviors, and their interrater reliability can be determined. Two early influential publications concerning rating scales and psychopharmacologic research in children were the *Psychopharmacology Bulletin's* special issue *Pharmacotherapy of Children* (1973) and its 1985 issue featuring "Rating scales and assessment instruments for use in pediatric psychopharmacology research" (Rating Scales, 1985).

Rating scales are being used in clinical practice with increasing frequency, particularly in primary care settings. They should not be used as a replacement for a complete diagnostic interview and observation of the patient, but they can be useful augmenters for the diagnostic interview. Many have been demonstrated to be sensitive to treatment effects, and measurement-based care is a growing means of monitoring and demonstrating effects of both pharmacologic and nonpharmacologic interventions. Table 2.1 provides a summary of some commonly used rating scales in clinical practice. More comprehensive reviews of rating scales are also available. Also see the Appendix for the scales that are available on the public domain.

The AIMS (Table 2.2) is a 12-item scale designed to record in detail the occurrence of dyskinetic movements as a potential adverse effect of some psychotropic medications. Abnormal involuntary movements are rated on a 5-point scale from 0 to 4, with 0 being none, 1 being minimal or extreme normal, 2 being mild, 3 being

TABLE 2.1 » Commonly Used Rating Scales

Screen	Forms and Factors	Ages	Psychometric Properties	Item Number	Time to Complete	Public Domain	References
ADHD							
Connors Rating Scale-Revised (CRS-R)	Parent: [a]7 factors: cognitive problems/inattention, hyperactivity, oppositional, anxious-shy, perfectionism, social problems, [a]psychosomatic	3–17	IC 0.75–0.94; 6–8 wk TR 0.13–0.78; IR parent–teacher 0.12–0.50; SENS 92%, SPEC 94%, PPP 94%, NPP 92%	80 items	20–30 min	N	Connors et al. (1998a, 1998b, 1997)
	Teacher: 6 factors	3–17	IC 0.73–0.94; 6–8 wk TR 0.47–0.88; SENS 78%, SPEC 91%, PPP 90%, NPP 81%	59 items	20–30 min	N	
	Adolescent: 6 factors	12–17	IC 0.74–0.92; 6–8 wk TR 0.73–0.89; IR adolescent–parent 0.13–0.53, IR adolescent–teacher 0.08–0.41; SENS 81%, SPEC 84%, PPP 83%, NPP 82%	87 items	20–30 min	N	
Vanderbilt ADHD Parent Rating Scale (VADPRS)	Six factors: inattention, hyperactivity/impulsivity, oppositional defiant/conduct, anxiety/depression, academic performance, behavioral performance	6–12	IC excellent for ADHD; TR >0.80, SENS 0.80, SPEC 0.75, PPV 0.19, NPV 0.98	43 items	10–15 min	Y	Bard et al. (2013)
Vanderbilt ADHD Teacher Rating Scale (VADTRS)	Six factors: inattention, hyperactivity/impulsivity, oppositional defiant/conduct, anxiety/depression, academic performance, behavioral performance	6–12	IC good to excellent; SENS 0.69, SPEC 0.84, PPV 0.32, NPV 0.96	43 items	10–15 min	Y	Wolraich et al. (2013)
ADHD Rating Scale-IV (ADHD-RS-IV)	Two factors: inattentive, hyperactive/impulsive; parent and teacher forms	5–18	IC 0.86–0.92; TR over 4 wk 0.78–0.86 (home) 0.88–0.90 (school); IR 0.40–0.45; parent reports with better SENS; teacher reports with better SPEC	18 items	5–10 min	N	DuPaul et al. (1998)
Depression							
Patient Health Questionnaire (PHQ)	PHQ-A	12–18	SENS 0.73; SPEC 0.94	13 items	5 min	Y	Johnson et al. (2002)
	PHQ-9		SENS 0.80; SPEC 0.92; PPV 10.12; NPV 0.22	9 items	5 min	Y	Gilbody et al. (2007)

(continued)

27

TABLE 2.1 » Commonly Used Rating Scales (*continued*)

Screen	Forms and Factors	Ages	Psychometric Properties	Item Number	Time to Complete	Public Domain	Reference
Beck Depression Inventory (BDI-II)	Self-administered	13+	IC 0.79–0.91; mild cutoff ≥14 SENS 0.89 SPEC 0.72; moderate cutoff ≥20 SENS 1.00 SPEC 0.77; severe cutoff ≥29 SENS 0.67 SPEC 0.83	21 items	10 min	N	Dolle et al. (2012)
Child Depression Inventory (CDI)	Five factors: dysphoric mood, acting out, loss of interest, self-deprecation, vegetative sxs	7–18	IC 0.59–0.88; TR 0.38–0.87	27 items	<20 min	N	Kovacs (1992, 1985)
Mania							
Child Mania Rating Scale (CMRS-P)	Parent-rated scale based on DSM-IV Manic episode criteria	5–17	IC 0.97; TR 0.96; cutoff = 20 SENS 0.84 SPEC 0.98 compared to healthy controls; SENS 0.82 SPEC 0.94 compared to ADHD	21 items	10–15 min	Y	Pavuluri et al. (2006)
Anxiety							
Multidimensional Anxiety Scale for Children (MASC)	Four factors: physical sxs, social anxiety, separation anxiety, harm avoidance	8–16	IC 0.60–0.90; TR 0.65–0.93; parent–child agreement low but better for observable sxs and mother-child dyads; validity moderate to good	39 items	<25 min complete and score	N	March et al. (1997)
Pediatric Anxiety Rating Scale (PARS)	Frequency and severity of separation anxiety, social phobia, generalized anxiety	6–17	IC 0.64; TR 0.55; IRR 0.97; shows sensitivity to treatment effects	50-item checklist; 7 item severity scale	Clinician admin: 30 min initial; 15 min follow-up	Y	Research Units on Pediatric Psychopharmacology Anxiety Study Group (2002)
Screen for Child Anxiety Related Emotional Disorders (SCARED)	Five factors: panic/somatic, generalized anxiety, separation anxiety, social phobia, school phobia	9–19	IC total 0.9, range 0.78–0.87; TR 0.70–0.90; parent–child correlation total 0.32, range 0.22–0.39; cutoff point = 25 SENS 71%, SPEC 67%–71%	41 items	<15 min to complete and score	Y	Birmaher et al. (1999, 1997)

Trauma

Scale	Description	Age	Reliability/Validity	Items	Administration		Reference
Child PTSD Symptom Scale (CPSS)	Three factors: reexperiencing, avoidance, arousal; additional items assess function	8–18	IC total 0.89, range 0.70–0.80; TR total 0.84, range 0.63–0.85	24 items	15 min to complete and score	Y	Foa et al. (2001)

OCD

| Children's Yale-Brown Obsessive Compulsive Scale (CY-BOCS) | Obsessions and compulsions with separate scales | 6–17 | IC 0.81–0.87; IR 0.66–0.91 | 17 item checklist; 10 item severity scale | Clinician admin: variable, up to 120 min to administer and score | Y | Scahill et al. (1997) |

Tics/Tourette's

| Parent Tic Questionnaire (PTQ) | Motor and vocal tic domains | 7–16 | IC motor 0.79–0.82, vocal 0.83–0.87, total 0.86–0.90; 2 wk TR motor 0.79, vocal 0.72, total 0.84 | 28 items rated on frequency and intensity | parent rated | Y | Chang et al. (2009) |

Aggression

| Modified Overt Aggression Scale (MOAS) | Four aggression subscales | 12–18 | Normative data unavailable | 16 items | 5 min | Y | Sorgi et al. (1991) |

Substance Use

| Stages of Change Readiness and Treatment Eagerness Scale (SOCRATES) | Three factors: recognition, ambivalence, taking Steps | 12–18 | IC 0.88 for recognition, 0.93 for taking steps; strong concurrent evidence for validity | 19 items (short form) | | Y | Maisto et al. (2003) and Miller and Tonigan (1996) |
| CRAFFT Brief Screen for Adolescent Substance Abuse | | 14–18 | Cutoff score 2+ any problem use/abuse/ dependence SENS 0.76, SPEC 0.94, PPV 0.83, NPV 0.91 | 6 items | <5 min | Y | Knight et al. (2002, 1999) |

[a]The fact that the Parent questionnaire includes a psychosomatic factor. The Teacher and Adolescent versions have the six factors listed, and the Parent version has those six factors plus this 7th factor.

ADHD, attention–deficit/hyperactivity disorder; IC, internal consistency; IR, interrater reliability; NPP, negative predictive power; NPV, negative predictive value; OCD, obsessive compulsive disorder; PPP, positive predictive power; PPV, positive predictive value; SENS, sensitivity; SPEC, specificity; sxs, symptoms; TR, test–retest reliability (timeframe indicated if available).

TABLE 2.2 » Abnormal Involuntary Movement Scale (AIMS)

INSTRUCTIONS: Complete Examination Procedure before making ratings. MOVEMENT RATINGS: Rate highest severity observed. Rate movements that occur upon activation one less than those observed spontaneously

		(Circle One)				
FACIAL AND ORAL MOVEMENTS	1. **Muscles of facial expression** (e.g., movements of forehead, eyebrows, periorbital area, cheeks; include frowning, blinking, smiling, grimacing)	0	1	2	3	4
	2. **Lips and perioral area** (e.g., puckering, pouting, smacking)	0	1	2	3	4
	3. **Jaw** (e.g., biting, clenching, chewing, mouth opening, lateral movement)	0	1	2	3	4
	4. **Tongue:** Rate only increase in movement both in and out of mouth, NOT inability to sustain movement	0	1	2	3	4
EXTREMITY MOVEMENTS	5. **Upper** (arms, wrists, hands, fingers): Include choreic movements (i.e., rapid, objectively purposeless, irregular, spontaneous), athetoid movements (i.e., slow, irregular, complex, serpentine). Do NOT include tremor (i.e., repetitive, regular, rhythmic)	0	1	2	3	4
	6. **Lower** (legs, knees, ankles, toes): For example, lateral knee movement, foot tapping, heel dropping, foot squirming, inversion and eversion of foot	0	1	2	3	4
TRUNK MOVEMENTS	7. **Neck, shoulders, hips** (e.g., rocking, twisting, squirming, pelvic gyrations)	0	1	2	3	4
GLOBAL JUDGMENTS	8. **Severity of abnormal movements**	None, normal Minimal Mild Moderate Severe				0 1 2 3 4
	9. **Incapacitation due to abnormal movements:** Rate only patient's report	None, normal Minimal Mild Moderate Severe				0 1 2 3 4
	10. **Patient's awareness of abnormal movements:** Rate only patient's report	No awareness Aware, no distress Aware, mild distress Aware, moderate distress Aware, severe distress				0 1 2 3 4

DENTAL STATUS

11. Current problems with teeth and/or dentures

No   0
Yes   1

12. Does patient usually wear dentures?

No   0
Yes   1

EXAMINATION PROCEDURE

Either before or after completing the Examination Procedure, observe the patient unobtrusively at rest (e.g., in waiting room).

The chair to be used in this examination should be a hard, firm one without arms.

1. Ask patient whether there is anything in his/her mouth (gum, candy, etc.) and, if there is, to remove it.
2. Ask patient about the current condition of his/her teeth. Ask patients if he/she wears dentures. Do teeth or dentures bother patient now?
3. Ask patient whether he/she notices any movements in mouth, face, hands, or feet. If yes, ask to describe and to what extent they currently bother patient or interfere with his/her activities.
4. Have patient sit in chair with hands on knees, legs slightly apart, and feet flat on floor. (Look at entire body for movements while in this position.)
5. Ask patient to sit with hands hanging unsupported. If male, between legs, if female and wearing a dress, hanging over knees. (Observe hands and other body areas.)
6. Ask patient to open mouth. (Observe tongue at rest within mouth.) Do this twice.
7. Ask patient to protrude tongue. (Observe abnormalities of tongue movement.) Do this twice.
8. Ask patient to tap thumb, with each finger, as rapidly as possible for 10–15 s; separately with right hand, then with left hand. (Observe facial and leg movements.)[a]
9. Flex and extend patient's left and right arms (one at a time). (Note any rigidity and rate on DOTES.)
10. Ask patient to stand up. (Observe in profile. Observe all body areas again, hips included.)
11. Ask patient to extend both arms outstretched in front with palms down. (Observe trunk, legs, and mouth.)[a]
12. Have patient walk a few paces, turn, and walk back to chair. (Observe hands and gait.) Do this twice.[a]

[a]Activated movements.

Code: 0, none; 1, minimal, may be extreme normal; 2, mild; 3, moderate; 4, severe.

DOTES, Dosage and Treatment-Emergent Symptoms Scale (Guy, 1976a).

Modified from Public Health Service, Alcohol, Drug Abuse, and Mental Health Administration, National Institute of Mental Health. Abnormal Involuntary Movement Scale (AIMS). https://dmh.mo.gov/docs/dd/forms/healthsafety/aims.doc. Accessed May 30, 2018.

moderate, and 4 being severe. If a procedure is used to activate the movements (e.g., having the patient tap his or her thumb with each finger as rapidly as possible for 10 to 15 seconds separately with the right and then the left hand), movements are rated one point lower than those occurring spontaneously. Seven of the items rate abnormal involuntary movements in specific topographies: four items concern facial and oral movements, two items concern extremity movements, and one item concerns trunk movements. Three items are global ratings: two by the clinician concern the overall severity of the abnormal movements and the estimated degree of incapacity from them and a third records the patient's own degree of awareness of the abnormal movements. Using the AIMS will also make it less likely that an area that should be assessed will be omitted inadvertently and will also provide quantitative ratings for following the clinical course. Having a baseline and subsequent AIMS ratings available is most helpful to the initial treating physician in assessing any changes in baseline abnormal involuntary movements and increases, decrements, or changes in topography during the course of active treatment with psychoactive medication, as well as during periods of withdrawal from medication. These ratings are often essential to differentiate preexisting abnormal involuntary movements from withdrawal dyskinesias. Such ratings are even more helpful when other physicians may assume the treatment of the patient at a future time.

Medicating the Patient: Selecting the Initial and Subsequent Medications

In general, it is recommended that a medication approved by the FDA—for the patient's age, diagnosis, and target symptoms—be chosen initially unless other, off-label agents that are equally or more clinically effective and safer regarding adverse effects are available and are regularly used in the practice of child and adolescent psychopharmacology (e.g., the atypical antipsychotics). Factors such as selecting the medication with the least risk of serious adverse effects; known previous response(s) of the patient to psychotropic medication; the responses of siblings, parents, and other relatives with psychiatric illnesses to psychotropic medication; family history (e.g., a history of Tourette disorder); and the clinician's previous experience in using the medication should also be weighed in choosing the initial and, if necessary, subsequent medications.

The Texas Children's Medication Algorithm Project published algorithms for the treatment of childhood major depressive disorder (Hughes et al., 2007) and childhood ADHD with and without common comorbid disorders (Pliszka et al., 2006) diagnosed by DSM-IV (APA, 1994) criteria. The algorithms and guidelines for their use were developed using expert consensus methodology on the basis of scientific evidence, when available, and clinical experience and opinion, when necessary, with the goal of synthesizing research and clinical experience for clinicians in the public health sector and thereby increasing the quality and consistency of their treatment strategies.

Six of the Texas Children's Medication Algorithms are reproduced in Figures 2.1 to 2.6 as examples of the current state of the art in child and adolescent psychopharmacology research. To fully appreciate the thinking behind these and before using them, the complete publications should be read carefully. Algorithms serve only as a guide and these are presented as an example; clinicians will modify them to suit the individual clinical needs of their patients. Psychotherapeutic and psychosocial interventions, which are important to varying degrees with different patients, are not specifically integrated with these algorithms, but remain essential components of any comprehensive treatment program.

Generic Versus Trade Preparations

There has been controversy in the literature on the merits of brand-name agents, usually the initial, patented preparations of a medication, and generic preparations that typically enter the market after exclusive patent rights expire, and cost considerably less than the brand-name product. Although the active ingredients in the various preparations should be pharmaceutically equivalent, the inert ingredients and

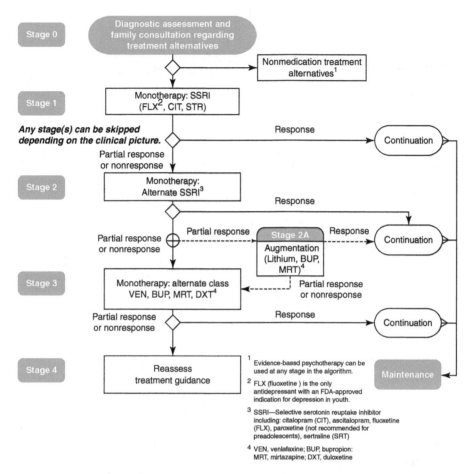

FIGURE 2.1 Medication algorithm for treating children and adolescents who meet DSM-IV criteria for major depressive disorder. FDA, U.S. Food and Drug Administration. (Revised based on Hughes et al. [1999]; Adapted from Hughes et al. 2007.)

the manufacturing processes may vary; therefore, the bioavailability of a medication may be significantly different among various preparations.

Many states now permit substitution of generic medications for the brand name under specified conditions. New York State, for example, requires all prescription forms to have imprinted: "This prescription will be filled generically unless prescriber writes 'daw' (dispense as written) in the box below." Pharmacists are directed to "substitute a less expensive drug product containing the same active ingredients, dosage form and strength" as the medication originally prescribed, if available (New York State Department of Health, 1988, p. iii). The book recognizes the differences in bioavailability among products.

The FDA Center for Drug Evaluation and Research publishes a book, *Approved Drug Products with Therapeutic Equivalence Evaluations* (the "Orange Book"), which lists medications, both prescription and nonprescription, approved by the FDA on the basis of safety and effectiveness. The list gives the FDA's evaluations of the therapeutic equivalence of prescription medications that are available from multiple sources. It classifies drug preparations into two basic categories: A and B ratings. A ratings are given to medication products that the FDA considers to be therapeutically equivalent to other pharmaceutically equivalent products for which there are no known or suspected bioequivalence problems or for which actual or potential problems are thought to have been satisfactorily resolved. B ratings are

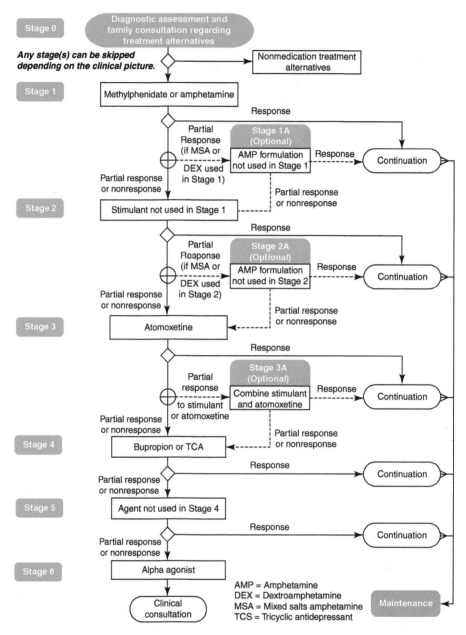

FIGURE 2.2 Algorithm for the psychopharmacologic treatment of attention-deficit/hyperactivity disorder without comorbid psychiatric disorder. (Adapted from Pliszka et al. 2006.)

given to medication products that the FDA does not at this time consider to be therapeutically equivalent to other pharmaceutically equivalent products.

These differences can have great clinical significance. For example, Dubovsky (1987) reported a case of severe nortriptyline intoxication due to changing from a generic to a trade preparation, which seemed to result from the significantly greater bioavailability of the trade preparation.

These comments are not a recommendation for any preparation over any other, but are meant to inform the clinician that different preparations of the same medication of the same strength may have different bioavailabilities; and that when they are

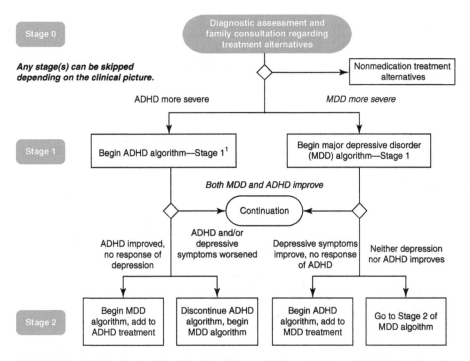

FIGURE 2.3 Medication algorithm for treating children and adolescents who meet DSM-IV criteria for major depressive disorder who also meet criteria for attention-deficit/hyperactivity disorder (ADHD). (Revised on the basis of Hughes et al. [1999]; Adapted from Hughes et al. 2007.)

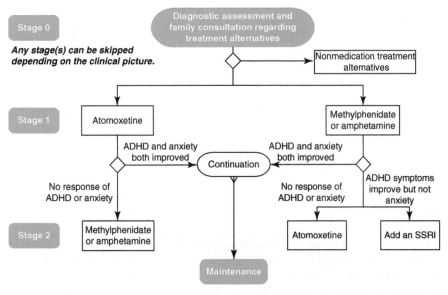

FIGURE 2.4 Algorithm for the psychopharmacologic treatment of ADHD and comorbid anxiety disorder. (Adapted from Pliszka et al. 2006.)

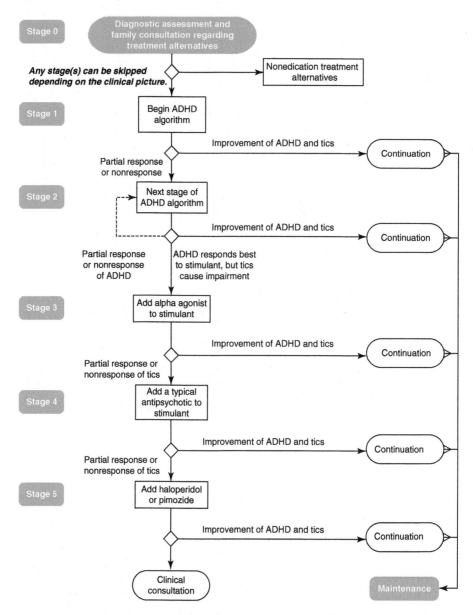

FIGURE 2.5 Algorithm for the psychopharmacologic treatment of ADHD and comorbid tic disorder. ADHD, attention-deficit/hyperactivity disorder. (Adapted from Pliszka et al. 2006.)

substituted for one another, there is a potential for significant clinical repercussions. If prescriptions that may be filled with various generic preparations are written, it is prudent for the physician to inform the patient or responsible adult that if the medication is different when refilled, to inform him or her and to note any changes in symptoms or feelings after switching to a new preparation. Although changes in manufacturer may occur at times even when prescriptions are filled at the same pharmacy, the likelihood of a change in manufacturer increases when different pharmacies are used. If a patient runs out of medication while traveling and must obtain the medication(s) from a new source, a change of manufacturer may be more likely. Hence, it is worthwhile to remember to ascertain that a patient has sufficient medication before going to summer camp or traveling.

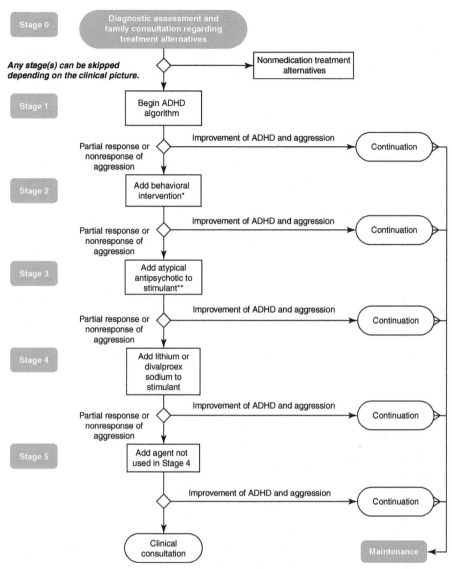

FIGURE 2.6 Algorithm for the psychopharmacologic treatment of attention-deficit/hyperactivity disorder (ADHD) and comorbid aggression. (Adapted from Pliszka et al. 2006.)

Standard (FDA-Approved) and Nonstandard (Off-label) Treatments

In this book, treatments approved by the FDA for advertising and interstate commerce will be considered standard treatments. This implies that the medication demonstrated clinical efficacy and that its use is substantially safe. The FDA's legal authority over how marketed medications are used, the dosages employed, and related matters is limited to regulating what the manufacturer may recommend and must disclose in the package insert or labeling. "The prescription of a drug for an unlabeled (off-label) indication is entirely proper if the proposed use is based on rational scientific theory, expert medical opinion, or controlled clinical studies" (AMA, 1993, p. 14).

Over the past five decades, a substantial body of clinical and investigational data has accumulated on using FDA-approved medications to treat children below the recommended age, using FDA-approved medications to treat children and adolescents for non–FDA-approved (off-label) indications (e.g., lithium to treat aggressive conduct disorder in any age group and TCAs to treat ADHD), and using medications before they were approved by the FDA for any indication (investigational medications) to treat psychiatric disorders in children and adolescents (e.g., clomipramine and fluvoxamine maleate).

Selective serotonin reuptake inhibitor (SSRI) antidepressants and atypical antipsychotics are at present the most clinically important FDA-approved medications used for nonapproved (off-label) indications in children and adolescents, although some SSRIs are approved for some indications in this age group. There is a growing consensus among child psychiatrists that the benefit/risk ratio of their use for non–FDA-approved indications is often preferable to that of some currently approved medications (e.g., a decreased risk of developing tardive dyskinesia). This is discussed in more detail in the specific medication section of this book.

Medication Interactions

Many psychoactive medications have significant interactions with other medications. It is essential to be aware of any medication, prescription, or otherwise that the patient may be taking concurrently and to evaluate the potential interaction.

As part of the medical history, enquiries should be made about all medications, including those prescribed by other physicians; over-the-counter medications; dietary supplements; and herbal preparations used even occasionally by the patient; and, as appropriate, alcohol and illicit or recreational drug use. Parents or caretakers and patients, as appropriate to their age and mental abilities, should be instructed to inform any physician who may treat them of the psychoactive medication(s) currently being taken. Similarly, patients whom the clinician is treating with psychoactive medication should be instructed to report at the next appointment whenever another physician prescribes any other medication for them or if they take any other drugs, over the counter or illicit, on their own initiative.

If substance abuse is known or suspected, screening of urine and/or blood for toxic substances may be indicated.

Drug interactions are discussed for each of the classes of psychoactive agents. An attempt has been made to emphasize the most important interactions and those interactions most likely to be encountered by the physician who is treating psychiatrically disturbed children and adolescents.

It is beyond the scope of this book to review all possible drug interactions. It is the prescribing physician's responsibility to attempt to determine any other medications his or her patient is taking and to assess any potentially adverse interactions of the medications before prescribing a new medication. The package insert, current *PDR*, current *Drug Interactions and Side Effects Index*, *Drug Facts and Comparisons*, *Drug Interactions in Psychiatry* (Ciraulo et al., 2006), or other suitable reference should be consulted. When appropriate and with the patient's consent, any other physicians treating the patient should be contacted so that a comprehensive treatment regimen that addresses both the psychiatric and the medical disorders of the patient safely may be mutually developed.

Regulating the Medication

Selecting the Initial Dosage

It is recommended in most cases that the treating physician initially prescribe a low dose, which will be either ineffective or inadequate for most patients. Although this cautious approach may lengthen the time necessary to reach a therapeutic dose, it is worthwhile for several reasons. First, pharmacokinetics vary not only among various age groups but also among individuals of a specific age. For genetic and other reasons, some individuals, for example, slow metabolizers, may be highly sensitive and responsive to a given medication, whereas others, namely, rapid metabolizers, may be relatively resistant or nonresponsive. By beginning with a low dose, the physician will avoid starting at a dose that is already in excess of the optimal therapeutic dose for a few patients, and those children and adolescents who are good responders at low dosages of medication will not be missed. If the initial dose is too high, the therapeutic range for these low-dose responders will not be explored and only adverse effects, which may at times even be confused with worsening of target symptoms, will be seen. Hence, a potentially beneficial medication may be needlessly excluded. For example, first, with stimulants a worsening of behavior may occur when optimal therapeutic doses for a specific patient have been exceeded. Second, with some medications (e.g., methylphenidate), there is no significant relationship between the serum level and clinical response. Third, excessive initial dosage may also cause behavioral toxicity, particularly in younger children. Behavioral toxicity has long been known to occur often before other adverse effects and includes symptoms such as worsening of target symptoms, hyperactivity or hypoactivity, aggressiveness, increased irritability, mood changes, apathy, and decreased verbal productions (Campbell et al., 1985). Fourth, some adverse effects of the medication may be eliminated or minimized; for example, acute dystonic reactions of antipsychotics and some adverse effects of lithium carbonate appear to be related in many cases to both serum levels and the rapidity of increase in serum level, and sedation may be less of a problem if dosage is increased gradually (Green et al., 1985).

The primary exceptions to gradual titration occur when an emergency situation exists, most often where there is danger or potential danger for injury to self, others, or property, and acute agitation or psychosis must be controlled as soon as possible.

Timing of Medication Administration

Scheduling Dosages

Times chosen for administration of the medication and the number of times it is administered per day should be related to its pharmacokinetics; for example, stimulants are most frequently given around breakfast and lunch, whereas antipsychotics may initially be given three or four times daily to reduce the risk of sedation and acute dystonic reactions. Once dosage is stabilized, it may be clinically more convenient and may increase adherence if medications with longer half-lives are administered only once or twice daily. Over the past 15 years, the number of long-acting, sustained, or extended-release preparations of medication increased significantly, increasing convenience to the patient. This is especially helpful for school children taking stimulant medication for ADHD who no longer require medication administration during school hours.

Pharmacokinetics and developmentally determined pharmacodynamic factors must still take precedence over convenience. For example, it may be possible to give the entire daily dose of an antipsychotic at bedtime to children and adolescents, whereas because younger children metabolize TCAs differently compared with adolescents and adults and they may be more sensitive to cardiotoxic effects, it is recommended that these medications continue to be administered to children and younger adolescents in divided doses.

Medication Holidays

Because of the adverse effects of medications and their known and unknown effects on the growth, maturation, and development of children and adolescents, it is universally agreed that it is prudent to use medication in as low a dose and for as short a time as is clinically expedient. For some children, "drug holidays" may be a useful means of minimizing the cumulative amount of medication taken over time. The feasibility and type of medication holidays vary with the diagnosis and severity of the disorder.

When stimulant medication is needed primarily to improve classroom functioning (increase attention span and decrease hyperactivity and sometimes conduct problems), as with some ADHD children, it is often possible to withhold medication on weekends and on school holidays and vacations, including the entire summer. This is particularly important if there appears to be evidence of any suppression of height and weight percentiles, because there may be catch-up or compensatory growth following discontinuation of stimulant medication.

Sometimes parents find that their hyperactive child is not a serious management problem without medication at home, but that difficulties arise when the child accompanies them on a shopping excursion or goes to a birthday party. In cases like this, when the parents' judgment can be trusted and medication is not used as a punishment, an understanding with the parents and child that medication may be used occasionally on weekends or vacations in situations that are particularly difficult for the child may be therapeutically indicated.

There is reasonable concern about the possibility of the development of an irreversible tardive dyskinesia in children and adolescents who receive long-term therapy with antipsychotic medication. There is some evidence that the development of tardive dyskinesia may be associated with both the total amount of antipsychotic agent ingested and the duration of treatment, although constitutional vulnerabilities to developing tardive dyskinesia also appear to play an important role (Jeste & Wyatt, 1982). Consequently, possible means of reducing the total amount of an antipsychotic agent ever taken may be clinically important in reducing the likelihood of developing tardive dyskinesia.

Both Newton et al. (1989) and Perry et al. (1989) reported studies of patients receiving first-generation antipsychotic medications, among whom medication holidays were not associated with differences either in symptom severity or adverse effects. Medication holidays require continued maintenance of clinical supervision and of observation by parents and caretakers, to document clinical changes and to circumvent relapses.

Dosage Increases

Changes in medication level should be based on the clinical response of the patient, and the rationale for each change should be documented in the clinical record. Knowledge of the characteristic time frame of response for a particular medication and diagnosis should influence these decisions. Therefore, the clinician may increase dosage once or twice weekly in some cases, when using stimulants or neuroleptics. On the other hand, the clinical efficacy of antidepressants may not be fully apparent for several weeks when used to treat a major depressive disorder. Once the total daily dose of an antidepressant has reached a level that is usually associated with clinical response, increasing the dose because of a failure to respond during the first 2 or 3 weeks of treatment is not sound psychopharmacologic practice unless serum medication levels are being monitored and are thought to be in the subtherapeutic range.

Titration of Medication

The goal of the clinician is to achieve meaningful therapeutic benefits for the patient with the fewest possible adverse effects. Here again, it is recommended that risks versus benefits be assessed. To do so scientifically, however, it is necessary to explore the dose range of a patient's response. Unless there are extenuating circumstances, it is usually advisable to continue raising the dose level until one of the following events occurs:

1. Entirely adequate symptom control is established.
2. The upper limit of the recommended dosage (or higher level if commonly accepted) is reached.

3. Adverse effects that preclude a further increase in dose occur.
4. After a measurable improvement in target symptoms, a plateau in improvement or a worsening of symptoms occurs with further increases in dose.

Unless this procedure is followed, an injustice may be done to the patient. This occurs most frequently when there is some behavioral improvement and the treating clinician stabilizes the dosage at that point. Further significant improvement that might have occurred had a higher dose been given is missed. It is recommended that the next higher dose be explored. If there is significant additional improvement, the therapist, in consultation with the patient and his or her parents, can make a judgment regarding whether the benefits outweigh the risks from the additional dosage.

Determining the Optimal Dose

Once the titration of the therapeutic dose to maximum clinical benefit is achieved for a specific patient, the lowest possible dose that produces the desired effects should be determined. This is considered the optimal dose for a specific patient. In clinical practice, this may sometimes require a compromise, and amelioration of target symptoms to an acceptable degree may occur only when some adverse effects are also present.

In those cases in which either no significant therapeutic benefit occurs or adverse effects prevent the employment of a clinically meaningful therapeutic dose, trial of a different medication must be considered. If there is a partial but meaningful clinical response, some clinicians would consider adding an additional medication (polypharmacy) rather than discontinuing the first medication and administering another. Whatever the case, clinician should not continue to prescribe medication in doses that do not result in significant clinical improvement.

Tolerability and Adverse Effects

All agents, including placebos, have adverse effects, or side effects. Actually, if one excludes allergic and idiosyncratic reactions, adverse effects are as much a characteristic of the pharmacologic makeup of a specific medication and are as predictable as its therapeutic effects. Simply put, medications have effects: some effects are desirable and some are not. Individual patients may vary as much in their experience of adverse effects of a medication as in their therapeutic responses to it. Adverse effects are important not only because of the immediate problematic effects they cause but also because they may be intimately related to issues of adherence, as discussed in the preceding text.

It is sometimes useful to think of adverse effects as the "unwanted effects" of the medication for the specific patient and therapeutic indication. For a different patient and situation, an adverse effect or a side effect will actually become the desired therapeutic action of the medication. For example, sedation, which may be an adverse effect when a benzodiazepine is prescribed for anxiolysis, is the desired result when a benzodiazepine is prescribed as a soporific. Similarly, appetite suppression is usually an undesired effect of stimulants prescribed for ADHD, but the action of choice when used to treat exogenous obesity.

Many adverse effects are related to dose or serum levels, but others are not. They may occur almost immediately (e.g., an acute dystonic reaction) or be delayed for years (e.g., tardive dyskinesia). They may be life threatening or fatal, or relatively innocuous. The adverse effects of a specific medication may differ according to the age and/or diagnosis of the subjects. For example, haloperidol produced excessive sedation in hospitalized school-age aggressive-conduct-disordered children on doses of 0.04 to 0.21 mg/kg/day (Campbell et al., 1984b), but not in preschoolers with autistic disorder on doses of 0.019 to 0.217 mg/kg/day (Anderson et al., 1984).

A thorough knowledge of the most important and frequent adverse effects of the medications considered is essential and will often play a decisive role in which medication is selected and/or when dosage is scheduled. For example, if a schizo-phrenic youngster has insomnia, the clinician may select a low-potency antipsychotic agent and adjust the dosage schedule so that any sedation will aid the child in falling asleep. As an added benefit, the risk of an acute dystonic reaction is lower than if a high-potency antipsychotic is chosen.

Likewise, the management of adverse effects is a vital component of pharmaco-therapy. In clinical practice, careful attention to adverse effects and flexibility about the time and amounts of specific doses may enable one to obtain a satisfactory clini-cal result with a minimal or acceptable level of adverse effects that is not possible if a fixed dosage schedule is used, as in some research protocols. Therefore, one can adjust medication levels slowly and in small increments or divide doses unequally over the day (e.g., giving more in the morning, more before bed, or the entire daily dose at bedtime).

The clinician must remember that the ability to understand adverse effects and verbalize unusual sensations, feelings, or discomfort not only varies among individual children but is also developmentally determined. Younger children spontaneously report adverse effects less frequently than do older children. Hence, the younger the child, the more essential it becomes for caretakers to be actively looking for adverse effects and for the physician to ask the patient about adverse effects using language appropriate to the child's level of understanding.

Many psychotropic medications may cause treatment-emergent sexual dysfunction–related adverse effects which are of significant concern to adolescents, especially those who may be sexually active. As many adolescents are uncomfortable in discussing such matters and do not spontaneously report them, it is particularly important for the clinician to routinely ask about such symptoms in a nonjudgmental, non-threatening way.

It is essential that the clinician examine the patient frequently for the develop-ment of adverse effects during the period when the medication is being regulated, at regular intervals during maintenance therapy, and during scheduled periodic with-drawals of the medication. For example, with antipsychotic medications, one should look particularly for sedation and extrapyramidal side effects, the development of abnormal movements, and, during medication withdrawal periods, any evidence of a withdrawal dyskinesia. Completion of the AIMS, as described earlier, is recom-mended as an aid in quantifying and following abnormal movements over time.

Monitoring of Serum Levels of Medications and/or of Their Metabolites

Morselli et al. (1983) and Gualtieri et al. (1984a) reviewed the pharmacokinetics of psychoactive medications used in child and adolescent psychiatry and the clini-cal relevance of determining their serum or blood levels. Determining the blood or plasma levels of medications and/or their metabolites is most useful when accurate measurements of all significant active metabolites are available and there is a known relationship between the clinical effects of the medication and serum concentration (Gualtieri et al., 1984a). Obviously, monitoring levels of medications whose toxicity is level-related, such as TCAs or lithium is crucially important for patient safety.

For many medications in current use in child and adolescent psychopharmacology, serum levels are not as clearly related to clinical effects or toxicity. Consequently, serum levels of stimulants, selective serotonin and norepinephrine reuptake inhibi-tors, and second-generation neuroleptics are not as commonly measured as those of older agents and are often of uncertain clinical utility. Still, there is a role for these measurements in some situations, especially when adherence is in question.

Clinically, the monitoring of serum levels is useful to verify adherence and to be certain that adequate therapeutic serum levels are available (i.e., that values fall within the therapeutic window) and thereby avoid discontinuing a trial of medication before clinically effective serum levels are reached or, conversely, avoid inadvertently reaching toxic serum levels.

School-aged children often have more efficient physiologic systems for metabolism and excretion than adults. As a result, doses comparable to those administered to adults, either on a total daily dose or on a dose-per-unit-weight basis, may result in subtherapeutic serum levels in children and younger adolescents. This could be one factor contributing to the clinical observation that children with schizophrenia, as a group, appear to show less dramatic clinical improvement than do adolescents and adults when administered neuroleptics (Green, 1989). It will be necessary to measure antipsychotic serum levels to determine whether this lack of improvement is due to subtherapeutic levels in some cases, because some children may also show clinical improvement at lower serum levels than do adults (Rivera-Calimlim et al., 1979).

Meyers et al. (1980) reported the case of a 13-year-old prepubescent boy diagnosed as having schizophrenia who required a dose of haloperidol of at least 30 mg/day to reach therapeutic serum neuroleptic levels. Monitoring serum levels of antipsychotics may therefore yield clinical information that is, at times, extremely useful. If a child or adolescent does not have a satisfactory response to usual doses of antipsychotics, serum neuroleptic levels should be determined, if available, before deciding to discontinue the medication.

In addition to age-related differences in pharmacokinetics, remarkable interindividual variations occur. For example, Berg et al. (1974) reported that a 14-year-old girl with bipolar manic-depressive disorder required up to 2,400 mg of lithium daily to maintain serum lithium levels of 1 mEq/L. Her father had the same disorder and also required unusually high doses of lithium to reach therapeutic levels.

Currently, regular determinations of serum levels should be considered mandatory when lithium carbonate, certain antiepileptic medications, or TCAs are used in treating children and adolescents. In current practice, monitoring of medication and metabolite serum levels is of considerable practical importance in the use of the TCAs. This monitoring is needed because there is minimal correlation between the dose and serum level, and serum levels are correlated significantly with the clinical response and/or potentially serious adverse effects (e.g., cardiotoxicity).

Similarly, Biederman et al. (1989b) reported that desipramine serum levels varied an average of 16.5-fold at four different dose levels in 31 children and adolescents diagnosed with attention-deficit disorder. These authors, however, found no significant linear relationship between the total daily dose or weight-corrected (mg/kg) daily dose and the steady-state serum desipramine level and any outcome measure, including clinical improvement. There was a tendency for serum desipramine levels in subjects who were rated very much or much improved on the Clinical Global Improvement Scale to average 60.8% higher than in unimproved subjects.

Morselli et al. (1983) also emphasized that monitoring plasma levels of haloperidol, chlorpromazine, imipramine, and clomipramine is particularly helpful in optimizing long-term treatment with these agents.

On the other hand, a detailed review of the pharmacokinetics and actions of methylphenidate concluded that "blood MPH (methylphenidate) levels are not statistically related to clinical response, nor are they likely to prove clinically helpful until this lack of correlation is understood" (Patrick et al., 1987, p. 1393).

When antiepileptics are used for control of aggression or as mood stabilizers, effective serum levels are thought to be in the same range as when they are used to control seizures. Monitoring of serum levels (both medication and significant metabolites) will become increasingly important for other medications used in child and adolescent psychiatry if and when their determinations become more readily available and correlations with clinical efficacy and adverse effects are established.

Discontinuation/Withdrawal Syndromes

Rapidly metabolized medications such as methylphenidate and amphetamines may be discontinued abruptly. However, with these agents, which have short half-lives, there may be some rebound effect during routine daily administration as serum levels decline during late afternoon or evening.

To minimize the likelihood of developing withdrawal syndromes, it is recommended that most medications be gradually reduced rather than stopped abruptly. The clinician should continue to complete the AIMS in patients who had preexisting abnormal movements before the initiation of medication that may have been masked or ameliorated or who are otherwise at risk for developing abnormal movements following withdrawal. If a withdrawal dyskinesia emerges upon discontinuing an antipsychotic medication, effort should be made to keep the patient off antipsychotics. Any abnormal movements should continue to be recorded on the AIMS.

Gualtieri et al. (1984b) reported both physical withdrawal symptoms (e.g., decreased appetite, nausea and vomiting, diarrhea, and sweating) and acute behavioral deterioration in approximately 10% of children and adolescents after their withdrawal from long-term treatment with first-generation antipsychotics. Both types of withdrawal symptoms ceased spontaneously within 8 weeks. It is extremely important that the clinician recognize that such symptoms may be expected withdrawal effects and that they are not necessarily a return of premedication symptoms. The symptoms must be monitored qualitatively and quantitatively over a sufficient period to see if they diminish, as would be expected with a withdrawal syndrome, or if they indicate that the underlying psychiatric disorder still requires medication for symptom amelioration.

When tricyclics are withdrawn abruptly or too rapidly, some children experience a flulike withdrawal syndrome resulting from cholinergic rebound. This characteristically includes gastrointestinal symptoms such as nausea, abdominal discomfort and pain, vomiting, and fatigue. Tapering the medication down over a 10-day period rather than abruptly withdrawing it will usually avoid this effect or significantly diminish the withdrawal syndrome. The clinician is cautioned that in patients with poor adherence, who in essence may undergo periodic self-induced acute withdrawals, the withdrawal syndrome may be confused with adverse effects, inadequate dose levels, or worsening of the underlying psychiatric disorder.

A withdrawal or discontinuation syndrome has also been identified for the SSRIs. Rosenbaum et al. (1998) reviewed the literature on discontinuation-emergent symptoms in adults taking SSRIs and noted that dizziness, headache, nausea, vomiting, diarrhea, movement disorders, insomnia, irritability, visual disturbances, lethargy, anorexia, tremor, electric shock sensations, and lowered mood have all been reported following SSRI discontinuation. There appeared to be a relationship between half-life and the development of discontinuation-emergent symptoms. Patients abruptly discontinued from medications with longer half-lives, for example, fluoxetine, developed fewer clinically significant effects than did patients who abruptly discontinued medications with short half-lives, for example, paroxetine or sertraline. Similar data are now emerging for children (Diler & Avci, 2002). A more detailed discussion of the discontinuation syndrome associated with SSRIs follows in Chapter 8.

Similarly, it is recommended that the alpha-adrenergic agonists, clonidine hydrochloride and guanfacine hydrochloride, be tapered gradually to reduce the likelihood of a hypertensive reaction and other symptoms, such as headache, nervousness, and agitation. This is more important for clonidine, as its half-life is significantly shorter than that of guanfacine.

In significant numbers of cases, after an initial treatment period of varying duration, medication may no longer be required or adequate symptom control can be maintained on a lower maintenance dose. In contrast, over time some patients may require higher doses to maintain gains. This may reflect a worsening of the psychiatric disorder per se or a developmental/maturational effect, as in a child with autistic disorder who becomes both stronger and more aggressive as he or she enters adolescence. In other cases, the need for increased medication may be a consequence of an individual's normal physiologic maturation altering the medication's pharmacokinetics and/or normal or excessive weight gain. In any case, ongoing regular clinical supervision of any child on medication is essential. This is both the responsibility and the privilege of the child and adolescent psychiatrist.

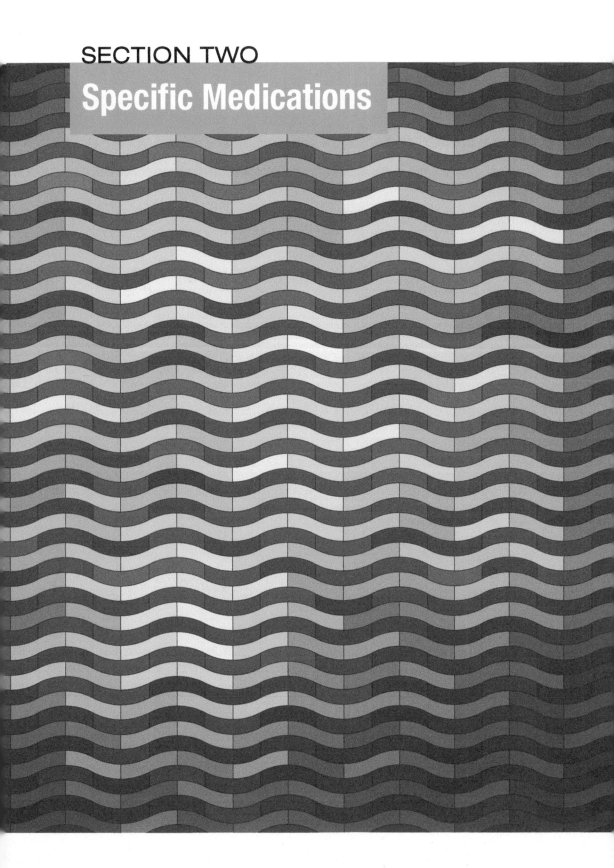

SECTION TWO
Specific Medications

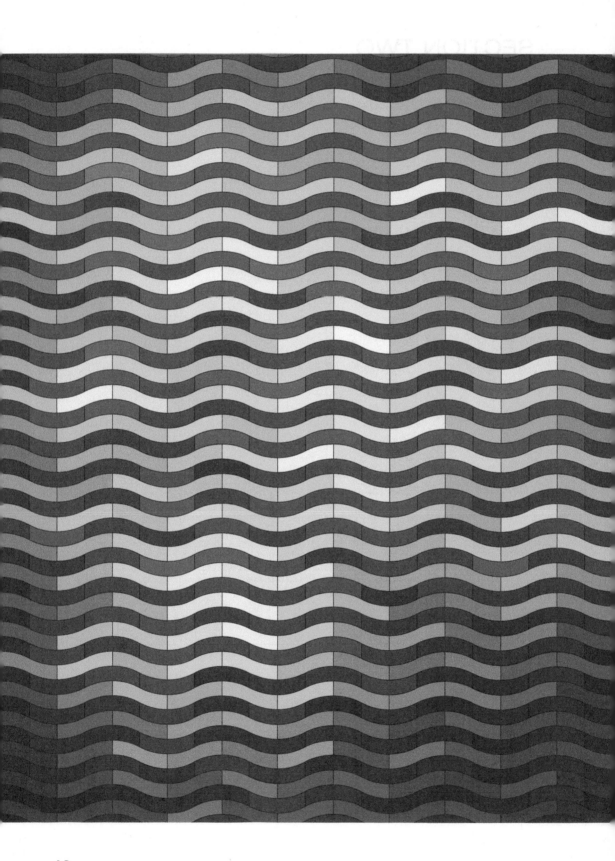

CHAPTER 3

Introduction

RYAN C. MAST AND RAVINDER S. SANDHU

INTRODUCTION

Child and adolescent psychopharmacology is a relatively new field, and the beginning of the modern era is usually considered to be Charles Bradley's 1937 publication that reported the effects of racemic amphetamine sulfate (Benzedrine) on 30 children (aged 5 to 14 years) who had various behavioral disturbances.

Bradley's publication in 1937 was followed by three papers from M. Molitch and coworkers. These papers detailed an investigation of amphetamine sulfate in children, including two placebo-controlled studies (Molitch & Eccles, 1937; Molitch & Polia-koff, 1937; Molitch & Sullivan, 1937). Two of the studies found that amphetamine sulfate improved the intelligence test scores of children, and one study reported that 86% of 14 boys with enuresis (who had not responded to placebo) were dry when given increasing doses of amphetamine sulfate and reverted to bedwetting within 2 weeks of the medication being discontinued.

Although these papers began the era in 1937, the first book concerned exclusively with child psychopharmacologic research was introduced over 20 years later. This text (*Child Research in Psychopharmacology*) evolved out of the 1958 Conference on Child Research in Psychopharmacology that was sponsored by the National Institute of Mental Health (Fisher, 1959). The book contains an annotated list of 159 references of studies on the effects of psychopharmacologic agents administered to children with various psychiatric problems.

Also, in the 1950s, the following classes of medications were introduced: the typical antipsychotics (chlorpromazine and other compounds), the antidepressants (imipramine), and lithium carbonate. The benzodiazepines, in particular diazepam and chlordiazepoxide, were introduced into clinical psychiatric practice in the early 1960s. Then, in the late 1980s and throughout the 1990s, the selective serotonin reuptake inhibitor antidepressants and the atypical antipsychotics (also referred to as second-generation antipsychotics [SGAs]) began to be introduced.

Certainly, the modern era of medication has been life-saving for many children and adolescents. Although children of today may live in an era where medication and therapy can be life changing, the use of daily medication remains a challenging concept for many children (and sometimes their families) to process. In fact, children may view any illness and the need for any medication as a defect. It is developmentally normal for many young children to see themselves as invincible and immortal, and therefore the need for a medication can cause them to view themselves as a "broken person." This is a significant consideration to address with patients in the clinic setting. As part of the therapy and education, it is often important to utilize the findings from research studies as part of this education.

There are certainly other barriers to address to maximize medication adherence. First, some children have difficulty swallowing pills, and this can be addressed in a variety of ways including the use of liquid formulations, chewables, melt-tabs, powder formulations that can be mixed into liquids, and transdermal patches, for instance.

Some children are not habituated to taking medication every day, so this remains one of the major benefits of taking a daily multivitamin. If a child has never taken a multivitamin, then taking a daily antibiotic or stimulant medication can be a foreign concept that will require additional education to improve adherence.

Concerns regarding medication adherence and safe administration also must be addressed by the clinician when the guardians express that they feel as though their 7-year-olds should be "mature enough" to remember to take the medications regularly on their own. Although it is important for children to develop maturity, it is not recommended that children manage their own medications for a host of reasons including the inherent dangers associated with this. First, children who have to self-administer medications will often forget to take the medication, and that can have significant consequences. Most adults inadvertently miss medication doses; and asking a child (particularly one with attention-deficit/hyperactivity disorder [ADHD]) to remember to take a medication is bound to end poorly. Also, it is developmentally normal for children of a certain age to be magical thinkers. The danger of magical thinking is: "Well, if one of these pills makes me better today, then I could take all 30 pills right now to cure me the whole month and maybe forever!" In addition, the patient's 4-year-old sibling might think that the medications are candy that will make him or her big and strong and give superpowers like the sibling. Proper storage and administration of medication is always to be underscored in the session.

Medication adherence is built in the clinician's office through active listening, developing rapport, and addressing questions and concerns. It therefore remains essential for the clinician to possess a strong foundational knowledge on the research related to the medication risks, benefits, potential side effects, and alternatives (including the potential consequences of not taking medications).

Although new medications are being both studied and introduced, the examination of medication effects on children generally has lagged behind studies in adult populations for a variety of reasons. Importantly, children have been recognized as a special population in medication research studies. As a result, early research has tended to focus more on adult populations due in part to the increased requirements when conducting psychopharmacologic research and in obtaining U.S. Food and Drug Administration (FDA) approval on the safety and efficacy of psychoactive medications in children and younger adolescents. Subsequently, the introduction of psychoactive medications into clinical practice for children has lagged behind that for adults. Weiner and Jaffe (1985) have written a brief but interesting overview of the earlier history of child and adolescent psychopharmacology.

As additional medications have been introduced and research studies published, texts focusing entirely or significantly on child and adolescent psychopharmacology have detailed those findings. These texts include those by Aman and Singh (1988), Bezchlibnyk-Butler and Virani (2004), Campbell et al. (1985), Gadow (1986a, 1986b), Klein et al. (1980), Kutcher (1997, 2002), Martin et al. (2003), Riddle (1995a, 1995b), Rosenberg et al. (1994, 2002), Walsh (1998), Weiner (1985), Werry (1978), Werry and Aman (1999), Trivedi and Chang (2012), and McVoy (2012). The reader who wishes an in-depth review of major issues of the past is referred to *Neuropsychopharmacology: The Fifth Generation of Progress* (Davis et al., 2002) and the fascinating *An Oral History of Neuropsychopharmacology: The First Fifty Years, Peer Interviews (Volumes 1–10)* (Ban, 2011). A review of these texts documents the massive growth of psychopharmacology as a component of the medical care of children and adolescents.

In most instances, a detailed review of the literature establishing the clinical efficacy and safety of early FDA-approved treatments for the psychiatric disorders of children and adolescents are not included in this book. Readers who wish to review the research data establishing these standard treatments will find such information to be accessible in the texts cited.

Section Two of this book not only summarizes the standard treatments but also focuses in greater detail on research into new and not yet approved uses of medications in child and adolescent psychiatry. Some knowledge of psychopharmacologic research principles and techniques is essential to critically evaluate the data that appear in the psychiatric literature and to make informed clinical decisions about whether a trial of a particular medication is warranted for a particular patient.

Most important psychopharmacologic research designs include a comparison of the medication being investigated with either placebo or with a medication approved as a standard treatment for the psychiatric disorder in question (head-to-head clinical trials). Hence it is important to have a basic understanding of placebos.

PLACEBOS

According to the *Oxford English Dictionary* (OED, 1989), the English word *placebo* was directly adopted from the Latin word meaning "I shall be pleasing or acceptable." By 1811, placebo was defined in *Hooper's Medical Dictionary* (OED, 1989) as "an epithet given to any medicine adapted more to please than benefit the patient." In 1982, the OED added the following definition of *placebo*, which fairly accurately described its current use in psychopharmacologic research: "A substance or procedure which a patient accepts as a medicine or therapy but which actually has no specific therapeutic activity for his condition or is prescribed in the belief that it has no such activity." Although placebos are often composed of substances thought to be inert, in psychopharmacologic research, placebos may also contain active ingredients chosen to simulate adverse effects of the medication to which the placebo is being compared. The purpose of this is to keep all participants "blind" by making it more difficult for patients and observers to distinguish between medication and placebo based solely on the medication's potential adverse effects.

Placebos play a crucial role in clinical psychopharmacologic research by providing nonspecific treatment effects for comparison with the medication under investigation. These nonspecific psychological and physiologic changes are not medication specific and may be measured by rating scales (Prien, 1988). These changes include both beneficial and adverse effects produced by the expectations that the patient and/or observers have about the medication. The changes in symptoms that a patient may notice may also include natural fluctuations in the clinical course of the disease, spontaneous alterations in the patient's condition that may have nothing to do with the illness under consideration, effects of the therapeutic relationship among the patient, therapist, and other medical staff, and other unknown effects.

Because of these nonspecific effects, even "inert" placebos have potential side effects. These may commonly include such symptoms as fatigue, anxiety, muscle aches, nausea, diarrhea, constipation, dry mouth, dysmenorrhea, and behavioral changes (such as increased or decreased aggressiveness, impulsivity, attention span, or irritability). These are often symptoms that might appear periodically in the general population. It is the difference in incidence and severity of these unwanted effects between placebo and medication that is important.

The psychological consequences of placebos have long been recognized. Recent research has explored the possibility that some placebo effects may be mediated by detectable neurobiologic processes, including endorphin activity (Zubieta et al.,

2005). A masterful review of the scientific and ethical consequences of our increased understanding of these issues has been produced by Finniss et al. (2010).

The most methodologically sound use of a placebo for testing a new medication is a double-blind, randomized, parallel-groups design (Prien, 1988). Stanley (1988) has written an interesting article concerning ethical and clinical considerations in the use of placebos that evaluated such factors as withholding medication during a placebo period and whether treatment may be ethically withheld in a placebo-controlled trial when a known treatment is available.

Head-to-head studies compare a new medication to a medication already recognized as effective and safe. This strategy/design can avoid the ethical conundrum of denying treatment to patients who would have been assigned placebo in a placebo-controlled study, and this is important when a delay in treatment that is known to be effective for a given diagnosis could result in serious harm to the patient. Prien (1988) offered six alternative study designs for use when it is not possible to use a double-blind, randomized, parallel-groups design and discussed some of their limitations. Regarding the use of placebos, White et al. (1985) edited a fascinating book concerning the theory, ethics, use in research and clinical practice, and mediating mechanisms of placebos.

EVALUATING RESEARCH STUDIES

Efficacy and safety are determined by a statistically significant benefit with acceptable adverse effects of the new medication compared with placebo. Statistics, however, inform us about groups of patients, not individuals. Hence, if etiologically dissimilar groups are subsumed under the same diagnosis, a few patients may truly benefit; but their improvement could be so diluted by the larger majority who did not benefit that the medication might show no statistically significant benefit. Some researchers now note whether there are strong individual responders in a medication study even when there is no statistical difference between experimental and control groups. Therefore, individual case reports, studies of relatively small numbers, and open studies should not be summarily dismissed.

In evaluating the literature on child and adolescent psychopharmacology, it is important to remember that a medication that is statistically and significantly better than another medication or placebo does not necessarily mean that the medication is the optimal treatment for a given condition or for a specific child or adolescent. The medication may be effective only in certain environments (e.g., in a laboratory) and cannot be generalized to more ordinary circumstances. In addition, the medication may improve only certain symptoms but not affect other major target symptoms to a clinically meaningful degree, and the overall improvement may be relatively modest with significant symptoms or deficits remaining. For example, Sprague and Sleator (1977) found that 0.3 mg/kg of methylphenidate produced optimal enhancement of learning short-term memory tasks in hyperkinetic children in the laboratory, but it was 1 mg/kg of methylphenidate that produced the maximum improvement of social behavior in the classroom setting as shown by ratings on the Abbreviated Conners Rating Scale. Another example is that although children with autism spectrum disorder have shown statistically significant improvements with several medications, the degree of their improvement is typically modest, with marked residual deficits remaining; and at present no medication is satisfactory for treatment of this condition (Green, 1988).

When reading and evaluating research, one must consider many factors including the diagnostic criteria used, the heterogeneity/homogeneity of the sample, the symptom severity of the patients included, and the clinical setting in which the medication was given. Importantly, the year in which the study was conducted is also important because, for instance, the diagnostic distinctions between schizophrenia (with childhood onset) and autistic disorder (or their equivalents) were not formalized until the publication of DSM-III (American Psychiatric Association, 1980a). Before that, both conditions were subsumed under the diagnosis of schizophrenia (childhood type). Many studies before that therefore included diagnostically heterogeneous samples or the composition of the sample could not be determined, rendering interpretation of those studies difficult or impossible (Green, 1989).

Gadow and Poling (1988) provide another relevant example. They noted that stimulant medication is not commonly prescribed for persons with intellectual disabilities in residential facilities where most of the patients are usually severely or profoundly disabled. They pointed out that some reviews suggested that stimulant use in this patient population might not be useful in treating behavior disorders and could even exacerbate attention deficit in these patients. However, they noted that the large majority of these individuals are not in institutions and that they are prescribed stimulants for management of disturbed behavior (particularly hyperactivity) much more frequently and with more favorable results than one might expect from reading the literature. In fact, these authors concluded that stimulants were highly effective in diminishing conduct problems and hyperactivity for some individuals with intellectual disabilities, whatever their intellectual quotient.

As psychiatric nosology and diagnosis become more refined and the etiopathogeneses of more homogeneous subgroups are delineated, more focused research may be undertaken and more specific and rational psychopharmacology will inevitably follow.

SPECIFIC MEDICATION TREATMENTS

In this section, psychopharmacologic agents are organized and discussed by class rather than according to the psychiatric diagnoses for which they are treatments. The rationale for this organization is related to several of the issues discussed in the first part of the book. At the present time, most diagnoses are based on phenomenology (i.e., constellations of clinical symptoms) rather than on any basic understanding of the etiopathogenesis of the condition. Therefore, a given medication may be used to treat several psychiatric diagnoses. Hence, repetition of facts under each diagnostic category and extensive cross-referencing are avoided.

Each class of medications is introduced with some general comments, including indications for use, contraindications, interactions with other medications, and the most common untoward effects. The basic pharmacokinetics are discussed, including approximations of time of peak serum levels, the medication's serum half-life, major metabolites, and excretion. Unless otherwise noted, all dosage recommendations are for oral administration.

Specific medications of each class are reviewed individually. Traditional or standard, FDA-approved treatments are discussed, and many treatments that are not approved for advertising by the FDA but that are reported to be efficacious in the literature and used clinically by practitioners are discussed as well.

Most of the studies cited in this book either illustrate a particular point or provide the reader with some of the evidence for using off-label treatments. This evidence ranges from convincing to merely suggestive of a possible alternative for a seriously disturbed patient who has not responded satisfactorily to any prior treatment attempts. Some diagnoses have a clearer treatment algorithm than other diagnoses, and treatment always includes a risk–benefit analysis on the part of the clinician, the patient, and the caregivers. Excellent and extensive literature reviews of the standard psychopharmacologic treatments discussed later are readily accessible in the additional texts on child and adolescent psychopharmacology referenced earlier in this chapter.

Although always important, informed consent and assent (preferably written) are particularly important if FDA-approved medications are used for non-approved indications. If standard approved treatments for a seriously disabling disorder have been tried with little or no success, a clinical trial of a non-approved or even an investigational medication is much more easily justified. The physician has the responsibility to become thoroughly familiar with the official package labeling information provided by the manufacturer of the medication or the relevant entry in the latest edition and supplements of the *Physicians' Desk Reference* before prescribing any medication.

Table 3.1 lists the most common psychiatric diagnoses in children and younger adolescents for which psychopharmacotherapy may be therapeutically indicated and the medications that have been used in treating that disorder. Whenever a specific medication or class of medications is generally preferred for a particular condition, an attempt has been made to rank them in order of usual preference if possible; however, for some diagnoses, there are many medications for which there is no clear order of preference. The listing of a medication indicates that it is discussed or reports of interest are summarized in the text; such a listing does not necessarily imply that the medication is a recommended treatment.

TABLE 3.1 » Diagnoses in Childhood and Adolescence for Which Psychopharmacotherapy May Be Therapeutically Indicated and Medications Discussed in the Text

Attention-deficit/hyperactivity disorder
 Methylphenidate preparations
 Amphetamine preparations
 Atomoxetine
 Clonidine
 Guanfacine
 Bupropion
 Tricyclic antidepressants
 Haloperidol[a]
 Atypical (second-generation) antipsychotics[a]
 Fluoxetine[a]
 Clomipramine[a]
 MAOIs[a]
 Venlafaxine[a]
 Modafinil[a]
Autism spectrum disorder, accompanied by agitation or aggression
 Risperidone and other atypical (second-generation) antipsychotics
 Haloperidol
 Fluphenazine
 Naltrexone
 Methylphenidate preparations
 Amphetamine preparations
 Clomipramine
 Buspirone
 Clonidine
Bipolar disorder/mania
 Lithium
 Atypical (second-generation) antipsychotics (risperidone, quetiapine, aripiprazole, olanzapine, ziprasidone)
 Valproic acid
 Carbamazepine
 Oxcarbazepine
 Topiramate
 Lamotrigine[a]

Conduct disorder (severe, aggressive)
 Atypical (second-generation) antipsychotics
 Haloperidol; other first-generation antipsychotics
 Methylphenidate
 Lithium
 Buspirone
 Propranolol
 Valproic acid
 Carbamazepine
 Trazodone
 Clonidine
 Molindone
Encopresis
 Lithium
Enuresis
 Desmopressin (DDAVP)
 Imipramine
 Benzodiazepines
 Carbamazepine
 Amphetamines
 Clomipramine
 Desipramine
Generalized anxiety disorder (overanxious disorder of childhood)
 Diphenhydramine
 Fluoxetine
 Buspirone
 Hydroxyzine
 Benzodiazepines
Intermittent explosive disorder
 Propranolol
Major depressive disorder
 Antidepressants
 Lithium augmentation
 Lithium for prophylaxis

TABLE 3.1 » Diagnoses in Childhood and Adolescence for Which Psychopharmacotherapy May Be Therapeutically Indicated and Medications Discussed in the Text (*continued*)

Intellectual disability (with severe behavioral disorder and/or self-injurious behavior)
  Atypical (second-generation) antipsychotics
  Haloperidol
  Chlorpromazine
  Lithium
  Propranolol
  Naltrexone
Obsessive-compulsive disorder
  Sertraline
  Fluoxetine
  Paroxetine
  Fluvoxamine
  Clomipramine
  Clonazepam
Panic disorder
  Sertraline
  Paroxetine
  Alprazolam
  Clonazepam
  Tricyclic antidepressants
Post-traumatic stress disorder
  Sertraline
  Propranolol
  Prazosin
Schizophrenia
  Atypical (second-generation) antipsychotics
  Typical (first-generation) antipsychotics
Selective mutism
  Fluoxetine
  Sertraline
Separation anxiety disorder
  Fluoxetine
  Chlordiazepoxide
  Buspirone
  Clomipramine
  Imipramine
  Clonazepam

Sleep disorders
  Primary insomnia
    Melatonin
    Diphenhydramine
    Hydroxyzine
    Clonidine
    Benzodiazepines
  Circadian-rhythm sleep disorder
    Diphenhydramine
    Melatonin
    Hydroxyzine
    Benzodiazepines
  Sleep terror disorder
    Diazepam
    Alprazolam
    Imipramine
    Carbamazepine
  Sleepwalking disorder
    Diazepam
    Imipramine
Tourette disorder
  Haloperidol
  Pimozide
  Clonidine
  Desipramine
  Guanfacine
  Bupropion
  Nortriptyline
  Fluoxetine

[a]These are agents for which there are limited clinical data, which have problematic untoward effects, or which are otherwise seldom used.

MAOIs, monoamine oxidase inhibitors.

Deprescribing: The Prescription for Polypharmacy in the Child and Adolescent Psychiatric Population

RONNE J. PROCH AND CHRISTINA G. WESTON

POLYPHARMACY

There has been increasing attention given to the rates of psychotropic use in children and in special populations within child psychiatry not only within clinical practice but also among the public. In 2014, Alan Schwarz of the New York Times published an article highlighting the concern that patients aged 2 to 3 years were being diagnosed with attention-deficit/hyperactivity disorder (ADHD) and medicated with psychotropics such as stimulants. This chapter was based on a report produced by the Centers for Disease Control and Prevention which found that in 2014, more than 10,000 toddlers were being medicated for ADHD and a vast majority of these children were part of the Medicaid population. Public concern over this topic has the potential to bring unwanted scrutiny to our profession. For this reason, the discussion of polypharmacy and its anecdote known as deprescribing is a necessary discourse for professionals prescribing to and treating these populations.

In its most generic form, polypharmacy is considered the "simultaneous use of multiple drugs to treat a single ailment or condition." Most commonly described and understood in the elderly population, polypharmacy has become a concern among medical professionals across the spectrum of patients accessing health care. However, it is especially alarming in vulnerable populations including not only the elderly but also children and adolescents being treated for psychiatric conditions. All of these populations have in common a limited or impaired capacity for decision making, which makes them especially susceptible to overzealous prescribing practices.

Environment also plays an integral role in the prevalence of polypharmacy because these patients are often placed in extended care facilities, foster care, juvenile detention centers, or group homes where disruptive behavior is especially disconcerting and can lead to dangerous situations for patients and staff members alike. All of these factors together contribute ostensibly to the likelihood that these particular patients will be managed with polypharmacy and therefore subjected to the practice's risks and benefits.

WHAT IS IT?

The purpose of this chapter is to focus on polypharmacy in the child and adolescent psychiatric population and provide some clinical suggestions to help reduce the incidence of polypharmacy in the patients we treat without sacrificing improved clinical outcomes. Although there are no official standardized parameters for what is polypharmacy and what is not, there are some generally accepted concepts that have been listed. Many of these parameters are written to give credence to the patient's age, the type of medication, and the total number of medications prescribed. Multiple studies and statewide prescription monitoring programs have found the following five principles to be criteria which should alert the provider that their patients may be prescribed unneeded medications that can have untoward effects on their health.

1. **Patient is prescribed four or more psychotropic medications.** Although not specific to child and adolescent psychopharmacology, Mojtabai and Olfson found in 2010 that already the rates of prescribing two or more psychotropics in the outpatient office had increased to 59.8% in 2005 to 2006 from 42.6% in 1996 to 1997. Office visits resulting in psychotropic prescriptions totaling three or more rose from 16.9% in 1996 to 1997 to 33.2% in 2005 to 2006. Extrapolating this data to present prescribing conditions likely would show a general increase in patients being prescribed four or more medications, thus meeting criteria for psychotropic polypharmacy.
2. **Patient is a child under the age of 1 who is prescribed any psychotropic medication.** Most prudent clinicians should be hesitant to prescribe psychotropic medication to any child under 1 year. Sound treatment principles in this age group involve interventions that include evaluation of the caregivers and provide treatments aimed at improving the behavioral management of an infant's challenging behaviors.
3. **Patient is a child under the age of 6 prescribed an antipsychotic/mood stabilizing medication.** Wei et al. (2017) looked at the health consequences experienced by preschool age patients who were prescribed antipsychotics both short and long term. Extrapyramidal symptoms (EPS) and obesity were by the far most common deleterious side effects, with 57 cases and 19 cases out of 1,000 combined treatment years of multiple patients, respectively. Both of these side effects were significantly more prevalent in patients taking the medications for 1 to 7 years (long term) as opposed to less than 1 year (short term). These side effects are both concerning for and distressing to the patient and could have long-term health effects on patients, thus highlighting the need for caution when prescribing to this population. A careful evaluation of the risk–benefit ratio should be made before deciding to use antipsychotics in this age group.
4. **Children of any age prescribed two or more antipsychotic/mood stabilizing medications.** Kreider et al. (2014) estimated a 22% increase in the prescription of antipsychotics between the years of 2004 and 2008 in Medicaid youth, a population known to be at higher risk for polypharmacy. More broadly, Olfson et al. (2006) found that there has been a sharp increase (201,000 office visits in 1993 to 1,224,000 in 2002) in prescription antipsychotics in

patients under the age of 20 in the outpatient setting. Patients in this study were being treated for diagnoses of disruptive behavior disorders (37.8%), mood disorders (31.8%), pervasive developmental disorder or mental retardation (17.3%), and other psychotic disorders (14.2%). In 2002, 92.3% of office visits for antipsychotics included prescription of a second-generation antipsychotic (SGA) that may or may not have substantial empiric evidence of benefit in this population. Verdoux et al. (2010) found a similar increase in the number of SGAs being prescribed outside of psychotic disorders in both the adult and pediatric population. Some of this use is for U.S. Food and Drug Administration (FDA)-approved indications such as mood stabilization in bipolar disorder and for severe irritability associated with autistic spectrum disorder; however, these medications are often used for other indications. Both of these studies show a general trend in prescribers attempting to treat behavioral disorders outside of psychosis with antipsychotics, which many consider an alarming trend.

5. **Children of any age prescribed two or more psychotropic medications from the same class or for the same psychiatric or behavioral condition.** Zonfrillo et al. (2005) found that the practice of using two or more psychotropics for the same condition was on the rise, although the literature describing and examining these patterns was not yet abundantly available. The study found it alarming that this practice would be increasing despite the lack of evidence-based medicine supporting it. Not surprisingly, Mojtabai and Olfson found in 2010 that prescribing of two or more medications in the same class (i.e., antidepressants, sedative hypnotics, antipsychotics, and mood stabilizers) is directly correlated with diagnoses of major depressive disorder, anxiety disorders, schizophrenia, and bipolar disorder, respectively. On the basis of these correlations, patients with multiple diagnoses would be even more likely to be prescribed four or more psychotropics, thus meeting criteria for #1 and #5.

HOW AND WHERE DOES IT HAPPEN?

There are many reasons why polypharmacy can occur among child psychiatrists. The American Academy of Child and Adolescent Psychiatry (AACAP, 2009) practice parameter on the use of psychotropic medication in children and adolescents highlights several situations where this can occur. In some situations it can be difficult to know the exact cause of a behavioral symptom in a child. Often trauma is under-recognized as a cause of behavioral symptoms when a child is evaluated. In some areas, access to quality psychosocial treatments is not available or unfeasible for families to participate in. Often, prescribers will react to a behavioral crisis by adding a new medication that may not be necessary in the long term. In many situations, especially when a patient moves from one care provider to another, the lack of continuity contributes to overprescribing. The new provider often has little knowledge of which prescribed medications are helpful and which may not be necessary and just continues them. As is often the case for children in foster care with frequent changes in care providers, history is often lacking and environmental changes can contribute to brief behavioral problems that may lead to medications being prescribed for long periods, which are not necessary.

Rates of reported polypharmacy are highly variable among studies and treatment settings, the most basic dichotomy of treatment settings being outpatient versus inpatient and residential treatment environments. Chen et al. (2011) estimated polypharmacy in the outpatient setting to be as high as 28.8% in the short term (multiple psychotropics overlapping in a 14-day period), but this figure dropped to 20.9% in the long term (multiple psychotropics overlapping in a 60-day period). Duffy et al. (2005) examined patients across multiple settings and found rates of concomitant pharmacotherapy to be as high as 52%. Connor et al. (1997) found rates of polypharmacy to be as high as 60.3% in the residential treatment center. Chen et al. (2011) argued that some of these discrepancies are due to a lack of standardized stringent criteria extrapolated in the long term; however, data for a 60-day period in a residential treatment center would likely be uncommon and highly biased because of the severity of mental health problems that often comprise that patient population.

Beyond the distinction between inpatient versus outpatient settings, other variables influence rates of polypharmacy. For instance, Duffy et al. (2005) found that of the youths treated with concomitant polypharmacy, 87% had been diagnosed with bi-polar disorder. Other risk factors included having co-occurring Axis I or II disorders, comorbid medical conditions, or current inpatient hospitalization (consistent with abovementioned data). Connor et al. (1997) found that treatment with combined pharmacotherapy was also correlated to lifetime number of psychiatric placements, direct admission from inpatient psychiatric facility into residential treatment facility, lifetime number of psychiatric diagnoses, nonseizure neuropsychiatric comorbidity, aggression, and neuroleptic use.

Discrepancies in polypharmacy also exist between demographic classes. Youths enrolled in Medicaid are among the most vulnerable population to experience poly-pharmacy. Subclasses of Medicaid-enrolled youth include patients from low-income families, youths with disabilities, and youths in foster care. Fontanella et al. (2014) studied these three groups within the larger umbrella of youths enrolled in Ohio Medicaid from 2002 to 2008. They found that when these three subgroups were analyzed, polypharmacy in low-income youths increased from 8.8% to 11.5% from 2002 to 2008 and rates increased from 18.0% to 24.9% in the disabled youth for the same period. Most concerning of all was an increase in polypharmacy from 19.8% in foster care youths in 2002 to 27.3% in 2008. However, this trend is not specific to Ohio. Across the country there has been growing concern among multiple state agencies and large organizations regarding prescribing policies in state-funded patients, especially children in foster care.

A report from the Government Accountability Office published December 2011 suggested that children in foster care are prescribed psychotropics at rates 2.7 to 4.5 times higher than children enrolled in Medicaid who are not in foster care. Zito et al. (2008) found that among foster care youth aged 0 to 19 years in a south-western state in 2004, 72% were receiving medications from two or more classes, whereas 41.3% were receiving medications from three or more classes. In response to these alarming reports, multiple agencies have published guidelines and practice parameters suggesting ways of detecting, monitoring, and addressing polypharmacy in the foster care population. Many states have also developed programs to moni-tor prescribing practices and limit polypharmacy with prior authorizations or child psychiatric consultation programs.

The National Center for Youth Law published guidelines in February 2016 sug-gesting ways that the "overmedication problem" could be addressed and potentially resolved. In 2015 Pennsylvania Department of Human Resources published their response to the in-depth analysis conducted by PolicyLab identifying trends in psychotropic prescription practices in the Medicaid population. PolicyLab found that among youths aged 6 to 18 years enrolled in Medicaid in 2012, 43% of youths enrolled in foster care were prescribed psychotropic medications as compared to 16% in the Pennsylvania Medicaid population as a whole. Multiple recommenda-tions and action plans were proposed in an effort to address the problem. In 2016, the Texas Department of Family and Protective Services published its fifth version of practice parameters detailing the appropriate use of psychotropic medications with respect to this population and red flags suggesting that more review of care is necessary. The U.S. government followed suit when the Congressional Research Service published its extensive report regarding psychotropic prescribing practices for children in foster care in 2015. Finally, the AACAP published guidelines for the treatment of this particular population in 2015.

The problem of polypharmacy is not exclusive to psychiatrists because much of the mental health treatment provided to children and adolescents is administered by primary care providers or general practitioners rather than a psychiatrist or psychiatric specialist. Burcu et al. (2016) found that as many as 71% of behavioral health-related visits were provided by a non-psychiatrist. More specifically, Olfson et al. (2014) found that only 27.4% of outpatient child visits and 47.9% of outpatient adolescent visits resulting in a psychiatric diagnosis were actually performed by psychiatrists. Although the adolescent group is more likely to be diagnosed by a psychiatrist than adults (36.6%), they found that the rate of mental health diagnoses and psychiatric visits increased more rapidly among youths than adults between the years of 1995 and 1998 and 2007 and 2010.

There is significant concern among practitioners about the regulation of psychotropic medications, especially antipsychotics, by all prescribers but especially those with limited professional experience using these medications in children. While Burcu et al. (2016) found that psychiatrists do prescribe more antipsychotics on average than non-psychiatrists (24.2% of all antipsychotics), still 4.6% of antipsychotics prescribed to youth are prescribed by non-psychiatrists. This percentage is likely to continue rising as the practice of antipsychotic prescribing increases in frequency. Most at risk is Medicaid youth who was predicted by this study to be twice as likely to receive antipsychotics than youth with private insurance. However, regardless of insurance coverage, patients requiring antipsychotics typically are more difficult and behaviorally disturbed patients, thus requiring a higher level of care and typically are at higher risk for polypharmacy. It was also found that one of every three youths being prescribed antipsychotics was also being prescribed two or more other psychotropic medication classes concurrently, thus meeting the aforementioned criteria for polypharmacy.

Antipsychotic prescription in youth for illnesses other than schizophrenia or bipolar disorder remains a controversial practice for many reasons. Most notably, there is limited data on the efficacy of antipsychotics in the pediatric population because research in this population is more heavily regulated than that in adults. Antipsychotics are often used to control the symptoms of aggression present in many disorders and are often caused by environmental factors. Moreover, both generations of antipsychotics are known to have many side effects that can have deleterious and long-term effects on patients. First-generation antipsychotics are more commonly associated with causing EPS, tardive dyskinesia, progressive brain cell degeneration, and hyperprolactinemia, whereas SGAs have been found to cause lipid dysregulation, hyperglycemia, and obesity in adult populations. Although both classes of medication have significant side effects, those of the second generation are often considered less severe. Thus, SGAs are more frequently used in the pediatric population and these side effects are still significant.

Metabolic syndrome describes a cluster of symptoms known to increase risk of diabetes, heart disease, and stroke in the long term. These symptoms include high blood pressure, hyperglycemia, increased abdominal waist circumference (secondary to increased visceral adipose), and abnormal lipids. Fleischhacker et al. (2008) highlighted the well-known association between SGAs and an increased incidence of obesity (contributing to hypertension), hyperglycemia, and hyperlipidemia, although these effects were known long before 2008. In 2004, the American Diabetes Association (ADA) and the American Psychiatric Association (APA) acknowledged these well-known effects and called for metabolic screening including monitoring of weight, body mass index, waist circumference, blood pressure, fasting serum glucose, and lipid profiles of patients receiving SGAs. Despite the knowledge of these effects and recommendations set forth by the ADA and APA, Mitchell et al. (2012) found that only 42% to 48% of adult patients taking SGAs received routine screening for cholesterol, glucose, and weight. The incidence of surveillance is even more dismal in the pediatric population. Morrato et al. (2010) found that 1 year after the recommendation from the ADA and APA, only 31.6% of youth on SGAs were receiving glucose screening, whereas only 13.4% were undergoing lipid screening during a review of Medicaid participants between the years of 2004 and 2006. When compared with control patients receiving albuterol, youth receiving SGAs were nearly twice as likely (8.9/1,000 children vs. 4.9/1,000) to develop glucose abnormalities and more than twice as likely (9.7/1,000 vs. 4.6/1,000) to develop lipid abnormalities. Wei et al. (2017) found that long-term use of these medications was more likely to result in obesity than short-term use in the pediatric population. Thus, the use of SGAs in children is not benign and should be monitored carefully.

The motivation behind the use of these medications has also become a topic of scrutiny. There is growing concern among providers that antipsychotics are being used in lieu of therapy or nonpharmacologic behavioral therapies because these are more time and money consuming. Access to these services is often limited to patients, although it would likely be more beneficial in the long term than chemical behavior management. In a study performed by Finnerty et al. (2016), it was found that only 48.8% of youth received any psychosocial treatment in the 3 months preceding the initiation of SGA therapy. Olfson et al. (2014) found that psychotherapy visits only increased from 2.25 to 3.17 per 100 patients, whereas psychiatric visits as a whole increased from 2.86 to 5.7 per 100 patients for youth between 1995 and 1998 and 2007 and 2010. This figure supports the notion of the general population that psychiatry has shifted from a therapy- and medication-based practice to a medication-based practice only which was highlighted in a National Public Radio talk in October 2012 featuring Dr. Richard Friedman (Director, Psychopharmacology Clinic, Weill Cornell Medical College) and Dr. Steve Balt (psychiatrist and editor-in-chief, the Carlat Psychiatry Report).

However, the practice of psychotropic polypharmacy may not be completely without merit. There are some trials that suggest that dual psychotropic treatment could be beneficial for aggressive and volatile patients such as youth diagnosed with ADHD. Aman et al. (2014) suggested that there may have been some improvement in aggressive and disruptive behaviors in patients receiving both a stimulant and risperidone. Aggressive behaviors are especially disruptive to a patient's ability to function or be placed in a therapeutic environment. Lack of treatment can often result in patients being removed from their homes or, at worst, becoming incarcerated for behavioral disruption. However, as Blader (2014) pointed out, many trials suggesting efficacy with treatment by multiple psychotropic classes are fraught with possible procedural biases that may influence results because the patients are getting treatment that they never previously received and subjective symptoms are reported by parents with no quantitative measures. Baker et al. (2017) highlights the complexity of navigating the multitude of literature both supporting and negating the utility of polypharmacy in youth. Thus, it becomes apparent that some guidelines are needed to help prescribers understand and utilize these complicated treatment regimens.

DEPRESCRIBING

A new discourse has risen among providers in the child and adolescent population regarding how providers should prevent polypharmacy or, in the event that it has already taken place, decipher a way to reduce polypharmacy. This practice has become known as deprescribing, a phrase initially coined in the literature with respect mostly to the geriatric population. However, the concept has been gaining traction in the world of psychiatry and has been more specifically described by Gupta and Cahill (2016) as "a process of pharmacologic regimen optimization through reduction or cessation of medications for which benefits no longer outweigh risks." They also pointed out that the nature of psychiatry has presented its own specific challenges to employing deprescription because the art of prescribing in psychiatric patients is not well defined. For instance, there is a lack of diagnostic and therapeutic precision mostly due to the heavy focus on symptomatology rather than clinical outcomes, subjective reporting of symptoms by patients rather than methodic quantification, and difficulty maintaining continuity of care in therapeutic and community relationships. Bellonci et al. (2016) and the AACAP have been proposing ways to extend deprescription as a concept into the field of child psychiatry. The subspecialty of child and adolescent psychiatry further complicates this practice given the variation in the patient's ability to express and report symptoms in conjunction with the parent's perspective on the patient's progress.

In cases where a patient is already prescribed multiple psychotropics and meeting the parameters of polypharmacy listed earlier in this chapter, there is an increasing but still small amount of literature aimed at guiding prescribers in tapering and reducing medication use in a methodic way. Discourse among professionals has yielded some general principles that could help inform clinicians of a method for deprescribing in the child and adolescent psychiatric population.

1. Start with a comprehensive evaluation that includes a review of previous records, development of a biopsychosocial formulation, and analysis of current medications and how they may or may not be contributing to or relieving symptoms. The 2009 AACAP Practice Parameter, "Prescribing Psychotropic Medication to Children" details a comprehensive way of performing an adequate assessment on a child before starting psychotropic medications.
2. Appropriate diagnosis is important because it dictates the modality and length of treatment course that can inform which medications to continue or discontinue. When a patient has failed several medication trials for the initial diagnosis, it is often helpful to take a step back and reconsider the possibility that another diagnosis may be present which would require a different treatment plan.
3. Any recommendation to taper or discontinue a psychotropic medication should be done while engaging in developmentally appropriate shared decision making with the youth and caregiver. Assent from the youth and consent from the caregiver should be obtained after the appropriate risks, benefits, and alternatives are discussed. If the youth is in foster care, consent needs to be obtained from the person who is authorized in that state or county to provide consent for psychotropic medication decisions. These principles are outlined in "A Guide for Public Child Serving Agencies on Psychotropic Medications for Children and Adolescents" (AACAP, 2012, pp. 8–9).
4. Avoid using SGAs to aid sleep unless the patient has as a diagnosis of bipolar disorder. Sleep hygiene techniques should always be considered first-line treatment. If sleep agents must be used, then they should be tapered during school and summer breaks with an appropriate washout period.
5. Stability is defined as showing significant symptom reduction. Signs of stability could be decreased incidence of scoring in the clinical range on standardized rating scales, lack of hospitalizations, and no recent placement disruptions.
6. For youth on monotherapy, deprescribing would typically consist of reducing the dose and observing for a return of the target symptoms for which the medication was originally prescribed. If the youth is prescribed more than one medication concurrently, the first medications to be considered for tapering could meet the criteria given here:
   a. Has the least evidence of efficacy and/or greatest evidence of side effects or risk of side effects, for example, SGAs
   b. Is prescribed at a supratherapeutic (higher than standard) dose without obvious justification
   c. Is prescribed at doses that are subtherapeutic
   d. Has limited or no evidence of effectiveness for the condition for which it is prescribed

7. During the medication trial, the youth should be receiving an evidence-based psychosocial therapy teaching skills to manage the target symptoms for the prescribed medication. If target symptoms recur in the course of a medication taper or discontinuation, the first intervention should be to provide refreshers of the skills that were taught or booster sessions of the therapy before considering restarting the medicine or increasing the dose except in cases of severe symptomatology.

8. Although this practice parameter focuses on deprescribing, youth should also be systematically screened and evaluated for medication-responsive conditions. Treating some medication-responsive conditions with medication may facilitate deprescribing of other medications, especially those with less supported indications. Combined psychotropic and psychosocial interventions are sometimes more effective than either treatment alone. For some diagnosis such as post-traumatic stress disorder, the evidence base for psychotherapy alone is superior to that for medications in children.

9. Once the youth is discontinued from all prescribed psychotropic medications, the clinician should remain available to the family as needed for support should a resumption of symptoms occur. It is best for the child to also continue in therapy for a period of several months to ensure there is no relapse.

10. If discontinuation of a medication is being prompted by abnormal laboratory values or concerning side effects, the youth should be observed to see whether the side effects have remitted following medication discontinuation and/or follow-up laboratory studies should be completed to document normalization of any abnormal laboratory values. If normalization does not occur or there is active symptomatology, the youth should be referred to the appropriate health care professional for treatment.

More recently, studies such as Hulvershorn et al. (2017) are demonstrating that applying deprescription principles such as reducing medication and focusing on diagnosis have resulted in positive outcomes even in the most severe psychiatric patients. This study suggests that discontinuation of atypical antipsychotics with diagnosis as the guiding principle resulted in both metabolic and psychiatric improvement in patients hospitalized in state facilities. Although the evidence is just recently becoming available, it is likely that deprescription will and should become a typical strategy in the toolbox of prescribers.

CASE EXAMPLE

Given here is an example of a case in which the child benefited from some of the strategies for deprescribing described earlier.

> BACKGROUND: Joshua is an 8-year-old boy in foster care who endured severe physical abuse and neglect by his biological family. Since being removed from his parents, he was placed with multiple different families and in several foster care situations, which were all disrupted because of his behavior. He was eventually placed into a residential treatment center after eight or more failed placements. At the time of his evaluation, he was recently released from the residential treatment center and placed into a two-parent foster home without any other children.
>
> DIAGNOSES: ADHD, reactive detachment disorder, previous diagnosis of unspecified bipolar disorder
>
> ADDITIONAL CONCERNS: Bedwetting, intermittent drooling, falling asleep at school, intermittent outbursts with minimal provocation
>
> MEDICATION LIST:
> Lithium 300 mg PO BID
> Methylphenidate HCl 54 mg QAM

Methylphenidate 10 mg after school
Risperidone 0.5 mg PO TID
Sertraline 25 mg PO QAM
Clonidine 0.05 mg TID and 0.1 mg QHS
Desmopressin (DDAVP) 0.2 QHS
NONPHARMACOLOGIC INTERVENTION: Foster parents were highly motivated to decrease the amount of medications that the patient was on to better his overall health and were willing to partake in behavioral modification strategies rather than medication intervention only. The patient was home schooled and began seeing a reactive attachment disorder (RAD) therapist twice a week.

DEPRESCRIPTION STRATEGY

1. Lithium was tapered and discontinued. Enuresis resolved.
2. DDAVP was discontinued and bedwetting did not recur.
3. Sertraline was discontinued. Mood was stable and patient did not experience an increase in anxiety.
4. Clonidine was discontinued. Patient's ability to focus was unchanged. Some sleep difficulties remained, but the family managed them with behavioral strategies.
5. Risperidone was tapered and eventually discontinued without any episodes of aggression.
6. Methylphenidate after school was discontinued and patient had improved ability to sleep.
7. Methylphenidate HCl was tapered down to 18 mg QAM, but had to be increased back to 36 mg QAM after patient became hyperactive and had difficulty concentrating.

Overall, it took a year for the deprescribing process to be completed. When it was over, the patient was taking only 36 mg methylphenidate in the morning for ADHD.

RESULTS: Joshua was able to finish his therapy sessions with the RAD specialist and then eventually was enrolled in a regular elementary school taking only methylphenidate 36 mg QAM. He was formally adopted by his foster parents. After a year of stability on one medication, his care was transferred to a primary care physician for continued management of his stimulant medication.

FUTURE DIRECTIONS

Concern over the increasing rates of psychotropic medication in youth has caused many involved parties such as insurers, health care systems, child welfare agencies, state governments, and national agencies to express concern that there is inappropriate prescribing. This has led to the creation of psychotropic medication oversight programs. Schmid and colleagues (2015) report that at least 31 state Medicaid divisions have chosen to implement some form of prior authorization policy for antipsychotic use in youth. States have adopted different ages, dose, and medication use situations which institute a prior authorization or clinical consultation with an academic child psychiatrist for continued coverage.

The field of pharmacogenetics is also another interesting possibility that may have an effect on polypharmacy because it may be able to better inform prescribing practices in the first place, thus preventing or at least decreasing polypharmacy. Lohoff and Ferraro (2010) acknowledged that although there has not yet been much utility for pharmacogenetics in the field of psychiatry, there is a very good possibility that pharmacogenetics could change prescription practices altogether.

CONCLUSION

Overall polypharmacy is of growing concern in the field of medicine and, more specifically, in psychiatry. The reasons for polypharmacy are multifactorial; often caregivers do not have time or willingness to attend therapy or have the availability of competent therapists. In these situations, they turn to prescribers and medication to solve their children's behavior problems. In some instances, a new provider has little knowledge of how the current medication regimen was developed and does not know which, if any, medications made a significant improvement in a child's symptoms. Especially with children in foster care, past history is often unavailable. Multiple studies and statewide agendas have highlighted the overwhelming prevalence of the practice, the lack of supporting evidence, and the potential harms. Deprescribing aims at solving the problem of polypharmacy and may be able to improve clinical outcomes for patients in the long run. It is important for prescribers to stop medications that have not had successful trials before adding new ones as well as carefully reassess the continued need for medications when episodic illnesses have resolved.

5

Sympathomimetic Amines, Central Nervous System Stimulants, and Executive Function Agents

RYAN C. MAST, BETHANY L. HARPER, AND KAITLYN T. POLLOCK

INTRODUCTION

In the treatment of attention-deficit/hyperactivity disorder (ADHD), there are both stimulant and non-stimulant medications to consider. Of these medication types, both immediate-release (IR) and sustained-release versions of many stimulant and non-stimulant medications are available. Owing in part to their better efficacy, stimulant medications are considered the first-line agents unless there is a compelling reason to avoid their use.

Agents that modulate dopamine and/or norepinephrine seem to have an impact on ADHD symptomatology. Due in large part to their effects on dopamine, stimulant medications can have a profound effect on ADHD symptoms. Of the non-stimulant medications, atomoxetine is a selective norepinephrine reuptake inhibitor (SNRI) that is approved by the U.S. Food and Drug Administration (FDA) for the treatment of ADHD; however, head-to-head comparisons suggest that stimulants are more effective than atomoxetine in improving hyperactivity, impulsivity, and inattention in such subjects (Starr & Kemner, 2005; Wigal et al., 2005; this is further reviewed later in this chapter under the section "Atomoxetine versus Stimulants in the Treatment of Attention-Deficit/Hyperactivity Disorder in Children and Adolescents").

Long-acting forms of non-stimulant medications include the alpha-2 adrenergic agonists guanfacine and clonidine that have FDA approval for the treatment of ADHD. These agents can be used either as monotherapy or as adjunctive therapy to stimulant medications. Although the long-acting versions of both clonidine and guanfacine have FDA approval for the treatment of ADHD, their short-acting forms do not (however, the short-acting forms are effective off-label treatment for ADHD).

In addition to IR (short-acting) clonidine and guanfacine, there are other medications whose use in the treatment of ADHD is considered off-label use because they do not have FDA approval for the treatment of ADHD. Tricyclic antidepressants (TCAs) and bupropion are also used off-label in the treatment of ADHD; and although this chapter covers the majority of common ADHD medications, certain medications that can treat multiple disorders (e.g., TCAs and bupropion) are included in other sections of this text. Amantadine (AMT) is a novel agent whose actions on the dopamine system are indirect and appear to be involved more as a modulator of dysfunction in the dopamine system. AMT seems to have utility for individuals with brain injury from various causes who have moderate to severe intellectual disability (ID) and exhibit behavioral problems. Modafinil (Provigil) is prescribed to patients with narcolepsy, shift-work sleep disorder, and obstructive sleep apnea, but it has been used in the treatment of ADHD when other agents have failed.

STIMULANT MEDICATIONS

Sympathomimetic amines and central nervous system (CNS) stimulants are commonly referred to as stimulants. Two of these agents (methylphenidate [MPH] and amphetamine) are the medications of choice in the treatment of ADHD. Particularly, the extended-release formulations of these medications may be preferable in situations where there are concerns about poor medication adherence and/or potential for medication abuse or diversion.

Many stimulants have been in use for many decades. Bradley's (1937) report on the use of racemic amphetamine sulfate (Benzedrine) in children with behavioral disorders is usually cited as the beginning of child psychopharmacology as a discipline. Since this initial report, more research has been published on ADHD (and stimulants) than on any other childhood disorder. Double-blind, placebo-controlled studies have consistently found that stimulants are significantly superior to placebo in improving attention span and in decreasing hyperactivity and impulsivity. Although most of the earlier studies were in children, two double-blind studies in 1988 confirmed the clinical efficacy of MPH in treating adolescents diagnosed with attention-deficit disorder (ADD) who also had ADD as children (Klorman et al., 1988a, 1988b). Since then, many more studies on the use of stimulants in adolescents and adults (particularly the use of extended-release stimulant formulations) have been published.

MAJOR LANDMARK STUDIES ON STIMULANT MEDICATION

With ADHD affecting between 5% and 12% of children worldwide, it is not surprising that new medications are frequently developed and researched. Thousands of studies have been conducted, and two influential studies include PATS (Preschool ADHD Treatment Study) and MTA (Multimodal Treatment Study of Children with ADHD).

PATS is a multicenter, randomized trial examining the efficacy and safety of MPH use in preschoolers (aged 3 to 5 years) with severe ADHD who were unresponsive to a 10-week psychosocial intervention. The study was designed to evaluate MPH's efficacy over the short term (5 weeks) and its safety over the long term (40 weeks). The study results demonstrated that low-dose MPH over the short term is safe and effective, but that close monitoring remains critical. A subsequent follow-up occurred 6 years later with the same children. From the follow-up, the authors concluded that ADHD in preschoolers is a generally stable diagnosis over time, suggesting that it is a chronic condition even with medication. Therefore, it is important to develop multiple strategies to help this patient population (Riddle et al., 2013).

The MTA is a multisite study that was designed to evaluate the long-term safety and efficacy of leading treatments for ADHD (behavior therapy, medications, and the combination of the two). The study included 579 children (ages 7 to 9.9 years old). The MTA study examined safety and efficacy of medication and behavior therapy for ADHD for up to 14 months. By comparison, previous studies only examined short-term safety and efficacy. The children in the study were randomly assigned to one of four treatment arms: (1) intensive medication management alone; (2) intensive behavioral treatment alone; (3) medication plus behavioral treatment; or (4) routine community care (this was the control group). All four groups improved; but for most ADHD symptoms, the children in the medication and combination groups improved significantly more than those in the intensive behavior treatment and standard community care groups. Core ADHD symptoms improved equally with the combined treatment or with medication alone; however, the combined therapy may have provided modestly better outcomes for non-ADHD symptoms (e.g., oppositional and aggressive symptoms) and positive functioning (MTA Cooperative Group, 1999a, 1999b).

Many other studies comparing MPH with other medications and therapy have occurred in the years that followed. Storebø et al. (2015) performed a review of 38 parallel-group trials (5,111 participants randomized) and 147 crossover trials (7,134 participants randomized). Their findings affirmed the clinical efficacy of MPH in the treatment of ADHD in children and adolescents.

In addition to treating the impulsivity and hyperactivity symptoms of ADHD, several investigators have reported that MPH also improved academic performance and/or peer interactions (e.g., Pelham et al., 1985, 1987; Rapport et al., 1994). Whalen et al. (1987) reported on 24 children between 6 and 11 years of age who were diagnosed with ADD or attention-deficit disorder with hyperactivity (ADDH) and who received either placebo, 0.3 mg/kg MPH daily, or 0.6 mg/kg MPH daily, in random order so that all children received each dosage level for a total of 4 days. The authors reported that all children showed decrements in negative social behaviors when rated during relatively unstructured outdoor activities at the 0.3-mg/kg level, compared with placebo. The youngest 12 children showed further improvement in social behavior at the higher dose.

Rapport et al. (1994) evaluated the acute effects of four dose levels of MPH (5, 10, 15, and 20 mg) on classroom behavior and academic performance of 76 children diagnosed with ADHD in a double-blind, placebo-controlled, within-subject (crossover) protocol. Compared with baseline, the subjects showed a nearly linear increase in normalization of behavior as the dose of MPH increased. On the Abbreviated Conners Teacher Rating Scale (CTRS), scores improved in 16% and normalized in 78% of the subjects. Attention (measured by on-task behavior) improved in 4% and normalized in 72% of the subjects. Academic efficiency (measured by the percentage of academic assignments completed correctly) improved in 3% and normalized in 50% of the subjects. Hence, there are several different clinically significant subsets of children: (1) those who improve in all domains; (2) those who improve in the behavioral and attention domains but do not improve in the academic domain and require additional interventions (e.g., tutoring); (3) those who show behavioral improvement but no significant improvement in attention or academic ratings; and (4) those who do not benefit from MPH in any of the three domains.

Approximately 75% of children with ADHD treated with stimulants will show favorable responses (Green, 1995). Among these favorable responses, there will be a spectrum. Some children will respond extremely well, whereas others will benefit but to a lesser degree.

Also, some children with ADHD (or an earlier equivalent diagnosis such as ADD or ADDH) will respond favorably to one stimulant medication but less favorably, not at all, or unfavorably to another. For example, Arnold et al. (1976) conducted a double-blind crossover study of the D-amphetamine enantiomer, the L-amphetamine enantiomer, and placebo in 31 children with minimal brain dysfunction (MBD). Both isomers were statistically superior to placebo and did not differ significantly from each other. Interestingly, of the 25 children with positive responses, 17 responded well to both isomers, 5 responded favorably to the D-isomer only, and 3 responded favorably to the L-isomer only (Arnold et al., 1976).

In a double-blind crossover study, Elia et al. (1991) compared MPH, dextroamphetamine, and placebo in treating 48 males (age range, 6 to 12 years; mean, 8.6 ± 1.7 years) with a history of hyperactive, inattentive, and impulsive behaviors that interfered with functioning both at home and at school. Following a 2-week baseline period, the subjects were assigned randomly for 3-week periods, during each week of which the dosage was increased (unless untoward effects prevented it) to one of three regimens: (a) MPH doses were given at 9 AM and 1 PM. The mean dosage for all subjects was 0.9 mg/kg for week 1; 1.5 mg/kg for week 2; and 2.5 mg/kg for week 3. (b) Dextroamphetamine doses were given at 9 AM and 1 PM. The mean dosage for all subjects was 0.4 mg/kg during week 1; 0.9 mg/kg for week 2; and 1.3 mg/kg for week 3. (c) Placebo—owing to untoward effects, for 19 subjects (40%) (including 7 on MPH, 7 on dextroamphetamine, and 5 on both medications) the dosage was held at the preceding week's level, increased (but to a lower dosage than mandated by the next level), or decreased. The authors reported that 38 (79%) subjects responded to MPH and that 42 (88%) responded to dextroamphetamine; overall, 46 (96%) of the 48 subjects had a positive clinical response to one or both stimulants as rated on the Clinical Global Impressions (CGI) Scale and, in particular, for restless and inattentive behaviors. Eight subjects did not respond to MPH, four did not respond to dextroamphetamine, and two did not respond to either medication. Elia et al. (1991) distinguished between behavioral nonresponse and untoward effects, which few investigators had previously done. They noted that although behavioral nonresponse to stimulants is rare, when a wide range of doses is given, most subjects had some untoward effects. When behavioral nonresponders were combined with subjects having untoward effects, the rate of nonresponse was similar to that reported in the literature. The authors noted that making a definitive clinical decision regarding improvement was often difficult because behavioral improvements had to be balanced against untoward effects, and different symptoms responded independently to dosage, setting, and subject (Elia et al., 1991).

Children who have a diagnosis of ADHD many times have comorbid conditions that may include oppositional defiant disorder (ODD), conduct disorder, major depressive disorder (MDD), anxiety, tics, and substance use disorders. In a double-blind, placebo-controlled study of 40 children (age range, 6 to 12 years; mean, 8.6 ± 1.3 years) who were diagnosed with ADHD and treated with MPH, DuPaul et al. (1994) found that subjects ($N = 12$) who had additional internalizing symptoms such as anxiety or depression and who had high scores on the internalizing scale of the Child Behavior Checklist (CBCL) were significantly less likely to benefit from MPH at three different doses (5, 10, and 15 mg) in school, as evidenced by teachers' ratings and in the clinic setting compared with subjects with borderline ($N = 17$) or low ($N = 11$) scores on the CBCL. There was a significant deterioration in functioning on MPH among some children. In particular, 25% of the subjects in the high internalizing group were rated on the Teacher Self-Control Rating Scale as showing a worsening in classroom behavior, compared with 9.1% in the low and none in the borderline internalizing groups. On the same scale, however, 50% of the high, 93.75% of the borderline, and 72.7% of the low internalizing groups were rated as improved or normalized. It appears that the presence of anxiety or depression may hinder the effectiveness of stimulant treatment or the stimulant may even worsen behavior.

ADHD and conduct disorder may frequently coexist; and if either diagnosis is present, then the other diagnosis is commonly found. Psychostimulants also reduce some forms of aggression present in children diagnosed with ADHD (Allen et al., 1975; Klorman et al., 1988b). Amery et al. (1984) compared dextroamphetamine and placebo in 10 boys diagnosed with ADDH with a mean age of 9.6 ± 1.6 years. Dextroamphetamine was administered in doses of 15 to 30 mg/day. The authors reported that scores on the Thematic Apperception Test Hostility Scale, scores on the Holtzman Inkblot Test Hostility Scale, and observations of overt aggression in a laboratory free-play situation were reduced significantly ($P < .05$) during a 2-week period on dextroamphetamine, compared with a similar period on placebo. These data are important because ADHD and conduct disorder frequently coexist and stimulants are often not considered in treating children whose conduct disorders are the primary consideration.

Wender (1988) notes that development of tolerance to the therapeutic effects of stimulant medication is unusual, and when it occurs it progresses gradually over a period of 1 or 2 years. If this occurs, a trial of another stimulant is suggested, because complete cross-tolerance among the stimulants does not occur (Wender, 1988). There is a suggestion that the efficacy of stimulants typically decreases with age (Taylor et al., 1987).

Regarding stimulant use in the treatment of patients with ID, Gadow and Poling (1988) reviewed the literature on the use of stimulants in these patients, and they concluded that stimulants are highly effective in reducing symptoms of hyperactivity and conduct disorder in some individuals, regardless of the degree of their ID.

When given single doses of dextroamphetamine, normal prepubertal boys and college-aged men reacted similarly to patients diagnosed with ADHD; they exhibited decreased motor activity and generally improved attentional performance (Rapoport et al., 1978a, 1980a). Hence, earlier teachings that stimulants have a paradoxical effect in hyperactive children are incorrect, and a positive response to stimulant medication cannot be used to validate the diagnosis of ADHD (Pliszka et al., 2007).

PHARMACOKINETICS OF STIMULANTS

The stimulant medications undergo metabolism via enzymes in both the liver and the gastrointestinal tract, and these medication metabolites are then primarily excreted by the kidneys. Table 5.1 gives the site of metabolism, main metabolic products, time of peak plasma levels, serum half-lives, and routes of excretion of MPH and dextroamphetamine.

STANDARD STIMULANT PREPARATIONS COMPARED WITH LONG-ACTING OR SUSTAINED-RELEASE FORMS

Sustained-release preparations of stimulant medications make once-daily dosage possible. It is important to note that among the sustained-release medications, each has a specific time-release pattern. Within the MPH class, for example, Focalin XR has

TABLE 5.1 » Some Pharmacokinetic Properties of Stimulant Medications

Medication	Principal Metabolite(s)	Peak Serum Levels	Serum Half-life	Principal Route(s) of Excretion
Methylphenidate (Ritalin)	Liver → 75% ritalinic acid, which is pharmacologically inactive	1.9 h (range, 0.3–4.4 h); Ritalin SR, 4.7 h (range, 1.2–8.2 h)	2–2.5 h	Kidney excretes 70% to 80%, (primarily as ritalinic acid) in 24 h
Dextroamphetamine sulfate (Dexedrine)	Liver P-hydroxylation, N-demethylation, deamination, and conjugation	2 h for tablet; 8–10 h for spansule	6–8 h in children, 10–12 h in adults	May be excreted unchanged by kidney (amount varies according to urinary pH: from 2% to 3% in very alkaline urine, to 80% in acidic urine)

a time-release pattern of 50% IR and 50% delayed release. A Metadate CD capsule contains 30% IR and 70% extended release. This is an important consideration when evaluating the time of day when a child's symptoms are most impairing (e.g., do they need a larger quantity of active medicine in the morning or in the afternoon). These variations in time-release pattern were in part a response to early reports that found the clinical efficacy of sustained-release MPH occurred approximately 1 hour later than the IR form of MPH. In particular, two early studies of 22 boys with ADHD (Pelham et al., 1987) and a study by Birmaher et al. (1989) made note of this delay. These authors suggested that the relative inefficacy of sustained-release MPH at that time could result from differences in pharmacokinetics, absorption, or from tachyphylaxis.

Some subsequent studies, however, have reported significantly different results. Pelham et al. (1990) administered 10 mg of standard MPH every morning and noon; 20 mg of sustained-release MPH every morning; 10 mg of dextroamphetamine spansule (long-acting) every morning; 56.25 mg pemoline (pemoline has subsequently been withdrawn from the market), every morning; and placebo in random order for 3 to 6 days. Each double-blind, placebo-controlled, crossover study involved 22 boys (ages 8.08 to 13.17 years) diagnosed with ADHD. Midday placebos were given during the periods when long-acting medications were administered. Subjects were rated on measures of social behavior and classroom performance and on a continuous performance task. All four medication conditions had similar time courses (with effects evident between 1 and 9 hours after medication administration), and they were significantly (and approximately equally) better than placebo. The effects of the three long-acting preparations were as great, or almost as great, at 9 hours as at 2 hours after ingestion. Only 15 (68%) of the 22 patients improved sufficiently for the authors to recommend that they continue to receive stimulant medication. Of these 15 patients, dextroamphetamine spansules were recommended for 6, pemoline for 4, sustained-release MPH for 4, and standard MPH for 1. The clinical implications of this study are potentially very important because they suggest that the great majority (14 [93.3%] of 15 children with ADHD) derive more overall benefit from long-acting forms than from standard-release forms of stimulants. At the time of the study over 25 years ago, it was estimated that approximately 90% of children receiving medication for ADHD were prescribed MPH, and, of these, only approximately 10% received the sustained-release form. It should be noted that early forms of long-acting MPH such as Ritalin SR used an inferior wax-bead delivery system and were inconsistent in delivery and results. Later sustained-release MPH preparations such as Ritalin LA, Metadate CD, Focalin XR, and Concerta utilized more sophisticated delivery systems that seem to provide more consistent and prolonged stimulant effect.

Fitzpatrick et al. (1992) compared the efficacy of standard MPH, sustained-release MPH, and a combination of the two forms, in a double-blind, placebo-controlled study of 19 children (17 males and 2 females; age range, 6.9 to 11.5 years) diagnosed with ADD. Patients were rated on several scales by parents, teachers, and clinicians. All three active medication conditions were significantly better than placebo and were approximately equivalent in efficacy.

These studies alert the clinician to the likelihood that sustained-release preparations are more efficacious than thought initially, and they may be the preferred dosage forms for most children with ADHD, especially when considering adherence issues and abuse potential.

In the time since the preceding studies were published, several new stimulant preparations with increased duration of action have appeared in the market. Adderall XR, which is a preparation of four amphetamine salts, has a duration of action that increases significantly with increases in dose and is compared to MPH and reviewed later under the discussion of amphetamines. Vyvanse, a D-isomer amphetamine prodrug, has also been released. Extended-release forms of MPH in tablet, beaded

TABLE 5.2 » Duration of Action: ADHD Stimulant Medications			
	Onset of Action (min)	Duration of Action (h)
Short-Acting Stimulant Medications		
Amphetamine salts (Adderall)	30–60	4–6
Dextroamphetamine (Dexedrine)	30–60	4–6
Methylphenidate (Ritalin, Methylin)	30–60	3–5
Dexmethylphenidate (Focalin)	30–60	4–5
Intermediate- and Long-Acting Stimulant Medications		
Dextroamphetamine extended release (Dexedrine) Spansule)	30–60	6–10
Amphetamine salts extended release (Adderall XR)	30–90	8–12
Lisdexamfetamine (Vyvanse)	30–60	Up to 13
Methylphenidate long acting (Ritalin LA)	30–60	8–10
Methylphenidate extended release (Metadate ER)	30–60	6–8
Methylphenidate controlled delivery (Metadate CD)	30–60	8–12
Methylphenidate OROS (Concerta)	30–60	8–12
Methylphenidate transdermal patch (Daytrana)	120*	12 (dependent on when patch is removed)
Dexmethylphenidate extended release (Focalin XR)	30–60	6–10

ADHD, attention-deficit hyperactivity disorder; OROS, osmotic release oral system.
*Due to being a transdermal medication, the Daytrana patch should be placed on the skin 2 hours before desired effect is needed.

capsules, a patch, and an extended-release MPH preparation that uses an osmotic release oral system (OROS) of medication delivery combined with a semipermeable membrane to achieve a reported 12-hour duration of effect, have all been marketed. These medications are discussed later. Table 5.2 details the relative duration of effect for the more common stimulant medications.

SAFETY CONSIDERATIONS AND CONTRAINDICATIONS FOR STIMULANT ADMINISTRATION

Note: The FDA issued a black box warning for amphetamine and MPH formulations, and this warning states that stimulants "have a high potential for abuse. Administration of stimulants for prolonged periods of time may lead to drug dependence and must be avoided. Particular attention should be paid to the possibility of subjects obtaining stimulants for non-therapeutic use or distribution to others, and the drugs should be prescribed or dispensed sparingly. Misuse of stimulants may cause sudden death and serious cardiovascular adverse events."

These agents should therefore be prescribed cautiously to patients with a history of substance use disorders (including alcohol). Chronic, abusive use of stimulant medications can lead to marked tolerance and psychological dependence with varying degrees of abnormal behavior, whereas rare, frank psychotic episodes can occur, especially with parenteral abuse. Careful supervision is required during medication withdrawal from abusive use because severe depression may occur.

The risk of dependence with stimulant medications should be weighed against the benefits of prescribing the medication. In this risk–benefit–alternatives analysis, it should be noted here that for patients with a diagnosis of ADHD, the use of prescribed stimulants may actually prevent them from using illicit drugs for at least three reasons: (1) the treatment of ADHD usually improves impulsivity, and therefore the prescribed stimulant reduces the patients' risk of impulsively taking an illicit substance that is offered to them; (2) patients whose ADHD is adequately treated are less likely to self-medicate their ADHD symptoms with substances that might slow down their thoughts and hyperactivity (e.g., alcohol and cannabis); and (3) a patient with untreated or undertreated ADHD might develop depression, anxiety, and/or ODD, and these conditions may place them at a greater risk of developing a substance use disorder to self-medicate those symptoms and because they might be more likely to be friends with others who have ODD and conduct disorder who may have greater access to illicit substances.

At the intake session, some parents express concern that treatment with stimulants will predispose their child to later drug abuse or addiction. Most available evidence indicates that this is not the case. Although drug abuse itself is of major concern in our culture, children diagnosed with ADHD who have been treated with stimulants appear to be at no greater risk for drug or alcohol abuse as teenagers and adults than controls (Weiss & Hechtman, 1986). Past research looking for a link between ADHD medications and substance abuse has produced conflicting conclusions from no association, a protective effect, and an increased risk. However, many of those studies had methodological limitations to varying degrees, and not all of the studies followed their samples for a sufficient period of time into late adolescence and early adulthood. A National Institutes of Health–funded study at the Massachusetts General Hospital attempted to overcome the deficiencies of previous studies (Biederman et al., 2008). This was accomplished by following the study subjects up to a median age of about 22, including an assessment for psychiatric problems such as conduct disorder that are associated with substance abuse, and applying rigorous methods to accurately analyze the data. The research study team interviewed 112 young men (ranging in age from 16 to 27), previously diagnosed with ADHD, over a span of a decade about their use of alcohol, tobacco, and other psychoactive drugs. Seventy-three percent of the subjects had been medicated with stimulants at some time in their treatment, but only 22% were currently taking the stimulant medications. The study found no relationship between having ever received stimulant treatment and the risk of future alcohol or other substance abuse. The age at which stimulant treatment began and how long it continued also had no impact on substance use. Such data indicating low adherence of stimulant therapy during these critical years of late adolescence and young adulthood, however, begs the question: If stimulant medication adherence into young adulthood was greater, would substance abuse be less?

Wilens et al. (2009) performed a meta-analysis to examine whether stimulant treatment for ADHD begets later substance abuse. They reviewed six studies (two of which had follow-up in adolescence and four that had follow-up in young adulthood). The studies included subjects who were prescribed a medication ($N = 674$) and unmedicated subjects ($N = 360$). They were followed up for at least 4 years. They concluded that prescribed stimulant medication in childhood is actually associated with a reduction in the risk for subsequent drug and alcohol use disorders.

Overall, stimulant medications should not be prescribed to patients who have a history of drug abuse or where there is a likelihood that family members or friends would abuse the medication and/or sell it. In those cases where the family is unreliable but stimulants are still indicated, it is worthwhile to attempt to work out a way to dispense and store all of the stimulant medication at school because (for most children) coverage during the time in school is the foremost consideration. It should also be noted that compared to the IR agents, the sustained-release formulations (especially the prodrug lisdexamfetamine dimesylate [Vyvanse]) have less abuse potential. As is true for all medications, a careful risk–benefit analysis is an important consideration in the prescription of stimulant medications because there are both risks in prescribing and in not prescribing.

Sudden death has also been reported in association with CNS stimulant treatment at usual dosages in children and adolescents with structural cardiac abnormalities or serious heart problems. It is noted specifically for Adderall XR that "its misuse is associated with serious cardiovascular adverse events and may cause sudden death in patients with pre-existing cardiac structural abnormalities." The FDA does not recommend general use of stimulants in children or adults with structural cardiac abnormalities or other serious cardiac problems that may place them at increased vulnerability. It is recommended that a doctor be consulted right away if a child has any sign of heart problems such as chest pain, shortness of breath, or fainting while taking stimulant medications.

In the assessment of ADHD, it is therefore important to screen for a personal history of cardiac symptoms and disease (including dysrhythmias, murmurs, and syncope) and a family history of heart problems (including ventricular rhythms and sudden death [especially in a young person]). On the basis of the results of the screening, the following may be warranted before starting a stimulant medication: an electrocardiogram (ECG), echocardiogram, and referral to a pediatric cardiologist.

This issue must be taken seriously; and given the decline in prescriptions following the black box warning with SSRIs in 2004, some expressed concern about the effect the FDA's 2006 warning regarding stimulant use and cardiac risk might have. Barry et al. (2012) examined whether the FDA's 2006 stimulant warning had an impact on prescribing. The authors examined whether children (ages 0 to 20) filled a prescription for any ADHD medication during a given calendar year (from 2002 to 2008). They then analyzed news coverage of the issue in 10 high-circulation newspapers, on the 3 major television networks, and on a major cable news network in the United States. They reported finding no declines in stimulant medication use following FDA safety warnings overall or by parental education level. They added that the news media coverage was relatively balanced in its portrayal of the risks and benefits of ADHD medication use by children.

In addition to these, there exist other important contraindications to stimulant use. Known hypersensitivity to a stimulant medication and glaucoma are also significant contraindications. There are several other conditions such as tics, seizures, autism, and psychosis that were once considered absolute contraindications to the implementation of psychostimulant therapy. Indeed, such warnings are still cited in the manufacturers' product information literature that accompanies most psychostimulant products. However, more recent literature tends to qualify such conditions as relative contraindications depending on the clinical findings that many patients with these conditions still benefit markedly by the utilization of these agents even when these conditions are a comorbid health issue. Today, a review of the relevant literature suggests that if risks and benefits are carefully assessed and explained to the patient, it is reasonable to proceed with a trial of a psychostimulant (for patients with a relative contraindication to the medication) while carefully monitoring the patient. The following discussions of the literature will further clarify the "relative" nature of these contraindications as they apply to various comorbid conditions.

As mentioned earlier, children with ADHD can have a host of comorbidities, and one of these is tic disorder. It is important to note that a child with ADHD may have an undiagnosed and unnoticed tic disorder that becomes unmasked when a stimulant medication is prescribed. There is controversy over whether the stimulants should be given to children and adolescents with tic disorder, Tourette syndrome (TS), or a family history of such. Their use in autism spectrum disorder (ASD) and in TS or with tic disorders is discussed in greater detail later in this chapter.

Stimulants may also cause stereotypies and psychosis *de novo* in sensitive individuals or if given in high-enough doses. Stimulants are relatively contraindicated in children and adolescents with a history of schizophrenia or other psychosis, ASD, or borderline personality organization because stimulants appear to worsen these conditions in some cases. However, stimulants have been given to some patients with these diagnoses under conditions of close scrutiny with very beneficial results. If the patients are also being treated simultaneously with mood-stabilizer medications, then these risks may be diminished.

Stimulants may aggravate symptoms of marked anxiety, tension, and agitation; and are contraindicated when these symptoms are prominent (*Physicians' Desk Reference* [PDR], 2005, p. 2353). However, it is important to note that some children with untreated or undertreated ADHD develop anxiety as a result of always feeling unprepared and inattentive. Therefore, by treating ADHD with a stimulant, a patient's anxiety might, in fact, lessen. Stimulants therefore have the potential to either worsen or improve anxiety.

During the initial evaluation, it is important to screen for a personal and family history of bipolar disorder because stimulant medications (when no mood stabilizer is being prescribed) may induce a manic or mixed episode.

In 2005, magnesium pemoline was withdrawn from the market because its potential risks were greater than its potential benefits. Reports of acute hepatic failure, some of which were fatal and others which necessitated liver transplants, were the reason for this. The reader who wishes to have information regarding magnesium pemoline may consult the prior editions of this book.

INTERACTIONS OF STIMULANTS WITH OTHER MEDICATIONS

Stimulants have the potential to cause hypertensive crises when used with monoamine oxidase inhibitors (MAOIs). They should not be used concomitantly with an MAOI or within 14 days of an MAOI being discontinued.

In combination with TCAs, the actions of both the stimulant and the TCA may be enhanced.

Stimulants potentiate sympathomimetic medications (including street amphetamines and cocaine) and may counteract the sedative effect of antihistamines and benzodiazepines.

Lithium may inhibit the stimulatory effects of amphetamines.

Amphetamines may act synergistically with either phenytoin or phenobarbital to increase anticonvulsant activity.

On July 13, 1995, a National Public Radio broadcast reported that sudden deaths had occurred in three children taking a combination of MPH and clonidine, which caused alarm among parents and physicians of patients taking this combination of medications. Popper's editorial concerning this noted that the FDA had not publicized the data or informed clinicians, because it considered the "link between the deaths and the medications highly dubious." Detailed reviews of the medications and the three cases by Popper (1995) and Fenichel (1995) concluded that there was no convincing evidence of an adverse MPH–clonidine interaction in any of the cases. Popper (1995) and Swanson et al. (1995) concluded that combined clonidine–MPH treatment of ADHD is usually safe and that the available evidence did not support discontinuation of such therapy in patients experiencing significant clinical benefit. All authors also noted the lack of systematic studies of the efficacy and safety of combined MPH–clonidine treatment.

Swanson et al. (1995) noted in their review of untoward effects that when the combination of clonidine and a stimulant was given, sedation–hypotension–bradycardia would be most expected when the clonidine effect was at its peak and the stimulant's effect is decreasing and, conversely, that hypertension–tachycardia would be most expected when the stimulant is at its peak and clonidine's effect is waning.

In 1999, in a "Debate Forum" on "Combining methylphenidate and clonidine" published in the *Journal of the American Academy of Child and Adolescent Psychiatry (JAACAP),* Wilens and Spencer argued the affirmative ("A clinically sound medication option") and Swanson, Connor, and Cantwell argued the negative ("Ill-advised"). Before prescribing this combination, it is therefore recommended that the clinician reviews this literature and thoroughly discusses the risks and benefits with the parents/legal guardians and patient.

In addition to all of the potential drug–drug interactions listed here, many other medication interactions (which are less likely to be encountered in child and adolescent psychiatry than those mentioned in the preceding text) may occur.

ADVERSE EFFECTS OF STIMULANTS

There is some evidence that, overall, the untoward effects of MPH occur less frequently and with less severity than those from dextroamphetamine (Conners, 1971; Gross and Wilson, 1974). Gross and Wilson (1974) noted that side effects were infrequently severe enough to necessitate immediate discontinuation of the medication (1.1% of 377 patients for MPH and 4.3% of 371 patients for dextroamphetamine). With so many more stimulant medication options presently available, prescribers seem to be more willing to switch to another agent when a patient has a side effect to a medication. In one study, 50 of 684 children (7.3%) treated with IR Focalin experienced an adverse event that resulted in discontinuation of the medication, and the most common reasons cited for the discontinuation were twitching (vocal and motor tics), insomnia, loss of appetite, and tachycardia; PDR, 2015).

The most frequent and troublesome immediate untoward effects of stimulant medications include insomnia, loss of appetite, nausea, abdominal pain or cramps, headache, thirst, vomiting, lability of mood, irritability, sadness, weepiness, tachycardia, and blood pressure changes. Many of these symptoms diminish over a few weeks, although the cardiovascular changes may persist. Regarding the stimulants, it is said that amphetamine preparations are more likely than MPH to cause an increase in whininess/irritability.

It should be noted that patients with ADHD (even before treatment) generally do not sleep as well as those people without ADHD. Adding a stimulant as treatment can therefore make already poor sleep worse.

Since 1972, disturbances in growth—decrements in both height and weight percentiles—have been reported for both MPH and dextroamphetamine, and the long-term untoward consequences of these effects have been of particular concern (Safer et al., 1972). There has been controversy about the significance of these changes. Mattes and Gittelman (1983) reported significant decreases in height and weight percentiles over a 4-year period. A subsequent controlled study found a significant reduction in growth velocity during the period when stimulants are actively administered (Klein et al., 1988). Despite this adverse effect (AE) on growth during the active treatment phase, it appears that an accelerated rate of growth or growth rebound occurs once the stimulant is discontinued and that there is usually no significant compromise of ultimate height attained (Klein and Mannuzza, 1988). It seems likely, however, that some children are at greater risk for growth suppression than others, and serial heights and weights of any child receiving stimulant medication should be plotted carefully on a growth chart (e.g., the National Center for Health Statistics Growth Chart) (Hamill et al., 1976).

Vincent et al. (1990) reported no significant deviations from expected height and weight growth velocities in 31 adolescents diagnosed with ADHD who had received MPH continuously for a minimum of 6 months to a maximum of 6 years after their 12th birthdays. Mean age at the beginning of the study was 12.9 ± 0.8 years. The mean daily dose was 34 ± 14 mg or 0.75 ± 0.29 mg/kg and did not differ significantly with age or sex. The results suggested that early adolescent growth is not significantly adversely affected by MPH.

Nonetheless, patients taking stimulants may notice a decrease in appetite (especially during the school day), and they should be encouraged to eat healthy meals, and parents should not be alarmed to find that their child is suddenly very hungry at dinner (because their appetite has rebounded with the stimulant's effect having worn off). Regarding appetite, strategies can be developed to help. These include finding ways to get more healthy calories into a child's diet. Many insurance companies will cover the cost of nutritional supplements such as Pediasure if a prescription is written. Although medication holidays are generally not recommended, if there are significant concerns about appetite (but the patient needs a stimulant), then lower doses can be used on the weekend and in the summer if appropriate.

Faraone et al. (2005) reported on the long-term effects of extended-release mixed amphetamine salts (MAS XR) on growth in 568 children (mean age, 8.7 ± 1.8 years; age range, 6 to 12 years; 78% male, 73% White, 12% Black, 9% Hispanic), in a multicenter, open-label study. Subjects received doses of 10 to 30 mg/day for a period of 6 to 30 months. On the basis of the Centers for Disease Control and Prevention (CDC) norms, subjects experienced decreases in weight, body mass index (BMI), and height percentiles over the period of study; these decrements were greatest for the heaviest and tallest children; and these deficits occurred primarily during the first year. Decreases in weight, BMI, and height were not significant during the second year on medication. The height deficit was significant for subjects whose baseline heights were greater than the 25th percentile ($P = .001$ for the second quartile and $P < .0001$ for the third and fourth quartiles). The height loss was only 1.2 percentile points for the shortest children at baseline, whereas the tallest children at baseline experienced a 10 percentile decrease in height at the end of the study. The authors noted that monitoring growth parameters was essential; but that for most children, the decreases caused by MAS XR were not likely to be of clinical concern.

Charach et al. (2006) followed up 79 subjects (age range 6 to 12 years) who were diagnosed with ADHD by DSM-III-R criteria (APA, 1980a) and maintained on stimulant medication. They were followed up annually for up to 5 years to determine the long-term effects of stimulants on their height and weight. The subjects were taking various preparations of amphetamine and MPH. Small but statistically significant effects were found. On the basis of a statistical model, patients receiving the equivalent of >1.5 mg/kg/day of MPH show a decrease in expected weight gain after 1 year and subjects receiving >2.5 mg/kg/day have a decrease in expected height after 4 years on medication; the higher the dose, the greater the decrease in expected weight or height. Regular monitoring of height and weight is indicated for children and adolescents administered stimulants as a long-term treatment.

Stimulants successfully treat the symptoms of ADHD in part due to their effect of blocking dopamine reuptake into the presynaptic neuron. More dopamine effect in certain brain regions is clearly helpful in reducing ADHD symptoms, but excess dopamine in other brain regions can lead to auditory hallucinations (consistent with the dopamine hypothesis of schizophrenia). A few children treated with stimulants may develop a clinical picture resembling schizophrenia. This condition occurs most frequently when untoward effects such as disorganization are misinterpreted as a worsening of presenting symptoms and the dosage is further increased until prominent psychotomimetic effects occur. It may also occur when stimulants are administered to children with borderline personality disorders or schizophrenia (conditions in which stimulants are relatively contraindicated). In most such cases, the psychotic symptomatology improves rapidly after discontinuation of the medication (Green, 1989).

REBOUND EFFECTS OF STIMULANTS

Rebound effects may occur beginning approximately 5 hours after the last dose of short-acting MPH. Simply stated, ADHD symptoms often return after the effects of the stimulant have worn off. In some cases, the ADHD symptoms may even exceed baseline levels before administration of stimulants.

Rapoport et al. (1978a) reported that normal children who received short-acting dextroamphetamine also experienced behavioral rebound approximately 5 hours after a single acute dose. Symptoms included excitability, talkativeness, overactivity, insomnia, stomachaches, and mild nausea. Long-acting formulations of stimulants may reduce the risk of rebound effects, but may still occur albeit much later in the day when serum concentrations taper off approximately 8 to 12 hours after dosing.

STIMULANTS' RELATIONSHIP TO TICS AND TOURETTE SYNDROME

ADHD may be comorbid with many conditions including tic disorder. Stimulants may unmask a previously unnoticed and undiagnosed tic, and stimulants can also exacerbate existing tics. Owing to this, manufacturers state that the use of stimulants is contraindicated in patients with motor tics, a diagnosis of TS, or a family history of TS. Although this is the statement from the medication manufacturers, there is some disagreement among clinical experts regarding whether stimulants should be given to persons with tics, TS, or a family history of either condition.

Comings and Comings (1984) investigated the relationship between TS and ADDH. They found that ADDH was present in 62% of 140 males <21 years of age who were diagnosed with TS. A study of their family pedigrees suggested that the TS gene could be expressed as ADDH but without tics. The authors thought that their data implied that patients diagnosed with ADDH and treated with stimulants who subsequently developed tics had ADDH as a result of the TS gene and probably would have developed tics or TS even if they had not received stimulants.

In a study of 1,520 children diagnosed with ADDH and treated with MPH, Denckla et al. (1976) reported that existing tics were exacerbated in 6 cases (0.39%) and tics developed *de novo* in 14 cases (0.92%). After the discontinuation of MPH, all 6 of the tics that had worsened returned to their premedication intensity, and 13 of the 14 new tics completely remitted.

Shapiro and Shapiro (1981) reviewed the relationship between treating ADDH with stimulants and the precipitation or exacerbation of tics and TS. In addition, they treated 42 patients who had symptoms of both MBD and TS with a combination of MPH and haloperidol. Dosage of MPH ranged from 5 to 60 mg/day and was individually titrated for each patient. The authors also used MPH (dose range, 5 to 40 mg/day) in 62 additional patients with TS to counteract the untoward effects of haloperidol, such as sedation, amotivation, dysphoria, cognitive impairment, and dullness. The authors concluded that the evidence suggests that stimulants do not cause or provoke TS, although high doses of stimulants can cause or exacerbate tics in predisposed patients. Clinically, they noted that tics seemed less likely to be exacerbated by stimulants in patients who were also taking haloperidol for TS. When tics did increase in intensity, they remitted within 3 to 6 hours, which is the approximate duration of the usual clinical effects of MPH.

Lowe et al. (1982) noted that the early clinical signs of TS may be difficult to differentiate from ADDH. Shapiro and Shapiro (1981) noted that approximately 57% of children with tics or TS had concomitant MBD; however, most children with MBD do not develop either tics or TS.

Gadow et al. (1992) treated 11 boys (aged 6.1 to 11.9 years [mean, 8.3 ± 1.96 years]), diagnosed with comorbid tic disorder and ADHD, with MPH. The medication was administered under double-blind conditions; each subject was assigned to random 2-week periods of placebo and MPH in doses of 0.1, 0.3, and 0.5 mg/kg/day. The authors noted that MPH significantly decreased hyperactive and disruptive behaviors in the classroom and reduced physical aggression on the playground. Vocal tics were also significantly reduced in the lunchroom and classroom. On the basis of this and other studies cited in their report, the authors concluded that MPH is a safe and effective treatment for some children with comorbid ADHD and tic disorder over a short-term period; however, they cautioned that a risk of protraction or irreversible worsening of tics may exist for some individuals.

Gadow et al. (1995) conducted a double-blind, placebo-controlled, 8-week study in which 34 prepubertal children, 31 males and 3 females (6.08 to 11.9 years of age) diagnosed with ADHD and comorbid chronic motor tic disorder or TS by DSM-III-R criteria (APA, 1987) were treated with placebo and MPH in doses of 0.1, 0.2, and 0.5 mg/kg given twice daily (usually before school and at noon) for 2 weeks for each condition. Most children were additionally diagnosed with opposition defiant or conduct disorder. Tics were rated on five different scales by a clinician and on the Global Tic Rating Scale by parents and teachers. All 34 subjects responded with dramatic clinical improvement in hyperactivity and inattentive, disruptive, oppositional, and aggressive behaviors when treated with MPH. Teachers noted significant improvement in symptoms on the 0.1 mg/kg dose. There were no statistically or clinically significant AEs on the severity of tics with MPH treatment; but in the classroom, there was an increased frequency of motor tics on the 0.1 mg/kg dose compared with placebo and in the physician's 2-minute motor tic count on the 0.5 mg/kg dose. Teachers rated vocal tics as significantly less frequent on all three doses of MPH than on placebo. The authors concluded that MPH was a safe and effective treatment for most children diagnosed with comorbid ADHD and tic disorder. They also cautioned that it can be extremely difficult to determine whether MPH or natural fluctuations are responsible for observed changes in the frequency or intensity of tics and that MPH is reported to have a negative effect on tics in some children (Gadow et al., 1995).

Gadow et al. (1999) continued to follow up prospectively the 34 children who participated in their 1995 study at 6-month intervals for an additional 2 years of open treatment with MPH. There was no significant change in mean group scores rating severity or frequency of motor or vocal tics during the 2-year maintenance period compared with baseline or double-blind placebo ratings. Direct observations in the simulated classroom were almost identical at baseline, during the double-blind placebo protocol, and during the 2-year follow-up. Although there was no evidence that MPH maintenance therapy (for up to 2 years) exacerbated vocal or motor tics for their subjects as a group, the authors cautioned that their results do not rule out the possibility of this occurring in specific individuals. Behavioral improvements in ADHD symptomatology were maintained during the 2-year follow-up; however, behavioral problems associated with ODD and conduct disorder did not maintain their gains. Over the 2-year period, there was a significant increase of approximately 10 beats per minute in heart rate, which was not felt to be clinically significant, and slightly less weight gain (0.72 kg) and less height gain (0.67 cm) than expected, both of which are so small as to not be of concern for most children.

Castellanos et al. (1997) conducted a 9-week, double-blind, crossover, placebo-controlled treatment protocol (in three separate cohorts) with a total of 20 males (mean age 9.4 ± 2.0 years, range 6 to 13 years) diagnosed with comorbid ADHD and TS comparing MPH, Dexedrine (DEX), and placebo at various doses. Doses of stimulants were quite high at the upper range. Efficacy was determined by ratings on the Tourette Syndrome Unified Rating Scale and the Conners teachers' hyperactivity ratings. Medication was administered at breakfast and lunch daily. Because of the three separate cohorts, only a summary of the overall findings is given here. Target ADHD behaviors of all subjects improved on teachers' ratings on stimulants, and there was no significantly greater improvement at the higher doses. At the lowest dose (12.5 or 15 mg/dose for MPH and 5 or 7.5 mg/dose for DEX), there was no significant change of tic severity. At highest medication doses, tic severity was significantly increased, but DEX increased the severity significantly more than MPH or placebo did. Of particular clinical interest was the finding that the increases in tics that occurred at higher doses of MPH tended to diminish over time and return to placebo levels when MPH was maintained or increased; this occurred in 17 of the 20 subjects. This diminution in tic severity also occurred with DEX, but less significantly (in 9 of 20 subjects, $P < .01$). The authors concluded that of the stimulants, usually MPH is preferred, and lowest effective dose should be considered as a possible treatment for children with comorbid ADHD and TS. Some clinicians would advocate that the purified d-isomer of MPH may have theoretic and true clinical benefit in providing a less tic-promoting effect than the combined d- and l-MPH formulations.

To further investigate whether treatment with MPH causes tics *de novo* or worsens preexisting tics in children diagnosed with ADHD, Law and Schachar (1999) conducted a 1-year-long randomized, placebo-controlled, prospective study of 91 such children who had never received medication for ADHD or tics. Mean age was 8.35 ± 1.55 years. Inclusion criteria included the following: ADHD symptoms beginning before age 7 and of at least 6 months' duration; Full Scale Intelligence Quotient (FSIQ) >80; and no primary anxiety or affective disorder. Exclusion criteria were as follows: severe motor or vocal tic disorder or TS, because it was assumed that MPH would exacerbate such tics, but subjects with mild to moderate tics were permitted, because the authors assumed the risk of their worsening would be less and they would be more easily managed if they did occur. Of the 46 randomly assigned to the MPH group, 11 (23.9%) had preexisting tics; of the 45 randomly assigned to the placebo group, 16 (35.6%) had preexisting tics. Tics were rated on a 10-point scale: 0 = no tics, 1 to 3 = mild tics, 4 to 6 = moderate tics, and 7 to 9 = severe tics.

By the end of the study, 10 (19.6%) of the 52 subjects with *no preexisting tics* who received MPH and 2 (16.7%) of the 12 subjects remaining in the placebo group had developed clinically significant tics that were of moderate intensity or worse, including 1 child in the MPH group who developed TS-like symptoms. There was no significant difference in the development of tics *de novo* between the groups (*P* = .59). The 12 subjects who developed tics were managed by maintaining the dose of MPH at the level when tics emerged in 8 cases, reducing the MPH dose in 3 cases, and adding clonidine in 1 case. Among the 27 subjects with preexisting tics, 7 (33.3%) of the 21 receiving MPH had worsening of their tics, including 1 boy who developed TS-like symptoms; 2 (9.5%) experienced no change in their tics; 5 (23.8%) experienced improvement; and 7 (33.3%) had complete remission of their tics. Of the six such patients in the placebo group, two (33.3%) had worsening of tics and four had complete remission of their tics. Hence, in both the MPH and the placebo groups, 66.7% (14/21 and 4/6) of the subjects with preexisting tics experienced improvement or no change in their tics, and tics worsened in 33.3% of the subjects (7/21 and 2/6). There was no significant difference between the groups (*P* = .70).

Tics *de novo* developed throughout the 1-year treatment in both groups. In the MPH group, 20 subjects developed new tics: 12 (60%) within the first 4 months. In the placebo group, nine subjects developed new tics: one (11.1%) within the first 4 months. Only 12 of these 29 subjects who developed new tics were reported to still have tics at the end of the study, illustrating both the waxing and waning natural course of tics as well as the response to decreasing the dose of MPH in some cases. Law and Schachar (1999) concluded that titration of MPH to an optimal average maintenance dose of 0.5 mg/kg/day does not cause tics *de novo* or worsen preexisting tics of moderate severity or less, more often than placebo in children being treated for ADHD for up to 1 year.

Sverd (2000) reviewed the use of MPH to treat children with comorbid ADHD and tic disorders. Sverd concluded that the literature supports that ADHD is genetically related to TS in a substantial proportion of cases, that stimulants relatively infrequently cause tics *de novo* or exacerbation of tics, and that MPH may be safely used to treat children diagnosed with ADHD and comorbid tic disorder.

Cohen et al. (2015) performed a meta-analysis on the risk of tics with stimulant medication use. They reviewed 22 studies of ADHD (2,385 children). They noted that new-onset tics or worsening of tic symptoms were commonly reported (event rate = 5.7% for stimulants and event rate = 6.5% for placebo). They concluded that the risk of new onset or worsening of tics associated with stimulant medication was similar to that observed with placebo. They added that type of stimulant, dose, duration of treatment, and participant age did not affect risk of new onset or worsening of tics. The major conclusion that was underscored in their report was that their meta-analysis did not support an association between new onset or worsening of tics and stimulant use.

If a conservative approach is still preferred, then one could proceed with caution knowing that a review of the relevant literature suggests that if risks and benefits are carefully assessed, it is reasonable to attempt a trial with MPH or amphetamine in such patients if they are carefully monitored.

STIMULANT MEDICATIONS APPROVED FOR USE IN CHILD AND ADOLESCENT PSYCHIATRY

Stimulants are the most frequently prescribed psychiatric medications during childhood. In 1977, more than half a million children were being treated with MPH in the United States alone (Sprague & Sleator, 1977). By 1987, it was conservatively estimated that the number increased to 750,000 youth in the United States (Safer & Krager, 1988). In 1987, MPH accounted for 93% of the medications prescribed, and other stimulants accounted for another 6% for ADHD (Safer & Krager, 1988). In more recent times, the development of improved long-acting formulations of MPH and amphetamine-based products has resulted in a greater balance in the prescription of MPH versus amphetamine products.

Zuvekas and Vitiello's 12-year prospective study on stimulant medication use (2012) estimated that 3.5% of children in the United States in 2008 received stimulant medication. This was up from 2.4% in 1996. Data continues to suggest that more children today are prescribed stimulants than in previous decades.

Of the stimulants approved for use in the treatment of ADHD, broadly there are the MPH and the amphetamine classes. Of the MPHs, there are many medications that contain both the D and the L enantiomers. For each of the compounds, the D enantiomers shows greater pharmacologic activity than the L enantiomers, and so Focalin XR was created with this in mind (it contains only the D enantiomer). Focalin is therefore discussed in its own section. Of the amphetamine medications, there are MAS, amphetamines, levoamphetamine, dextroamphetamine, and lisdexamfetamine.

Methylphenidate Stimulant Medications Approved for Use in Child and Adolescent Psychiatry

D-L-Methylphenidate Hydrochloride (Ritalin, Ritalin LA, Methylin, Methylin ER, Metadate, Metadate ER, Metadate CD, Aptensio XR, Concerta, Quillivant XR, QuilliChew ER, Cotempla XR ODT, Daytrana)

Pharmacokinetics of D-L-Methylphenidate Hydrochloride

Administration of short-acting MPH with meals does not appear to adversely affect its absorption or pharmacokinetics and may diminish problems with appetite suppression (Patrick et al., 1987). Long-acting stimulant formulations may be affected by high-fat meals in more rapid absorption, resulting in faster efficacy and lower peak serum levels. Stimulant medications may be taken with or without food, but patients describe less gastrointestinal upset when the medications are taken with food. For this reason (and also because stimulants can reduce appetite), it is generally recommended that they be taken with food.

An improvement in target symptoms can be seen in as few as 20 minutes after a therapeutically effective dose of standard/IR preparation MPH is taken (Zametkin et al., 1985). Peak blood levels occur between 1 and 2.5 hours after administration of short-acting stimulants (Gualtieri et al., 1982), and the serum half-life is approximately 2.5 hours (Winsberg et al., 1982). The major metabolite is pharmacologically inactive. Between 70% and 90% of radiolabeled MPH is recovered in the urine within 24 hours.

Because of these pharmacokinetics, the most frequent times to administer standard/IR preparation MPH to children and adolescents are before leaving for school and during the lunch hour. This dosage schedule usually ensures adequate serum levels during school hours, which is the foremost consideration for most students; however, some students require after-school dosing to treat ADHD symptoms that would interfere with their abilities to concentrate for homework, sports, and/or employment.

Concerta was designed to have a 12-hour duration of effect and to be administered once daily in the morning. It is a long-acting MPH product that uses osmotic OROS medication-delivery technology to provide for the delivery of MPH at a controlled rate throughout the day. It has an osmotically active trilayer core surrounded by a semipermeable membrane that releases MPH gradually, and its over-coating of rapidly available MPH produces an initial peak plasma concentration in approximately 1 to 2 hours. Plasma concentration then continues to gradually increase to an ultimate peak level in approximately 6 to 8 hours, following which levels gradually decline. Serum half-life is 3.5 ± 0.4 hours. Although most patients will not require a dose larger than 54 or 72 mg/day, small clinical trials have documented the safety and efficiency of dosages up to 108 mg in appropriate patients (although doses above 72 mg/day are not FDA approved). Doses >2 mg/kg/day are not recommended for any age.

Adverse Effects and Adjustment of the Methylphenidate Hydrochloride Dose Schedule

Children who develop significant behavioral or attentional difficulties in the late afternoon or early evening may do so because of a return-to-baseline behavior as serum levels decline into subtherapeutic levels and/or because of a rebound effect as the medication wears off (Rapoport et al., 1978a). A third dose of medication given in the afternoon may be helpful for some such children. Johnston et al. (1988), however, suggested that psychostimulant rebound effects are not clinically significant for most children.

Insomnia may also occur. It is clinically important to distinguish those children whose insomnia is an untoward effect of the medication from those whose insomnia may be due to the recurrence of behavioral difficulties as the medication effect subsides and/or a rebound effect. For the first group of children, a reduction in milligram dosage of the last dose of the day may be necessary. For the latter group, an evening dose or a dose approximately 1 hour before bedtime may be helpful. Chatoor et al. (1983) prescribed late afternoon or evening dextroamphetamine sustained-release capsules to seven children who had strong rebound effects as their medication wore off and who developed marked behavioral problems and difficulty settling down and sleeping at bedtime. Parents reported significant behavioral improvement and markedly less bedtime oppositional behavior and increased ease in falling asleep. The authors compared sleep electroencephalograms (EEGs) in seven children recorded during periods on dextroamphetamine sustained-release capsules and on placebo. Compared with placebo, dextroamphetamine tended to delay onset of sleep slightly, significantly increase rapid eye movement (REM) latency (time to first REM period), and significantly decrease REM time (by approximately 14%) and the number of REM periods. Length of stage 1 and stage 2 sleep was significantly increased, and sleep efficiency (amount of time asleep during recording) decreased. Reduction in sleep efficiency was only 5%, which seemed minor compared with the significant behavioral improvement that occurred (Chatoor et al., 1983).

Stimulant Medications as Proconvulsants and Anticonvulsants

As Gualtieri discusses, stimulants (like almost all psychoactive drugs) can affect the seizure threshold if the dose is sufficiently high or abruptly changed, but the patient's inherent predisposition to seizures is likely much more important than the effect of the medication. In high dosages, stimulants can cause seizures; but at typical therapeutic low dosages, stimulants usually raise the seizure threshold and therefore improve seizure control (Gualtieri, 2002). Nonetheless, the manufacturer's package insert warns that there is some evidence that MPH may lower the seizure threshold. However, McBride et al. (1986) found only a single case report in the literature in which a child who was previously seizure-free had a seizure soon after treatment with MPH. The authors treated 23 children and adolescents, aged 4 to 15 years and diagnosed with ADD who had seizure disorders of various types ($N = 20$) or epileptiform EEG abnormalities ($N = 3$), with MPH. Fifteen of the children with documented seizure disorder received concomitant antiepileptic medications. Individual doses of 0.33 ± 0.13 mg/kg of MPH were administered with total daily doses of 0.63 ± 0.25 mg/kg from 3 months to 4 years. The authors found no evidence of increased frequency of seizures following MPH treatment in 16 children with active seizure disorders or in 4 children who had had active seizure disorders but who had been seizure-free and off antiepileptic medications from 2 months to 2 years. The three children with epileptiform abnormalities also did not develop seizures during the period they received MPH. This evidence suggests that MPH may not lower the seizure threshold to a clinically significant degree at usual therapeutic doses and that the presence of a seizure disorder in a child or adolescent with ADHD is not an absolute contraindication for a trial of MPH (McBride et al., 1986).

Crumrine et al. (1987) also reported that they had administered MPH 0.3 mg/kg twice daily to nine males (6.1 to 10.1 years of age) who had diagnoses of ADHD and seizure disorder. The boys had been previously stabilized on anticonvulsant medication and experienced no seizures or changes in EEG background patterns or epileptiform activity during 4-week, randomized, double-blind crossover trials of MPH or placebo. Also, subjects improved significantly on the Hyperactivity Index (HI) factors on the Conners Teacher Questionnaire (Crumrine et al., 1987).

These reports suggest that when clinically indicated, it is not unreasonable to undertake a trial of MPH in children and adolescents with coexisting seizure disorders and ADHD. Clearly, frequency of seizures should be carefully monitored; and if their frequency increases or seizures develop *de novo*, then the clinician may discontinue MPH.

Indications for Methylphenidate Hydrochloride in Child and Adolescent Psychiatry

Methylphenidate has FDA approval for treating ADHD (age 6 years and older) and narcolepsy.

Immediate-Release MPH Dosage Schedule

- *Children <6 years of age:* not FDA approved for use.
- *Children at least 6 years of age and adolescents up to 17 years of age:* start with 5 mg once or twice daily (usually about 7 AM and noon) and raise dose gradually to 5 to 10 mg/week. Maximum recommended total daily dosage is 60 mg. The usual optimal dose falls between 0.3 and 0.7 mg/kg administered two to three times daily (total daily dose range of 0.6 to 2.1 mg/kg; Duncan, 1990).
- *Adolescents at least 18 years of age and adults:* start with an initial daily dose of 5 mg two or three times daily, usually before meals, and titrate depending on clinical response. Average dose is 20 to 30 mg/day with a range of 10 to 60 mg/day.

Immediate-Release D- and L-Methylphenidate Hydrochloride Dose Forms Available

- *Tablets: (Ritalin, Methylin):* 5, 10 (scored), and 20 mg (scored)
- *Chewable tablets (Methylin chewable tablets, Methylphenidate HCL chewable tablets):* 2.5, 5, and 10 mg
- *Oral solution (Methylin oral solution):* 5 mg/5 mL, 10 mg/5 mL

Extended/Sustained-Release MPH Dosage Schedule

- *Children <6 years of age:* not approved for use.
- *Individuals at least 6 years of age:* Methylphenidate hydrochloride sustained-release tablets and extended-release capsules are administered once daily in the morning. Their duration of action is between 8 and 12 hours depending on the formulation and with some variation from person to person. Start with an initial dose of 10 to 20 mg once daily and increase by a maximum of 10 mg weekly to a maximum total daily dose of 60 mg. If a patient is already receiving immediate-release MPH, an equivalent milligram

(continued)

Indications for Methylphenidate Hydrochloride in Child and Adolescent Psychiatry (*continued*)

dose of a sustained-release preparation may be substituted for the total dose of standard-release MPH used during the same period. Extended-release tablets must be taken whole and not crushed or chewed; sustained-release capsules may be opened and sprinkled on applesauce.

Extended/Sustained-Release Methylphenidate Hydrochloride Dose Forms Available

- *Sustained-release tablets (Metadate ER 10 mg, 20 mg):* Sustained-release tablets of equivalent strength may be substituted for the total dose of the immediate-release form given over 8 hours.
- *Sustained-release capsules (Ritalin LA 10, 20, 30, and 40 mg; Metadate CD 10, 20, 30, 40, 50, and 60 mg; Aptensio XR 10 mg, 15 mg, 20 mg, 30 mg, 40 mg, 50 mg, 60 mg):* The recommended initial dose is 20 mg once daily in the morning for Metadate CD and Ritalin LA, but it is 10 mg for Aptensio XR. Dosage may be titrated upward in 10 mg increments weekly. The maximum total daily dose recommended is 60 mg. For each of these three medications, the capsules may be opened and sprinkled on applesauce and consumed immediately without chewing, which is advantageous for some younger children or if there is a question of adherence (swallowing the capsule).
- *OROS (Osmotic Release Oral System) methylphenidate hydrochloride (Concerta, OROS: 18, 27, 36, and 54 mg):* The maximum recommended once-daily dose is 54 mg in children and up to 72 mg/day (not to exceed 2 mg/kg/day) in adolescents. Concerta was designed to have clinical effects lasting approximately 12 hours. Swanson et al. (2000) have shown that OROS MPH can be initiated at 18 mg/day and then titrated weekly to a maximum recommended dose of 54 mg/day in children; that is, without prior titration on standard (immediate-release) MPH. Swanson et al. (2003) showed that OROS MPH remains clinically effective for at least 12 hours and that its efficacy is comparable to that of immediate-release MPH given three times daily.
- *Sustained-release MPH disintegrating tablets (Cotempla XR ODT 8.6 mg, 17.3 mg, 25.9 mg):* The recommended initial dose is 17.3 mg once daily in the morning. May adjust by 8.6 to 17.3 mg/day every 7 days. Maximum dose is 51.8 mg/day.
- *Sustained-release MPH chewable tablets (QuilliChew ER 20 mg, 30 mg, 40 mg):* The recommended initial dose is 20 mg once daily in the morning. May adjust by 10 to 20 mg/day every 7 days. Maximum dose is 60 mg/day.
- *Sustained-release liquid formulation (Quillivant XR SUSP, 25 mg per 5 mL):* The recommended initial dose is 20 mg once daily in the morning. May adjust by 10 to 20 mg/day every 7 days. Maximum dose is 60 mg/day.
- *MPH transdermal system (Daytrana, 10, 15, 20, and 30 mg patches):* Daytrana is approved for ages 6 to 17. Patch is to be applied by holding firmly in place with the palm of the hand for 30 seconds to clean dry skin in hip area (alternating location of placement daily). The patch should be placed 2 hours before effect is needed and should be removed 9 hours after application (or 3 hours before bedtime) to allow decrease in serum MPH concentrations so as not to disrupt sleep onset. Daytrana patches may be removed earlier than 9 hours if a shorter duration of effect is desired. This allows for variable control of duration of effect to accommodate for changing patient schedules. The recommended initial dose is the 10-mg patch, increasing to the next patch size weekly if clinically indicated and tolerated. The maximum FDA-approved dosage is the 30-mg patch daily. The patch has the typical stimulant side-effect profile in addition to not infrequent skin erythema at patch site to some degree with accompanying pruritus, especially during the winter months.

Reports of Interest

Methylphenidate Hydrochloride in the Treatment of ADHD

Wilens et al. (2005) conducted a long-term open-label study of OROS MPH in the treatment of 407 children (age range 6 to 13 years, mean age 9.2 ± 1.8 years). Of those enrolled, 229 subjects continued treatment to the 21/24-month endpoint. Subjects were prescribed 18 to 54 mg daily (the mean daily dose at baseline was 35.2 mg and at endpoint was 44.2 mg). Using last observation carried forward analyses, 85% of parents/caregivers and 92% of investigators rated a good or excellent response on the Global Assessment of Effectiveness. Regarding AEs, 282 (69.3%) reported at least one AE that investigators thought to be probably due to OROS MPH. The most frequent were headache (30.2%), insomnia (19.9%), decreased appetite (18.7%), abdominal pain (11.1%), and tics (0.8%). The authors concluded that OROS MPH was effective and tolerable in this population (for up to 24 months).

Garfinkel et al. (1983) compared efficacy of MPH with placebo, desipramine, and clomipramine in a double-blind crossover study of 12 males (mean age,

7.3 years; range, 5.9 to 11.6 years) diagnosed with ADD who required day hospital or inpatient hospitalization because of the severity of their impulsivity, inattention, and aggressiveness. MPH was significantly better in improving symptoms on the Conners Scale as rated by teachers ($P < .005$) and program child care workers ($P < .001$).

Swanson et al. (1986) reported on six children who developed behavioral and cognitive tolerance to their usual doses of MPH during long-term treatment. To maintain satisfactory clinical response, their pediatricians had to titrate the total daily doses to levels of 120 to 300 mg of MPH administered in as many as five individual doses of 40 to 60 mg. These children performed a cognitive task better at their usual high dose (average, 60 mg three times daily) than at a lower dose (average, 30 mg three times daily), confirming cognitive tolerance. Overall, these children had high serum levels compatible with the high doses, suggesting that neither metabolic tolerance nor differential absorption was responsible for the behavioral tolerance.

Methylphenidate Hydrochloride in the Treatment of ADHD in Preschoolers

As was discussed previously, PATS is a multicenter, randomized trial examining the efficacy and safety of MPH use in preschoolers (aged 3 to 5 years old) with severe ADHD who were unresponsive to a 10-week psychosocial intervention. PATS demonstrated that the MPH was safe and effective in short-term use, and the authors recommended close medication monitoring of this very young ADHD population.

In another study (a double-blind, placebo-controlled comparison of two doses (0.3 and 0.5 mg/kg/day) of MPH and placebo), Musten et al. (1997) treated 31 preschoolers (26 males, 5 females, mean age 58.07 ± 6.51 months, range 48 to 70 months) diagnosed with ADHD by DSM-III-R (APA, 1987) criteria. Twenty-six (84%) of the subjects were also diagnosed with comorbid ODD and six (19%) with conduct disorder. MPH significantly improved impulsivity on the Gordon Delay Task. Subjects made more correct responses on MPH than on placebo ($P < .05$) and there was no difference between the two doses of MPH. On the Gordon Vigilance Task (assessing sustained attention and impulsivity under conditions of high arousal and low feedback), there was significantly better performance on MPH than on placebo ($P < .01$), and there were no significant differences between the two doses of MPH. Parents ratings on the three subscales of the Conners Parent Rating Scale (CPRS)-R (Learning, Conduct, and HI) all showed MPH to be significantly better than placebo ($P = .001$). There was no difference in the two MPH doses for the Conduct or HI, but MPH 0.5 mg/kg/day was significantly better than MPH 0.3 mg/kg/day on the learning subscale. There was no evidence of improvement with MPH in children's adherence with parental directives on three laboratory tasks; however, MPH significantly improved the children's ability to stay on task in the 0.5 mg/kg dose but not in the 0.3 mg/kg dose. Subjects' productivity in a "cancellation task" was significantly improved on the 0.5 mg/kg dose only. The authors concluded that the treatment of their subjects with MPH resulted in improvement similar to that reported for older children. It significantly improved attention and parent-rated behaviors. Overall, the results on using 0.5 mg/kg/day were superior to using the lower dose and supported using an initial dose of 0.5 mg/kg/day in this age group. The authors also noted that their protocol had fixed doses and that optimal doses for some subjects may have been higher and resulted in further improvement (Musten et al., 1997).

In their review of stimulant medication, Wilens and Spencer (2000) reviewed seven earlier placebo-controlled studies of MPH in a total of 187 preschoolers, with mean age of 4.9 years and age range of 1.8 to 6 years. The studies were 3 to 9 weeks long; total mean MPH daily dose was 5 to 20 mg/day or 0.3 to 1.0 mg/kg/day. Overall, there was mild to moderate improvement in ADHD symptomatology in all the studies. They noted that subjects' adherence increased with higher doses, which tended to improve the mother–child relationship.

Handen et al. (1999) reported a 3-week, double-blind, placebo-controlled study of MPH in treating 11 preschool children (9 males and 2 females; mean age, 58.9 ± 8.2 months; age range, 4.0 to 5.9 years), 9 of the 11 were diagnosed with ADHD by DSM-III-R (APA, 1987) criteria and the other 2 had long-standing difficulty with inattention and overactivity. Two of the subjects with ADHD were diagnosed with comorbid ODD. Subjects had intelligence quotients (IQs) in the range of 40 to 78 (mean IQ, 60.0 ± 11.6). Receptive/expressive language functioning was consistent with IQ in most subjects. Although the children in the study were diagnosed with comorbid ID and ADHD, none were diagnosed with autism.

Subjects were administered MPH in 0.3 and 0.6 mg/kg doses or placebo for 1 week each. The three conditions were randomly assigned; but because of concern of untoward effects, the 0.3 mg/kg dose always preceded the 0.6 mg/kg dose. Efficacy was measured on the CTRS, the Preschool Behavioral Questionnaire (PBQ), the Side Effects Checklist, and several measures of behavior in the laboratory classroom (waiting task, resistance-to-temptation task, an 8-minute play session, compliance task, and cleanup task). One child experienced a significant increase in social withdrawal, irritability, tearfulness, whining, and anxiety on 0.3 mg/kg and further treatment with MPH was not recommended, so that child withdrew from the study.

Overall, 8 (73%) of the 11 subjects responded positively to MPH with a minimum of 40% decrease on the HI of the CTRS and/or the Hyperactive-Distractible subscale of the PBQ. Ratings on MPH, 0.6 mg/kg, compared with placebo on three of the CTRS indices (Hyperactivity [$P < .005$], Inattention-Passivity [$P < .05$], and HI [$P < .05$]) and the PBQ Hyperactive-Distractible subscale ($P < .005$) all showed significant improvement. In the "laboratory classroom," play intensity and movement during free play decreased significantly; and during the compliance and cleanup tasks, vocalization and disruptive behavior decreased and compliance increased significantly on the omnibus test while on MPH. Most children experienced a positive but not significant change on the MPH 0.3 mg/kg dose; the 0.6 mg/kg MPH dose was better for most of the variables, which showed significant improvement. Unfortunately, more clinically important untoward effects (e.g., social withdrawal and irritability) also occurred more frequently at the higher MPH dose. Overall, 45% of the 11 subjects developed untoward effects on MPH. The authors concluded that preschoolers with ADHD and ID responded to MPH similarly to typically developing children with ADHD. They also noted that children with developmental disabilities (e.g., intellectual disability) may be at greater risk for developing untoward effects on MPH, especially at higher doses, than are children without such disabilities.

Pearson et al. (2003, 2004a, 2004b) reported on the behavioral adjustment, cognitive functioning, and individual variation in treatment response in a 5-week, within-subject, crossover, placebo-controlled, double-blind study of 24 children (18 males, 6 females; mean age 10.9 ± 2.4 years) diagnosed by DSM-III-R (APA, 1987) criteria with ADHD and mental retardation (17 with a diagnosis of mild mental retardation; 7 with moderate mental retardation; estimated mean IQ of the 24 subjects using the *Stanford Binet Intelligence Scale*, fourth edition, was 56.5 ± 10.24). Subjects were treated with placebo or MPH in doses of 0.15, 0.3, and 0.6 mg/kg administered twice daily, before breakfast and at lunch time. During the first week, all subjects received placebo; during the following 4 weeks, they were randomly administered each of the four conditions for 1 week. None of the children had other comorbid psychiatric diagnoses.

Behavioral adjustment (Pearson et al., 2003) was assessed by rating scales completed by teachers and parents. Symptoms of inattention, hyperactivity, oppositional behavior, conduct problems, and asocial behavior declined steadily with increasing MPH doses. The most significant findings were reported by teachers for the 0.6 mg/kg dose as follows: attention ($P = .024$), hyperactivity ($P < .001$), and oppositional behavior ($P = .012$) compared with placebo on the ADDH CTRS and hyperactivity

($P < .001$), conduct problem ($P < .001$), emotional overindulgence ($P = .006$), asocial ($P = .009$), daydream-attention ($P = .022$), and HI ($P < .001$) on the CTRS. The only parent rating that showed significant improvement was Impulsive-Hyperactive ($P = .018$) on the CPRS. The only AEs reaching significance were insomnia and loss of appetite, which were dose related. Parents reported that 16.7% (4/24) of the subjects experienced insomnia and that 29.2% (7/24) experienced significantly decreased appetite at the 0.6 mg/kg bid dose. Subjects did not experience significant increases in staring, social withdrawal, or anxiety. The authors noted that their findings of increasing improvement with increasing dose in the 0.15 to 0.6 mg range were consistent with the MTA study findings (MTA Cooperative Group, 1999a). The authors also noted that their results suggest that, whenever possible, dose regulation should be done when feedback from subjects' teachers is available.

In the same subjects (diagnosed with ID and ADHD), Pearson et al. (2004b) investigated the effects of MPH on cognitive functioning as assessed by their performance on tasks of sustained attention (using a modified version of the Continuous Performance Test), visual sustained attention (using the Speeded Classification Task), auditory selective attention (using the Selective Listening Task), impulsivity/inhibition (using a Delay of Gratification Task and the Matching Familiar Figure Test), and immediate memory (using the Delayed Match to Sample [DMTS]) task. Overall, higher MPH doses were associated with significantly greater gains in cognitive task performance on all these measures except the DMTS, where no significant MPH effects were found. The 0.15 mg/kg bid dose was relatively ineffective compared with the 0.6 mg/kg bid dose. The authors noted that for subjects who could not tolerate the 0.6 mg/kg bid dose because of untoward effects such as appetite suppression or insomnia, 0.3 mg/kg bid also produced significant, but lesser gains.

Pearson et al. (2004a) also looked at their 24 subjects' individual variations in cognitive and behavioral responses to MPH. The authors reported that 57% of subjects on 0.15 mg/kg bid, 63% of subjects on 0.3 mg/kg bid, and 71% of subjects on 0.6 mg/kg bid showed gains in cognitive task performance. When "significant cognitive gains" (defined as >30% improvement relative to placebo on tasks where such a score was possible) were assessed, these percentages decreased to 31%, 37%, and 46%, respectively. The authors also looked at deterioration in cognitive task performance. The authors reported that 35% of subjects on 0.15 mg/kg bid, 29% of subjects on 0.3 mg/kg bid, and 23% of subjects on 0.6 mg/kg bid showed some deterioration in cognitive task performance. When "significant cognitive deterioration" (defined as >30% deterioration relative to placebo) was assessed, these percentages decreased to 14%, 15%, and 9%, respectively. The authors noted that these data suggest that MPH is not causing the deterioration, as fewer children exhibited cognitive deterioration as the MPH dose increased.

Regarding behavioral responses to MPH, Pearson et al. (2004a) reported that 45% of subjects on 0.15 mg/kg bid, 58% of subjects on 0.3 mg/kg bid, and 68% of subjects on 0.6 mg/kg bid showed (any) behavioral gains. When "significant behavioral gains" (defined as >30% improvement) were assessed, these percentages decreased to 25%, 38%, and 55%, respectively. The authors also looked at deterioration in behavior. The authors reported that 38% of subjects on 0.15 mg/kg bid, 24% of subjects on 0.3 mg/kg bid, and 13% of subjects on 0.6 mg/kg bid showed some degree of deterioration in behavioral functioning. When "significant behavioral deterioration" (defined as >30% deterioration relative to placebo) was assessed, these percentages decreased to 22%, 16%, and 9%, respectively.

Importantly, the authors noted that there was substantial independence between the effects of MPH on behavioral and cognitive changes, and they suggested that the clinician should monitor both responses when treating such children to determine the overall efficacy in a given child. The authors concluded that children with ADHD and ID show substantial improvement in cognitive and behavioral domains when treated with MPH, that the percentage of subjects who improve far outweighs subjects who substantially worsen, and that this favorable ratio improved as the study dose of MPH increased. They reported that at the 0.6 mg/kg bid dose, five times as many subjects showed substantial cognitive and behavioral gains compared with subjects who showed substantial declines in these domains. The authors concluded that treating children diagnosed with ADHD and mild to moderate mental retardation (MR) with MPH results in improvement in both cognitive and behavioral domains and that, on average, higher doses are more effective. The authors also noted that the response rate of children with ADHD and ID to MPH is not as favorable as in children with ADHD whose IQs are in the normal range (Pearson et al., 2004a).

MPH in Conduct Disorder with and without ADHD

Klein et al. (1997) conducted a double-blind, placebo-controlled study in which 84 children (age range, 6 to 15 years; mean, 10.2 ± 2.3 years; 74 males, 10 females) who were diagnosed with conduct disorder were randomly assigned to a 5-week trial of MPH ($N = 41$) or placebo ($N = 42$). (One subject dropped out before beginning treatment.) A comorbid diagnosis of ADHD consistent with DSM-IV criteria was made in 69% of the subjects. Medication was administered twice daily (morning and noon doses) and was gradually raised to a total of 60 mg/day unless untoward effects prevented this. Subjects received no psychosocial therapy; however, their parents were given weekly supportive counseling.

Seventy-four subjects completed the study (four taking MPH and five receiving placebo withdrew). The authors noted that 72 (97.3%) of the subjects completing the study had at least three symptoms of conduct disorder consistent with DSM-IV criteria and that 51 (69%) had comorbid ADHD. The average dose of MPH at the termination of the study was 41.3 mg/day or 1 mg/kg, with the morning and noon doses never varying >5 mg. Untoward effects were reported by 31 (84%) of the 37 subjects receiving MPH; the most common were decreased appetite and delay of sleep, with only a few instances of the latter being severe. Seventeen (46%) of the 37 subjects on placebo reported at least one untoward effect.

Compared with subjects receiving placebo, those taking MPH were rated significantly better by teachers and parents on all ratings of ADHD symptoms and all ratings of conduct disorder except socialized aggression (which measures severe delinquent behavior, such as membership in a gang, which was rare in this population). Teachers' ratings specifically noted significant reductions in: "obscene language, attacks others, destroys property, and deliberately cruel." Parents' ratings on "cruel to others, bad companions, and steals outside the home" showed significant decreases. Global improvement ratings of "improved or better" versus "slightly improved or worse" were statistically significant ($P < .001$) for subjects on MPH compared with those on placebo (teachers, 59% vs. 9%; mothers, 78% vs. 27%; and psychiatrists, 68% vs. 11%). Further analysis of the data showed that the significant improvements in symptoms of conduct disorder in subjects treated with MPH were not influenced significantly by the presence, absence, or severity of comorbid ADHD. The authors concluded that MPH had an independent positive influence on provocative, aggressive, mean behaviors and that MPH had a clinically significant effect in the treatment of conduct disorder that was independent of the presence or absence of ADHD.

MPH in the Treatment of Children Diagnosed with ASD with Symptoms of ADHD

MPH has been investigated in the treatment of children diagnosed with ASD who also have symptoms of ADHD. Although most of the earlier literature states that stimulants are contraindicated for children with autism and cause a worsening in behavior and/or stereotypies, several recent studies have reported that MPH is effective in treating some children with ASD who also exhibit such symptoms as hyperactivity, impulsivity, short attention spans, and aggression. Strayhorn et al. (1988) reported on two children with autism prescribed MPH: a 6-year-old boy and a preschool child. The 6-year-old child was reported to show improvement with

MPH in both attention and activity levels, less destructive behavior, and a decrease in stereotyped movements, but sadness and temper tantrums significantly worsened. The preschooler was said to have had similar results.

Birmaher et al. (1988) treated nine hyperactive children diagnosed with autism (aged 4 to 16 years) with 10 to 50 mg/day of MPH. Eight of the children improved on all rating scales; the oldest child improved on all scales except the one measuring behavior in school. In contrast, Realmuto et al. (1989), who treated two 9-year-old boys diagnosed with autism with 10 mg of MPH administered twice daily, found that one became fearful and unable to separate from significant adults, had a worsening of his hyperactivity, and developed a rapid pulse. The second child's baseline behaviors did not change significantly, although he developed mild anorexia.

Quintana et al. (1995) reported a 6-week, double-blind, placebo-controlled crossover study of monotherapy with MPH in the treatment of 10 children (6 males, 4 females; mean age, 8.5 ± 1.3 years; age range, 7 to 11 years) who were diagnosed with autistic disorder by DSM-III-R (APA, 1987) criteria. Subjects' mean developmental quotient was 64.3 ± 9.9. Efficacy was determined by ratings on the Childhood Autism Rating Scale (CARS; scores of ≤29 = nonautistic; 30 to 36.5 = mildly to moderately autistic; 37 to 60 = severely autistic) and the 10-item Conners Abbreviated Parent Questionnaire, the hyperactivity factor of the Conners Teacher Questionnaire (CTQ), the Aberrant Behavior Checklist (ABC), and three subscales of the ABC (I = irritability factor; III = stereotypies; and IV = hyperactivity factor). Untoward effects were rated on the Side Effects Checklist.

All subjects had previously been treated with neuroleptics but not with MPH; all were off medication for at least 1 month and completed a 2-week baseline rating period off medication. Subjects were then randomly assigned to 1 week of placebo or of MPH 10 mg twice daily (morning and noontime doses) with a dose range of 0.17 to 0.33 mg/kg/day followed by a second week of placebo or MPH 20 mg twice daily or 0.34 to 0.68 mg/kg/day. Subjects then crossed over to receive the treatment they had not received for the final 2 weeks of the study.

Ratings improved significantly over baseline, more so when subjects were taking MPH compared with placebo on the hyperactivity factor of the CTQ ($P = .02$), the ABC total score ($P = .04$), ABC irritability factor ($P = .01$), and the ABC hyperactivity factor ($P = .02$). However, all these ratings (except the ABC irritability factor) also improved significantly over baseline when on placebo, but the improvements were significantly less than when receiving MPH. There were no statistically significant differences in improvement between the two doses of MPH or any correlation with age or developmental quotient. Untoward effects were few and not statistically different from placebo; there was no significant change in ratings on the Abnormal Involuntary Movement Scale or on stereotypy ratings on the ABC stereotypic movement subscale. The authors concluded that MPH produced modest but significant improvement in hyperactivity in these patients without clinically significant untoward effects. They also recommended that hyperactive children diagnosed with ASD be given a trial of MPH before a neuroleptic is administered. In some cases, this may result in sufficient improvement so that a neuroleptic is not required; and in some other cases, a lower dose of neuroleptic may be effective if combined with MPH (Quintana et al., 1995).

Handen et al. (2000) conducted a double-blind, placebo-controlled crossover study of MPH in the treatment of 13 children (10 males and 3 females; mean age, 7.4 years; age range, 5.6 to 11.2 years), 9 of whom were diagnosed by DSM-IV criteria with autistic disorder and 4 of whom were diagnosed with pervasive developmental disorder not otherwise specified (PDD NOS). In addition to a diagnosis of either autism or PDD NOS, all had comorbid diagnoses of ADHD and/or ODD. IQs were in the following ranges: average ($N = 1$), mild mental retardation ($N = 4$), moderate mental retardation ($N = 5$), severe/profound mental retardation ($N = 3$). Seven children were in special education classes and six were inpatients or in an intensive day-treatment program. Subjects were administered MPH in 0.3 or 0.6 mg/kg doses or placebo for 1 week each. The three conditions were randomly assigned; but because of concern about untoward effects, the 0.3 mg/kg dose always preceded the 0.6 mg/kg dose. Doses were given to all subjects at breakfast and lunch times; 11 subjects were given an optional third dose at about 4:00 PM. Efficacy was assessed by ratings on the Conners Teacher Scale 10-item Hyperactivity Index (CTSHI), the IOWA CTRS, the ABC, the CARS, and the Side Effects Checklist.

Eight children (61.5%) were rated as responders (seven of the eight showed improvement on both doses of MPH, and the eighth only on the higher [0.6 mg/kg dose]). Significant improvements occurred on one or both doses of MPH on the CTSHI, the aggression subscale of the IOWA CTRS, and two (hyperactivity and inappropriate speech) of the five factors on the ABC. Significant change occurred on measures on the Stereotype and Inappropriate Speech subscales of the ABC, with the greatest improvements in "odd, bizarre behavior" and "repetitive speech." No significant changes in core features of autism were evident on the CARS (which is a global assessment of autistic symptoms). There were no significant differences in clinical response between the two doses of MPH and no correlation of response with age or IQ. The authors concluded that clinically significant behavioral gains were obtained on MPH at the lower 0.3 mg/kg dose and that children diagnosed with autism may be at greater risk for untoward effects, especially in the 0.6 mg/kg dose range. One child developed crying, tantrums, aggression, and skin picking on the 0.3 mg/kg dose and was dropped from the study without getting the 0.6 mg dose; two children on the 0.6 mg/kg dose were dropped during the week, one for severe staring spells and one for increased aggression in school. Other children developed increased levels or irritability and/or social withdrawal, especially at the higher dose. At the end of the study, eight children had benefited enough to continue to be prescribed MPH in doses of 0.2 to 0.6 mg/kg.

Sturman et al. (2017) conducted a meta-analysis on the use of MPH in children diagnosed with ASD. The authors included four crossover studies ($N = 113$ aged 5 to 13 years). Most of the subjects (83%) were boys. They concluded that short-term use of MPH improves symptoms of hyperactivity and, possibly, inattention in children with ASD who are tolerant of the medication. They noted that there was no evidence that MPH has a negative impact on the core symptoms of ASD.

Single-Isomer Dexmethylphenidate Hydrochloride (Focalin; Focalin XR)

Pharmacokinetics of Dexmethylphenidate Hydrochloride

Single Isomer

Dexmethylphenidate hydrochloride (D-MPH) is the D-threo-enantiomer, and this is the more pharmacologically active enantiomer of racemic methylphenidate hydrochloride (D,L-MPH). Dexmethylphenidate is thought to block the reuptake of norepinephrine and dopamine into the presynaptic neuron and increase the release of these monoamines into the extraneuronal space. The medication is well absorbed orally, and it may be taken with or without food. Peak plasma concentrations are reached in approximately 1 to 1½ hours after ingestion in the fasting state. When taken with a high-fat breakfast, peak plasma levels are about the same but take about twice as long to be reached. The medication is administered twice daily with at least 4 hours between doses. There is evidence that the therapeutic effects of D-MPH are of somewhat longer duration (approximately 5 to 6 hours) compared with a dose of D,L-MPH containing an equivalent amount of the D-isomer (D-MPH; Wigal et al., 2004).

Dexmethylphenidate is metabolized primarily to ritalinic acid, which has little or no pharmacologic activity and is excreted primarily by the kidneys. The mean plasma elimination half-life of dexmethylphenidate is approximately 2.2 hours.

Contraindications of Dexmethylphenidate Hydrochloride

Dexmethylphenidate is contraindicated in patients with marked anxiety, tension, and agitation because it may worsen such symptoms.

Dexmethylphenidate is contraindicated in patients with hypersensitivity to MPH or other components of the medication. It is also contraindicated in patients with glaucoma. It is recommended that patients with motor tics or with a family history or diagnosis of TS should not be prescribed dexmethylphenidate.

To avoid a potential hypertensive crisis, dexmethylphenidate should not be prescribed to patients who are taking MAOIs or within a minimum of 14 days of discontinuation of such medications.

Adverse Effects of Dexmethylphenidate Hydrochloride

In premarketing trials with a total of 684 children (age range 6 to 17 years) the most frequently reported untoward effects were stomach pain, fever, decreased appetite, and nausea. Other less frequent untoward effects included vomiting, dizziness, sleeplessness, nervousness, tics, allergic reactions, increased blood pressure, and psychosis (abnormal thinking or hallucinations). A total of 50 children (7.3%) experienced untoward effects that resulted in the medication's discontinuation. The untoward effects most frequently responsible for this were twitching (described as motor or vocal tics), anorexia, insomnia, and tachycardia (approximately 1% each).

Indications for Dexmethylphenidate Hydrochloride in Child and Adolescent Psychiatry

Dexmethylphenidate hydrochloride is FDA approved for the treatment of ADHD.

Dexmethylphenidate Dosage Schedule

Immediate-release dexmethylphenidate should be taken twice daily with at least a 4-hour interval between doses and may be taken with or without food.
- *Children <6 years of age:* not approved for use.
- *Children at least 6 years of age, adolescents, and adults who were not taking racemic MPH or who were on other (non-MPH) stimulants:* Start with 2.5 mg twice daily. Titrate at approximately weekly intervals in increments of 2.5 to 5.0 mg to a maximum of 20 mg daily.

Conversion Strategy

- *Children at least 6 years of age, adolescents, and adults who are currently taking racemic MPH:* Start with one-half the dose of racemic D- and L-methylphenidate to a maximum of 20 mg daily (10-mg doses administered approximately 4 hours apart).

    From time to time, a patient will need to switch from one stimulant to another. This may need to happen because of side effects, changing insurance plans, or national shortage of a medication. Table 5.3 can be used to find approximate dose equivalents so as to allow for a more smooth transition from one stimulant to another.

Single-Isomer Dexmethylphenidate Hydrochloride Dose Forms Available

- *Tablets:* 2.5, 5, and 10 mg (unscored)

Extended-release capsules (Focalin XR): 5, 10, 15, 20, 25, 30, 35, and 40 mg. The 35- and 40-mg dosages are approved for adults only. This preparation permits once-daily dosing and produces a bimodal plasma concentration-time profile of two distinct peaks—an initial IR and the second approximately 4 hours later. Doses >30 mg/day in pediatrics are not recommended. The capsule can be taken whole or the capsule contents can be sprinkled on applesauce and ingested without chewing the beads.

TABLE 5.3 » Stimulant Dosing Conversion Chart

Amphetamine Salts (Adderall IR)	Amphetamine Salts Extended Release (Adderall XR)	Lisdexamfetamine (Vyvanse)	Dexmethylphenidate Extended Release (Focalin XR)	Methylphenidate Long Acting (Ritalin LA)	Methylphenidate Controlled Delivery (Metadate CD)	Methylphenidate OROS (Concerta)	Methylphenidate Transdermal Patch (Daytrana)
2.5-5 mg bid	5-10 mg qAM	20-30 mg qAM	5-10 mg qAM	10 mg qAM	10 mg qAM	18-36 mg qAM	10 mg patch qAM
5 mg bid	10 mg	30 mg	10 mg	20 mg	20 mg	36 mg	10-15 mg
7.5 mg bid	15 mg	30-40 mg	15 mg	25 mg	25 mg	36 mg	15-20 mg
7.5-10 mg bid	13-20 mg	40 mg	15-20 mg	30 mg	30 mg	36-54 mg	20 mg
10 mg bid	20 mg	40-50 mg	20 mg	30 mg	30 mg	54 mg	20-30 mg
10 mg bid	20 mg	50 mg	20 mg	30-40 mg	30-40 mg	54 mg	30 mg
10-12.5 mg bid	20-25 mg	50 mg	20-25 mg	40 mg	40 mg	54-72 mg	30 mg
12.5 mg bid	25 mg	60 mg	25 mg	40 mg	40 mg	72 mg	30-40 mg
12.5 mg bid	25 mg	60 mg	25 mg	45-50 mg	45-50 mg	72 mg	40 mg
12.5-15 mg bid	25-30 mg	60-70 mg	25-30 mg	50 mg	50 mg	72-90 mg	40 mg
15 mg bid	30 mg	70 mg	30 mg	60 mg	60 mg	90 mg	50 mg
15-17.5 mg bid	30-35 mg	70-80 mg	30-35 mg	60-70 mg	60-70 mg	108 mg	50-60 mg
17.5 mg bid	35 mg	80 mg	35 mg	70 mg	70 mg	108 mg	60 mg
Dose forms available 5, 7.5, 10, 12.5, 15, 20, and 30 mg	5, 10, 15, 20, 25, 30 mg	10, 20, 30, 40, 50, 60, and 70 mg	5, 10, 15, 20, 25, 30, 35, and 40 mg	10, 20, 30, and 40 mg	10, 20, 30, 40, 50, and 60 mg	18, 27, 36, and 54 mg	10-, 15-, 20-, and 30-mg patch
Maximum FDA-recommended dose for kid 40 mg	40 mg	70 mg	30 mg	60 mg	60 mg	72 mg	30 mg

There are times when a patient must switch from one stimulant to another (either due to side effects, a national medication shortage, or the medicine no longer being covered by their insurance). In these instances, some clinicians prefer to cross-taper from one stimulant to another. Other clinicians always start at the starting dose, but many have found that using a chart similar to the one above is beneficial to their patients. For instance, if a person is taking lisdexamfetamine (Vyvanse) 50 mg, but they switch insurances and it is no longer covered (but Adderall XR 25 mg is covered), then using the chart, the clinician sees that a person taking Vyvanse 50 mg might need either 30 or 40 mg of 20 or 25 mg of Adderall XR. These clinicians generally choose the lower of the two doses (Adderall XR 20 mg), but they also give the patient a second script for Adderall XR 25 mg that they can fill in 7 days if the 20 mg is not enough.

OROS, osmotic release oral system

This chart is adapted from the work of Biederman J. Practical considerations in stimulant drug selection for the attention–deficit/hyperactivity. *Today's Therapeutic Trends.* 2002;20(4):311.

Reports of Interest

Dexmethylphenidate Hydrochloride in the Treatment of ADHD

Wigal et al. (2004) compared D-MPH and D,L-threo-methylphenidate (D,L-MPH) in a 5-week, multicenter, double-blind, placebo-controlled study of 132 subjects (age range, 6 to 17 years; mean 9.8 years; 116 male, 16 female), diagnosed by DSM-IV criteria with ADHD. Following a 1-week, single-blind placebo lead in, subjects received D-MPH ($N = 44$), D,L-MPH ($N = 46$), or placebo ($N = 42$) twice daily (between 7:00 AM and 8:00 AM and between 11:30 AM and 12:30 PM) for 4 weeks. Dosage was adjusted on a weekly basis. At endpoint, the average daily dose for the D-MPH group was 18.25 mg and that for the D,L-MPH group was 32.14 mg.

Primary efficacy was rated on the Swanson, Nolan, and Pelham (SNAP) Rating Scale completed by the teacher (Teacher SNAP) twice weekly in the afternoon. Secondary efficacy measures included the Parent SNAP (Saturdays and Sundays at 3:00 PM and 6:00 PM), Clinical Global Impressions Scale–Improvement (CGI-I), and a math test; these ratings were obtained at 6:00 PM to test the hypothesis that the duration of action of D-MPH would be longer than that of D,L-MPH.

On the Teacher SNAP, both the D-MPH group ($P = .0004$) and the D,L-MPH group ($P = .0042$) had significantly greater improvement than the placebo group; the effect size was large (1.0) and equal for both medications. Duration of significant efficacy was longer for the D-MPH group. On the CGI-I, 16.2% of subjects on placebo were rated "much improved" and 5.4% were "very much improved." Compared with the placebo group, 67% of D-MPH subjects were rated as either "much" (35.7%) or "very much improved" (31%) with $P = .0010$; 49% of D,L-MPH subjects were rated "much" (26.8%) or "very much improved" (22.0%) with $P = .0130$. The D-MPH group improved significantly more from baseline to endpoint than the placebo group ($P = .0007$); the D,L-MPH group's improvement did not quite reach significance compared with the control group ($P = .0589$).

On the 6:00 PM math test, the D-MPH group scored significantly better than the placebo group. The placebo group worsened from baseline with an average of 3.9 fewer correct answers, whereas the D-MPH group got an average of 12.5 more problems correct ($P = .0236$). The D,L-MPH group scores on the 6:00 PM math test were not significantly different from those of the placebo group.

No patients experienced serious AEs. Headache, abdominal pain, nausea, and diminished appetite were the most frequently reported AEs. Abdominal pain was reported more frequently in the D-MPH group compared with the D,L-MPH group ($P = .0252$). Clinically significant changes occurred in the vital signs of 13 subjects (3 D-MPH, 8 D,L-MPH, and 2 placebo). Significant weight loss (ranging from 5% to 18% of baseline weight) was reported for four subjects in the D-MPH group, six subjects in the D,L-MPH group, and two subjects in the placebo group.

The authors concluded that D-MPH (mean dose, 18.25 mg) and D,L-MPH (mean dose, 32.14 mg) have similar efficacy and safety in treating ADHD, similar large effect sizes, and suggest that D-MPH has a longer duration of action than D,L-MPH after twice-daily dosing (Wigal et al., 2004).

As part of a multicenter study, Arnold et al. (2004) administered D-MPH to 89 subjects (72 males, 17 females; mean age 10.1 ± 2.9 years, age range 6 to 16 years) who were diagnosed with ADHD; 71.9% were treatment naive. The first phase of the study was an open-label, dose-titration study of 6-week duration; this was followed by a 2-week, double-blind, randomized, placebo-controlled withdrawal phase.

Efficacy was measured on the CGI-I Scale, the SNAP–ADHD-RS, and a "Math Test," which was used as a measure of "duration of effect" of the medication. The CGI-Severity (CGI-S) Scale was used to assess the severity of each subject's illness.

During the first 4 weeks, medication was titrated upward to a maximum total dose of 20 mg daily or until AEs prevented increase or until a CGI-I score of 1 ("very much improved") or 2 ("much improved") was achieved. During weeks 5 and 6, the dose was held constant.

Of the 89 subjects, 76 completed the 6-week open-label phase. The 13 dropouts were because of therapeutic failure (4), AEs (4), lost to follow-up (3), withdrawn consent (1), and protocol violation (1). Seventy-three of the completers (82% of the subjects) were rated 1 or 2 on the CGI-I; 89.2% were rated "normal to mildly ill" on the CGI-S Scale versus only 1.1% at baseline ($P < .001$). A total of 77 patients (86.5%) experienced AEs. Of the four subjects who were discontinued because of AEs, one was due to rambling speech and tremor, one due to labile mood, one with moderate headaches, and one with sleep terrors with somnambulism. Eight subjects had reduction in dosage because of tremor and anergy, gastrointestinal distress (including nausea, emesis, and diarrhea), headache, insomnia, unusual sensory experience, and irritability. Except for insomnia, these AEs remitted with dose reduction.

Seventy-five of the subjects entered the subsequent 2-week withdrawal phase; 35 were assigned to D-MPH and 40 to placebo; 1 dropped out from each group. At the time of assignment, 88.6% of the subjects in the D-MPH group and 87.5% of those in the placebo group were rated as showing only mild to no ADHD symptoms. Similarly, 70.6% of the D-MPH group and 80% of the placebo group were taking 10 mg of dexmethylphenidate twice daily. The placebo group showed significantly more treatment failures than the D-MPH group on the CGI-I, deterioration in the 3:00 PM Math Test and the 6:00 PM Math Test, Teacher SNAP-ADHD, and the Parent SNAP-ADHD scores at 3:00 PM and at 6:00 PM.

The authors also noted that AEs were similar to those of other stimulants and that score on the Math Tests at 3 and 6 hours after the noon dose confirmed the earlier reported duration of efficacy for dexmethylphenidate to be at least 6 hours after the second daily dose (Arnold et al., 2004).

Silva et al. (2006) reported a multicenter, 2-week, double-blind, placebo-controlled, crossover study that consisted of 54 subjects (age range 6 to 12 years, mean age 9.4 ± 1.6 years) who were diagnosed with ADHD by DSM-IV criteria. All subjects had been stabilized on a total daily dose of 20 to 40 mg of D,L-MPH for a minimum of 1 month before beginning the study. Subjects were randomly assigned to treatment for a 7-day period, which consisted of a 20-mg dose of D-MPH-ER (extended release) for 5 days, a day off medication, then on the seventh day, ratings in the (period 1) classroom laboratory setting on D-MPH-ER followed by another 7-day period consisting of placebo for 5 days, a day off medication, and then on the seventh day ratings in the (period 2) classroom laboratory setting on placebo (sequence A) or the reverse order (sequence B).

Ratings were done at post-dose hours 1, 2, 4, 6, 8, 9, 10, 11, and 12. The authors estimated the duration of effect of D-MPH-ER to be from 1 to 12 hours post-dose. Scores on the SKAMP-Attention (SKAMP = Swanson, Kotkin, Agler, M-Flynn, and Pelham rating scale) and SKAMP-Deportment Scales were significantly better with D-MPH-ER than with placebo at all timepoints. Overall, the authors concluded that in this group of subjects, D-MPH-ER was both safe and effective in treating ADHD. Its duration of action may last for up to 12 hours (Silva et al., 2006).

Amphetamine Stimulant Medications Approved for Use in Child and Adolescent Psychiatry

Amphetamine (Evekeo; Adzenys XR-ODT; Adzenys ER liquid, Dyanavel XR liquid); Methamphetamine (Desoxyn); Dextroamphetamine (Dexedrine, ProCentra, Zenzedi, Dexedrine Spansules); Mixed Amphetamine Salts (Adderall, Adderall XR, Mydayis); Lisdexamfetamine (Vyvanse)

Amphetamines are non-catecholamine sympathomimetic amines with CNS activity. Amphetamine's two enantiomers (dextro [D-] and levo- [L-]) have very different levels of pharmacologic activity. The D-isomer is biologically more active than the L-isomer.

However, as noted in the preceding text, some individuals respond positively to the L-isomer and not to the D-isomer (Arnold et al., 1976).

The medications listed here as "amphetamine" contain both the D and L enantiomers. Medications listed as "dextroamphetamine" contain only the D enantiomer. Adderall XR (which is a mixed salt amphetamine formulation) contains 25% dextroamphetamine sulfate, 25% amphetamine sulfate, 25% dextroamphetamine saccharate, and 25% amphetamine aspartate monohydrate.

In the treatment of ADHD, all of these medications may be prescribed: amphetamine medications, dextroamphetamine medications, MAS, methamphetamine medication, and lisdexamfetamine (a prodrug). Although a methamphetamine medication (Desoxyn) is available to prescribe for ADHD, some authorities such as Timothy Wilens, believe it to be potentially neurotoxic to dopamine neurons in the brain on the basis of animal studies. It also carries a high potential for abuse. Many caution against its use, and Desoxyn is therefore not recommended as a first-line agent in the treatment of ADHD.

Dextroamphetamine sulfate (Dexedrine) is the dextro [D-] isomer of racemic amphetamine sulfate, and Dexedrine was historically the first stimulant studied in child and adolescent psychopharmacology (Bradley, 1937).

Pharmacokinetics of Dextroamphetamine Sulfate

Regarding the pharmacokinetics, maximal dextroamphetamine plasma concentrations occur approximately 3 hours after oral ingestion. Average plasma half-life is approximately 12 hours.

Contraindications for the Administration of Dextroamphetamine Sulfate

The administration of dextroamphetamine sulfate is contraindicated in individuals with symptomatic cardiovascular disease, moderate to severe hypertension, hyperthyroidism, hypersensitivity to the sympathomimetic amines, or glaucoma. Sudden death has been reported in children with structural cardiac abnormalities who were treated with amphetamines at usual therapeutic doses.

Individuals who are in an agitated state or who have a history of drug abuse should also not be prescribed this medication. As discussed earlier, both MPH and dextroamphetamine medications have a black box warning regarding the risk of dependence with these medications.

Amphetamines should not be prescribed during or within 14 days of the administration of an MAOI to avoid the risk of a hypertensive crisis.

Amphetamines should be used with caution in individuals who have motor or vocal tics, TS, or a family history of such. This is discussed in more detail in the introductory section of this chapter.

Untoward Effects of Dextroamphetamine Sulfate

Dextroamphetamine sulfate elevates the systolic and diastolic blood pressure and has weak bronchodilator and respiratory stimulant action. Tachycardia may occur. The most frequent and troublesome immediate untoward effects include insomnia, anorexia, nausea, abdominal pain or cramps, vomiting, constipation or diarrhea, headache, dry mouth, thirst, lability of mood, irritability, sadness, weepiness, tachycardia, and blood pressure changes. Many of these symptoms diminish over a few weeks, although the cardiovascular changes may persist.

Owing to amphetamine's effects on dopamine, clinical experience suggests that behavioral symptoms and thought disorder in children with psychosis may be worsened by the administration of amphetamines.

Amphetamines may cause short-term suppression of growth. Their long-term effects on growth inhibition are uncertain, and growth should be monitored during their administration. This was discussed in more detail in the introductory part of this chapter.

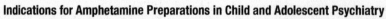

Indications for Amphetamine Preparations in Child and Adolescent Psychiatry

Dextroamphetamine sulfate is FDA approved for treating ADHD, narcolepsy, and obesity. (Lisdexamfetamine has FDA approval in the adult population for treating moderate to severe binge-eating disorder.)

Immediate-Release Amphetamine Sulfate Dosage Schedule for Treating ADHD

The serum half-life for standard-preparation dextroamphetamine sulfate is approximately 6 to 8 hours in children. This half-life makes it possible for some children to take the medication before leaving for school and maintain clinical effectiveness for the duration of the school day without taking a noontime dose (which is required when the standard-preparation MPH is used).

- *Children <3 years of age:* not approved for use.
- *Children 3 through 5 years of age:* begin with 2.5 mg daily; raise by 2.5-mg increments once or twice weekly; titrate for optimal dose.
- *Patients 6 years and older:* begin with 5 mg daily; raise by 5-mg increments once or twice weekly; the usual maximum dose is 40 mg/day or less.

The usual optimal individual dose falls between 0.15 and 0.5 mg/kg for each dose (Duncan, 1990), administered two to three times daily (total daily dose range, 0.3 to 1.5 mg/kg/day).

MAS (Adderall), which is a combination of equal parts of dextroamphetamine saccharate, amphetamine aspartate, dextroamphetamine sulfate, and amphetamine sulfate, is also approved for the treatment of narcolepsy. Peak plasma concentration occurs approximately 3 hours after ingestion. The manufacturer states that its plasma half-life is 7 to 8 hours, based on the amphetamine component. Usually, the first dose is given soon after awakening or before leaving for school; this may be followed by an additional one or two doses at 4- to 6-hour intervals. Whether this combination has clinically significant benefits compared with standard- or extended-release dextroamphetamine sulfate is uncertain at present.

Immediate-Release Preparations, Dosage Schedule, and Available Dose Forms for Treating ADHD

Immediate-Release Dextroamphetamine Preparations Available

- *Tablets (Dexedrine):* 5, 10 mg; *(Zenzedi):* 2.5, 5, 7.5, 10, 15, 20, 30 mg
- *Liquid formulation (ProCentra):* 5 mg/5 mL

Immediate-Release Mixed Amphetamine Salt Preparations Available

- *Tablets (Adderall):* 5, 7.5, 10, 12.5, 15, 20, and 30 mg

Immediate-Release Amphetamine Preparations Available

- *Tablets (Evekeo):* 5, 10 mg

Immediate-Release Methamphetamine Preparations Available

- *Tablets (Desoxyn):* 5 mg

Extended-Release Preparations, Dosage Schedule, and Available Dose Forms for Treating ADHD

Extended-Release Dextroamphetamine Preparations Available

- *Sustained-release capsules (Dexedrine spansules):* 5, 10, and 15 mg

The maximum dextroamphetamine plasma concentrations of Dexedrine spansules occurs approximately 8 hours after oral ingestion of the sustained-release capsule. The plasma half-life is approximately 12 hours, similar to that of the immediate-release form. The manufacturer also noted that this "formulation has not been shown superior in effectiveness over the same dosage of the standard, noncontrolled-release formulation given in divided doses" (*PDR*, 2005, p. 1465).

Extended-Release Mixed Amphetamine Salt Preparations Available

- *Sustained-release capsules (Adderall XR):* 5, 10, 15, 20, 25, 30 mg; *(Mydayis):* 12.5, 25, 37.5, 50 mg.

The average time to maximum serum levels of Adderall XR is approximately 7 hours. Its duration of action is roughly equivalent to taking two doses of immediate-release Adderall of the same total dose 4 hours apart. The capsule can be opened and sprinkled on applesauce without significantly changing its rate of absorption.

Indications for Amphetamine Preparations in Child and Adolescent Psychiatry (*continued*)

Extended-Release Amphetamine Preparations Available

- *Sustained-release tablets (Adzenys XR-ODT):* 3.1, 6.3, 9.4, 12.5, 15.7, 18.8 mg
- *Sustained-release liquids (Adzenys ER liquid):* 1.25 mg/mL; (*Dyanavel XR liquid):* 2.5 mg/mL

Extended-Release L-Lysine-Dextroamphetamine Preparations Available

- *Sustained-release capsules (Vyvanse):* 10, 20, 30, 40, 50, 60, and 70 mg. Originally approved in February 2007. Vyvanse is approved for ADHD in children 6 to 17 years old as well as adults.

L-Lysine-Dextroamphetamine (also known as lisdexamfetamine) is the first stimulant prodrug that is therapeutically inactive until it is converted to active D-amphetamine in the body upon cleavage of the lysine portion of the molecule. It was originally developed with the intention of creating a longer lasting and more difficult to abuse version of dextroamphetamine, because the requirement of conversion into dextroamphetamine via enzymes in red blood cells increases its duration, regardless of the route of ingestion.

When first released, it was recommended for pediatric patients either beginning treatment or switching from another medication, to initiate treatment at 30 mg once daily in the morning. Later a 20-mg capsule was released to allow another option to initiate treatment at a lower dosage, and subsequently a 10-mg capsule is now available. Dosage may be adjusted in increments of 10 or 20 mg at approximately weekly intervals up to maximum dose of 70 mg/day. The capsules may be taken whole or may be opened and the entire contents dissolved in a glass of water and consumed immediately.

The plasma half-life is 12 to 13 hours and time to maximum concentration (T_{max}) of Vyvanse is consistent with little interpatient variability at 3.5 hours post-dose. After oral administration, lisdexamfetamine is rapidly absorbed from the gastrointestinal tract. Lisdexamfetamine is converted to dextroamphetamine and L-lysine primarily in the blood because of the hydrolytic activity of red blood cells. *In vitro* data demonstrated that red blood cells have a high capacity for metabolism of lisdexamfetamine via hydrolysis. Lisdexamfetamine is not reportedly metabolized by cytochrome P450 enzymes.

Vyvanse demonstrated significant improvement in attention for up to 13 hours in a pediatric analog classroom study utilizing SKAMP-A scores. In a 12 month effectiveness and safety study conducted by Findling, et al (2008), greater than 80% of subjects at endpoint (and more than 95% of completers at 12 months) were rated as "improved" based on Clinical Global Impression-Improvement scale scores.

Adverse Effects of Lisdexamfetamine

The most common AEs reported during the dose-optimization phase of regulatory studies were decreased appetite, insomnia, headache, upper abdominal pain, irritability, and affect lability.

The most common side effects reported in studies of Vyvanse were as follows:

- Anxiety
- Decreased appetite
- Diarrhea
- Dizziness
- Dry mouth
- Irritability
- Nausea
- Trouble sleeping
- Upper stomach pain
- Vomiting
- Weight loss

Reports of Interest

Vyvanse demonstrated a significantly lower abuse-related liking effect (Drug Rating Questionnaire-Subject [DRQ-S] scores) than an equivalent oral dose of D-amphetamine in an abuse liability study. Oral administration of 150 mg/day of Vyvanse produced increases in positive subjective responses that were statistically indistinguishable from the positive subjective responses produced by 40 mg/day of oral IR D-amphetamine (data on file, LDX009. Shire US Inc.; Vyvanse [package insert], 2007).

Studies conducted by Jasinski and Krishnan (2009a) seem to indicate that lisdexamfetamine dimesylate is less addictive than its counterparts (such as MAS [Adderall] and OROS MPH [Concerta]) because of its unique formulation. There is no increased onset of effect as occurs with intravenous administration of dextroamphetamine compared with oral use of lisdexamfetamine. Intravenously administered lisdexamfetamine produced likability effects similar to that of placebo, which the authors contend affirmed the medication's ability to reduce abuse potential (Jasinski & Krishnan, 2009b).

Dextroamphetamine in the Treatment of ADHD

Dextroamphetamine sulfate and Adderall (a preparation of four amphetamine salts) are two amphetamines commonly used to treat ADHD in the United States, and they are the only stimulants currently in use that are approved by the FDA for administration to children as young as 3 years of age. Hence, they are officially the standard treatment for children up to age 6 years; however, many clinicians do prescribe MPH for some patients <6 years of age because there is considerable clinical experience and literature (PATS) supporting this. If MPH does not provide satisfactory benefit in controlling symptoms of ADHD, it is recommended that an amphetamine product be tried before moving on to another class of medications. MPH (Desoxyn) is approved for use in children older than 6 years; however, as in the author's experience, it is infrequently prescribed and is not discussed in this book. In addition, some clinicians have expressed concern that it may be neurotoxic and is well known to have high abuse potential.

Reports of Interest

Amphetamines in Treatment Involving Seizures or Electroconvulsive Therapy

Amphetamines may obtund the maximal electroshock seizure discharge and have been reported to prevent typical three-per-second spike-and-dome petit mal seizures and to abolish the abnormal EEG pattern in some children (Weiner, 1980). Amphetamine preparations may therefore be the stimulants of choice for individuals who have seizures or who are at risk for developing them; although, as noted earlier, MPH does not appear to increase the frequency of seizures or their development *de novo* when administered in usual therapeutic doses.

Amphetamine Sulfate in the Treatment of ADHD

Gillberg et al. (1997) reported a 12-month, randomized, double-blind, placebo-controlled study in which 62 subjects (52 males and 10 females; mean age, 9.0 ± 1.6 years; range, 6 to 11 years), diagnosed by DSM-III-R criteria with severe ADHD (26 [42%] of whom had various comorbid disorders) were treated with (racemic) amphetamine sulfate. Seventy-two subjects entered the study, and the entire 18-month-long protocol was preceded by a 1-month baseline evaluation. During months 1 through 3, they were administered amphetamine sulfate in a single-blind manner beginning with initial daily doses of 5 mg at breakfast and 5 mg at lunchtime. Subsequent dose regulation permitted a maximum total daily dose of 60 mg. Ten subjects dropped out during this period because of untoward effects or lack of clinical response. The remaining 62 subjects all improved significantly. The 4th through 15th months consisted of the double-blind, placebo-controlled administration of amphetamine sulfate or placebo. The mean amphetamine sulfate dose of the 62 participating subjects at the beginning of this portion was 17 mg/day (or 0.52 mg/kg/day), with a range of 5 to 35 mg/day (or 0.2 to 1.1 mg/kg/day). During the double-blind portion, dosage was increased for 11 subjects and decreased for 8 subjects. Although 24 of the 32 [75%] on active medication completed the 12-month double-blind, placebo-controlled portion of the protocol, only 8 of the 30 [27%] receiving placebo did. Most of the subjects assigned to the placebo group required switching to open treatment with amphetamine before the completion of the double-blind portion. Months 16 through 18 consisted of administration of single-blind placebo. Efficacy was assessed by ratings on Conners Parent and Teacher Scales and the Wechsler Intelligence Scale for Children–Revised (WISC–R).

During the 12-month placebo period, the group assigned to amphetamine retained the improvements achieved during the 3-month period on amphetamine, but the group assigned to placebo experienced re-exacerbation of ADHD symptoms, as shown by comparison of ratings on the Conners Parent Scale. When comparing baseline WISC-R scores to those at 15 months, the 35 subjects taking amphetamine for ≥9 months showed a mean increase of 4.5 ± 4.7 points in FSIQ versus a mean increase of 0.7 ± 7.2 for the 8 subjects taking placebo for ≥6 months ($P < .05$). With the exception of decreased appetite for the amphetamine group, there were no significant differences in untoward effects for the placebo and amphetamine groups during the double-blind portion of the study. Four males developed hallucinations during the study; three were on active medication and one was on placebo. On stopping medication or with dose reduction, the hallucinations rapidly ceased. This long-term study of amphetamines suggests that the medication is safe and effective in treating children with ADHD for up to 15 months. Interestingly, when amphetamine was replaced with placebo during the 16th to 18th months of the study, there was no change in parent ratings and only a nonsignificant decline in teachers' ratings, suggesting that behavioral improvements were being maintained without the active medication.

Dextroamphetamine Sulfate in the Treatment of ADHD in Children Diagnosed with ASD

Geller et al. (1981) reported that dextroamphetamine administered to two children with PDD and ADDH improved their attention spans with no significant worsening of behavior.

Lisdexamfetamine in the Treatment of Binge-Eating Disorder

In the adult population, lisdexamfetamine (Vyvanse) has an indication for treating moderate to severe binge-eating disorder. Reinblatt et al. (2015) wondered about a possible link between ADHD in childhood and binge-eating disorder. To examine this, they looked at inhibitory control in children with loss of control eating syndrome (LOC-ES). Their study consisted of 79 children (aged 8 to 14 years) who were over the fifth weight percentile. They used the Eating Disorder Examination for Children and the Standard Pediatric Eating Episode Interview to assess LOC-ES. ADHD diagnosis was determined by the Schedule for Affective Disorders and Schizophrenia for children and Conners-3 (Parent Report) DSM-IV Scales of Inattention and/or Hyperactivity. To assess impulse control, they used the Go/No-Go Task and the Behavior Regulation Inventory of Executive Function.

Their reported results were that the odds of LOC-ES were increased 12 times for children with ADHD; suggesting that ADHD and binge-eating disorder have impulse control deficits at their core. The question then remains: will a stimulant prescription that helps with impulse control therefore treat both ADHD and prevent binge-eating disorder?

Adderall

Adderall (MAS) is composed of equal proportions of four amphetamine salts (D-amphetamine saccharate, D-amphetamine sulfate, D,L-amphetamine sulfate, and D,L-amphetamine aspartate), resulting in a 3:1 ratio of D-isomer to L-isomer.

Two double-blind placebo-controlled studies (the 4-week multicenter study of Biederman et al. [2002] in naturalistic home and school settings with an N of 584, and the 6-week analog classroom study of McCracken et al. [2003] with an N of 51) reported that an extended-release formulation of MAS (Adderall XR) was effective and safe in treating children 6 to 12 years of age who were diagnosed with ADHD. In 2005, McGough et al. reported on the long-term tolerability and effectiveness of once-daily MAS XR in a 24-month, multicenter, open-label extension of these two studies. A total of 568 subjects who had completed one of the double-blind studies with no significant AEs or had withdrawn for reasons other than AEs entered the long-term study. MAS XR was initiated in all subjects at a once-daily morning dose of 10 mg; 10-mg increases were permitted at weekly intervals during the first month to a maximum of 30 mg/day. The primary measure of effectiveness was the 10-item Conners Global Index Scale, Parent version (CGIS-P). A total of 273 subjects (48%) completed the 24-month extension. The major reasons for discontinuing prematurely were as follows: withdrew consent (87, 15.3%), AEs (84, 14.8%), and lost to follow-up (74, 13%). The mean once-daily dose for completers was 22.4 ± 6.9 mg. Improvement of >30% in CGIS-P scores was maintained over the duration of the study ($P < .001$). Most AEs were of mild or moderate severity. The most frequent AEs responsible for withdrawal from the study were weight loss (27 of the 568 subjects in the study [4.8%]), anorexia/decreased appetite (22, 3.9%), insomnia (11, 1.9%), depression (7, 1.2%), and emotional lability (4, 0.7%). Mean systolic and diastolic blood pressure increased by 3.5 and 2.6 mm Hg, respectively; heart rate increased by 3.4 beats per minute. There were no clinically significant changes in laboratory test values. The authors concluded that MAS XR in once-daily doses of between 10 and 30 mg was well tolerated and resulted in significant clinical benefits over the 24-month extension period in children diagnosed with ADHD (McGough et al., 2005).

Adderall Versus Methylphenidate

Several studies have compared Adderall and MPH in the treatment of children and adolescents diagnosed with ADHD.

Swanson et al. (1998) conducted a 7-week, double-blind, placebo-controlled, crossover study of placebo, MPH, and Adderall in doses of 5, 10, 15, and 20 mg. All subjects had prior significant clinical responses to MPH (average total daily dose was 31.06 ± 13.59 mg divided into three doses), and each subject received an initial dose of MPH identical to that he or she had been taking (average dose was 12.5 mg) during the week on that condition. Each subject was on one of the six conditions for a week; during the seventh week, one of the conditions was repeated randomly, or if one condition had been missed, the medication appropriate for that week was given.

Findings of particular clinical interest were as follows: peak clinical effects of MPH occurred at an average of 1.88 hours, more rapidly than Adderall at usual doses, where peak clinical effects occurred at 1.5, 2.6, and 3 hours for the 5-, 10-, and 20-mg doses, respectively.

MPH had a shorter duration of action that ended rather abruptly at an average of 3.98 hours. The duration of action of Adderall was dose dependent, increasing with the dose; duration of action was 3.52, 4.83, 5.44, and 6.40 hours for the 5-, 10-, 15-, and 20-mg doses, respectively.

Adderall was efficacious in the treatment of ADHD, and there were no unexpected or serious untoward effects; those that occurred were typical of stimulants.

Manos et al. (1999) compared the efficacy of MPH given twice daily (breakfast and lunch times) with a single breakfast-time dose of Adderall in a 4-week, double-blind titration, placebo-controlled study of 84 subjects (66 males and 18 females; mean age, 10.1 years; range, 5 to 17 years) diagnosed with ADHD by DSM-IV (APA, 1994) criteria. Each child's physician decided which active medication the child would be prescribed; parents and clinicians were aware of which active medication their child would receive, but not of the dose titration or when placebo would be given. All subjects received 7 days of treatment with placebo, and 5-, 10-, and 15-mg doses of either MPH or Adderall. The four conditions were assigned randomly except that the week of the 10-mg dose had to precede the week of the 15-mg/day dose. Seven children on MPH and four on Adderall did not receive the 15-mg/day dose because their physician thought they were too young or weighed too little and had made an assessment that the optimal dose had already been achieved.

Efficacy was determined by the following: the ADHD-RS, the Conners Abbreviated Symptoms Questionnaire, Composite Ratings, School Situations Questionnaire–Revised, and the Side Effect Behavior Monitoring Scale. The average optimal dose of MPH was 19.5 mg/day and of Adderall was 10.6 mg/day, suggesting that Adderall is clinically about twice as potent as MPH. There were no significant differences between parent and teacher ratings of subjects on MPH or Adderall. There were no clinically or statistically significant medication effects at any dose for pulse, blood pressure, or weight.

The authors concluded that their data showed that the efficacy of a single morning dose of Adderall was comparable to that of morning and noon doses of MPH and that a single morning dose of Adderall can therefore eliminate the need for a noontime dose in school and simplify the medication management of such children. Of additional clinical interest, all 15 of the Adderall subjects who had previously tried MPH without clinical benefit (7 were nonresponders and 8 had serious untoward effects) showed clinical improvement on Adderall. The only two subjects who showed no clinical improvement in the study were both receiving Adderall.

Pliszka et al. (2000) conducted a 3-week, double-blind, placebo-controlled, parallel-group study comparing placebo, Adderall, and MPH in the treatment of 58 children, mean age 8.2 ± 1.4 years diagnosed with ADHD. A flexible dosing algorithm was devised to permit blind titration of the dose at the end of the first and second weeks depending on clinical response. At the end of the study, the mean dose of Adderall was 12.5 ± 4.1 mg/day and the mean dose of MPH was 25.2 ± 13.1 mg/day. The most important clinical findings of the study were that both medications were superior to placebo. The positive effects of Adderall on behavior lasted longer than those of MPH. No subject receiving Adderall required a noon dose; however, 7 of the 13 MPH responders also did not require a noon dose. There was a greater tendency for the children on Adderall to have more stomachaches and to manifest a sad mood than for those receiving MPH.

Faraone et al. (2002) concluded in their meta-analysis of four studies of Adderall versus MPH that they were both efficacious, with Adderall possibly having a slight advantage.

Before we embark on an examination of the literature supporting non-stimulants in the treatment of ADHD, Table 5.4 presents a comprehensive list of the medications that are FDA approved in the treatment of ADHD (both stimulants and non-stimulants).

NON-STIMULANT MEDICATIONS FOR THE TREATMENT OF ADHD IN CHILD AND ADOLESCENT PSYCHIATRY

Although evidence points out that stimulant medications are superior to non-stimulants in the treatment of ADHD, there remain clear indications for the administration of non-stimulant medications. These indications include either as monotherapy when the use of stimulants are contraindicated or as adjuncts to stimulants when symptoms necessitate a non-stimulant. Of the non-stimulant medications used in the treatment of ADHD, several have FDA approval for this indication, and these medications include atomoxetine (Strattera), long-acting guanfacine (Intuniv), and long-acting clonidine (Kapvay). While the short-acting forms of guanfacine and clonidine lack FDA approval for the treatment of ADHD, they are prescribed frequently for this off-label use. Bupropion (Wellbutrin) is also frequently prescribed off-label for the treatment of ADHD. Less frequently prescribed are TCAs (imipramine and nortriptyline), modafinil (Provigil), and armodafinil (Nuvigil). In addition, lipirinen (Vayarin) is described as a prescription medical food (containing phosphatidylserine-omega 3) for the dietary management of ADHD.

TABLE 5.4 » FDA-Approved Stimulant and Non-stimulant Medications for the Treatment of ADHD

Stimulant Medication	Dose Forms	Typical Starting Dose	FDA Maximum Daily Dose	Medication Comments
Amphetamine Preparations				
Short-Acting Agents				
Dextroamphetamine, amphetamine (Adderall)	5-, 7.5-, 10-, 12.5-, 15-, 20-, 30-mg tablets	3–5 y: 2.5 mg daily ≥6 y: 5 mg daily-bid	40 mg 40 mg	Short-acting stimulants are often used as initial treatment in small children (<16 kg). As a result, they may require bid and tid dosing for symptom management; however, this split dosing may result in reduced med adherence.
Dextroamphetamine (Dexedrine)	5-, 10-mg tablets	3–5 y: 2.5 mg daily ≥6 y: 5 mg daily-bid	40 mg 40 mg	
Dextroamphetamine (Zenzedi)	2.5-, 5-, 7.5-, 10-, 15-, 20-, 30-mg tablets	3–5 y: 2.5 mg daily ≥6 y: 5 mg daily-bid	40 mg 40 mg	
Dextroamphetamine (ProCentra)	5 mg/5-mL liquid	3–5 y: 2.5 mg daily ≥6 y: 5 mg daily-bid	40 mg 40 mg	Children < 6 y are more susceptible to side effects, so prescribe cautiously. Adderall may also increase whininess.
Amphetamine (Evekeo)	5-, 10-mg tablets	3–5 y: 2.5 mg daily ≥6 y: 5 mg daily-bid	40 mg 40 mg	Although Desoxyn has FDA approval for ADHD in ages 6 y and older, there remain serious concerns regarding neurotoxicity and higher risk for abuse potential. It should therefore not be considered a first-line agent.
Methamphetamine (Desoxyn)	5-mg tablet	≥6 y: 5 mg daily-bid	25 mg	
Long-Acting Agents				
Dextroamphetamine, amphetamine extended release (Adderall XR)	5-, 10-, 15-, 20-, 25-, 30-mg capsules	≥6 y: 5–10 mg daily	6–12 year-old: 30 mg 13–17 year-old: 40 mg	Adderall XR capsule may be opened and sprinkled on soft food (e.g., yogurt, pudding).
Dextroamphetamine, amphetamine extended release (Mydayis)	12.5-, 25-, 37.5-, 50-mg capsules	≥13 y: 12.5 mg	25 mg	Longer acting stimulants offer greater convenience, confidentiality, and adherence (because of single daily dosing), but they may have a greater effect on evening appetite.
Dextroamphetamine (Dexedrine Spansule)	5-, 10-, 15-mg capsules	≥6 y: 5 mg daily-bid	60 mg	
Amphetamine ER (Adzenys XR-ODT)	3.1-, 6.3-, 9.4-, 12.5-, 15.7-, 18.8-mg ODT	6–12 y: 6.3 mg qAM 13–17 y: 6.3 mg	18.8 mg 12.5 mg	
Amphetamine ER (Adzenys ER liquid)	1.25 mg/mL liquid	6–12 y: 6.3 mg qAM 13–17 y: 6.3 mg	18.8 mg 12.5 mg	
Amphetamine ER (Dyanavel XR liquid)	2.5 mg/mL liquid	≥6 y: 2.5–5 mg qAM	20 mg	

Drug	Formulations	Starting Dose	Maximum Dose	Comments
Lisdexamfetamine (Vyvanse)	20-, 30-, 40-, 50-, 60-, 70-mg capsules	≥6 y: 30 mg daily	70 mg	To minimize stimulant abuse and misuse, consider using lisdexamfetamine or non-stimulants.
Methylphenidate Preparations				
Short-Acting Agents				
Methylin	5-, 10-, 20-mg tablets; 2.5-, 5-, 10-mg chewable tablets; 5 mg/mL, 10 mg/mL liquid	≥6 y: 5 mg bid	60 mg	Short-acting stimulants are often used as initial treatment in small children (<16 kg). As a result, they may require bid and tid dosing for symptom management; however, this split dosing may result in reduced medicine adherence.
Ritalin	5-, 10-, 20-mg tablets	≥6 y: 5 mg bid	60 mg	
Intermediate-Acting Agents				
Metadate ER	10-, 20-mg tablets	≥6 y: 10 mg qAM	60 mg	Longer acting stimulants offer greater convenience, confidentiality, and adherence (because of single daily dosing), but they may have a greater effect on evening appetite.
Ritalin SR	20-mg tablets	≥6 y: 20 mg	60 mg	
Metadate CD	10-, 20-, 30-, 40-, 50-, 60-mg capsules	≥6 y: 20 mg qAM	60 mg	Metadate CD, Ritalin LA, and Focalin XR may be opened and sprinkled on soft food.
Ritalin LA	10-, 20-, 30-, 40-mg capsules	≥6 y: 10 mg	60 mg	
Long-Acting Agents				
Concerta	18-, 27-, 36-, 54-mg tablets	≥6 y: 18 mg qAM	6–12 year-old: 54 mg >13 year-old: 72 mg	Do not open Concerta (swallow it whole with liquids). Concerta has a nonabsorbable tablet shell that may be seen in stool.
Aptensio XR	10, 15, 20, 30, 40, 50, 60 mg	≥6 y: 10 mg	60 mg	To minimize stimulant abuse and misuse, consider the use of lisdexamfetamine or non-stimulants.
Cotempla XR ODT	8.6, 17.3, 25.9 mg	≥6 y: 17.3 mg	51.8 mg	
QuillivantXR	25 mg/5 mL liquid	≥6 y: 20 mg qAM	60 mg	
QuilliChew ER	20, 30, 40 mg	≥6 y: 20 mg qAM	60 mg	
Daytrana (patch)	10-, 15-, 20-, 30-mg patches	≥6 y: Begin with 10-mg patch daily, then titrate up weekly by patch strength	30 mg	Daytrana patch may cause skin irritation. Place patch on skin 2 h before desired effect. Wear patch for 9 h, then remove it. Effects of patch may persist 5 h after patch is removed.

(continued)

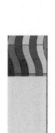

TABLE 5.4 » FDA-Approved Stimulant and Non-stimulant Medications for the Treatment of ADHD (*continued*)

Stimulant Medication	Dose Forms	Typical Starting Dose	FDA Maximum Daily Dose	Medication Comments
Dexmethylphenidate Preparations				
Short-Acting Agent				
Focalin	2.5-, 5-, 10-mg tablets	2.5 mg bid	20 mg	
Long-Acting Agent				
Focalin XR	5-, 10-, 15-, 20-, 30-, 35-, 40-mg tabs	5 mg qAM	30 mg	

Non-Stimulant Medication	Dose Forms	Typical Starting Dose	FDA Maximum Daily Dose	Medication Comments
Selective Norepinephrine Reuptake Inhibitor				
Atomoxetine (Strattera)	10-, 18-, 25-, 40-, 60-, 80-, 100-mg capsules	Children and adolescents <70 kg: 0.5 mg/kg/d for at least 3 d; then 1 mg/kg/d for 3 d; then 1.2 mg/kg/d >70 kg: 40 mg for at least 3 d, then 80 mg daily	Lesser of 1.4 mg/kg or 100 mg	Consider atomoxetine if there is active substance use or severe side effects with stimulants (mood lability, tics). Give qAM or divided doses (bid). Do not open capsule. Monitor for suicidal symptoms, clinical worsening, or unusual changes in behavior. (Black box warning regarding SI) Monitor for signs of liver injury such as jaundice or dark urine.
Alpha 2-Adrenergic Agonists				
Long-Acting Agents				
Clonidine (Kapvay)	0.1, 0.2 mg	6–17 y: 0.1 mg	0.4 mg	Can be used as adjunctive therapy with stimulants. Clonidine is generally more sedating than guanfacine.
Guanfacine (Intuniv)	1-, 2-, 3-, 4-mg tablets	6–17 y: 1 mg qAM	7 mg	Taper when discontinuing (0.1 mg for Clonidine every 3-7 d (and 1 mg for Guanfacine every 3-7 d)). Abrupt discontinuation or nonadherence may result in rebound hypertension.

ADHD, attention–deficit hyperactivity disorder.
Table adapted from AACAP ADHD Practice Parameters.

Selective Norepinephrine Reuptake Inhibitors

Atomoxetine Hydrochloride (Strattera)

Atomoxetine hydrochloride is an SNRI that selectively inhibits the presynaptic norepinephrine transporter, and this is the primary mechanism of action by which atomoxetine treats the symptoms of ADHD. In 2002, atomoxetine gained FDA approval for the treatment of ADHD, and it remains one of the few non-stimulant medications with this FDA-approved indication. As an SNRI, however, it can take time for this medication to begin treating ADHD symptoms (which is in stark contrast to the rapid efficacy of stimulant medications).

Although stimulant medications are generally considered to be the first-line agents in the treatment of ADHD, stimulants are not well tolerated by some patients. For instance, stimulant medications may cause clinical worsening of anxiety and tics. Patients with ADHD that is comorbid with either anxiety and/or tics may therefore benefit from a trial of atomoxetine. Once treatment with atomoxetine is initiated for the treatment of ADHD, individuals with comorbid anxiety and/or tics may also notice an improvement in those symptoms; however, in rare instances tics and anxiety have been worsened by the initiation of atomoxetine.

Atomoxetine may also be considered a first-line agent in patients who have a history of illicit substance use. Cases where there is a concern about medication diversion (either by the patient or the patient's family members) are often good candidates for a trial of a non-stimulant such as atomoxetine.

In addition, atomoxetine is often used as either a second-line agent or as an augmentation strategy. For patients who have failed one or more stimulants, a trial of atomoxetine is often considered. In other cases, atomoxetine can be used as an augmenting agent for those patients whose stimulant dose has been maximized. In addition, if a patient has an unpleasant medication side effect with a stimulant, the stimulant dose can be reduced and atomoxetine can be added to the regimen.

Atomoxetine can have profound effects on the symptoms of ADHD. An additional benefit of atomoxetine is that it can provide 24-hour treatment of ADHD symptoms (which is not feasible with stimulants because of their effect on sleep). Atomoxetine generally does not worsen sleep, tics, or anxiety, and it can be taken at any time of the day. Atomoxetine has less abuse potential than stimulants; and because it is not a Schedule II medication, prescriptions can be written with refills and/or called in to the pharmacy.

Although atomoxetine is an SNRI, its only FDA-approved indication is for the treatment of ADHD. Although it does not have FDA approval for other diagnoses, some patients who take it for ADHD have noticed improvements in their symptoms of depression, anxiety, and/or tics. The literature suggests that between 25% and 35% of children with ADHD have a comorbid anxiety disorder. Geller et al. (2007) conducted a study to determine the effects of atomoxetine in children with ADHD and comorbid anxiety. This double-blind study compared atomoxetine with placebo in patients aged 8 to 17 years. The subjects were randomized to 12 weeks of atomoxetine ($N = 87$) or placebo ($N = 89$). Geller concluded from the results that atomoxetine was effective in reducing ADHD symptoms in patients with ADHD and comorbid anxiety, and also noted that there was also a significant reduction in independently assessed symptoms of anxiety (using clinician-rated and self-rated measures).

Atomoxetine can have a significantly positive impact on ADHD symptoms and on patients' lives, but patients must be aware of atomoxetine's black box warning regarding suicidal ideation (discussed at the end of this section). They should also be aware that because atomoxetine is an SNRI, it can take at least 6 weeks for its full effects to be realized. However, some benefits may be noticed after the first dose. Because it takes time to build up in the body, it can also take time to wash out. As a consequence of this, if there is an adverse event with atomoxetine, it could possibly take longer to resolve than an adverse event with a stimulant.

Pharmacokinetics of Atomoxetine Hydrochloride

Taken orally, atomoxetine hydrochloride is rapidly absorbed, with maximal plasma concentrations being reached in approximately 1 to 2 hours. Absorption is minimally affected by food, but taking it with meals does result in a 9% lower maximum plasma concentration in children and adolescents. Mean elimination half-life is approximately 5.2 hours. At standard doses, 98% of atomoxetine in plasma is protein bound (mostly to albumin). Atomoxetine is metabolized primarily via oxidative metabolism through the CYP2D6 enzymatic pathway followed by glucuronidation. The major metabolite is 4-hydroxyatomoxetine, which is equipotent to atomoxetine but circulates at a much lower plasma concentration. Atomoxetine is excreted primarily as 4-hydroxyatomoxetine-O-glucuronide (about 80% of which is excreted in urine and 17% in feces). Less than 3% of atomoxetine is excreted unchanged.

About 7% of Caucasians and 2% of African Americans are poor metabolizers of atomoxetine because of a reduced ability to metabolize CYP2D6 substrates. Such individuals have a net increase in the maximum plasma concentration of atomoxetine of 500% compared with extensive (normal) metabolizers of the medication. These poor metabolizers therefore have roughly five times as much medication in their system. The elimination half-life of atomoxetine for poor metabolizers is approximately 24 hours (nearly five times that of extensive metabolizers). Laboratory testing is available to determine if someone is a poor metabolizer of CYP2D6 medications. Atomoxetine itself neither inhibits nor induces the CYP2D6 pathway (Atomoxetine, 2012).

Interactions of Atomoxetine with Other Medications

The current or recent use of nonselective MAOIs is contraindicated with atomoxetine (discussed subsequently). Both nonselective and selective MAOIs should be avoided.

Medications such as quinidine, fluoxetine (Prozac), and paroxetine (Paxil), which inhibit CYP2D6, can result in significant increases in plasma levels of atomoxetine. Fluoxetine and paroxetine may increase the maximum plasma concentration of atomoxetine by up to three or four times in extensive (normal) metabolizers. Coadministration of atomoxetine with these medications will therefore require downward adjustment of the dose of atomoxetine (Michelson et al., 2007).

Patients taking blood pressure medications (either pressors or antihypertensives) will need close monitoring with any dosing changes of atomoxetine due to atomoxetine's effects on blood pressure (because of its effect on norepinephrine). Coadministration of atomoxetine and beta-2 agonists (e.g., Albuterol) can result in clinically significant increases in blood pressure and heart rate.

Changes in gastric pH do not affect the bioavailability of atomoxetine, so no dosing adjustments need to be made if a patient is also being treated for gastro-esophageal reflux.

Contraindications for Atomoxetine Administration

Atomoxetine is contraindicated in patients with known hypersensitivity to the medication. It should not be taken concomitantly with an MAOI or within 2 weeks of discontinuing an MAOI. In addition, an MAOI should not be administered within the 2-week period of discontinuing atomoxetine.

Atomoxetine is also contraindicated in individuals with narrow-angle glaucoma because atomoxetine use in clinical trials was associated with an increased risk of mydriasis. Atomoxetine is contraindicated in patients with a history of pheochromocytoma and in people who have severe cardiovascular disorders that may deteriorate with the increases in heart rate and blood pressure that often occur from atomoxetine's effect on norepinephrine. In placebo-controlled registration studies with pediatric patients, the mean heart rate increase with atomoxetine was 5 beats per minute. Overall, 5% to 10% of pediatric patients taking atomoxetine have clinically important changes in blood pressure (≥15 to 20 mm Hg) and/or heart rate (≥20 beats per minute).

It is important to note that the coadministration of MPH and atomoxetine did not increase cardiovascular effects beyond those seen with MPH alone.

Warnings and Precautions

Atomoxetine carries the black box warning regarding the risk of suicidal ideation. It is therefore recommended that the patient be monitored closely for suicidality, worsening of symptoms, and unusual behavioral changes (particularly during the initiation phase and during any changes in medication dosing).

Atomoxetine has also been associated with severe liver injury in some cases. The medication should be stopped and not restarted if the patient develops jaundice or has laboratory values consistent with liver injury. Patients with signs of possible liver dysfunction (e.g., dark urine, pruritis, jaundice, unexplained flulike symptoms, or right-upper-quadrant pain) should have liver enzyme levels tested. It should be noted that routine labs before starting atomoxetine are not required; however, baseline labs are recommended at the psychiatric intake.

Sudden death has been reported in association with atomoxetine treatment (at usual doses) in children and adolescents with structural cardiac abnormalities or other serious heart problems. In adults, sudden death, myocardial infarction, and stroke have been reported in association with atomoxetine treatment (particularly in individuals with preexisting cardiovascular ailments). Atomoxetine should generally not be used in children and adolescents with known serious structural cardiac abnormalities, serious heart rhythm abnormalities, cardiomyopathy, or other serious cardiovascular problems that may worsen with an increase in norepinephrine. Before starting atomoxetine, it is therefore important to screen for both a personal and family history of cardiac disease (including a family history of sudden death or ventricular arrhythmia). An ECG and echocardiogram are not considered a part of the routine ADHD workup unless there is a personal or family history of concerning cardiovascular ailments. Blood pressure and heart rate should be monitored routinely, and questions about syncope and orthostasis should be asked. Patients who develop unexplained syncope, exertional chest pain, or other symptoms of possible cardiac disease should have a prompt cardiac evaluation.

With the administration of atomoxetine, it is also important to monitor both height and weight in children because this medication has been shown to have some effects on appetite and growth. In general, gains in both height and weight for patients taking atomoxetine are less than expected (on the basis of population norms) for the first 9 to 12 months of medication use. After approximately 12 months, gains in height and weight stabilize with them approaching expected norms.

Children and adolescents should also be monitored for increases in aggressive behavior and possible mania/hypomania. Other potential side effects include that some adults have developed urinary hesitancy and retention, priapism, and/or sexual side effects with this medication. Individuals may also develop a rash with atomoxetine.

In some cases of overdose of atomoxetine, seizures have occurred. Because atomoxetine is mostly protein bound, dialysis is not thought to be useful for atomoxetine overdose. Treatment of an atomoxetine overdose is mostly symptomatic (including monitoring for and treatment of cardiovascular symptoms [changes in blood pressure, heart rate, and QTc prolongation]).

Untoward Effects of Atomoxetine

In clinical trials, the most common untoward effects of atomoxetine in children and adolescents (with an incidence of ≥5% and occurring at least twice as frequently as in patients treated with placebo) were nausea, vomiting, fatigue, abdominal pain, decreased appetite, and somnolence. If a child experiences drowsiness as a side effect of atomoxetine, it is generally recommended to move the administration to bedtime.

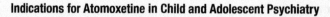

Indications for Atomoxetine in Child and Adolescent Psychiatry

Note: Review the black box warning at the end of this section or in the package insert before prescribing.

   Atomoxetine is FDA approved for the treatment of ADHD in individuals at least 6 years of age.

Atomoxetine Hydrochloride Dosage Schedule

- *Children <6 years of age:* Not recommended. The safety and efficacy of atomoxetine have not been established for this age group.
- *Children and adolescents ≥6 years of age and who weigh <70 kg:* Atomoxetine should be administered as a single morning dose or in two divided doses (in the morning and late afternoon/early evening). The initial total daily dose should be approximately 0.5 mg/kg. After a minimum of 3 days, the dose should be increased to reach a total target daily dose of 1.2 mg/kg. No additional benefit has been demonstrated for doses over 1.2 mg/kg/day, and the maximum recommended total daily dose should not exceed 1.4 mg/kg or 100 mg, whichever is less. Table 5.5 presents a detailed dosing chart for atomoxetine depending on the patient's weight (kilograms or pounds).
- *Children and adolescents ≥6 years of age and who weigh ≥70 kg and adults:* Atomoxetine should be administered as a single morning dose or in two divided doses (in the morning and late afternoon/early evening). The initial total daily dose should be 40 mg. After a minimum of 3 days, the dose should be increased to reach a total target daily dose of approximately 80 mg. After 2 to 4 additional weeks, the dose may be increased to a maximum of 100 mg.

   Dosing adjustments should be made for individuals who have hepatic impairment, are taking CYP2D6 inhibitors (fluoxetine, paroxetine), or are CYP2D6 poor metabolizers.

Atomoxetine Hydrochloride Dose Forms Available and Instructions for Administration

- *Capsules:* 10, 18, 25, 40, 60, 80, 100 mg.
- Capsules should not be opened because the contents of the capsule may be an ocular irritant.
- Capsules can be taken with or without food, but should be taken with at least a glass of water.
- Patients should be instructed to use caution when driving a car or operating heavy machinery until they are reasonably certain that their performance is not adversely affected by atomoxetine.
- Atomoxetine may be discontinued without a taper, although a taper may be recommended.

TABLE 5.5 » Atomoxetine (Strattera) Dosing Chart for Children and Adolescents

Weight (kg)	Weight (lb)	FDA Start Dose (mg; 0.5 mg/kg/d for 3 d)	Next Dose (mg; 1 mg/kg/d for 3 d)	Next Dose (mg; 1.2 mg/kg/d) (the FDA Target Dose)	FDA Maximum Dose (mg; 1.4 mg/kg/d)
20	44	10	20	24	28
25	55	12.5	25	30	35
30	66	15	30	36	42
35	77	17.5	35	42	49
40	88	20	40	48	56
45	99	22.5	45	54	63
50	110	25	50	60	70
55	121	27.5	55	66	77
60	132	30	60	72	84
65	143	32.5	65	78	91

For children >70 kg, start at 40 mg for at least 3 days, then increase to 80 mg daily. Maximum dose of atomoxetine is the lesser of 1.4 mg/kg or 100 mg. Dose forms for atomoxetine are 10-, 18-, 25-, 40-, 60-, 80-, and 100-mg capsules.

Reports of Interest

Atomoxetine Versus Stimulants in the Treatment of ADHD in Children and Adolescents

In head-to-head studies, stimulant medications have been more efficacious than atomoxetine in the treatment of ADHD. In a multicenter, randomized, double-blind, forced-dose-escalation laboratory school study, Wigal et al. (2005) compared MAS XR (Adderall XR) to atomoxetine in 203 children aged 6 to 12 years who were diagnosed with ADHD (combined or hyperactive/impulsive type). The MAS XR group ($N = 102$) demonstrated significantly greater improvement from baseline than did the atomoxetine group ($N = 101$). The authors noted that AEs were similar in both groups and that their data suggested that with its extended duration of action and greater therapeutic efficacy, MAS XR was more effective than atomoxetine in children diagnosed with ADHD.

Hanwella et al. (2011) published a meta-analysis comparing the efficacy and acceptability of MPH and atomoxetine in the treatment of ADHD in children and adolescents. Nine randomized trials with a total of 2,762 subjects were included. The authors concluded from their analysis that atomoxetine and IR MPH have comparable efficacy in the treatment of ADHD; however, OROS MPH was considered to be more effective than atomoxetine. Regarding all-cause discontinuation, the authors noted that there was no significant difference between MPH and atomoxetine.

Kemner et al. (2005) reported on the treatment outcomes for African American children who participated in the Formal Observation of Concerta versus Strattera (FOCUS) study (funded by the maker of OROS MPH). Within the study, 183 children (13.8%) were African American. Of the 183, 125 were assigned to OROS MPH and 58 to atomoxetine. The authors noted that both medications were associated with significant improvement in ADHD symptoms from baseline, but the group receiving OROS MPH demonstrated significantly greater improvement in total ADHD symptoms, inattentiveness, and CGI-I ratings.

Atomoxetine in the Treatment of ADHD in Children and Adolescents

In 2009, Newcorn et al. published their findings from the Integrated Data Exploratory Analysis study. In this retrospective analysis of six randomized controlled trials, there were 1,069 subjects (age range from 6 to 18 years of age). The authors reported that atomoxetine's effect on ADHD symptoms were that 47% of patients were much improved, 13% had a minimal response, and 40% did not respond. They suggested that there seemed to be a bimodal response to atomoxetine (e.g., responders and nonresponders). They noted that most of the responders had at least some improvement in symptoms by week 4 of treatment. They suggested that perhaps any patient who is a nonresponder at week 4 should either have another agent added to the atomoxetine regimen or should be switched from atomoxetine to another medication.

Wehmeier et al. (2010) published the results of a meta-analysis of five atomoxetine trials. In all, there were 794 subjects (611 children and 183 adolescents). Atomoxetine was shown to be effective in improving some aspects of health-related quality of life (HR-QoL) in both children and adolescents (including in the achievement domain [academic performance and peer relations] and the risk avoidance domain).

Michelson et al. (2001) showed in a randomized, placebo-controlled, dose-response study that atomoxetine was effective and safe in treating ADHD in children and adolescents when administered twice daily. In 2002, Michelson et al. conducted a study showing that (for most patients) atomoxetine could also be administered once daily with good clinical results. They reported a 6-week, double-blind, placebo-controlled study of once-daily treatment with atomoxetine in 171 children and adolescents (age range 6 to 16 years) who were diagnosed with ADHD. The treatment effect size (0.71) was noted to be similar to those observed in studies that used twice-daily atomoxetine dosing. The authors noted that this study suggested that once-daily dosing with atomoxetine is an effective treatment for ADHD. Despite its relatively short half-life, beneficial effects of one morning dose lasted into the evening for many subjects.

Weiss et al. (2005) also studied once-daily dosing of atomoxetine. In this multicenter, randomized, placebo-controlled, 7-week study in the school setting, 153 subjects (123 male and 30 female) were enrolled (age range 8 to 12 years). At its conclusion, 69% of the atomoxetine group versus 43% of the placebo group were rated as responders. Safety and tolerability were examined, and the authors concluded that once-daily dosing of atomoxetine was safe and effective in the treatment of ADHD.

Two studies by Wehmeier et al. examined possible gender differences in atomoxetine treatment of ADHD. This 2011 study was a pooled analysis of gender differences in five atomoxetine trials. Data from 136 girls and 658 boys were pooled. It was concluded that atomoxetine was effective in improving some aspects of the HR-QoL in both genders without any significant difference across genders.

Atomoxetine in the Treatment of ADHD with Comorbid ODD or Conduct Disorder in Children and Adolescents

ADHD and ODD are frequent comorbidities. Newcorn et al. (2005) reported on the effects of atomoxetine on 293 subjects (8 to 18 years old) who were diagnosed with either ADHD-only ($N = 178, 61\%$) or ADHD comorbid with ODD ($N = 115$, 39%). This was a 13-site, outpatient-only, approximately 8-week, randomized, double-blind, placebo-controlled study. At the conclusion of the study, in the ADHD/ODD group, atomoxetine was superior to placebo in reducing ADHD symptoms only for the 1.8 mg/kg/day dose (and not for the lower doses that were studied). The authors concluded that atomoxetine resulted in statistically and clinically significant improvements. They also stated that their results suggested that higher doses are required when ODD is comorbid with ADHD.

Wehmeier et al. (2010) conducted a study on the effects of atomoxetine on patients with ADHD and comorbid ODD or conduct disorder. The 9-week study of 180 patients showed that atomoxetine improved quality of life as measured by the KINDL-R scores on emotional well-being, self-esteem, friends, and family. However, there were no significant effects on family burden in these children and adolescents with ADHD and either ODD or conduct disorder.

Atomoxetine in the Treatment of Children and Adolescents Diagnosed with Comorbid Anxiety Disorder

Geller et al. (2007) reported that 25% to 35% of children with ADHD have comorbid anxiety disorders. Their 12-week, double-blind study of patients (age 8 to 17 years old) with ADHD and comorbid generalized anxiety disorder, separation anxiety disorder, and/or social phobia showed that atomoxetine was efficacious in reducing both ADHD symptoms and anxiety symptoms. The medication was reported to be well tolerated in this population.

Atomoxetine in the Treatment of Children and Adolescents Diagnosed with ASD

Harfterkamp et al. (2012) published a study which included 97 patients between the ages of 6 and 17 with an ASD and ADHD-like symptoms. This 8-week, double-blind study showed that hyperactivity improved significantly with atomoxetine compared with placebo. AEs (mostly nausea, decreased appetite, fatigue, and early morning awakening) were reported in 81.3% of patients receiving atomoxetine and 65.3% of patients receiving placebo. The authors concluded that atomoxetine moderately improved ADHD symptoms and was generally well tolerated in this group. It has generally been noted that the effects of medications on the treatment of ADHD-like symptoms associated with an ASD are less robust than the effects of medications on patients with ADHD-only.

Two studies (one by Mazzone et al. [2011] and another by Fernández-Jaén et al. [2010]) examined the use of atomoxetine in patients with ADHD and lower-than-average IQ. Mazzone's study included children with both low and normal IQs (IQs ranged from 43 to 117). The authors' conclusion at the completion of the study was that children and adolescents with IQs <85 were less likely to respond to atomoxetine than children and were adolescents with IQs ≥85. Fernández-Jaén reported that patients with ID and ADHD-like symptoms did show clinically significant improvements in their ADHD-like symptoms with the use of atomoxetine.

Review of Atomoxetine's Black Box Warning

Atomoxetine increased the risk of suicidal ideation in short-term studies in children or adolescents with ADHD. Anyone considering the use of atomoxetine in a child or adolescent must balance this risk with the clinical need. Comorbidities occurring with ADHD may also be associated with an increase in the risk of suicidal ideation and/or behavior. Patients who start atomoxetine should be monitored closely for suicidality (suicidal thinking and behavior), clinical worsening, and unusual changes in behavior. Families and caregivers should be advised on the need for close observation and communication with the prescriber.

Pooled analyses of short-term (6 to 18 weeks), placebo-controlled trials of atomoxetine in children and adolescents (a total of 12 trials involving more than 2,200 patients, including 11 trials in ADHD and 1 trial in enuresis) have revealed a greater risk of suicidal ideation early during treatment in those receiving atomoxetine compared with placebo. The average risk of suicidal ideation in patients receiving atomoxetine was 0.4% (5/1,357 patients), compared with none in placebo-treated patients (851 patients). There was 1 suicide attempt among the 2,200 patients. No suicide completions occurred in these trials (Bangs et al., 2008).

All reactions were reported to have occurred in children 12 years of age and younger. All reactions occurred in the first month of treatment.

A similar analysis in adult patients treated with atomoxetine for either ADHD or MDD did not reveal an increased risk of suicidal ideation or behavior in association with the use of atomoxetine.

ALPHA-ADRENERGIC AGONISTS

Although the dopamine system is believed to be innately involved in frontal lobe executive functioning and manifests in the syndrome of ADHD when impaired, the norepinephrine system also appears to be important in causing behavioral and cognitive abnormalities, in at least some individuals with ADHD.

Clonidine Hydrochloride Extended Release (Kapvay), Clonidine Hydrochloride (Catapres), Clonidine (Catapres-Transdermal Therapeutic System)

Clonidine is a centrally acting antihypertensive agent. The only formulation that has a pediatric indication for ADHD is clonidine hydrochloride extended release (CXR), which is indicated for the treatment of ADHD as monotherapy and as adjunctive therapy to stimulant medications. The only therapeutic indication that IR clonidine has been approved by the FDA is the treatment of hypertension in older adolescents and adults; its safety and efficacy in children have not been established, although it is frequently prescribed off-label for the treatment of ADHD, anxiety, insomnia, tics, and aggression.

Clonidine is an alpha-2-adrenergic receptor agonist whose binding is independent of norepinephrine levels. There are three different subtypes of alpha-2 adrenoceptors in humans: the 2A, 2B, and 2C. The 2A and 2C subtypes have wide distributions in the brain, most importantly for ADHD in the prefrontal cortex (PFC), whereas the 2B receptors are most concentrated in the thalamus. Both the A and C subtypes are localized in the PFC, with the A subtype being more prevalent. Differential binding of alpha-2 receptors in these varying brain areas may account for their effects on cognitive as well as emotional functioning. It is theorized that alpha-2 agonists exhibit their therapeutic effects by strengthening (PFC) regulation of attention and behavior through direct stimulation of postsynaptic alpha-2A adrenoceptors (Arnsten et al., 2007). Alpha-2 agonists have been shown to bind to the alpha-2B and alpha-2C receptors as well. All three alpha-2-adrenoceptors subtypes are associated with sedative effects; in addition, hypotensive effects have been associated with subtype 2C (Arnsten et al., 2007; Franowicz and Arnsten, 2002). Clonidine appears to bind to all three alpha-2-receptor subtypes fairly equally, whereas guanfacine appears to be 15× to 20× more selective for the alpha-2A-receptor subtype.

Pharmacokinetics of Clonidine Hydrochloride Extended Release

The pharmacokinetic profile of CXR administration was evaluated in an open-label, three-period, randomized, crossover study of 15 healthy adult subjects who received three single-dose regimens of clonidine: 0.1 mg of CXR under fasted conditions, 0.1 mg of CXR following a high-fat meal, and 0.1 mg of clonidine IR (Catapres) under fasting conditions. Treatments were separated by 1-week washout periods.

After administration of CXR, maximum clonidine concentrations (C_{max} pg/mL) were approximately 50% of the Catapres maximum concentration means (443 pg/mL) and T_{max} occurred approximately 5 hours later (6.8 hours) relative to Catapres (2.07 hours). Similar elimination half-lives (T_{max} hour) were observed at 12 hours and total systemic bioavailability (area under the curve [AUC]) following CXR was approximately 89% of that following Catapres.

Food had no effect on plasma concentrations, bioavailability, or elimination half-life.

Pharmacokinetics of Clonidine Hydrochloride Immediate Release

Peak plasma levels of clonidine occur between 3 and 5 hours after ingestion of the IR form of clonidine, and plasma half-life is between 12 and 16 hours (package insert). Leckman et al. (1985), however, give different pharmacokinetic values for children and adolescents, stating that clonidine's half-life is approximately 8 to 12 hours in adolescents and adults, whereas in prepubertal children it is considerably shorter at approximately 4 to 6 hours. Between 40% and 60% of the medication is excreted unchanged by the kidneys within 24 hours of oral ingestion, and approximately 50% is metabolized by the liver (package insert).

Contraindications for Clonidine Hydrochloride Administration

Known hypersensitivity to clonidine hydrochloride is a contraindication. Significant cardiovascular disease is a relative contraindication; if clonidine is used in patients with such conditions, careful and frequent monitoring is required.

A careful risk/benefit analysis should be considered in the administration of clonidine to children and adolescents with depressive symptomatology, a past history of depression, or family history of mood disorder. Hunt et al. (1990) reported that clonidine worsened or induced depressive symptomatology in 5% of children.

Interactions of Clonidine Hydrochloride with Other Medications

TCAs may decrease the effects of clonidine, necessitating higher doses.

The CNS depressive effects of alcohol, barbiturates, and other medications and illicit drugs may be enhanced by simultaneous administration with clonidine. Owing to a potential for additive effects such as bradycardia and atrioventricular (AV) block, caution is warranted in patients receiving clonidine concomitantly with agents known to affect sinus node function or AV nodal conduction (e.g., digitalis, calcium channel blockers, and beta-blockers). Interactions with additional medications have been reported.

Clonidine and MPH

On July 13, 1995, a National Public Radio broadcast reported that sudden deaths had occurred in three children taking a combination of MPH and clonidine. The ramifications of this were discussed earlier in this chapter in the section "Safety Considerations and Contraindications for Stimulant Administration." Detailed reviews of the three cases and the medications by Popper (1995) and Fenichel (1995) concluded that there was no convincing evidence of an adverse MPH–clonidine interaction in any of the cases. Popper (1995) and Swanson et al. (1995) concluded that combined clonidine–MPH treatment of ADHD is usually safe and that the available evidence did not support discontinuation of such therapy in patients experiencing significant clinical benefit. All authors also noted the lack of systematic studies of the efficacy and safety of combined MPH–clonidine treatment.

Swanson et al. (1995) noted in their review of untoward effects that when the combination of clonidine and a stimulant was given, sedation–hypotension–bradycardia would be most expected when the clonidine effect was at its peak and the stimulant's effect is decreasing and, conversely, that hypertension–tachycardia would be most expected when the stimulant is at its peak and clonidine's effect is waning. Before prescribing this combination, it is recommended that the clinician reviews this literature and thoroughly discusses the risks and benefits with the parents/legal guardian and patient.

Untoward Effects of CXR

The most common side effects of CXR include the following:

- Sleepiness
- Tiredness
- Irritability
- Sore throat
- Trouble sleeping (insomnia)
- Nightmares
- Change in mood
- Constipation
- Stuffy nose
- Increased body temperature
- Dry mouth
- Low blood pressure and low heart rate

It is advised that the treating practitioner should check heart rate and blood pressure before starting treatment and regularly during treatment with CXR.

Sleepiness may be an early and bothersome side effect.

Somnolence and sedation were commonly reported adverse reactions in clinical studies. In patients who completed 5 weeks of therapy in a controlled fixed-dose pediatric monotherapy study, 31% of patients treated with 0.4 mg/day and 38% treated with 0.2 mg/day reported somnolence as an adverse event (compared with 7% of placebo-treated patients reported somnolence). In patients who completed 5 weeks of therapy in a controlled flexible-dose pediatric adjunctive to stimulants study, 19% of patients treated with Kapvay + stimulant versus 8% treated with placebo + stimulant reported somnolence.

The incidence of "sedation-like" AEs (somnolence and fatigue) appeared to be independent of clonidine dose or concentration within the studied dose range in the titration study.

Suddenly stopping clonidine may cause withdrawal symptoms, including increased blood pressure, headache, increased heart rate, lightheadedness, "tightness" in the chest, and nervousness.

Results from the add-on study showed that clonidine body weight normalized clearance (CL/F) was 11% higher in patients who were receiving MPH and 44% lower in those receiving amphetamine compared with subjects not on adjunctive therapy.

Untoward Effects of Clonidine Hydrochloride Immediate Release

Hunt et al. (1991) reported that sedation is the most frequent and troublesome untoward effect of clonidine in treating children. Cardiovascular untoward effects, including hypotension, were not usually clinically significant.

Clonidine worsened or induced depressive symptomatology in approximately 5% of children (Hunt et al., 1991). McCracken and Martin (1997) reported the case of an 8-year-old boy with ASD who developed an apparent severe depressive reaction on a total daily dose of 0.2 mg of clonidine, and there was rapid improvement following discontinuation of clonidine. They cautioned clinicians to monitor for depressive reactions secondary to clonidine that could be mistaken for worsening of the primary disorder.

Levin et al. (1993) reported the onset of precocious puberty in two 7-year-old girls with mild mental retardation (ID) who were being treated with clonidine for aggressivity; of note, discontinuation of clonidine halted the progression of puberty in both cases.

Swanson et al. (1995) reviewed briefly 20 MedWatch adverse-event reports concerning subjects <19 years of age who were taking clonidine and added three additional cases, one of which was fatal. Of the 23 cases, 4 were fatalities. Eleven cases were treated with clonidine only, 11 with combined clonidine–MPH therapy, and 1 with combined clonidine–Dexedrine therapy. In 12 cases, the untoward effect occurred after a change in medication protocol (e.g., prescribed dose change, accidental change, or nonadherence). In 10 of the 19 nonfatal cases, hypotension and/or bradycardia was reported, and in 5 cases hypertension and/or tachycardia was reported. (See also the preceding discussion on clonidine–MPH under medication interactions.)

Effects of CXR and Clonidine Hydrochloride Immediate Release on the Electrocardiograms of Children and Adolescents

In the CXR studies, there were no changes on ECGs to suggest a medication-related effect.

Several studies have looked at cardiac issues when using IR clonidine hydrochloride. Kofoed et al. (1999) reviewed relevant literature and conducted a retrospective study of the effects of clonidine alone ($N = 12$) and clonidine combined with stimulants (MPH [$N = 14$], dextroamphetamine [$N = 13$], or magnesium pemoline [$N = 3$]) on 12-lead ECGs of 42 children and adolescents (36 males and 6 females; age range, 4 to 16 years). The mean clonidine dose was 0.16 ± 0.075 mg/day (dose range, 0.05 to 0.3 mg/day). The mean daily MPH dose was 60 mg; the mean daily dextroamphetamine dose was 40 mg; and the mean daily magnesium pemoline dose was 112 mg. The authors stated that their data should be able to detect a difference of 0.012 second between baseline and post-clonidine treatment PR intervals and of 0.015 second between pretreatment and post-clonidine treatment for the QTc interval. Their data should also detect differences between clonidine only and clonidine plus a stimulant of 0.020 second for the PR interval and 0.024 second for the QTc interval. Two pediatric cardiologists, blinded to treatment condition, evaluated all ECGs.

Six (14%) of the 42 subjects had ECG abnormalities before medication treatment (3 sinus bradycardia, 2 ectopic atrial rhythm, and 1 short PR interval), and 7 (17%)

had ECG abnormalities after medication. The abnormal ECGs of two subjects normalized on medication and three subjects with normal pretreatment ECGs developed abnormal ECGs on medication ($P = .50$, not significant), suggesting spontaneous variability rather than medication effect. Except for a 10-year-old boy with a short PR interval who later required ablation of an accessory atrial pathway, all subjects had normal PR, QRS, and QTc intervals, suggesting that clonidine alone or in combination with stimulants has no significant effect on these ECG parameters.

The authors emphasized the importance of pretreatment ECGs, because 14% of their subjects had abnormalities on their ECGs, some of which could have been attributed to clonidine if baseline data were not available. They also noted that spontaneous variations in ECGs that were not caused by medication occurred over time. Such variations in QTc occur randomly with changes in the balance of sympathetic/parasympathetic input to the heart and possibly due to diurnal variations that have been reported in adults. The authors made the valuable suggestion that each subject's pre- and posttreatment ECGs should be recorded at the same time of day to minimize some of these possible confounding spontaneous variations. The authors concluded that clonidine alone or in combination with stimulants had no systematic cardiac effects on these behaviorally disturbed children, but that rare idiosyncratic responses could occur.

Guidelines for the Administration of CXR to Children and Adolescents

The dose of CXR, whether administered either as monotherapy or as adjunctive therapy to a psychostimulant, is the same. Dosing should be initiated with one 0.1-mg tablet at bedtime, and the daily dosage should be adjusted in increments of 0.1 mg/day at weekly intervals until the desired response is achieved. Doses should be taken twice a day, with either an equal or a higher split dosage being given at bedtime. Note that IR clonidine hydrochloride and CXR have different pharmacokinetic characteristics; dose substitution on a milligram-for-milligram basis will result in differences in exposure. A comparison across studies suggests that the C_{max} is 50% lower for CXR compared with IR clonidine hydrochloride.

Guidelines for the Administration of Clonidine Hydrochloride Immediate Release to Children and Adolescents

Hunt et al. (1990) recommend beginning clonidine administration with bedtime doses to utilize the usual initial sedative effect to facilitate sleep. Sedation is most severe during the first 2 to 4 weeks, after which tolerance usually develops (Hunt et al., 1991). Because of its short serum half-life, clonidine is sometimes administered three to four times daily and at bedtime. Hunt et al. have reported that some children have shown a loss of therapeutic effect or withdrawal symptoms when it is administered less frequently; CXR or transdermal patches eliminate this difficulty.

Cantwell et al. (1997) expressed additional concern about untoward effects and the lack of methodologically sound studies on using combined clonidine/stimulant treatment for behavioral disturbances in children. The following is a summary only of their suggested guidelines for clonidine:

- *Screening:* Preexisting cardiac or vascular disease is a contraindication for clonidine therapy for behavioral reasons. Sinus node and AV node disease and renal disease are relative contraindications.
- *Pulse and blood pressure:* Pulse rate and blood pressure should be obtained to provide a baseline, should be done weekly during titration, and should be repeated every 4 to 6 weeks on maintenance dosage. A thorough evaluation of "new-onset treatment-emergent" symptoms (especially if exercise-related) is essential.
- *ECG:* Baseline bradycardia or impaired AV conduction indicating first-degree, second-degree, or complete heart block or QRS interval >120 ms necessitates

cardiac consultation for medical clearance. Baseline ECG should be compared with an ECG recorded on full dose of clonidine.

- *Dose titration:* Clonidine should be titrated gradually and not exceed a 0.05-mg increment every 3 days. Medication termination should be by gradual tapering off of dose to minimize withdrawal effects.

Clonidine Administration with the Transdermal Therapeutic System

Hunt (1987) found that when transdermal patches were used in treating subjects diagnosed with ADHD, their efficacy wore off and that they had to be replaced in 50% of subjects after 5 days rather than the 7 days stated by the manufacturer. He also noted that, to achieve the same degree of symptom control, three of his eight subjects whose daily oral dose was 0.2 mg/day had to have their doses increased to 0.3 mg/day when clonidine was administered transdermally. Comings (1990), who has extensive clinical experience with patients with TS, stated that he found that clonidine administered using a patch may work even when oral clonidine is ineffective. Comings also found it convenient and useful to adjust the dose of clonidine by using scissors to cut the patch to the necessary size.

Indications for Clonidine Hydrochloride in Child and Adolescent Psychiatry

CXR (Kapvay) released in 2011 was the second alpha-2A-receptor agonist FDA indicated for the treatment of ADHD in children and adolescents aged 6 to 17 as monotherapy and as adjunctive therapy to stimulant medications. CXR was initially shown to be efficacious in the treatment of ADHD in two controlled trials (one monotherapy and one adjunctive to stimulant medication) in children and adolescents aged 6 to 17 who met DSM-IV criteria for ADHD hyperactive or combined hyperactive/inattentive subtypes. In the adjunctive study, CXR was administered to patients who had been on a stable regimen of either MPH or amphetamine (or their derivatives) and who had not achieved an optimal response. The effectiveness of CXR for longer term use (more than 5 weeks) has not been systematically evaluated in controlled trials.

Previously, clonidine IR had been investigated in many clinical studies for the treatment of children and adolescents diagnosed with ADHD and/or TS who have not responded to standard treatments for these disorders. Studies of these uses and the doses employed by the researchers are summarized later for each of these conditions.

CXR and Clonidine Discontinuation/Treatment Withdrawal

When discontinuing CXR, the total daily dose should be tapered in decrements of no more than 0.1 mg every 3 to 7 days.

IR clonidine should be gradually reduced over a period of 2 to 4 days to avoid a possible hypertensive reaction and other withdrawal symptomatology such as nervousness, agitation, and headache (package insert).

Clonidine Hydrochloride Dose Forms Available

- *CIR tablets (single scored):* 0.1, 0.2, and 0.3 mg
- *CXR tabs:* 0.1, 0.2 mg—tablets must be swallowed whole and never crushed, cut, or chewed.
- *Transdermal therapeutic system (TTS):* Programmed delivery by skin patch of 0.1 mg (Catapres-TTS 1), 0.2 mg (Catapres-TTS 2), or 0.3 mg daily (Catapres-TTS 3) for 1 week.

Safety and Efficacy Studies Involved in FDA Approval of CXR

Two placebo-controlled CXR ADHD clinical studies (Study 1 and Study 2) evaluated 256 patients who received active therapy with primary efficacy endpoints at 5 weeks.

Study 1: Fixed-Dose CXR Monotherapy

Study 1 was an 8-week, multicenter, randomized, double-blind, fixed-dose, placebo-controlled study. Its primary efficacy endpoint was at 5 weeks. The study examined two fixed doses (0.2 or 0.4 mg/day) of CXR in children and adolescents aged 6 to 17 ($N = 236$) who met DSM-IV criteria for ADHD (either hyperactive or combined inattentive/hyperactive subtypes). Patients were randomly assigned to one of the following three treatment groups: CXR 0.2 mg/day ($N = 78$), CXR 0.4 mg/day ($N = 80$), or placebo ($N = 78$).

Dosing for the CXR groups started at 0.1 mg/day and was titrated in increments of 0.1 mg/week to their respective dose (as divided doses). Patients were maintained at their dose for a minimum of 2 weeks before being gradually tapered down to 0.1 mg/day in the last week of treatment. At both doses, improvements in ADHD symptoms were superior in CXR-treated patients compared with placebo-treated patients at the end of 5 weeks as measured by the ADHDRS-IV total score.

Thirteen percent of patients receiving CXR discontinued from the study because of AEs, compared with 1% in the placebo group. The most common adverse reactions leading to discontinuation of CXR monotherapy–treated patients were somnolence/sedation (5%) and fatigue (4%).

Study 2: Flexible-Dose CXR as Adjunctive Therapy to a Psychostimulant

Study 2 was an 8-week, multicenter, randomized, double-blind, placebo-controlled study (with primary efficacy endpoint at 5 weeks). The study examined a flexible dose of CXR as adjunctive therapy to a psychostimulant in children and adolescents 6 to 17 years old ($N = 198$) who met DSM-IV criteria for ADHD (hyperactive or combined inattentive/hyperactive subtypes). Patients had been treated with a psychostimulant (MPH or amphetamine) for 4 weeks with inadequate response. Patients were randomly assigned to one of two treatment groups: CXR adjunct to a psychostimulant ($N = 102$) or psychostimulant alone ($N = 96$). The CXR dose was initiated at 0.1 mg/day, and doses were titrated in increments of 0.1 mg/week up to 0.4 mg/day, as divided doses, over a 3-week period depending on tolerability and clinical response. The dose was maintained for a minimum of 2 weeks before being gradually tapered to 0.1 mg/day in the last week of treatment. ADHD symptoms were statistically significantly improved in CXR plus stimulant group compared with the stimulant-alone group at the end of 5 weeks as measured by the ADHD-RS-IV total score.

In Study 2, the most common adverse reactions (defined as events that were reported in at least 5% of medication-treated patients and at least twice the rate as in placebo patients) during the treatment period were somnolence, fatigue, upper respiratory tract infection, irritability, throat pain, insomnia, nightmares, emotional disorder, constipation, nasal congestion, increased body temperature, dry mouth, and ear pain. The most common adverse reactions reported during the taper phase were upper abdominal pain and gastrointestinal virus.

In both of the studies, CXR treatment was not associated with any clinically important effects on any laboratory parameters. Mean decreases in blood pressure and heart rate were seen (see "Warnings and Precautions"). There were no changes on ECGs to suggest a medication-related effect.

Reports of Interest

Clonidine Immediate Release in the Treatment of ADHD

Hunt et al. (1982) reported on an open pilot study in which clonidine 3 to 4 µg/kg/day was administered orally for 2 to 5 months to four children between 9 and 14 years of age diagnosed with ADDH. Improvement was noted by parents and teachers. The authors noted that distractibility often persisted, but that the children were nevertheless more able to return to tasks and complete them.

Hunt et al. (1985) later conducted a double-blind, placebo-controlled crossover study of 12 children (mean age, 11.6 ± 0.54 years) who were diagnosed with ADDH. Ten children completed the study. Seven subjects had previously received stimulant medication; in four cases, stimulants had been discontinued because of significant untoward effects. Clonidine was begun at 0.05 mg and increased every other day until a dose of 4 to 5 µg/kg/day (approximately 0.05 mg four times daily) was attained. Parents, teachers, and clinicians all noted statistically significant improvements on clonidine for the group as a whole. The best responders were children who had been overactive and who were uninhibited and impulsive, which, in turn, had impaired their opportunities to use their basically intact capacities for social relatedness and purposeful activity. During the placebo period, parents, teachers, and clinicians noted significant deterioration in overall behavior for the group, with symptoms usually returning between 2 and 4 days after discontinuing the medication (Hunt et al., 1985).

The most frequent untoward effect seen in this study was sedation (occurring approximately 1 hour after ingestion and lasting 30 to 60 minutes). In all but one case, tolerance to this effect developed within 3 weeks. Mean blood pressure also decreased approximately 10%.

Hunt et al. (1990, 1991) have reported that children diagnosed with ADHD and treated with clonidine have been maintained on the same dose for up to 5 years without diminution of clinical efficacy. However, approximately 20% of such children require an increase in dose after several months of treatment, probably secondary to autoinduction of hepatic enzymes (Hunt et al., 1990).

Hunt (1987) compared the efficacies of clonidine (administered both orally and transdermally) and MPH in an open study of 10 children diagnosed with ADDH, all of whom had ratings by both parents and teachers of >1.5 SD above normal on Conners Behavioral Rating Scales. Eight subjects (seven males, one female; mean age, 11.4 ± 0.6 years; range, 6.7 to 14.4 years) completed the protocol. Subjects received either placebo, low-dose (0.3 mg/kg) MPH, or high-dose (0.6 mg/kg) MPH. Each of these conditions was randomized for a period of 1 week. All subjects then received an open trial of clonidine 5 µg/kg/day administered orally for 8 weeks. Eight subjects completed the open trial with positive results and were then switched from tablets to transdermal clonidine skin patch. Both clonidine and MPH were significantly more effective than placebo, and clonidine in both dosage forms was as effective as MPH (Hunt, 1987). Children reported that they felt more "normal" on clonidine than on MPH. Transdermal administration was preferred to oral administration by 75% of the children and their families, not only because the embarrassment of taking pills at school was avoided but also because it was more convenient. Skin patches caused localized contact dermatitis (usually presenting with itching and erythema) in approximately 40% of children and at times this limited their usefulness (Hunt et al., 1990).

Hunt (1987) noted that in contrast to the stimulants, clonidine appears to increase frustration tolerance, but does not decrease distractibility. He noted that an additional small dose of MPH may be safely added to help focus attention, and added that this combination frequently permits a much lower dose of MPH than would be required if it were the only medication used (Hunt, 1987).

In a review of clonidine use in child and adolescent psychiatry, Hunt et al. (1990) explained more specifically the differences between clonidine and MPH in treating ADHD and their possible synergistic use in treating ADHD. Stimulants (MPH) improve attentional focusing and decrease distractibility, whereas clonidine decreases hyperarousal and increases frustration tolerance and task orientation.

The authors found that children with ADHD who respond best to clonidine often have an early onset of symptoms, are extremely energetic or hyperactive (hyperaroused), and have a concomitant diagnosis of conduct disorder or oppositional disorder. Such children often respond to clonidine treatment with increased frustration tolerance and consequent improvement in task-orientated behavior; more effort, compliance, and cooperativeness; and better learning capacity and achievement. Clonidine was also efficacious in nonpsychotic inpatient adolescents with ADHD who were aggressive and hyperaroused (Hunt et al., 1990).

Unlike stimulants, clonidine in the original studies did not seem to directly improve distractibility; hence, stimulants were recommended preferable to IR clonidine for children with mild to moderate hyperactivity who had significant deficits in distractibility and attentional focus. The combination of clonidine and MPH was found to be helpful for children who were diagnosed with coexisting conduct or oppositional disorder and ADHD and who had both high arousal and were very distractible (Hunt et al., 1990). The combined use of these medications may permit the effective dose of MPH to be reduced by approximately 40%, making it potentially useful for patients with ADHD in whom significant motor hyperactivity persists, or in whom rebound symptoms or dose-limiting side effects such as aggression, irritability, insomnia, or decrements in weight or height gain have occurred with stimulant treatment (Hunt et al., 1990).

Steingard et al. (1993) published a retrospective chart review of 54 patients (age range, 3 to 18 years; mean, 10.0 ± 0.5 years) who were diagnosed with ADHD-only ($N = 30$) or ADHD and comorbid tic disorder ($N = 24$) and treated with clonidine. Clonidine was initiated at a low dose and titrated upward until a positive clinical result occurred or untoward effects prevented further increase. Mean optimal daily dose for all subjects was 0.19 ± 0.02 mg/day (range, 0.025 to 0.6 mg/day). There was no significant difference in mean daily dose between subjects with and without tics, responders and nonresponders, or subjects less and more than 12 years of age. Although 72% (39) of 54 subjects were rated as improved on the Clinical Global Improvement Scale subset of items for ADHD symptoms, a significantly greater proportion ($P = .0005$) of subjects with a comorbid tic disorder (23 [96%] of 24) improved than did subjects with ADHD-only (16 [53%] of 30). On Clinical Global Improvement Scale items pertinent to tics, 75% (18 of 24) showed improvement.

At present, clonidine immediate release may be regarded as a possible alternative monotherapy treatment for ADHD or as an adjunct. It may eventually prove useful in treating, in particular, a subgroup of children with ADHD who do not respond well to stimulants. Clonidine may also be a useful alternative treatment for some children with ADHD who have chronic tics or who develop side effects of sufficient severity as to preclude the use of stimulants (Hunt et al., 1985; Steingard et al., 1993).

Connor et al. (1999) reviewed the literature from 1980 to 1999 on the use of clonidine in the treatment of ADHD with and without comorbid diagnoses of conduct disorder, tic disorder, or developmental delay. Eleven of the 39 reports provided data sufficient to be used in a meta-analysis. The authors reported the overall effect size of clonidine for symptoms of ADHD to be moderate. It was similar to the effect size for TCAs but less than the large effect size for stimulants. The authors concluded that clonidine in doses of 0.1 to 0.3 mg/day was moderately effective in ameliorating common symptoms of ADHD and should be considered as a second-tier treatment. They also noted that clonidine's use is associated with many untoward effects, in particular, sedation, irritability, and, when administered by transdermal patch, skin irritation and rash.

Clonidine in the Treatment of Sleep Disturbances in Children and Adolescents Diagnosed with ADHD

Wilens et al. (1994) reported their experience in using the sedation that clonidine often produces to treat more than 100 patients diagnosed with ADHD who also had spontaneous or medication-induced sleep difficulties. The effect has allowed some children who responded very well to stimulants, but who could not tolerate them because of significant insomnia to be treated successfully with them. Typically, an initial dose of 0.05 mg of clonidine for patients between 4 and 17 years of age was given about half an hour before bedtime and was increased by 0.05-mg increments to a maximum of 0.4 mg. A few very young or underweight children required only 0.025 mg, whereas a few other children required >0.4 mg. Patients and parents reported better sleep, and there were decreased familial conflicts around sleep activities and fewer ADHD-like symptoms after treatment. Some of the latter improvement is likely to result from the fact that clonidine is also effective in treating ADHD independent of its sleep-enhancing qualities. Clonidine should be tapered gradually when it is discontinued, even if it is used only at night for insomnia.

Clonidine in the Treatment of Chronic Severe Aggressiveness

Kemph et al. (1993) treated openly with clonidine 17 outpatients (14 males and 3 females; age range, 5 to 15 years old; mean age, 10.1 years) diagnosed with conduct disorder or ODD. All subjects had a history of chronic and violent aggressiveness in multiple settings that had not responded to behavioral management. Clonidine was begun at an initial dose of 0.05 mg/day. After 2 days, it was increased to 0.05 mg twice daily, and on day 5 it was increased to 0.05 mg three times daily, following which it was titrated as clinically indicated on an individual basis. The maximum effective dose was 0.4 mg daily administered in divided doses. A comparison of mean baseline and follow-up scores on the Rating of Aggression against People and/or Property Scale showed significant improvement on medication ($P < .0001$). Drowsiness was the major untoward effect most frequently reported (usually occurring during the first weeks of treatment), and most patients developed tolerance to it. There were no significant changes in blood pressure or cardiovascular parameters. The authors noted that plasma gamma-aminobutyric acid (GABA) levels increased significantly ($P < .01$) in five of the six children for whom it was available at follow-up, suggesting that GABA plasma levels may be correlated with childhood aggressiveness and may also be useful to verify adherence. Clonidine may be a useful agent in the control of aggression in children and adolescents and merits further study.

Clonidine in the Treatment of ASD Accompanied by Inattention, Impulsivity, and Hyperactivity

Jaselskis et al. (1992) treated eight males (age range, 5.0 to 13.4 years; mean, 8.1 ± 2.8 years) diagnosed with ASD who also had significant inattention, impulsivity, and hyperactivity who had not responded to prior psychopharmacotherapy (e.g., MPH or desipramine). These patients received clonidine in a double-blind, placebo-controlled, crossover protocol. Clonidine or placebo was titrated over the initial 2 weeks to a daily total of 4 to 10 µg/kg/day (0.15 to 0.20 mg/day) divided into three doses; this regimen was maintained for the next 4 weeks. During the seventh week, subjects were tapered off clonidine or placebo. At week 8, subjects were crossed over to the other condition for 6 weeks. Parents' ratings on the Conners Abbreviated Parent–Teacher Questionnaire showed significant improvement while their children were on clonidine. Teachers' ratings on the ABC were significantly better during clonidine treatment for irritability ($P = .03$), hyperactivity ($P = .03$), stereotypy ($P = .05$), and inappropriate speech ($P = .05$). ADDH: Comprehensive Teacher's Rating Scale scores improved significantly only for oppositional behavior ($P = .05$). Although significant, improvement was modest. Clinician ratings at the end of each 6-week period showed no significant differences between clonidine and placebo. Untoward effects included significant drowsiness and hypotension requiring reduction of dosage in three subjects.

Clonidine in the Treatment of Tourette Syndrome

Cohen et al. (1980) reported that clonidine was clinically effective in at least 70% of 25 patients between 9 and 50 years of age diagnosed with TS who either did not benefit from haloperidol or could not tolerate the untoward effects of that medication. Dosage was begun at 1 to 2 µg/kg/day (usually 0.05 mg/day) and gradually titrated up to a maximum of 0.6 mg/day. Most patients did best with small doses three to four times daily. Comings (1990) recommended a starting dose of 0.025 mg/day (one-fourth of a tablet) and sometimes found it necessary to administer as many as five divided doses daily for best results. He found it to be an excellent medication for the approximately 60% of his patients who responded, and noted that it ameliorated oppositional, confrontational, and obsessive-compulsive behaviors and symptoms of ADHD when these were also present. In contrast, Shapiro and Shapiro (1989) noted that, in their experience, clonidine was only rarely effective in treating unselected patients with tics and TS.

Cohen et al. (1980) delineated five phases of treatment response to clonidine:

Phase I: Within hours or days, patients felt calmer, less angry, and more in control.

Phase II: Approximately 3 to 4 weeks after initiation of clonidine (usually coinciding with a therapeutic dose of 3 to 4 µg/kg/day [0.15 mg/day]), the patient recognized progressive benefits characterized by decreased compulsive behavior, further behavioral control, and decreased phonic and motor tics.

Phase III: A plateauing of improvement started at about the third month.

Phase IV: Five or more months after beginning, an increase in dosage up to 4 to 6 µg/kg/day (0.3 mg/day) of clonidine was needed to maintain clinical improvement.

Phase V: Further tolerance to clonidine may occur at a dose considered too high to increase further.

Leckman et al. (1991) reported a 12-week, double-blind, placebo-controlled trial of clonidine completed by 40 subjects (age range, 7 to 48 years; mean, 15.6 ± 10.4 years; 31 of the subjects were younger than 18 years) diagnosed with TS. Clonidine was titrated gradually during the first 2 weeks to a total daily dose of 4 to 5 µg/kg/day (maximum, 0.25 mg/day) and administered in two to four divided doses per day, depending on the total dose. Mean clonidine dose at the end of the 12 weeks for the 21 subjects randomly assigned to clonidine was 4.4 ± 0.7 µg/kg/day (range, 3.2 to 5.7 µg/kg/day). Clonidine serum levels (available for 19 subjects) ranged from 0.24 to 1.0 ng/mL, with a mean of 0.48 ± 0.23 ng/mL. Subjects receiving clonidine were rated as significantly more improved than those receiving placebo: on the Tourette Syndrome Global Scale for motor tics ($P = .008$) and total score ($P = .05$); on the anchored Clinical Global Impressions Scale for TS (TS-CGI); on the Shapiro Tourette Severity Symptom Scale for decrease in "tics noticeable to others"; and on the Conners Parent Questionnaire for total score ($P = .02$) and the impulsive/hyperactive factor ($P = .01$). Untoward effects most frequently reported were sedation/fatigue (90%), dry mouth (57%), faintness/dizziness (43%), and irritability (33%). Although clonidine is not as effective in controlling tic behavior as the D_2-dopamine receptor-blocking agents, haloperidol, aripiprazole, and pimozide, its more favorable untoward-effect profile should prompt the clinician to consider a trial of clonidine (or guanfacine) before using antipsychotic medications in milder cases (Leckman et al., 1991).

Bruun (1983) has provided useful guidelines for prescribing clonidine for TS. She suggests initiating daily dosage at 0.025 mg twice daily for small children and at 0.05 mg twice daily for older children and adolescents. Medication is titrated upward gradually, with increases of no greater than 0.05 mg/week; this slow pace often prevents untoward effects from interfering with the treatment. The usual optimal daily dose is between 0.25 and 0.45 mg. Doses above 0.5 mg/day may be required, but untoward effects (e.g., drowsiness, fatigue, dizziness, headache, insomnia, and increased irritability) become more troublesome. Bruun (1983) noted that drowsiness may occur at very low doses, and suggested that no further increases in dosage be made until the drowsiness subsides. Some patients note a decrease in beneficial effects 4 to 5 hours after their last dose, and treatment is usually more effective for all patients with total daily dosage administered in three or four smaller doses (Bruun, 1983).

Although presently not an approved treatment, there is evidence that some children and adolescents with TS respond favorably with significant symptom reduction when treated with clonidine. Clonidine may be regarded as a possible treatment for those youngsters with TS who have not responded satisfactorily or who have intolerable untoward effects to standard treatments.

Clonidine in the Treatment of Children Who Stutter

Althaus et al. (1995) reported that clonidine was *not effective* in the treatment of 25 children 6 to 13 years of age diagnosed with stuttering by DSM-III-R (APA, 1987) criteria. In a 28-week, double-blind, placebo-controlled crossover study, medication or placebo was gradually increased for 1 week, followed by maintenance for 8 weeks; dosage was then tapered for 4 days followed by 4.5 weeks of washout before beginning the other condition or at the end of the study before the final ratings. Clonidine was given in a total dose of 4 µg/kg/day divided into three equal portions over the day. Efficacy was determined by ratings of repetitions, prolongations, blockades, and interjections at baseline, before first dose reduction, after first washout period, before second dose reduction, and after the final washout. There was no significant improvement in any of the measures used. Parents and teachers also rated no significant difference between placebo and clonidine and improvement of children's stuttering, but they did notice significant behavioral improvements in hyperactivity, task orientation, and greater approachability. The authors concluded that clonidine was not a useful medication for treating children diagnosed with stuttering.

Guanfacine Hydrochloride

Guanfacine hydrochloride is a centrally acting antihypertensive agent, and the extended-release formulation (Intuniv) has FDA approval for the treatment of ADHD. The only other FDA-approved indication for guanfacine hydrochloride is the treatment of hypertension. Guanfacine is not a CNS stimulant, and it therefore has no known potential for abuse.

Since Guanfacine extended release (GXR) is the only FDA-approved formulation of guanfacine for pediatric ADHD, it is highlighted and preferentially discussed versus the guanfacine immediate-release (GIR) formulation, which is not FDA approved for the treatment of ADHD. It is important to note that both GXR (Intuniv) and (GIR) Tenex have been shown to often be useful in the treatment of ADHD. Both GXR and GIR are also sometimes prescribed off-label for the treatment of anxiety, tics, and aggression.

Although both guanfacine and clonidine are alpha-2 agonists, guanfacine acts as a selective alpha-2A-adrenergic receptor agonist that has a 15 to 20 times higher affinity for this receptor subtype than for the alpha-2B or alpha-2C subtypes (compared with clonidine affinities). Guanfacine and clonidine may be similar in many ways, but there is one notable difference: clonidine is known to be more sedating than guanfacine, and this can be useful when considering which agent to use for a child who has both ADHD and insomnia.

Guanfacine Extended-Release (Intuniv)

Although GIR may be administered two or three times per day, GXR is a once-daily, extended-release formulation of guanfacine hydrochloride (HCl) in a matrix tablet formulation. Intuniv, released in 2009, was the first alpha-2A-receptor agonist FDA indicated for the treatment of ADHD in children and adolescents ages 6 to 17. The efficacy of GXR tablets as a monotherapy treatment for ADHD was first based on results of two 8- to 9-week studies in children and adolescents aged 6 to 17. In 2011, GXR tablets received additional FDA approval as adjunctive therapy to stimulant medications in 6- to 17-year-olds with ADHD who had a suboptimal response to stimulant monotherapy based on a 9-week trial.

Guanfacine Pharmacokinetics

In vitro studies with human liver microsomes and recombinant CYPs demonstrated that guanfacine was primarily metabolized by CYP3A4. In pooled human hepatic microsomes, guanfacine did not inhibit the activities of the major cytochrome P450 isoenzymes (CYP1A2, CYP2C8, CYP2C9, CYP2C19, CYP2D6, or CYP3A4/5).

Guanfacine is a substrate of CYP3A4/5 and exposure is affected by CYP3A4/5 inducers/inhibitors.

GXR tablets were developed with rate-limiting excipients in its matrix to slow guanfacine absorption, thereby reducing the peak-to-trough fluctuations (Shojaei et al., 2006). Peak plasma levels occur from 4 to 8 hours (mean, 6 hours) after ingestion. Average plasma half-life is approximately 18 ± 4 hours. However, younger subjects tend to metabolize GIR more rapidly. The long-acting formulation of guanfacine results in a much lower (60%) C_{max} (ng/mL) of 1.0 versus 2.5 for GIR and thus provides a slower rise to maximum concentration compared with GIR. Steady-state blood levels usually occur within 4 days. GXR is a unique formulation of guanfacine; therefore, one cannot substitute for GIR tablets on a milligram-for-milligram basis because of the differing pharmacokinetic profiles. Guanfacine and its metabolites are excreted primarily by the kidneys.

Contraindications for Guanfacine Hydrochloride Administration

GXR tablets should not be used in patients with a history of hypersensitivity to guanfacine or any of its inactive ingredients or by patients taking other products containing guanfacine.

Interactions of Guanfacine Hydrochloride with Other Medications

The depressive effects of alcohol, barbiturates, and other medications and illicit drugs on the CNS may be enhanced by simultaneous administration of guanfacine. Interactions with additional medications have been reported.

Untoward Effects of Guanfacine Hydrochloride

Untoward effects include those typical of the central alpha-2-adrenoreceptor agonists such as dry mouth, sedation, fatigue, dizziness, low blood pressure, constipation, weakness/asthenia, irritability, and upper abdominal pain. Most are mild and transient if treatment is continued. Adverse reactions in GXR studies 301 and 304 that were dose related include somnolence, abdominal pain, dizziness, hypotension/decreased blood pressure, dry mouth, and constipation.

Horrigan and Barnhill (1998) reported five cases in which intense activation with a cluster of signs and symptoms resembling an acute-onset manic episode occurred within 3 days of the administration of guanfacine (GIR). These cases were from a series of 95 outpatients who were treated with guanfacine (GIR) during a 12-month period. However, it should be noted that all five patients were reported to have personal and family risk factors for bipolar disorder.

Indications for Guanfacine Hydrochloride in Child and Adolescent Psychiatry

Intuniv, released in 2009, was the first alpha-2A-receptor agonist FDA indicated for the treatment of ADHD in children and adolescents aged 6 to 17.

Hirota et al. (2014) conducted a meta-analysis of studies examining the efficacy of alpha-2 agonists in the treatment of attention-deficit/hyperactivity disorder in youth. They reviewed 12 studies ($N = 2,276$), and they concluded that monotherapy and (possibly to a lesser extent) co-treatment were significantly superior to placebo in the treatment of hyperactivity and inattention, but they noted that a risk/benefit analysis should acknowledge potential side effects that include fatigue, somnolence, hypotension, bradycardia, and possible QTc prolongation.

GXR Tablet Dosage Schedule

GXR is an extended-release tablet and should be dosed once daily. Tablets should not be crushed, chewed, or broken before swallowing because this will increase the rate of guanfacine release. Prescribing instructions advise to not administer with high-fat meals (C_{max} approximately 75% and AUC approximately 40%). One

(continued)

Indications for Guanfacine Hydrochloride in Child and Adolescent Psychiatry (*continued*)

cannot substitute GXR for GIR tablets on a milligram-for-milligram basis because of differing pharmacokinetic profiles. It is recommended to begin at a dose of 1 mg/day and adjust in increments of no more than 1 mg/week. The dose is recommended to be kept within the studied range of 1 to 4 mg once daily, depending on clinical response and tolerability. In the initial clinical trials, patients were randomized to doses of 1, 2, 3, or 4 mg and received GXR once daily in the morning when used as monotherapy. Later adjunctive therapy studies demonstrated the efficacy of GXR when dosed either in the morning or evening when combined with stimulant therapy dosed in the morning.

In the monotherapy studies, clinically relevant improvements were observed beginning at doses in the range of 0.05 to 0.08 mg/kg once daily. Efficacy increased with increasing weight-adjusted dose (mg/kg). If well tolerated, doses up to 0.12 mg/kg once daily seemed to provide additional benefit. Dosages above 4 mg/day have been found to be helpful for some patients including up to 7 mg/day for patients weighing at least 58.5 kg.

GIR Dosage Schedule

- *Children up to 11 years of age:* Not recommended. Efficacy and safety have not been established in this age group. Hunt et al. (1995) conducted a study where they initiated guanfacine at a dose of 0.5 mg/day and, on the basis of clinical response, individually titrated guanfacine in 0.5-mg increments every 3 days to a maximum of 4 mg/day, which appears to be appropriate in the treatment of ADHD in this age group.
- *Adolescents ≥ 12 years of age and adults:* For the treatment of hypertension, an initial dose of 1 mg at bedtime is recommended to minimize the impact of any initial sedation that may occur. If clinically indicated, higher doses may be administered.

Medication Interactions

Coadministration of guanfacine and valproic acid can result in increased concentrations of valproic acid. Both guanfacine (via a phase I metabolite, 3-hydroxy guanfacine) and valproic acid are metabolized by glucuronidation, possibly resulting in competitive inhibition. In such cases, patients should be monitored for potential additive CNS effects and consideration given to monitoring serum valproic acid concentrations. Adjustments in the dose of valproic acid may be indicated when coadministered with guanfacine.

It is recommended to use caution when guanfacine is administered to patients taking ketoconazole and other strong CYP3A4/5 inhibitors, because elevation of plasma guanfacine concentrations increases the risk of AEs such as hypotension, bradycardia, and sedation.

When patients are taking guanfacine concomitantly with a CYP3A4 inducer such as rifampin, an increase in the dose of guanfacine within the recommended dose range may be indicated and considered.

Guanfacine Discontinuation/Treatment Withdrawal

Because of possible rebound phenomena, including nervousness and anxiety (from relative increases in catecholamines) and increases in blood pressure to over baseline, GIR should be tapered gradually when discontinued. When discontinuing GXR formulations, it is recommended to taper the dose in decrements of no more than 1 mg every 3 to 7 days. Owing to guanfacine's relatively long half-life, if rebound is to occur, it usually does so 2 to 4 days after abrupt withdrawal. Although rebound hypertension can occur, it is infrequent and blood pressure usually returns to pretreatment levels over 2 to 4 days.

GXR Dose Forms Available

- *Extended-release tablets:* 1, 2, 3, and 4 mg

Guanfacine Hydrochloride (GIR) Dose Forms Available

Tablets: 1 and 2 mg

CLINICAL STUDIES

Safety and Efficacy Studies Involved in FDA Approval of GXR

Studies 1 and 2: Fixed-Dose GXR Monotherapy

The efficacy of GXR in the treatment of ADHD was established in two placebo-controlled trials in children and adolescents aged 6 to 17 years. Study 1 evaluated 2, 3, and 4 mg of GXR dosed once daily in an 8-week, double-blind, placebo-controlled, parallel-group, fixed-dose design (N = 345). Study 2 evaluated 1, 2, 3, and 4 mg of GXR that was dosed once daily in a 9-week, double-blind, placebo-controlled, parallel-group, fixed-dose design ($N = 324$). In both Studies 1 and 2, patients were randomized to a fixed dose of GXR. Doses were titrated in increments of up to 1 mg/week. The lowest dose of 1 mg used in Study 2 was assigned only to patients <50 kg (110 lb). Patients who weighed <25 kg (55 lb) were not included in either study.

Signs and symptoms of ADHD were evaluated on a once-weekly basis using the clinician-administered and scored ADHD-RS–IV, which includes both hyperactive/impulsive and inattentive subscales. In both studies, the primary outcome was the change from baseline to endpoint in mean ADHD-RS scores.

The mean reductions in ADHD-RS scores at endpoint were statistically significantly greater for GXR compared with placebo for Studies 1 and 2. Placebo-adjusted changes from baseline were statistically significant for each of the 2-, 3-, and 4-mg GXR randomized treatment groups in both studies, as well as the 1-mg GXR treatment group (for patients 55 to 110 lb) that was included only in Study 2.

Interestingly, dose-responsive efficacy was evident (particularly when data were examined on a weight-adjusted [milligram/kilogram] basis). When evaluated over the dose range of 0.01 to 0.17 mg/kg/day, clinically relevant improvements were observed beginning at doses in the range 0.05 to 0.08 mg/kg/day. Doses up to 0.12 mg/kg/day were shown to provide additional benefit and some clinicians consider this to be a "sweet spot" for dosing, but each patient must be individualized on a risk/benefit ratio.

Subgroup analyses were performed to identify any differences in response depending on gender or age (6 to 12 vs. 13 to 17). Analyses of the primary outcome did not suggest any differential responsiveness on the basis of gender. Analyses by age subgroup revealed a statistically significant treatment effect only in the age 6 to 12 subgroup. Owing to the relatively small proportion of adolescent patients (ages 13 to 17) enrolled into these studies (approximately 25%), these data may not be sufficient to demonstrate efficacy in the adolescent subgroup. In these studies, patients were randomized to a fixed dose of Intuniv rather than optimized by body weight. Therefore, it is likely that some adolescent patients were randomized to a dose that resulted in relatively low plasma guanfacine concentrations compared with the younger subgroup. More than half (55%) of the adolescent patients received doses of 0.01 to 0.04 mg/kg.

In studies in which systematic pharmacokinetic data were obtained, there was a strong inverse correlation between body weight and plasma guanfacine concentrations.

Study 3: Flexible-Dose GXR as Adjunctive Therapy to Psychostimulants

Study 3 (PDR) evaluated 1, 2, 3, and 4 mg of Intuniv dosed once daily in a 9-week, double-blind, placebo-controlled, dose-optimization study. This study evaluated the safety and efficacy of GXR (dosed either in the morning or in the evening) compared with placebo, when given in combination with a psychostimulant, in children and adolescents aged 6 to 17 years with a diagnosis of ADHD who had a suboptimal response to stimulants ($N = 455$). Subjects were started at the 1-mg GXR dose level and were titrated weekly over a 5-week dose-optimization period to an optimal GXR dose (not to exceed 4 mg/day) depending on tolerability and clinical response. The dose was then maintained for a 3-week dose-maintenance period before entry to 1 week of dose tapering. Subjects took GXR either in the morning or in the evening while maintaining their current dose of psychostimulant treatment given each morning. Allowable psychostimulants in the study were Adderall XR, Vyvanse, Concerta, Focalin XR, Ritalin LA, Metadate CD, or the FDA-approved generic equivalents.

Symptoms of ADHD were evaluated on a weekly basis by clinicians using the ADHD-RS-IV, which includes both hyperactive/impulsive and inattentive subscales. The primary efficacy outcome was the change from baseline to endpoint in ADHD-RS-IV total scores. Endpoint was defined as the last post-randomization treatment week before dose tapering for which a valid score was obtained (up to week 8).

Mean reductions in ADHD-RS-IV total scores at endpoint were significantly greater for GXR given in combination with a psychostimulant compared with placebo given with a psychostimulant for Study 3, for both morning and evening GXR dosing. Nearly two-thirds (64.2%) of the subjects reached optimal doses in the 0.05 to 0.12 mg/kg/day range.

Controlled adjunctive long-term efficacy studies (>9 weeks) have not been conducted.

Pearls

Study 3 was a dose-optimization study and thus theoretically more clinically relevant to actual prescribing practices. Although previous experience with short-acting alpha-2 agonists led many clinicians to perceive guanfacine and clonidine as primarily useful for hyperactive and emotional impulsivity/anger features of ADHD, Study 3 seemed to demonstrate that GXR was beneficial for both hyperactive and inattentive symptoms of ADHD. This adjunctive medication study also indicated that the combination of stimulant and GXR was more efficacious than each agent given alone. GXR appeared to have very similar efficacy whether dosed in the morning or in the evening. The fact that evening dosing is effective is useful as one of the more common dose related side effects of GXR is sedation, which may allow sleep-onset complaints by patients to be addressed successfully utilizing evening administration of GXR. Although GXR is only FDA approved for once-a-day dosing, clinicians sometimes utilize bid dosing to address efficacy issues or side-effect issues such as daytime sedation.

Reports of Interest Using GIR Tablets

Guanfacine in the Treatment of ADHD

Guanfacine appears to have potential advantages over clonidine in the treatment of ADHD because it has both a longer plasma half-life and it appears to be less sedating than clonidine (Hunt et al., 1995).

Hunt et al. (1995) treated 13 subjects (11 males and 2 females; age range, 4 to 20 years; mean, 11.1 years) who were diagnosed with ADHD. They were treated with guanfacine at a start dose of 0.5 mg/day and individually titrated by 0.5-mg increments every 3 days to achieve optimal clinical response to a maximum of 4 mg/day. Mean therapeutic dose was 3.2 mg/day (0.091 mg/kg/day). Medication was usually administered in four divided doses (with the morning, noon, and approximately 4:00 PM doses being somewhat less than the bedtime dose). Parental ratings on the Conners 31-item Parent Questionnaire at baseline and after 1 month of treatment with guanfacine showed a significant improvement on guanfacine in total average score ($P < .015$). Headaches and stomachaches were reported by approximately 25% of subjects, but resolved within 2 weeks except in one patient. Decreased appetite occurred initially in 16% of the subjects, but stabilized within 2 weeks. No subject had clinically significant changes in blood pressure.

Guanfacine in the Treatment of ADHD and Tics and/or Tourette Syndrome

Chappell et al. (1995) reported an open study of 10 subjects (aged 8 to 16 years) who were diagnosed with ADHD and TS and treated with guanfacine. Two subjects received other psychoactive medications concurrently. An initial bedtime dose of 0.5 mg of guanfacine was titrated upward in 0.5-mg increments every 3 to 4 days and was given in two or three divided doses. Daily doses ranged from 0.75 to 3 mg; optimal daily dose was 1.5 mg for seven of the subjects. Although analysis of the group data did not show significant improvement in ADHD symptoms, three subjects had moderate and one had marked improvement based on ratings on the 48-item CPRS. Group means measuring the severity of motor and phonic tics decreased in ratings by clinicians and patients themselves. The most common untoward effects were lethargy or fatigue (60%), headache (40%), insomnia (30%), and dizziness or lightheadedness (20%); these symptoms usually remitted over 3 to 4 days. No child experienced clinically significant exacerbation of tics. Guanfacine may be a useful medication for some children and adolescents who have comorbid ADHD and a chronic tic disorder.

Horrigan and Barnhill (1995) administered guanfacine to 15 treatment-resistant boys (age range, 7 to 17 years; mean, 13.3 years) diagnosed with ADHD. Most subjects also were diagnosed with comorbid psychiatric disorders, including TS ($N = 8$) and specific developmental disorders ($N = 11$). Subjects failed to respond satisfactorily to a mean of 2.0 prior medications, including dextroamphetamine, MPH, clonidine, imipramine, fluoxetine, carbamazepine, lithium, haloperidol, thyroid hormone, tryptophan, and biotin. Guanfacine was initiated with a 0.5-mg dose at bedtime and increased every 5 to 7 days by 0.25- to 0.5-mg increments as clinically indicated. Because the pediatric population metabolizes guanfacine more rapidly than do adults, it was administered in two divided doses. After 10 weeks, the range of optimal doses was from 0.5 mg to 3 mg/day (with 0.5 mg twice daily being the most frequent optimal dose). Thirteen subjects received guanfacine only; 1 subject additionally received lithium carbonate 1,800 mg/day, and another received fluoxetine 10 mg/day.

Overall, guanfacine produced a significant clinical response in the patients with ADHD and these comorbidities. Parental ratings (made 4 to 8 weeks after the dose was stabilized on the 13 subjects who completed the study) showed decreases on the Conners Parent–Teacher Scale (short form) of 11.1 points (from 19.9 to 8.8); on the Edelbrock CAP Inattention Subscale of 4.85 points; and on the Edelbrock CAP Overactivity Subscale of 3.23. The authors noted that the greater improvement in inattention compared with overactivity is the opposite of the pattern often seen with clonidine; they thought that this reversal might be explained by guanfacine having a greater affinity for alpha-2 adrenoreceptors in the prefrontal areas compared with clonidine having a greater affinity for the alpha-2 adrenoreceptors in more basal regions (Horrigan & Barnhill, 1995). One subject did not complete the trial because his mother discontinued the medication citing lack of improvement and another because he developed symptoms of overactivation/overarousal. The only other untoward effects noted were initial mild sedation in five boys. No patient experienced a significant change in blood pressure or pulse.

Scahill et al. (2000) conducted an 8-week, randomized, double-blind, placebo-controlled trial of guanfacine in the treatment of 34 subjects (31 males, 3 females; mean age, 10.4 ± 2.01 years; age range, 7 to 14 years) diagnosed with ADHD and either comorbid TS ($N = 20$), chronic motor tic disorder ($N = 12$), or stimulant-induced tic disorder ($N = 2$). Eleven subjects (32%) were medication naive; 19 of the other 23 subjects who had previous trials on at least one stimulant medication had experienced worsening of tics on stimulants. Subjects were assigned randomly to guanfacine ($N = 14$) or placebo ($N = 14$). Efficacy was determined by ratings on the DuPaul ADHD Rating Scale (Teacher), the CGI-I Scale (CGI-I), the Total Tic Score of the Yale Global Tic Severity Scale (YGTSS), and the HI of the Parent Conners. On the CGI-I, nine subjects receiving guanfacine were rated 1 ("very much improved") or 2 ("much improved") at endpoint compared with no such ratings on placebo ($P < .001$). Subjects on guanfacine improved by 38% on the ADHD-RS versus only 8% improvement for subjects on placebo ($P < .001$). Total Tic Score on the YGTSS for subjects on guanfacine decreased by 30% versus no change in the placebo group ($P < .05$). There was no significant difference between placebo and guanfacine on HI scores. There were no clinically significant changes in pulse or blood pressure; one subject on guanfacine discontinued the study after 4 weeks because of sedation.

Other Non-approved FDA Medications/Substances Used for Enhancement of Frontal Lobe Executive Function in Child and Adolescent Psychiatry

Bupropion (Wellbutrin, Wellbutrin SR, Wellbutrin XL)

Bupropion is a medication with FDA approval for the treatment of MDD in adults, but it is also used off-label for the treatment of MDD in children. Owing to its use as an antidepressant, bupropion's use is discussed extensively in that chapter (Chapter 8: Antidepressant Medications).

Bupropion acts as a norepinephrine-dopamine reuptake inhibitor and a nicotinic receptor antagonist, so it is not surprising that bupropion is also prescribed off-label for the treatment of both ADHD symptoms and nicotine dependence in children and adolescents. For the treatment of ADHD, it may be used either as an adjunct to a stimulant medication or as monotherapy.

As an antidepressant medication, bupropion's ability to reduce ADHD symptoms may take weeks, and it also carries the black box warning regarding suicidal ideation. Contraindications to its use include seizure disorder, anorexia, and bulimia.

Tricyclic Antidepressants (Amitriptyline, Imipramine, and Nortriptyline)

TCAs act on many receptors and therefore are able to treat many conditions. TCAs have proven efficacy in the treatment of MDD, anxiety, insomnia, migraine prophylaxis, abdominal pain, nocturnal enuresis, and ADHD. For the patient who has all of these symptoms, there is the prospect that one medication might treat all of their symptoms, but TCAs are not without drawbacks.

Although TCAs work on many neurotransmitter systems, this also means that patients experience significant side effects (including anticholinergic side effects, but importantly [in overdose] coma, convulsions, cardiac dysrhythmias, and death). They also carry the black box warning regarding suicidal thinking. For these reasons, TCAs are not used much in child and adolescent psychiatry. The curious reader may refer to previous editions for more detailed discussion on TCAs.

Narcolepsy Medications (Modafinil and Armodafinil)

Modafinil (Provigil) is prescribed to patients with narcolepsy, shift-work sleep disorder, and obstructive sleep apnea; but it has been used in the treatment of ADHD when other agents have failed. Armodafinil (Nuvigil) is also sometimes prescribed off-label when other options have been exhausted.

Caffeine

Caffeine is a mild stimulant with some clinical suggestions that it may be useful in treating some aspects of frontal lobe functioning. Two reviews of the relevant literature concluded that caffeine is not therapeutically useful in the treatment of ADHD (Klein, 1987; Klein et al., 1980).

Bernstein et al. (1994) investigated the effects of caffeine on learning, performance, and anxiety in 21 prepubescent normal children (12 males and 9 females aged 8 through 12 years old [mean age, 10.6 $\pm$ 1.3 years]) who ingested a minimum of 20 mg/day of caffeine in their usual diets (average daily caffeine consumption by subjects was 50.9 $\pm$ 52.2 mg/day or 1.3 mg/kg/day). Children who were excluded from the study included those with a significant medical condition and also those who had a diagnosis of ADHD.. Subjects were enrolled in a double-blind, placebo-controlled, crossover study in which they were seen for four 2-hour sessions spaced approximately 1 week apart. The four rated conditions were baseline, placebo, low-dose (2.5 mg/kg) caffeine, and high-dose (5 mg/kg) caffeine. Caffeine intake was restricted for 12 to 15 hours before the sessions. Children reported feeling less "sluggish" after receiving caffeine, and their performances improved significantly on two of four measures of attention and a test of manual dexterity for the dominant hand. Self-reported anxiety level showed a trend to increase.

Magnesium Pemoline (Cylert)

Between the second (1995) and third (2001) editions of this book, the situation regarding magnesium pemoline changed significantly. The manufacturer noted in the package insert that Cylert was associated with life-threatening hepatic failure and that 15 cases of acute hepatic failure had been reported to the FDA since it was first marketed in 1975. This was 4 to 17 times the rate expected in the general population. Twelve of the cases resulted in death or liver transplantation, usually within 4 weeks of onset of signs of liver failure.

Pemoline was withdrawn from the market (in 2005) after it was determined by the FDA that the overall risk of liver toxicity from pemoline magnesium outweighed its potential benefits. The interested reader may consult the prior editions if he/she requires further information.

Amantadine Hydrochloride

Gualtieri (2002) in his book *Brain Injury and Mental Retardation* promoted that AMT is an "excellent drug for agitation during coma recovery and disinhibition, behavioral instability, abulia, and hypoarousal after severe TBI." It is thought that most medications that have therapeutic value in the treatment of TBI do so by some direct or indirect effect on the dopamine system.

This issue of TBI is not of small significance in the field of child and adolescent psychiatry. Child and adolescent psychiatrists have always assumed a major role in the treatment of children with primary prominent cognitive delays or outright clear ID from known and (more commonly) unknown causes. The advances in prenatal and neonatal medicine have also made it possible for infants with marked prematurity or profound medical illness (such as severe strokes) to now live after birth in numbers never before realized. Unfortunately, many of these early "premies," multiple birth cohorts, and infants with profound fetal alcohol syndrome have marked brain damage and cognitive impairment. Although many of these children demonstrate frontal lobe executive function deficits and may receive a diagnosis of ADHD, this is not classic or mainstream ADHD. Neuropsychologists have, for instance, previously diagnosed such children and adults with "cognitive disorder NOS secondary to static encephalopathy due to frontal lobe impairment from fetal alcohol effects." This lengthy but descriptive diagnosis is useful in capturing the true etiology of the underlying brain damage, but does not aid the treating clinician in being able to call upon a wealth of clinical data to guide treatment especially in the psychopharmacology realm.

AMT is a water-soluble acid salt that is FDA approved as an antiviral agent for the prophylactic treatment of influenza A and for Parkinson disease. It also can be used for neuroleptic-induced side effects such as extrapyramidal symptoms (EPS), pseudoparkinsonism, akathisia, and neuroleptic malignant syndrome. It is comparable to anticholinergic agents or benztropine for EPS but with fewer side effects (such as memory impairment).

Clinical experience indicates AMT may have utility for a number of other neuropsychiatric conditions. It was originally thought that AMT acted as a pure dopamine agonist, that is, effecting dopamine (DA) neurotransmission by presynaptically enhancing DA release and inhibiting DA reuptake and/or postsynaptically directly effecting DA receptors in some manner such as facilitating the effects of endogenous DA agonists. However, as Gualtieri explained, it now believed that AMT acts as a weak antagonist of the N-methyl-D-aspartate–type glutamate receptor-ion channel which may mitigate the excitotoxic damage of glutamatergic hyperactivity. Its actions on the dopamine system are indirect and appear to be involved more as a modulator of dysfunction in the dopamine system. It also may function as an anticholinergic and is specifically a nicotinic alpha-7 antagonist like the similar pharmaceutical agent memantine which is approved for the treatment of moderate-to-severe Alzheimer disease.

Pharmacokinetics of Amantadine Hydrochloride

Plasma half-life is 16 ± 6 hours with negligible metabolism before it is renally excreted basically unchanged in the urine. Across studies, the time to C_{max} (T_{max}) averaged about 2 to 4 hours after a 100-mg dose.

Contraindications for AMT

AMT is contraindicated in patients with known hypersensitivity to amantadine hydrochloride or to any of the other ingredients in AMT.

Untoward Effects of Amantadine

CNS side effects include nervousness, anxiety, agitation, insomnia, difficulty in concentrating, and exacerbations of preexisting seizure disorders and psychiatric symptoms in patients with schizophrenia and Parkinson disease. Clinically, it exhibits anticholinergic-like side effects such as dry mouth, urinary retention, and constipation. A small number of suicide attempts (some of which have been fatal) have been reported in adult patients treated with AMT. Patients with a history of epilepsy or other "seizures" should be observed closely for possible increased seizure activity.

Overdosage

Deaths have been reported from overdose with AMT. The lowest reported acute lethal dose was 1 g. Acute toxicity may be attributable to the anticholinergic effects of AMT.

Indications for AMT in Child and Adolescent Psychiatry

There are no approved uses of AMT for psychiatric symptoms in children and adolescents.

Reports of Interest

There have been anecdotal reports that low-dose AMT has been successfully used to treat ADHD (Hallowell & Ratey, 2005).

Limited data have shown that AMT may help to relieve SSRI-induced sexual dysfunction (Balogh et al., 1992).

In a 2012 study, 184 patients with severe TBI were treated with AMT or placebo for 4 weeks. In this study, the medication accelerated functional brain recovery (Giacino et al., 2012).

For patients with symptoms of agitation and aggression during coma-recovery treatment or problems with disinhibition, behavioral instability, abulia, and hypoarousal after severe TBI, treatment with AMT for several months can be very efficacious. For an indirect dopamine agonist such as AMT to work, it requires an intact presynaptic neuron, which is not the case in patients with brain stem injuries who may benefit from a direct agonist agent such as bromocriptine. AMT can be used in combination with low to moderate dosages of MPH or amphetamine stimulant agents as well. True stimulants appear to be better for patients with normal IQs, milder brain injuries such as postconcussion syndromes, or in later stages of TBI recovery. AMT seems to have the greatest response for individuals with moderate-to-severe ID. The adult dosing strategy can be modified for use in pediatrics using AMT syrup to initiate treatment at 25 to 50 mg and increase the dosage every 4 days to effect in a range of 50 mg bid to 400 mg/day. AMT is not typically sedating and has a favorable side-effect profile; but if behavioral toxicity develops, it can be readily addressed by discontinuation of AMT. It should be noted that AMT should not be discontinued abruptly if coadministered with neuroleptics because toxicity in the form of neuroleptic malignant syndrome and catatonia can ensue. For a much more in-depth discussion of this area, one may read Gualtieri's chapter on these agents.

Omega-3 Fatty Acids (Lipirinen)

Lipirinen (Vayarin) is described as a prescription medical food (containing phosphatidylserine-omega 3) for the dietary management of ADHD. A number of clinical studies have noted a possible connection between low levels of omega 3 fatty acids and ADHD symptoms. Three studies by Glade & Smith (2015), Antalis et al. (2006), and Manor et al. (2012) examined the use of omega-3 as it relates to cognitive function. Also examined were the safety and efficacy of omega-3 in the treatment of ADHD. Beyond the treatment of ADHD, omega-3 fatty acids have been studied for the treatment of all psychiatric conditions.

To their credit, omega-3 fatty acids are well tolerated and have caused no known serious reactions. Bozzatello et al. (2016) performed a review of data from clinical trials, systematic reviews, and meta-analyses that were published between 1980 and 2015. They concluded that although many studies have been conducted, an overall consensus about the efficacy of omega-3 fatty acids is still lacking. They note that differences in methods, dosing, and type of supplement administered have resulted in findings that remain inconclusive in aggregate.

Vitamin D

Vitamin D is also another natural compound whose potential relationship with all psychiatric diagnoses is being evaluated. Khoshbakht et al. (2018) conducted a meta-analysis on the possible association between vitamin D and ADHD. They identified 13 observational studies (9 case-control or cross-sectional studies and 4 prospective studies). An analysis of the 10,334 children and adolescents in the nine case-control or cross-sectional studies showed that those children with ADHD had lower serum concentrations of 25-hydroxyvitamin D than their healthy counterparts (kids with no ADHD diagnosis).

Prospective studies conducted in 4,137 subjects indicated that perinatal suboptimal vitamin D concentrations were significantly associated with a higher risk of ADHD in later life. However, the overall effect sizes were small, and the authors note that the association should be considered equivocal at this time. More research is needed. That being said, many families reason that the potential side effects of vitamin D are minimal, and vitamin D is a supplement that they can buy over the counter.

First-Generation (Typical) Antipsychotic Medications

RYAN C. MAST AND ROBERT P. CUSSER

INTRODUCTION

In the 1950s, chlorpromazine and other antipsychotic medications (also commonly referred to as *neuroleptics* or *major tranquilizers*) began to be introduced into clinical practice, and these medications showed significant efficacy in reducing the positive symptoms of schizophrenia (e.g., auditory hallucinations and delusions). Chlorpromazine and other medications in this class have come to be known as the first-generation (typical) antipsychotics (FGAs). Although their benefits were significant, they were also not without potential side effects (including extrapyramidal symptoms [EPS]).

Approximately 40 years after chlorpromazine entered clinical practice, the introduction of clozapine ushered in the era of the second-generation (atypical) antipsychotics (SGAs). These SGAs also have demonstrated efficacy in treating the positive symptoms of schizophrenia, but they have the additional benefit of improving the negative symptoms of schizophrenia (e.g., apathy and anhedonia). Compared to the FGAs, the SGAs carry a lower risk of EPS as a side effect, but research has shown that they do carry the risk of metabolic side effects.

Although both classes of antipsychotic medications are often prescribed to both adults and children to treat psychoses, they have been shown to also effectively treat other common nonpsychotic psychiatric disorders including autism spectrum disorder, bipolar disorder, and Tourette disorder. Owing to their use in nonpsychotic disorders, some clinicians prefer to refer to the class as neuroleptics (instead of as antipsychotics), and this is a worthy consideration especially when explaining the use of these medications to patients and their caregivers. Still other practitioners include them in the category of mood stabilizers.

Regarding the use of these medications in the treatment of schizophrenia in children, it is important to note that there is some evidence that antipsychotics are not as clinically effective in the treatment of schizophrenia with childhood onset as they are in treating schizophrenia occurring in later adolescence and adulthood

(Green et al., 1984). Meyers et al. (1980) noted that serum neuroleptic levels of 50 ng/mL of chlorpromazine equivalents correspond to the threshold for clinical response in adult patients with schizophrenia and suggest that similar therapeutic serum levels are necessary in children. Because children may metabolize and excrete antipsychotic medications more efficiently than do adults, determination of serum neuroleptic levels, if they are available, is recommended before a trial of an antipsychotic is deemed a failure.

The choice of whether to prescribe an FGA versus an SGA in early-onset psychotic disorders remains controversial. The TEOSS (treatment of early-onset schizophrenia spectrum disorders; Sikich et al., 2008) noted that molindone appeared to have efficacy similar to that of SGAs, but with more benign metabolic effects. Families often enquire about side-effect profiles, medication efficacy, and cost of medications when deciding on a treatment. Given their different side-effect profiles (as well as the higher financial cost of the second-generation agents), it is important for clinicians to be familiar with FGAs because they remain relevant in clinical practice for these reasons. Of the FGAs, haloperidol and (to a lesser extent) chlorpromazine remain the most relevant in clinical practice.

It should be further noted that Kumar et al. (2013) reviewed 13 randomized controlled trials (RCTs; with a total of 1,112 participants aged 13 to 18 years old). They concluded that there was no convincing evidence to suggest that SGAs were superior to FGAs in the treatment of adolescents with psychoses. However, they did add that adolescents may prefer SGAs because of fewer symptomatic adverse effects felt in the short term. Because bothersome side effects lead to medication nonadherence, it is important to weigh this consideration when prescribing neuroleptics to teenagers and children. Of significant importance to children and adolescents are sedation and weight gain, and many patients have also seen television commercials regarding the potential side effect of elevated prolactin levels and gynecomastia (particularly with risperidone and paliperidone). This has led many teenagers (especially boys) and their families to ask for a switch from this medication. Although this chapter is chiefly concerned with FGAs, there will be some discussion of SGAs; however, an in-depth discussion of SGAs follows this chapter.

In addition to the use of antipsychotics in the treatment of psychosis, Shapiro and Shapiro (1989) concluded that antipsychotics were also the medications of choice for treating chronic motor or vocal tic disorder and Tourette disorder when psychosocial, educational, and/or occupational functioning was so impaired that medication was required. SGAs are now often used in the treatment of tic disorders (including aripiprazole which is approved by the U.S. Food and Drug Administration [FDA] for tic disorders in children), but FGAs (including haloperidol and pimozide) remain common agents (Roessner et al., 2012; Singer, 2010). Both FGAs and SGAs can lead to increases in body mass index in patients with tic disorders, with resultant metabolic effects.

Antipsychotic medications are also clinically effective in children with severely aggressive conduct disorders, and some are approved for use in such children. Lithium is also effective in some such children (perhaps more so when an explosive affect is present), and lithium generally has fewer clinically significant untoward effects than do neuroleptics. However, because lithium is still not approved for use either in children younger than 12 years or for this indication, and because of the necessity of monitoring serum lithium levels, many clinicians prefer to prescribe antipsychotic medications to patients with severely aggressive conduct disorders.

The use of antipsychotics in patients with intellectual disability (ID) continues to be controversial, but they are prescribed frequently, especially for institutionalized patients. In optimal doses, antipsychotics are effective in decreasing irritability, sleep disturbances, hostility, agitation, and combativeness, and they may improve concentration and social behavior in agitated individuals with severe intellectual disabilities (American Medical Association, 1986). Aman and Singh (1988) cautioned that the influential studies of patients with ID by Breuning, which showed significant detrimental effects on cognition resulting from antipsychotic use, appear to have been fabricated. However, concerns pertaining to the overuse and misuse of these medications in this population continue, especially as psychosocial resources are threatened. Of particular concern is the use of prn ("as needed") doses of antipsychotic medications for patients with ID in group homes and other institutions, because without clear instructions for when it may be administered, there exists the very real possibility that a staff member may feel compelled (especially when short-staffed) to too quickly administer an "as needed" dose of an antipsychotic medication before an adequate trial of behavioral intervention has been attempted. Consequently, some group homes do not allow the use of any "as needed" doses of antipsychotic medications. When some group homes do allow it, the instructions for the "as needed" dose must often contain very specific language such as "one tablet may be given as needed every 8 hours for severe agitation, aggression, or self-harm only if 30 minutes of verbal re-direction is unsuccessful." All of this can leave the prescriber to wonder at what point should an "as needed" dose of a medication become a scheduled dose. Is it two incidents per month? Five? And of what severity? This threshold becomes a case-by-case analysis of benefit versus risk.

In the treatment of all patients (but especially children), it is preferred to use the lowest dose possible, and therefore considerations related to when to attempt a dose reduction are important. Polypharmacy should also be minimized when possible.

ANTIPSYCHOTIC MEDICATIONS IN THE TREATMENT OF ATTENTION-DEFICIT/HYPERACTIVITY DISORDERS

Some antipsychotic agents (e.g., haloperidol) have been approved for treating children with symptoms such as excessive motor activity, impulsivity, difficulty sustaining attention, and poor frustration tolerance, which would be found in most children diagnosed with attention-deficit/hyperactivity disorder (ADHD). In fact, double-blind, controlled studies have shown antipsychotic medications to be effective in treating children who would meet the criteria for ADHD. However, studies comparing antipsychotic medications with stimulants almost always show that, overall, stimulants are statistically more effective clinically than antipsychotics in the treatment of ADHD (Gittelman-Klein et al., 1976; Green, 1995). In addition, many clinicians are reluctant to use antipsychotics to treat patients with ADHD because to help with clarification the risk that an irreversible tardive dyskinesia (TD) might develop, the possibility of adverse metabolic effects, and the worry that the sedative effects of antipsychotics may interfere significantly with cognition and learning. Owing to such factors, antipsychotics should be thought of as third-rank medications to be used primarily in the treatment of ADHD that is severely disabling and that has not responded to stimulants and other medications with untoward effects of more acceptable risk (e.g., clonidine, atomoxetine, and guanfacine).

Although these caveats in using antipsychotics are not to be dismissed, data moderating these dictums should be cited: (a) as stated previously, the studies of Breuning and colleagues (which showed that there were significant detrimental effects on cognition in patients with ID treated with antipsychotic medications) appear to have been fabricated (Aman & Singh, 1988); (b) other studies have reported minimal impairment of cognition in subjects diagnosed with ADHD who were treated with appropriate doses of antipsychotics (Klein, 1990/1991); and (c) Sallee et al. (1994) examined the effects of haloperidol and pimozide in patients with Tourette disorder, including subjects with ADHD, and found no decrement in cognition associated with FGA use.

In a randomized, crossover, double-blind study, Weizman et al. (1984) noted that the combination of a stimulant plus antipsychotic may be useful in some children who do not respond adequately to stimulants alone. Clinically, this may be a potentially useful option for a small subgroup of children who do not respond adequately to stimulants or to other medications alone. The combination of stimulant and antipsychotic would presumably achieve a satisfactory result that might otherwise not be achieved by the antipsychotic alone or would require higher doses of antipsychotics, which would carry an increased risk of untoward effects, such as TD and cognitive dulling.

PHARMACOKINETICS OF FIRST-GENERATION ANTIPSYCHOTIC MEDICATIONS

Dosing of antipsychotic medications in children remains complicated partly because of the changes in a child's body weight over time with growth, as well as medication metabolism rates by the liver. Rivera-Calimlim et al. (1979) reported plasma chlorpromazine levels in a total of 24 children aged 8 to 16 years who were treated with chlorpromazine for psychiatric disorders (including various psychoses, ID with aggression, hyperactivity, self-injurious behavior, and mood disorders with anxiety). The authors reported wide interpatient variations in chlorpromazine plasma levels for a given dose; for example, nine children receiving 0.8 to 2.9 mg/kg/day achieved mean plasma levels of 6.6 ng/mL, with a range from undetectable to 18 ng/mL. One child receiving 9.8 mg/kg/day showed only trace levels of plasma chlorpromazine.

In addition, children and adolescents had chlorpromazine plasma levels that were two to three-and-a-half times lower than those for adults, for a given dose per kilogram of body weight. Clinical improvement in these children usually began when plasma chlorpromazine concentration was at least 30 ng/mL and optimal levels ranged between 40 and 80 ng/mL; suggested optimal plasma levels for adults treated with chlorpromazine were higher, between 50 and 300 ng/mL. A final, clinically important observation was that plasma chlorpromazine levels declined over time in most patients who were on fixed doses (Rivera-Calimlim et al., 1979). It was suggested that one possible reason might be autoinduction of enzymes that metabolize chlorpromazine.

Although much of this chapter focuses on oral formulations of these medications, it is important to note that several also come in the form of short-acting intramuscular injections, long-acting injections, and intravenous (IV) formulations.

CONTRAINDICATIONS FOR THE ADMINISTRATION OF ANTIPSYCHOTIC MEDICATIONS

Known hypersensitivity to the medication and toxic central nervous system depression or comatose states are absolute contraindications. If a severe adverse event develops (e.g., agranulocytosis, neuroleptic malignant syndrome [NMS], TD, or a withdrawal dyskinesia), then children and adolescents should be managed without antipsychotics if at all possible.

Neuroleptics may lower the seizure threshold. Therefore, they should be used cautiously in patients with seizure disorders, and chlorpromazine probably should not be prescribed at all in such patients.

INTERACTIONS OF FIRST-GENERATION ANTIPSYCHOTIC MEDICATIONS WITH OTHER MEDICATIONS

For FGAs, the most frequent clinically important drug–drug reactions are with other central nervous system depressants (such as alcohol, sedatives and hypnotics, benzodiazepines, antihistamines, opiates, and barbiturates) in which an additive central nervous system depressive effect occurs.

Antipsychotic medications also have varying degrees of anticholinergic effects. When combined with another anticholinergic (antiparkinsonian) agent (such as when one is prescribed prophylactically to prevent acute dyskinesia, pseudoparkinsonism, or akathisia), then central nervous system symptoms of cholinergic blockade may result. These symptoms may include confusion, disorientation, delirium, hallucinations, and worsening of preexisting psychotic symptoms. Of clinical importance, this picture may be mistaken for inadequate treatment or a worsening of the psychosis, rather than an untoward effect.

The combination of antipsychotic medications and lithium carbonate (particularly if high doses are used) may lead to an increased incidence of central nervous system toxicity, including NMS.

The combined use of antipsychotic medications with tricyclic antidepressants (TCAs) or monoamine oxidase inhibitors (MAOIs) may increase plasma levels of these antidepressants.

Neuroleptics may also have noteworthy interactions with many other medications. Given today's easy access to databases of medication interactions, a review of all possible interactions in every patient receiving these medications should be standard clinical practice.

UNTOWARD EFFECTS OF FIRST-GENERATION ANTIPSYCHOTIC MEDICATIONS

Although FGAs may have numerous serious untoward effects, those of greatest concern in children and adolescents are the effects of sedation, on cognition, and the extrapyramidal syndromes, in particular the possible development of irreversible TD with the standard antipsychotics. We note that even older references documenting these effects remain current and unchallenged.

Agranulocytosis

Agranulocytosis is a major concern in patients treated with clozapine (an SGA), and it is discussed in more detail later. However, agranulocytosis has also been reported with some FGAs. It usually occurs relatively early in treatment (e.g., for chlorpromazine, usually between the 4th and 10th weeks). Guardians and older patients should be warned to report indications of sudden infections (such as fever and sore throat) to the physician. White blood cell count (including absolute neutrophil count) should be determined immediately, and if it is significantly depressed, medication should be stopped and therapy instituted.

Untoward Cognitive Effects

Regarding the FGAs, they are often categorized by potency (e.g., high-potency, low-potency). Low-potency antipsychotic medications require higher doses to achieve the same effect as high-potency agents. Notably, however, both high-potency and low-potency antipsychotic agents are effective when given in equivalent doses, but they differ in the frequency and severity of their untoward effects. Low-potency agents are more likely to cause sedation, and high-potency agents are more likely to produce EPS (movement disorders). The lower potency antipsychotic medications cause greater sedation, more autonomic side effects, and fewer extrapyramidal effects (Baldessarini, 1990). Because of the great importance of minimizing any cognitive dulling in schoolchildren and in patients with ID (whose cognition is already compromised), the high-potency, less-sedative antipsychotic medications are often preferred. Over a period of days to weeks, however, considerable tolerance often develops to the sedative effects of high-dose, low-potency antipsychotic medications, and thus they are still useful when untoward effects are carefully monitored (Green, 1989). Haloperidol is a high-potency agent, and chlorpromazine is a low-potency agent.

Extrapyramidal Syndromes

Significant numbers of children and adolescents receiving FGAs develop extrapyramidal syndromes. Baldessarini (1990) has enumerated six types of extrapyramidal syndromes associated with the use of antipsychotic medications. The risk of extrapyramidal syndromes with clozapine and other SGAs (with the possible exception of risperidone) appears to be considerably reduced compared with that of FGAs.

Adverse Effects Usually Appearing during First-Generation Antipsychotic Administration

Acute Dystonic Reactions

The period of maximum risk of developing an acute dystonic reaction is within hours to 5 days of initiation of FGA therapy. There may also be an increased risk following increases in dose. High-potency, low-dose antipsychotic medications (e.g., haloperidol) are more likely to precipitate an acute dystonic reaction than are low-potency, high-dose antipsychotic medications; and young males, both children and adolescents, may be at increased risk (American Psychiatric Association [APA], 1980b). Untreated acute dystonic reactions may last from a few minutes to several hours, and they may recur. Symptoms may be painful and frightening (particularly if the patient does not understand what is happening) and include muscular hypertonicity; tonic contractions (spasms) of the neck (torticollis), mouth, and tongue that may make speaking difficult; oculogyric crisis (eyes rolling upward and remaining in that position); and opisthotonos (spasm in which the spine and extremities are bent with an anterior convexity). Acute dystonic reactions respond rapidly to anticholinergic and antiparkinsonian medications, such as 25 to 50 mg diphenhydramine (Benadryl) orally or intramuscularly, or 1 to 2 mg benztropine (Cogentin) intramuscularly. (The manufacturer of benztropine cautions that [because of its atropine-like untoward effects] its use is contraindicated in children younger than 3 years of age and that it should be used with caution in older children [*Physicians' Desk Reference* (PDR), 2017].) If the dystonia is very severe, administering either 25 mg of diphenhydramine or 1 to 2 mg of benztropine intramuscularly will reverse the dystonia within a few minutes. The prophylactic use of anticholinergic and antiparkinsonian agents to prevent acute dystonic reactions is discussed following the section on "Akathisia (Motor Restlessness)."

Parkinsonism (Pseudoparkinsonism)

Symptoms of parkinsonism include tremor, cogwheel rigidity, drooling, decrease in facial expressive movements (masklike or expressionless facies), and akinesia (slowness in initiating movements). These symptoms respond to antiparkinsonian medications. For example, benztropine (Cogentin) 1 to 2 mg given two or three times daily usually provides relief within a day or two. Antiparkinsonian medication may be withdrawn gradually after 1 or 2 weeks to see whether it is still necessary for symptomatic relief.

The period of maximum risk for developing parkinsonism is 5 to 30 days after initiation of neuroleptic therapy. The risk for development of parkinsonism appears to be greater in women and appears to increase with age. It is rarely seen in preschool children treated with therapeutic doses of neuroleptics, but it occurs with some regularity in school-aged children and adolescents (Campbell et al., 1985). Richardson et al. (1991) reported that 21 (34%) of 61 hospitalized children and adolescents (of whom only 7 were diagnosed with psychotic or affective disorders) who were taking neuroleptics at the time of evaluation exhibited symptoms of parkinsonism when rated on several movement disorder scales. Three (14.3%) of the 21 children were rated as having parkinsonism despite the fact that they were concurrently receiving antiparkinsonian medications. Development of parkinsonism was significantly ($P = .05$) associated with a longer duration on medication at the time of evaluation (mean of 117 days for patients with parkinsonism and mean of 34 days for patients without parkinsonism).

Akinesia is perhaps the most severe form of parkinsonism, and it is defined by Rifkin et al. (1975) as a "behavioral state of diminished spontaneity characterized by few gestures, unspontaneous speech and, particularly, apathy and difficulty with initiating usual activities." It may be particularly difficult to differentiate akinesia caused by medication from the negative symptoms of schizophrenia (such as apathy and blunting). Van Putten and Marder (1987) suggested that akinesia might be the most toxic behavioral side effect of antipsychotic medications. The authors noted that a subjective sense of sedation or drowsiness, excessive sleeping, and a lack of any leg-crossing during an interview of approximately 20 minutes correlated with the presence of akinesia. Akinesia also interferes with social adjustment, and the patient may appear to have a "postpsychotic depression." Patients with akinesia are often less concerned with any psychotic symptoms and report that everything is fine; they may experience an absence of emotion and appear emotionally dead (Van Putten & Marder, 1987). Although antiparkinsonian medications may be helpful, in some cases they do not adequately control symptoms of akinesia. There is some evidence that antiparkinsonian medications become less effective at higher daily dosages of antipsychotics (Van Putten & Marder, 1987).

The prophylactic use of anticholinergic and antiparkinsonian agents to prevent pseudoparkinsonism is discussed following the section on "Akathisia (Motor Restlessness)."

Akathisia (Motor Restlessness)

Although akinesia might not be particularly bothersome to most patients, akathisia is. Symptoms include constant uncomfortable restlessness, a feeling of tension in the lower extremities often accompanied by a strong or irresistible urge to move them, inability to sit still, and foot-tapping or pacing. Clinically, a blunted affect, emotional withdrawal, and motor retardation may also be observed (Van Putten & Marder, 1987). The period of maximum risk for developing akathisia is 5 to 60 days after initiation of neuroleptic therapy, but it has been reported to occur in as few as 6 hours after an oral dose of a neuroleptic (Van Putten et al., 1984).

Van Putten and Marder (1987) noted the dual nature of akathisia: a subjective experience of restlessness and an observable motor restlessness. In their clinical experience, all patients with moderate or severe akathisia exhibited either rocking from foot to foot or walking on the spot. Akathisia was also strongly associated with depression, dysphoria, and, at times in severe and treatment-resistant cases, exacerbation of psychotic symptoms, and homicidal and suicidal ideation and behavior (Van Putten & Marder, 1987). Of particular clinical importance, patients who have unpleasant, untoward effects (especially akathisia) with antipsychotics are more likely to be nonadherent and to unilaterally discontinue medication early in treatment (Van Putten & Marder, 1987).

Fleischhacker et al. (1989) published a rating scale for akathisia that includes two subjective items: "a sensation of inner restlessness" and "the urge to move," and three items that characterize the frequency and magnitude of observed akathisia phenomena.

Akathisia may or may not respond to antiparkinsonian medications such as trihexyphenidyl (Artane), but there are medications that can help. Propranolol may be helpful in ameliorating akathisia (Adler et al., 1986); benzodiazepines and clonidine have also been reported to be effective in some cases. Clonazepam was administered to 10 adolescents with first-break psychosis (8 of whom were diagnosed with schizophrenia, paranoid subtype) between 16 and 19 years of age who experienced distressing akathisia following treatment with antipsychotics (Kutcher et al., 1987). Nine of the patients had also been receiving benztropine concomitantly with their antipsychotic medication. All patients reported subjective improvement in their akathisia symptoms, and scores on an akathisia subscale decreased significantly after 1 week's treatment with 0.5 mg/day of clonazepam.

In some cases, reduction in dose of the antipsychotic may be necessary. Neppe and Ward (1989) recommend that if only akathisia develops (i.e., without accompanying parkinsonism), a beta-blocker be used rather than an anticholinergic agent.

Prophylactic Use of Antiparkinsonian Agents for Acute Dystonic Reaction, Parkinsonism, and Akathisia

The use of antiparkinsonian (anticholinergic) agents prophylactically to minimize the likelihood of the patient developing an acute dystonic reaction, parkinsonism, or akathisia from antipsychotic medication use is controversial. Some of the reasons relate to the side effects caused by the anticholinergic agents themselves. Anticholinergic agents may adversely affect cognition and may aggravate psychotic symptomatology. In addition, there is some suggestion that at least part of the effectiveness of these agents is that they may lower the serum concentration of the antipsychotic medication (Rivera-Calimlim et al., 1976). Because of their reluctance to give an additional medication that itself may have untoward effects, many clinicians choose to minimize the risk of these extrapyramidal effects by beginning with a low dose and titrating the medication slowly. If an acute dystonic reaction should occur, it may be treated with diphenhydramine and the dosage of antipsychotic lowered temporarily if necessary. Conversely, some clinicians routinely prescribe an agent such as benztropine for approximately 4 to 6 weeks, covering the period of maximal risk for the development of both acute dystonic reactions and parkinsonian untoward effects. Another option for outpatients is to prescribe a small amount of an anticholinergic (e.g., diphenhydramine) with an explanation of how it is to be administered should a dystonic reaction occur (e.g., "take one capsule should such a reaction begin, and may take another dose in 20 to 30 minutes if there is no improvement, and to go to an emergency room if the reaction is severe, and alert the physician to the medication being taken").

In their review of the management of acute extrapyramidal syndromes induced by neuroleptics, Neppe and Ward (1989) note that anticholinergics can significantly reduce the rate of acute dystonias especially in the highest risk group (males younger than 30 years of age treated with high-potency antipsychotic agents). However, because acute dystonic reactions tend to be transient, prophylactic treatment for more than 2 weeks is not usually indicated. These authors recommend no prophylaxis for parkinsonism and akathisia because they rarely present as dramatically or emergently as acute dystonia. The parents/guardians and/or patient, as appropriate, should be carefully informed about the possibility of these conditions arising, to aid in their early detection. The clinician can then decide how best to treat the particular symptom in the particular patient (Neppe & Ward, 1989).

Van Putten and Marder (1987) point out that prophylactic use of antiparkinsonian medications may not fully prevent symptoms of akinesia from developing and that some patients with schizophrenia who have been stabilized using antiparkinsonian medication may experience increased anxiety, depression, general dysphoria, and suffering when the anticholinergics are withdrawn.

The clinician should decide on a case-by-case basis about which of the preceding possibilities is best for a given patient. This decision will be based on such factors as whether a high- or low-potency neuroleptic is given, how rapidly the dose is increased, previous experience of the patient, whether it is administered to an outpatient or an inpatient (who has ready access to clinical staff), how such a reaction might affect the relationship with the patient and/or the parents and subsequent adherence, and the patient's environment. For example, it can be particularly difficult for a patient and family if the patient develops an acute dystonic reaction while attending school.

Neuroleptic Malignant Syndrome

NMS is life threatening and can occur after a single dose, but it occurs most frequently within 2 weeks of initiation of neuroleptic therapy or an increase in dosage; males and younger individuals appear to be most often affected (for a review, see Kaufmann & Wyatt, 1987). Symptoms include severe muscular rigidity, altered consciousness, stupor, catatonia, hyperpyrexia, labile pulse and blood pressure, and occasionally myoglobinemia. Most patients have elevated creatine phosphokinase levels. NMS can persist for up to 2 weeks or longer after medication is discontinued and can be fatal.

Treatment of NMS consists of immediate cessation of the antipsychotic medication and hospitalization, under intensive care, with supportive treatment. Dopaminergic agonists (e.g., bromocriptine and amantadine) and/or dantrolene have also been reported to reduce the mortality rate significantly (Sakkas et al., 1991). Antiparkinsonian medications are not useful treatments for NMS.

Latz and McCracken (1992) conducted an extensive literature search and reported a total of 49 cases of NMS in patients 18 years or younger. The youngest reported case was that of an 11-month-old. Five (83%) of the six preschoolers developed NMS after a single dose of neuroleptic that either was an accidental overdose or was prescribed for a nonpsychiatric illness. Overall lethality for all cases reviewed was 16.3% (8 of 49). However, the death rate for patients 12 years of age or younger was 27% (3 of 11), more than twice the death rate of 13% (5 of 38) for adolescents 13 to 18 years old.

Steingard et al. (1992) also published a review with detailed summaries of 35 cases of NMS in patients younger than 19 years of age. Fever, rigidity, altered mental status, and tachycardia were present in >70% of the cases. Five (14%) of the patients died; however, only one of these died within the past two decades, and that was a 2-year-old who had ingested chlorpromazine accidentally. Croarkin et al. (2008) reported on 16 cases of NMS in subjects 18 years old and younger from 1991 through 2007, mostly male, all of whom survived. These data suggest that the standard of care for these patients has improved, but do not address reporting bias.

Late-Appearing Syndromes (after Months or Years of Treatment)

Tardive Dyskinesia

Definitions and descriptions of TD and related dyskinesias (withdrawal, masked dyskinesias) vary. Perhaps the most influential definition at present is the research diagnostic criteria proposed in 1982 by Schooler and Kane. They note that, if possible, the absence of abnormal involuntary movements before beginning pharmacotherapy should be documented. Schooler and Kane's (1982) research diagnostic criteria for TD proposed three prerequisites for making the diagnosis:

1. Exposure to neuroleptic medications for a minimum total cumulative exposure of 3 months
2. The presence of at least "moderate" abnormal involuntary movements in one or more body areas (face, lips, jaw, tongue, upper extremities, lower extremities, and trunk) or at least "mild" movements in two or more body areas
3. Absence of other conditions that might produce abnormal movements

Once these prerequisites have been met by a patient, Schooler and Kane (1982) proposed six diagnostic categories of TD: probable TD (either with "concurrent neuroleptics" or "neuroleptic-free"), masked probable TD, transient TD, withdrawal TD, persistent TD (either with "concurrent neuroleptics" or "neuroleptic-free"), and masked persistent TD.

Four additional diagnostic criteria were suggested by the American Psychiatric Association Task Force on TD (APA, 1992):

1. The abnormal movements are exacerbated or may be provoked by a decrease or withdrawal of an antipsychotic drug. Increasing the dose of antipsychotic will suppress (or dampen) the movements at least temporarily.
2. Anticholinergic medication does not ameliorate and may worsen the movements.
3. Emotional stress may worsen the movements.
4. The movements decrease or disappear during sleep.

TD develops while actively receiving a neuroleptic medication, as opposed to a withdrawal dyskinesia which occurs when a neuroleptic is withdrawn or its dose is decreased. TD, which may be both severely disabling and irreversible, is the most clinically significant common long-term untoward effect of FGA use. Baldessarini (1990) notes that in some cases, especially in younger patients, TD will disappear over the course of weeks to as much as 3 years. It is believed that the risk of developing irreversible TD increases with both total cumulative dose and duration of treatment. Older females appear to be at increased risk. It has been reported that fine, wormlike (vermicular) movements of the tongue may be an early sign of TD and that discontinuation of the medication when this occurs may prevent further development of the syndrome (PDR, 1995). Symptoms of TD most typically include involuntary choreoathetotic movements that affect the face; tongue; perioral, buccal, and masticatory musculature; and neck. However, the torso and extremities may also be involved.

Atypical and less common forms of TD, such as tardive akathisia (a persisting restlessness) and tardive dystonia, also occur. Burke et al. (1982) reported 42 cases of tardive dystonia that they diagnosed by the following criteria:

1. The presence of chronic dystonia
2. History of antipsychotic drug treatment preceding or concurrent with the onset of dystonia
3. Exclusion of known causes of secondary dystonia by appropriate clinical and laboratory evaluation
4. A negative family history for dystonia

Symptoms of tardive dystonia began after as few as 3 days and up to 11 years after initiation of antipsychotic medication. The incidence of tardive dystonia was more frequent in younger male patients than in older patients; was characterized by sustained abnormal postures accompanied by torticollis, torsion of the trunk and extremities, blepharospasm, and grimacing; and was incapacitating in severe cases. Spontaneous remission occurred in a few patients, but dystonia persisted for years in most. Of the many medications used to ameliorate tardive dystonia, the most helpful were tetrabenazine (which improved symptoms in 68% of patients) and anticholinergics (which were helpful in 39% of patients) (Burke et al., 1982). In 2017, two alterations of the tetrabenazine molecule, valbenazine and deutetrabenazine, were approved for the treatment of TD in adults, and studies in the pediatric population are under way. These newer agents are equally as efficacious as tetrabenazine, but with a much reduced side-effect profile. These agents are discussed in detail in Chapter 12.

In TD and other choreoathetotic syndromes, emotional stress typically causes a worsening of the movements, and drowsiness or sedation causes them to diminish (with sleep causing them to disappear; APA, 1980b). Antiparkinsonian medications may worsen the condition (for review, see APA, 1980b, 1992). There is evidence, however, that the atypical antipsychotic medication clozapine not only produces little or no TD when it is the only neuroleptic ever used but it also significantly decreases or eliminates existing symptoms of TD during the period it is prescribed (Birmaher et al., 1992; Mozes et al., 1994; Small et al., 1987). Upon its discontinuation, however, the dyskinetic movements that were suppressed by clozapine rapidly returned in 18 of 19 patients (Small et al., 1987).

Vitamin E and Tardive Dyskinesia

Vitamin E has also been reported to be helpful in treating TD in adults. Adler et al. (1999) note that although several short-term, controlled studies found vitamin E to be helpful, these studies were from a single site, had relatively small numbers, and treatment duration was short. To further investigate the effectiveness of vitamin E, the authors conducted a prospective, randomized, nine-site, double-blind, placebo-controlled study. They found no significant differences between vitamin E and placebo on any of the rating scales at the end of the study and concluded that vitamin E is not effective in treating TD in patients who are actively being treated with neuroleptics.

Withdrawal Dyskinesia

A withdrawal dyskinesia may emerge when neuroleptic medication is withdrawn or the dose is reduced. Withdrawal-emergent dyskinesias can occur for two different reasons. First, antidopaminergic medications (including antipsychotics) can suppress TD; thus, a decrease in their serum levels can "unmask" ongoing TD. Second, Baldessarini (1990) points out that a "disuse supersensitivity" to dopamine agonists may also occur following withdrawal of antidopaminergic medications. He suggests that this phenomenon may explain withdrawal dyskinesias that resolve within a few weeks.

The reported prevalence of neuroleptic-induced TD and withdrawal TD in children and adolescents has ranged from 0% to 51% (Wolf & Wagner, 1993). It is thought that the risk of developing TD that will become irreversible increases with both total cumulative dose and duration of treatment. The longest neuroleptic-free persistent TD was reported to last 4.5 years. Usually, withdrawal dyskinesias resolve within a few weeks to a few months of discontinuation of the neuroleptic (Wolf & Wagner, 1993).

Richardson et al. (1991) reported that 5 (12%) of 41 hospitalized children and adolescents (mean age, 15.5 years), of whom only 10 were diagnosed with psychotic or affective disorders, who had taken neuroleptics for at least one period of 90 continuous days before the time of evaluation exhibited symptoms of treatment-emergent TD (occurring while receiving neuroleptics) when rated on the Simpson Abbreviated Dyskinesia Scale. The five patients who developed TD were significantly more likely to have had a history of assaultive behavior ($P = .003$) and a first-degree relative who had been hospitalized for a psychiatric disorder ($P = .009$) compared to patients who did not develop TD. Using the more stringent research criteria of Schooler and Kane (1982), three (7%) were diagnosed with TD. McDonagh et al. (2010) reported a Cochrane review that disclosed that risperidone (an SGA) resulted in an increased risk of new-onset TD (3% compared with 1% to 2% for others).

If TD develops, every effort should be made to discontinue or at least reduce the dose of the antipsychotic medication as much as possible. The dyskinesia should be monitored with serial ratings on the Abnormal Involuntary Movement Scale (AIMS). If the severity of the psychiatric disorder precludes discontinuation of antipsychotic medication (e.g., in a patient diagnosed with autism spectrum disorder who exhibits severe self-injurious behavior and aggressiveness and who has not responded adequately to other medications such as lithium or propranolol), the clinician must carefully document the rationale for reinstituting antipsychotic medication and verify that the legal guardians (and patient, when appropriate) have given their informed consent/assent. Reinstating or increasing the dose of antipsychotic may suppress or mask TD.

Because of such risks, antipsychotic agents should be given only to children and adolescents for whom no other potentially less harmful treatment is available; for example, although effective in some children diagnosed with ADHD, antipsychotic medications should not be used unless stimulant medications and other non-stimulant medications with safer untoward-effect profiles have been treatment failures (Green, 1995).

Although antipsychotics are the only medications that result in persistent TD in a significant proportion of patients, a number of different medications may cause dyskinesias after short- or long-term treatment. Jeste and Wyatt (1982) note that the dyskinesia produced by L-DOPA most closely resembles the TD resulting from antipsychotics and that, typically, the dyskinesias caused by most other medications are usually acute effects and almost always remit when the medication is discontinued. Among the medications used in child and adolescent psychopharmacotherapy for which dyskinesias have been reported are: amphetamines, methylphenidate, MAOIs, TCAs, lithium, antihistamines, benzodiazepines, and antiepileptic medications (Jeste & Wyatt, 1982).

Rabbit syndrome (perioral tremor), which may be a late-onset variant of parkinsonism, is uncommon. Its name derives from the fact that these patients make rapid chewing movements similar to those of rabbits (Villeneuve, 1972). It may respond to antiparkinsonian medication.

Other Untoward Effects of First-Generation Antipsychotic Medications

Table 6.1 presents a compilation of most of the reported untoward effects of chlorpromazine (the prototype FGA antipsychotic medication). Most of these untoward effects have also been reported to occur to a greater or lesser degree with other FGAs.

REPRESENTATIVE FIRST-GENERATION (TYPICAL) ANTIPSYCHOTIC MEDICATIONS

Table 6.2 summarizes representative FGA medications commonly used in child and adolescent psychiatry, as well as clozapine (an SGA). This table compares their relative potencies and expected potential sedative, autonomic, and extrapyramidal

TABLE 6.1 » UNTOWARD EFFECTS OF CHLORPROMAZINE

Allergic
  Mild urticaria
  Photosensitivity, exfoliative dermatitis
  Asthma
  Anaphylactoid reactions
  Laryngeal edema
  Angioneurotic edema
Autonomic nervous system
  Antiadrenergic effects
  Orthostatic hypotension
  Ejaculatory disturbances
Anticholinergic effects
  Decreased secretion, resulting in dry mouth, dry eyes, nasal congestion
  Blurred vision, mydriasis
  Glaucoma attack in patients with narrow-angle closure
  Constipation, paralytic ileus
  Urinary retention
  Impotence
Cardiovascular
  Postural (orthostatic) hypotension
  Tachycardia
  ECG changes
  Sudden death due to cardiac arrest
Central nervous system
  Neuromuscular effects
  Dystonias
  Akasthisia (motor restlessness)
  Pseudoparkinsonism
  Tardive dyskinesia
  Seizures, lowering of seizure threshold
  Drowsiness, sedation
  Behavioral effects
  Increased psychotic symptoms
  Catatonic-like states

Dermatologic
  Photosensitivity
  Skin pigmentation changes in exposed areas
  Rashes
Endocrinologic
  Elevated prolactin levels
  Gynecomastia
  Amenorrhea
  Hyperglycemia, glycosuria, and hypoglycemia
Hematologic
  Agranulocytosis
  Eosinophilia
  Leukopenia
  Hemolytic anemia
  Aplastic anemia
  Thrombocytopenic purpura
  Pancytopenia
Hepatologic
  Jaundice
Metabolic
  Weight gain, increased appetite
Ophthalmologic
  Blurred vision
  Precipitation of acute glaucoma attack in persons with narrow-angle glaucoma
  Deposition of pigmented material and star-shaped opacities in lens
  Deposition of pigmented material in cornea
  Pigmentary retinopathy
  Epithelial keratopathy
  Teratogenic effects possible (seen in animal studies)
Other
  Neuroleptic malignant syndrome
  Sudden death, which may be related to cardiac failure or suppression of cough reflex

ECG, electrocardiogram.

TABLE 6.2 » Representative First-Generation (Typical) Antipsychotic Medications and Clozapine (a Second-Generation Antipsychotic)

Antipsychotic Medication/ Trade Name	Chemical Classification	Therapeutically Equivalent Oral Dose in Milligrams	Effects			Approved Age for Use
			Sedation	Autonomic[a]	Extrapyramidal Reaction[b]	
Chlorpromazine/ Thorazine	Phenothiazine: aliphatic compound	100	+++	+++	++	Over 6 mo
Clozapine/ Clozaril	Dibenzodiazepine	75	+++	+++	0?	16 y
Mesoridazine/ Serentil	Phenothiazine: piperidine compound	50	+++	++	+	12 y
Loxapine/ Loxitane	Dibenzoxazepine	15	++	+/++	++/+++	16 y
Molindone/ Moban	Dihydroindolone	10	++	+	+	12 y
Perphenazine/ Trilafon	Phenothiazine: piperazine compound	10	++	+	++/+++	12 y
Trifluoperazine/ Stelazine	Phenothiazine: piperazine compound	5	++	+	+++	6 y
Thiothixene/ Navane	Thioxanthene	5	+	+	+++	12 y
Fluphenazine/ Permitil, Prolixin	Phenothiazine: piperazine compound	2	+	+	+++	16 y
Haloperidol/ Haldol	Butyrophenone	2	+	+	+++	3 y
Pimozide[c]/Orap	Diphenyl-butylpiperidine	10	+	+	+++	Over 12 y

[a]Alpha-antiadrenergic and anticholinergic effects.

[b]Excluding tardive dyskinesia, which appears to be produced to the same degree and frequency by all agents except clozapine with equieffective antipsychotic doses. Clozapine has produced agranulocytosis; therefore, recommendations for its use are limited (see text).

[c]Only indicated for Tourette disorder that has not responded to other standard treatments; not approved for use in psychoses.

Adapted from American Medical Association. *Drug Evaluations Annual 1994.* Chicago, IL: American Medical Association; 1994.

untoward effects with chlorpromazine (the prototype of the antipsychotics). We note the deletion of thioridazine from this table because of its well-documented adverse effects including cardiac conductivity disturbance related to QT-interval elongation and retinal pigmentation leading to blindness.

Considerations about Dosage

The antipsychotic effects of neuroleptic agents evolve gradually. The depolarization inactivation of dopaminergic neurons, which is necessary for antipsychotic efficacy, takes approximately 3 to 6 weeks to develop. Hence, it is important to have a trial of adequate duration of an antipsychotic medication at usual therapeutic doses rather than rapidly increasing the dose, because a rapid dose increase could lead to the erroneous clinical impression that a much higher dose than necessary was responsible for the patient's clinical improvement. Studies have also suggested that there is a therapeutic window of approximately 300 to 1,000 mg of chlorpromazine or its equivalent for most adult patients with psychosis. Patients receiving <300 mg tend to improve less, and those receiving >1,000 mg of chlorpromazine or its equivalent show no increased benefit (for a review, see Levy, 1993). It is usually recommended that antipsychotic agents initially be administered in divided doses, most frequently three or four times daily. Once the optimal dose is established, however, their relatively long serum half-lives usually permit either once-daily dosage (e.g., before bedtime) or twice-daily dosage (in the morning and before bedtime).

FIRST-GENERATION (TYPICAL) ANTIPSYCHOTIC MEDICATIONS

Chlorpromazine Hydrochloride (Thorazine)

Indications for Chlorpromazine Hydrochloride in Child and Adolescent Psychiatry

In addition to being approved for uses similar to those for adults (including psychotic disorders), chlorpromazine is approved for the treatment of severe behavioral problems in children, marked by combativeness and/or explosive hyperexcitable behavior. It is also noted that dosages >500 mg/day are unlikely to further enhance behavioral improvement in severely disturbed patients with ID.

Chlorpromazine may lower the threshold to seizures; therefore, another antipsychotic medication should be chosen for seizure-prone individuals.

Chlorpromazine Dosage Schedule for Children and Adolescents

- *Infants younger than 6 months of age:* not recommended.
- *Children aged 6 months to 12 years with severe behavioral problems or psychotic conditions:*

  Oral: 0.25 mg/kg every 4 to 6 hours as needed. Titrate upward gradually. In severe cases, daily doses of 200 mg or higher may be required.
  Rectal: 1 mg/kg every 6 to 8 hours as needed.
  Intramuscular: 0.5 mg/kg every 6 to 8 hours as needed. Maximum daily intramuscular dose for a child younger than 5 years or below 22 kg is 40 mg; for a child 5 to 12 years of age or 22 to 45 kg, maximum daily intramuscular dose is 75 mg.

- *Adolescents:* depending on severity of symptoms, begin with 10 mg three times to 25 mg four times daily. Titrate upward with increases of 20 to 50 mg twice weekly. For severely agitated patients, 25 mg may be given intramuscularly and repeated if necessary in 1 hour. Any subsequent intramuscular medication should be at 4- to 6-hour intervals.

Chlorpromazine Hydrochloride Dose Forms Available

- *Tablets:* 10, 25, 50, 100, and 200 mg
- *Spansules (extended release, not recommended for children):* 30, 75, and 150 mg
- *Syrup:* 10 mg/5 mL
- *Oral concentrate:* 30 and 100 mg/mL
- *Suppositories:* 25 and 100 mg
- *Injection (intramuscular):* 25 mg/mL

Reports of Interest

Chlorpromazine in the Treatment of Children and Adolescents Diagnosed with Attention-Deficit/Hyperactivity Disorder

Werry et al. (1966) reported that chlorpromazine was significantly superior to placebo ($P = .005$) in reducing hyperactivity in a double-blind, placebo-controlled, 8-week study of 39 hyperactive children (mean age, 8.5 years; intelligence quotient, 85 or greater), a large number of whom had additional symptoms of distractibility, irritability, and specific cognitive defects. Intellectual functioning and symptoms of distractibility, aggression, and excitability did not appear to have been significantly affected by the medication. The authors concluded that chlorpromazine could be used for behavioral symptoms in therapeutic doses (mean dose was 106 mg/day with a maximum daily dose of 5 mg/kg or 150 to 200 mg) without fear of significantly impairing learning. The most frequent untoward effects were mild sedation and mild photosensitization of the skin (Werry et al., 1966).

Weiss and her colleagues (1975) reported that 5 years after initial diagnosis, there were no differences on measures of emotional adjustment, antisocial behavior, and academic performance among a group of hyperactive children treated with chlorpromazine for 1.5 to 5 years, a similar group treated for 3 to 5 years with methylphenidate, and a group whose medication was discontinued after 4 months because of poor response.

Haloperidol (Haldol)

Pharmacokinetics of Haloperidol

Morselli et al. (1983) noted that steady-state haloperidol plasma levels in children may vary up to 15-fold at a given milligram/kilogram daily dosage, but for a given individual the relationship between dosage and plasma level is fairly consistent. Most children had haloperidol plasma half-lives that were shorter than those of adolescents and adults. However, the authors also emphasized that despite their more rapid metabolism of haloperidol, children did not require proportionally higher daily doses because they also appear to be more sensitive to both the therapeutic and the untoward effects of haloperidol at lower plasma concentrations than were older adolescents and adults (Morselli et al., 1983).

Indications for Haloperidol in Child and Adolescent Psychiatry

Haloperidol is indicated for the treatment of acute and chronic psychotic disorders and for the control of tics and vocal utterances in Tourette disorder. Only after the failure of treatment with psychotherapy and non-antipsychotic medications has haloperidol been approved for treating children with severe behavioral disorders (e.g., "combative, explosive hyperexcitability [which cannot be accounted for by immediate provocation]" [package insert]) and for the short-term treatment of hyperactive children with coexisting conduct disorders, who exhibit such symptoms as "impulsivity, difficulty sustaining attention, aggressivity, mood lability, and poor frustration tolerance."

Haloperidol Dosage Schedule for Children and Adolescents with Psychotic Disorders, Tourette Disorder, or Severe Nonpsychotic Behavioral Disorders

- *Children younger than 3 years of age:* not recommended.
- *Children 3 to 12 years of age (weight: 15 to 40 kg):* begin with 0.5 mg daily; titrate upward by 0.5-mg increments at 5- to 7-day intervals. Therapeutic dose ranges are usually from 0.05 to 0.075 mg/kg/day for nonpsychotic behavioral disorders and Tourette disorder; for children with psychosis, the upper range is usually 0.15 mg/kg/day, but may be higher in severe cases. Morselli et al. (1983) reported good therapeutic results in children with tics and Tourette disorder associated with haloperidol plasma levels in the range of 1 to 3 ng/mL. Higher haloperidol plasma levels, usually between 6 and 10 ng/mL, were necessary for significant improvement in psychotic conditions.
- *Adolescents:* depending on severity, 0.5 to 5 mg two or three times daily. Higher doses may be necessary for more rapid control in some severe cases.

Haloperidol Dose Forms Available

- *Tablets:* 0.5, 1, 2, 5, 10, and 20 mg
- *Oral concentrate:* 2 mg/mL
- *Injectable immediate release (IR) (intramuscular):* Haloperidol lactate (Haldol IR injection): 5 mg/mL. Safety has not been established for children and younger adolescents. If necessary in acutely agitated older adolescents, an initial dose of 2 to 5 mg may be given intramuscularly. Additional medication may be given every 1 to 8 hours as determined by ongoing evaluation of the patient.
- *Injection, long-acting (intramuscular), haloperidol decanoate 50 and 100 mg:* Haldol Decanoate Injection 50 and Haldol Decanoate Injection 100 contain 50 and 100 mg of haloperidol (present as 70.52 and

(continued)

Indications for Haloperidol in Child and Adolescent Psychiatry (*continued*)

141.04 mg of haloperidol decanoate), respectively. The safety and efficacy of haloperidol decanoate has not been established for children and younger adolescents, and it is currently used primarily for treating adults diagnosed with chronic schizophrenia. However, in some severely disturbed adolescents, particularly when medication adherence is a major therapeutic issue, haloperidol decanoate may be indicated. Peak plasma concentration is reached approximately 6 days after injection and plasma half-life is approximately 3 weeks. The usual interval between doses is 4 weeks, but this may need to be adjusted for some patients.

- *Intravenous:* The use of IV haloperidol in children and adolescents is not FDA approved. In fact, the FDA has issued a warning regarding the risk of sudden death from cardiac reasons (including QTc prolongation) with the use of IV haloperidol. When clinicians do use IV haloperidol in adults, it is typically seen in the setting where the adult patient is on a cardiac monitor (such as in the intensive care unit).

Reports of Interest

Haloperidol in the Treatment of Schizophrenia with Childhood Onset

Green et al. (1992) administered haloperidol on an open basis to 15 hospitalized children younger than 12 years of age diagnosed with schizophrenia. They reported the optimal dose to range between 1 and 6 mg/day. Acute dystonic reactions occurred in approximately 25% of the children despite low initial doses and gradual dose increases of the medication.

Spencer et al. (1992) administered haloperidol to 12 patients (9 males and 3 females aged 5.5 to 11.75 years) in an ongoing, double-blind, placebo-controlled study of hospitalized children diagnosed with schizophrenia. Optimal haloperidol dose ranged from 0.5 to 3.5 mg/day (range, 0.02 to 0.12 mg/kg/day; mean, 2.02 mg/day). Haloperidol was significantly better than placebo on staff Global Clinical Judgments ($P = .003$) and on four of the eight Children's Psychiatric Rating Scale items selected for their pertinence to schizophrenia: ideas of reference ($P = .04$), persecutory ($P = .01$), other thinking disorders ($P = .04$), and hallucinations ($P = .04$). Two children (16.7%) experienced acute dystonic reactions. All 12 improved on haloperidol and were discharged on that medication.

In a double-blind, head-to-head comparison of haloperidol and clozapine, Kumra et al. (1996) reported that clozapine was significantly superior to haloperidol in treating treatment-resistant adolescents with childhood-onset schizophrenia. Because of its severe untoward-effect profile, however, clozapine is not a first-line therapeutic medication for schizophrenia. This study is reviewed in detail later under clozapine.

Haloperidol in the Treatment of Tourette Disorder

Shapiro and Shapiro (1989) concluded that the most effective neuroleptics in the treatment of tics and Tourette disorder were pimozide (Orap), haloperidol, fluphenazine (Prolixin, Permitil), and penfluridol (Semap, an investigational medication). Studies by Shapiro and Shapiro (1984), Shapiro et al. (1983), and Sallee et al. (1997) comparing haloperidol and pimozide found pimozide to be more efficacious and to have significantly less severe untoward effects in treating Tourette disorder. These studies are reviewed later under pimozide. Dysphoria upon withdrawal of haloperidol in treatment of Tourette disorder has been reported (Braña-Berríos et al., 2011).

Haloperidol in the Treatment of Autism Spectrum Disorder

Haloperidol is the most well-studied FGA used in the treatment of autism spectrum disorder. In a study of 40 children with autism aged 2.33 to 6.92 years, haloperidol in optimal doses of 0.5 to 3 mg/day yielded global clinical improvement, and it significantly decreased the symptoms of withdrawal, stereotypies, abnormal object relationships, hyperactivity, fidgetiness, negativism, and angry and labile affect (Anderson et al., 1984). However, a high rate of dyskinesias remains a problem. Significant numbers of children with autism (22%, or 8 of 36) developed TD or withdrawal dyskinesia in a prospective study in which 0.5 to 3 mg/day of haloperidol was administered for periods ranging from 3.5 to 42.5 months; thus, close monitoring is necessary (Perry et al., 1985).

In autism spectrum disorder, stereotypies existing at baseline may be suppressed by the administration of haloperidol. When the medication is withdrawn, there is the potential for confusion between the reappearance of stereotypies and a withdrawal dyskinesia; this is of special concern when a physician who is unfamiliar with the child at baseline assumes treatment responsibilities for the child while he or she is on maintenance medication.

Joshi et al. (1988) administered fluphenazine or haloperidol to 12 children aged 7 to 11 years who were hospitalized and diagnosed with childhood onset or atypical pervasive developmental disorders (PDDs) (i.e., approximately equivalent to the DSM-III-R [APA, 1987] diagnoses of autistic disorder with childhood onset and PDD not otherwise specified). The children responded with remarkable improvement in peer interactions and reality testing and decreases in autistic-like behavior, aggressiveness, impulsivity, and hyperactivity. Seven of the 12 children were able to return home rather than be admitted for residential treatment as had been planned. Haloperidol was initiated at a dose of 0.02 mg/kg/day and titrated depending on behavioral response, with increases at 3- to 5-day intervals. Mean optimal dose of haloperidol was 0.04 ± 0.01 mg/kg/day. Untoward effects were remarkably infrequent. Drowsiness occurred initially in some children, but it was transient and did not interfere with their later cognitive performance. Two children receiving haloperidol developed some rigidity and cogwheeling that responded to oral diphenhydramine during the first few days of treatment, and the EPS did not recur when the diphenhydramine was discontinued.

Haloperidol in the Treatment of Aggressive Conduct Disorder

In a double-blind, placebo-controlled study of 61 treatment-resistant hospitalized children, aged 5.2 to 12.9 years, with undersocialized aggressive conduct disorder, both haloperidol and lithium were found to be superior to placebo in ameliorating behavioral symptoms (Campbell et al., 1984b). Optimal doses of haloperidol ranged from 1 to 6 mg/day. The authors reported that, at optimal doses, the untoward effects of haloperidol appeared to interfere more significantly with the children's daily routines than did those of lithium.

Haloperidol in the Treatment of Attention-Deficit/Hyperactivity Disorder

Werry and Aman (1975) investigated the effects of methylphenidate and haloperidol on attention, memory, and activity in 24 children (ages 4.11 to 12.4 years), more than half of whom were diagnosed with hyperkinetic reaction and the remainder with unsocialized aggressive reaction. Each child received one of four medication conditions—placebo, methylphenidate (0.3 mg/kg), low-dose haloperidol (0.025 mg/kg), or high-dose haloperidol (0.05 mg/kg)—in a double-blind, placebo-controlled, crossover (within-subject) design. For all statistically significant measures of cognitive functions of vigilance and short-term memory, the rank order of the means was methylphenidate, haloperidol (low dose), placebo, and haloperidol (high dose). The data suggested that methylphenidate and low-dose haloperidol (although to a lesser degree) improved these cognitive functions, whereas high-dose haloperidol appeared to cause them to deteriorate (Werry & Aman, 1975). The clinical importance of observing this biphasic effect is that it is the dose of haloperidol (not the medication itself) that may cause cognitive improvement or impairment. On the basis of this study, most children and adolescents treated for ADHD with haloperidol should receive doses between 0.5 and 2.0 mg/day (i.e., 0.025 mg/kg for a weight range of 20 to 80 kg).

Pimozide (Orap)

Pimozide is an antipsychotic of the diphenyl-butylpiperidine series. It is indicated for the suppression of motor and phonic tics in patients with Tourette disorder who have failed to respond to standard treatment (e.g., haloperidol). It is not intended as a treatment of first choice, and it is seldom used as a psychotropic medication.

However, it remains in use and some studies suggest that it may be more efficacious that other FGAs (Roessner et al., 2012). Wijemanne et al. (2014) performed a retrospective chart review of the use of pimozide in 268 patients (mean age of 15.8 ± 10.7 years) for the treatment of Tourette disorder and concluded that it was both an effective and safe treatment with no reported cases of TD. Rizzo et al. (2012) compared the metabolic effects of aripiprazole and pimozide in children diagnosed with Tourette disorder ($N = 25$ prescribed aripiprazole, $N = 25$ prescribed pimozide, $N = 25$ with no medication). Both the aripiprazole and the pimozide groups showed treatment efficacy but also had subsequent metabolic symptoms.

A "Dear Health Care Provider" letter dated September 1999, from the manufacturer warned that sudden, unexpected deaths have occurred in patients taking pimozide at doses >10 mg/day.

Indications for Pimozide in Child and Adolescent Psychiatry

Pimozide is indicated only in the treatment of patients diagnosed with Tourette disorder whose development and/or daily life function is severely compromised by the presence of motor and phonic tics and who have not responded satisfactorily to or cannot tolerate standard treatments, such as haloperidol. Pimozide should not be considered a medication of first choice.

Unexplained deaths, perhaps cardiac related, and grand mal seizures have occurred in patients taking high doses of pimozide (>20 mg/day) (PDR, 1995). In September 1999, the manufacturer reported that sudden, unexplained deaths had occurred with doses >10 mg/day.

The usual start dose for patients 12 years and older is 0.05 mg/kg. Maximum dose for these patients is 0.2 mg/kg/day (with an absolute maximum of 10 mg/day).

Thioridazine Hydrochloride (Mellaril)

In July 2000, Novartis, the manufacturer of Mellaril (thioridazine hydrochloride), issued major changes in their labeling. The FDA Black Box Warning (PDR, 2006) states, "Thioridazine has been shown to prolong the QTc interval in a dose-related manner, and drugs with this potential, including thioridazine, have been associated with torsade de pointes–type arrhythmias and sudden death. Because of its potential for significant, possibly life-threatening proarrhythmic effects, thioridazine should be reserved for use in the treatment of schizophrenic patients who fail to show an acceptable response to adequate courses of treatment with other antipsychotic medications, either because of insufficient effectiveness or the inability to achieve an effective dose due to intolerable adverse effects from those drugs."

Currently, thioridazine no longer has FDA approval for treating severe behavioral problems marked by combativeness and/or explosive hyperexcitable behavior, or for the short-term treatment of hyperactive children who show excessive motor activity with accompanying conduct disorders consisting of some or all of the following symptoms: impulsivity, difficulty sustaining attention, aggression, mood lability, and poor frustration tolerance. The use of thioridazine in child and adolescent psychiatry would not only be "off-label" but also would ignore the current recommendations and warnings, and therefore cannot be recommended.

Trifluoperazine Hydrochloride (Stelazine, Vesprin)

Indications for Trifluoperazine Hydrochloride in Child and Adolescent Psychiatry

One manufacturer has a specific disclaimer that trifluoperazine has not been proved effective in the management of behavioral complications in patients with ID and recommends it only for the treatment of individuals with psychosis and for the short-term treatment of nonpsychotic anxiety in individuals with generalized anxiety disorder who have not responded to other medications.

(continued)

Indications for Trifluoperazine Hydrochloride in Child and Adolescent Psychiatry (*continued*)

Trifluoperazine Dosage Schedule

- *Children younger than 6 years of age:* not recommended.
- *Children aged 6 to 12 years of age:* a starting dose of 1 mg once or twice daily with gradual upward titration is recommended. Dosages in excess of 15 mg/day are usually required only by older children with severe symptoms.
- *Adolescents:* 1 to 5 mg twice daily. Usually the optimal dose will be 15 to 20 mg/day or less; occasionally, up to 40 mg/day will be required. Titration to optimal dose can usually be accomplished within 2 to 3 weeks.
- *Tablets:* 1, 2, 5, and 10 mg
- *Oral concentrate:* 10 mg/mL
- *Injection (intramuscular):* 2 mg/mL (One manufacturer notes that there is little experience using intramuscular trifluoperazine with children and recommends 1 mg intramuscularly once daily [or maximally twice daily] if necessary for rapid control of severe symptoms.)

Thiothixene (Navane)

Indications for Thiothixene in Child and Adolescent Psychiatry

Thiothixene use is indicated in the management of symptoms of psychotic disorders. It has not been evaluated in the management of behavioral disturbances in individuals with intellectual disabilities nor is its use recommended in children younger than 12 years of age because safe conditions for its use in that age group have not been established (PDR, 2000).

Loxapine Succinate (Loxitane)

Indications for Loxapine Succinate in Child and Adolescent Psychiatry

Loxapine is a dibenzoxazepine compound with antipsychotic properties used in treating psychotic disorders. The manufacturer does not recommend its use in persons younger than 16 years of age.

Molindone Hydrochloride (Moban)

Molindone hydrochloride is a dihydroindolone compound with antipsychotic properties; it is structurally unrelated to the phenothiazine, butyrophenone, and thioxanthene antipsychotics. Its clinical action resembles that of the piperazine phenothiazines (e.g., perphenazine [Trilafon]) (*Drug Facts and Comparisons*, 1995). Molindone is rapidly absorbed from the gastrointestinal tract, and peak blood levels of unmetabolized medication are achieved approximately 1.5 hours after ingestion. Molindone has many metabolites, and pharmacologic effects from a single dose may last up to 36 hours (PDR, 2000). Although molindone has been associated with sinus tachycardia, it is one of the few antipsychotics that have no warning of increased QTc intervals in the package insert (Gutgesell et al., 1999).

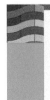

Indications for Molindone Hydrochloride in Child and Adolescent Psychiatry

Molindone hydrochloride is approved for the treatment of psychotic disorders. Its use in children younger than 12 years of age is not recommended because its efficacy and safety have not been established for use in that age group (PDR, 2000). However, its use in the TEOSS study (Sikich et al., 2008) suggests that it may

(*continued*)

Indications for Molindone Hydrochloride in Child and Adolescent Psychiatry
(*continued*)

have utility in the treatment of early-onset schizophrenia. It was found to have equal efficacy to risperidone and olanzapine, while conveying a lower metabolic risk.

Molindone Dosage Schedule

- *Children younger than 12 years of age:* not recommended.
- *Adolescents and adults:* the usual starting dose for treatment of psychotic symptoms is 50 to 75 mg/day, with an increase to 100 mg/day in 3 to 4 days. The medication should be titrated according to symptom response; up to 225 mg/day may be required in severely disturbed patients.

Molindone Hydrochloride Dose Forms Available

- *Tablets:* 5, 10, 25, 50, and 100 mg
- *Oral concentrate:* 20 mg/mL

Reports of Interest

Molindone Hydrochloride in the Treatment of Children Diagnosed with Conduct Disorder

Greenhill et al. (1985) compared molindone and thioridazine in the treatment of 31 hospitalized boys (ages 6 to 11 years) who were diagnosed with undersocialized conduct disorder, aggressive type. Children were assigned randomly to either medication in an 8-week, double-blind, parallel-design study. Subjects were medication-free for the baseline week and were on placebo the second week of the study. During week 3, the medication was raised until it produced sedation; this was followed by a fixed dose of medication during weeks 4 through 6. The final 2 weeks of the study were again with placebo. The mean dose of molindone over the 4-week treatment period was 26.8 mg/day (1.3 mg/kg/day), and the mean dose of thioridazine was 169.9 mg/day (4.64 mg/kg/day).

The groups were similar on baseline ratings, which showed these patients to be severely aggressive. In fact, the initial or terminal placebo periods had to be shortened for 11 of the 31 subjects and medication begun because of their severe symptomatology. Symptoms improved significantly during the 4 weeks on either medication compared with the placebo periods. On Clinical Global Impressions (CGI), nurses rated the severity of illness at the end of the study as less in the molindone group ($P < .08$) and the degree of improvement as significantly greater ($P < .035$). Untoward effects differed, although not significantly, between the medications; acute dystonic reactions occurred more frequently in the molindone group (23.5% vs. 6.1%), whereas sedation and gastrointestinal symptoms were more frequent among subjects treated with thioridazine. The authors concluded that molindone is relatively safe for inpatient children and adolescents and thought its efficacy in this population was similar to the more commonly used neuroleptics. (Note: as mentioned earlier, thioridazine is no longer to be used with children.)

Indications for Fluphenazine Hydrochloride in Child and Adolescent Psychiatry

Fluphenazine hydrochloride is approved for the treatment of psychotic disorders. It is not approved for administration to children younger than 12 years of age because of a lack of studies proving its efficacy and safety in this age group. A manufacturer notes that it has not been shown to be effective in treating behaviorally disturbed patients with intellectual disabilities.

(*continued*)

Indications for Fluphenazine Hydrochloride in Child and Adolescent Psychiatry (*continued*)

Fluphenazine Dosage Schedule

- *Children younger than 12 years of age:* safety and efficacy have not been established; however, United States Pharmacopeial Dispensing Information (USPDI, 2005) recommends 0.25 to 0.75 mg one to four times daily for psychotic disorders in children.
- *Adolescents and adults:* the manufacturer recommends an initial daily total dose of 2.5 to 10 mg for adults, divided and administered every 6 to 8 hours. One should be at least this conservative in adolescents (see also Joshi et al., 1988).

Fluphenazine Hydrochloride Dose Forms Available

- *Tablets:* 1, 2.5, 5, and 10 mg
- *Elixir:* 0.5 mg/mL (2.5 mg/5 mL)
- *Oral concentrate:* 5 mg/1 mL
- *Injectable preparation (intramuscular):* 2.5 mg/mL
- *Long-acting preparations for parenteral administration:* fluphenazine enanthate, 25 mg/mL, and fluphenazine decanoate, 25 mg/mL, are available. (They are used primarily in treating adults diagnosed with chronic schizophrenia. However, USPDI [2005] suggests an intramuscular or subcutaneous dose of between 3.125 and 12.5 mg every 1 to 3 weeks as needed and tolerated in children aged 5 to 11 years. In children aged 12 years and older, an initial dose of 6.25 to 18.75 mg is suggested with a subsequent increase to 12.5 to 25 mg, with injections every 1 to 3 weeks.)

Fluphenazine Hydrochloride (Prolixin, Permitil)

Report of Interest

Fluphenazine Hydrochloride in the Treatment of Children Diagnosed with Autism Spectrum Disorder

As discussed earlier for haloperidol, Joshi et al. (1988) found fluphenazine to be efficacious in treating children diagnosed with childhood-onset PDD or atypical PDD. Fluphenazine was begun at 0.02 mg/kg/day and increased at 3- to 5-day intervals depending on behavioral responses. Mean optimal dose of fluphenazine was 1.3 ± 0.7 mg/day. Untoward effects of fluphenazine were remarkably infrequent. Initial drowsiness occurred in some children, but it was transient.

Second- and Third-Generation Antipsychotic/Mood Stabilizer Medications

RICK T. BOWERS

"ATYPICAL" ANTIPSYCHOTIC/MOOD STABILIZER MEDICATIONS

Before these various medications are discussed in detail as to their relevance and application in the practice of child and adolescent psychiatry, it may be prudent to briefly and simplistically address the various generations of antipsychotic/mood stabilizers and the parameters that have been set in the field in an attempt to give some differentiation to these groups of medications.

First-generation (typical) antipsychotic/mood stabilizers (FGAs) block dopamine D_2 receptors. Second-generation (atypical) antipsychotic/mood stabilizers (SGAs) block dopamine D_2 receptors and 5-HT_{2A} (serotonin) receptors. Third-generation (atypical) antipsychotic/mood stabilizers (TGAs) block dopamine D_2 receptors, 5-HT_{2A} (serotonin) receptors, and cause partial dopamine agonism at various dopamine D receptors.

Class of Antipsychotic/Mood Stabilizers	Mechanism of Action	Antipsychotic/Mood Stabilizer Examples
First-generation (typical) antipsychotic/mood stabilizers (FGAs)	Block dopamine D_2 receptors	Chlorpromazine, haloperidol, thioridazine, fluphenazine, perphenazine
Second-generation (atypical) antipsychotic/mood stabilizers (SGAs)	Block dopamine D_2 receptors and 5-HT_{2A} receptors	Clozapine, olanzapine, quetiapine, risperidone, ziprasidone, paliperidone
Third-generation (atypical) antipsychotic/mood stabilizers (TGAs)	Block dopamine D_2 receptors, 5-HT_{2A} receptors, partial dopamine agonism at various dopamine D receptors	Aripiprazole, brexpiprazole, cariprazine

The simultaneous blocking of D_2 and S_2 receptors in the brain is thought to account for the increased efficacy of these SGA/TGA medications in modestly improving "negative" symptoms of schizophrenia as well as the decreased incidence of extra-pyramidal untoward effects that occur with the atypical antipsychotic medications compared with standard antipsychotic medications (Borison et al., 1992; *Physicians' Desk Reference [PDR]*, 2000). These SGA medications may also have a positive therapeutic effect when administered to some patients with preexisting tardive dyskinesia (TD; Birmaher et al., 1992; Chouinard et al., 1993; Mozes et al., 1994).

For the sake of simplicity, the second- and third-generation antipsychotic/mood stabilizers are combined and referred to as SGAs throughout the chapter because they do share many commonalities. Because prepubertal children and adolescents diagnosed with schizophrenia or bipolar disorder (BPD) differ from their adult counterparts in some significant parameters and frequently respond less satisfactorily to treatment with standard antipsychotics and mood stabilizers, specific randomized controlled (RTC) trials of the various atypical antipsychotic/mood stabilizers have been conducted resulting in child and adolescent U.S. Food and Drug Administration (FDA) indications for schizophrenia as well as BPD.

Neuroprotection and Neurogenesis

It is now apparent that several psychiatric disorders such as schizophrenia, BPD, and recurrent major depression demonstrate atrophic brain changes. The recent discovery that some psychotropic medications used in treating those disorders are neuroprotective in some manner and induce new nerve growth or neurogenesis has brought about a new understanding of the causes and the methods of healing neuropsychiatric diseases. The concept of *neuroprotection* now needs to be considered in the risk–benefit analysis when considering medication therapy in the treatment of these chronic psychiatric conditions.

A series of brain neuroimaging studies by Thompson et al. (2001) led clinicians to associate the clinical and functional deterioration in schizophrenia with the progressive neurodegeneration that was found in this brain disorder. Neuroimaging studies in childhood-onset schizophrenia (COS) revealed a subcortical gray matter and cortical volume loss estimated at 1% to 3% per year during the first 5 years. This is a very significant finding because Fox et al. (2000) reported a mean rate of brain atrophy in Alzheimer disease, on the basis of magnetic resonance imaging measures of total cerebral volumes, to also be about 1% to 3% per year compared with 0.5% to 1% per year in matched elderly controls. That schizophrenia and Alzheimer disease share a similar rate of brain atrophy is a startling and alarming finding. Researchers began to explore the pathogenesis of brain tissue loss in schizophrenia and discovered several interrelated causes. These include the following:

- Dopaminergic overstimulation that can lead to cell death
- Glutamate excitotoxicity and oxidative stress (similar to Alzheimer disorder)
- A decline in protective growth factors or neurotropins such as nerve growth factor (NGF), which stimulate brain-derived neurotropic factor (BDNF) production. These neurotropins, which are critical in brain development, neuroplasticity, and synaptic connectivity, are reduced in treatment-naive schizophrenia.

FGAs and SGAs have different effects on neurotropins in schizophrenia.

The FGAs never gave a promising neurogenesis signal in atrophic brain regions in schizophrenia such as the cerebral cortex or the hippocampus (Chakos et al., 1995). Several studies indicate that not only does haloperidol fail to stimulate neurogenesis in rats but it also appears to be neurotoxic by inducing apoptotic cell death (Wang et al., 2004).

This appears to occur in part due to the decline of neurotropins, such as BDNF. Nasrallah et al. (2004) found via neuroimaging that geriatric patients on FGAs for a long term experienced greater progressive brain loss and higher mortality rates, with haloperidol being the worst offender. Haloperidol causes pronounced reductions in NGF and BDNF, which is reversed by SGAs. FGAs induce caudate nucleus hyperplasia, which may be related to development of TD. The SGAs do not induce caudate hyperplasia (Corson et al., 1999) and, in fact, may reverse it (Chakos et al., 1995). The SGAs reduce whole-brain gray matter volume loss compared with FGAs. SGAs stimulate the genesis of glial cells, which create the myelin covering that pervades brain white matter. White matter deficits have been widely documented in schizophrenia. SGAs and mood stabilizers are known to have neuroprotective properties such as promotion of new nerve cell development and regeneration of cortical gray matter.

The role of neurotransmitters in neurogenesis is important, and the SGAs seem to have an advantage in this area as well. All the leading neurotransmitters that have been implicated in schizophrenia play a role in neurogenesis:

- Dopamine: D_3 receptor stimulation has been shown to promote neurogenesis; however, the role of the D_2 receptor is unclear.
- Serotonin: The $5\text{-}HT_{1A}$ receptor has been implicated in selective serotonin reuptake inhibitor–induced adult neurogenesis, and the $5\text{-}HT_{2A}$ and $5\text{-}HT_{2C}$ receptors have been definitely linked to neurogenesis.
- Gamma-aminobutyric acid (GABA): GABA plays a pivotal role in adult neurogenesis, which is evidenced by the fact that GABA precedes all other neurotransmitters in innervating newborn neurons.
- Glutamate: Group I metabotropic glutamate receptors promote adult neurogenesis; however, stimulation of the N-methyl-D-aspartate (NMDA) or aminomethylphosphonic acid receptors leads to a reduction in neurogenesis.

Now that the important potential benefit of neuroprotection associated with SGAs has been discussed, it is appropriate to contrast this with some of the serious side effects that may occur when these medicines are prescribed. The following table summarizes the comparative risks of the current SGA agents in relation to issues of weight gain, metabolic and hormonal syndromes, as well as cardiac functioning. Informed consent for medication therapy involves a discussion between the clinician and patient that addresses these pros and cons in a risk/benefit analysis each time a medication is prescribed or changed.

Risk of Weight Gain/Metabolic/Diabetes/Prolactin/QTc Issues with Atypical Antipsychotic/Mood Stabilizer Medications

| Medication (Trade Name) | Weight Gain | Risk for Significant Elevation | | | |
		Cholesterol/ Dyslipidemia	Diabetes Type 2	Prolactin Elevation	QTc Prolongation[a]
Clozapine	High	High	High	Low	Moderate
Olanzapine	High	High	High	Low	Low to moderate
Quetiapine	Moderate	Moderate	Low to moderate	0 to Low	Low to moderate
Risperidone	Moderate	Low to moderate	Moderate	Moderate	Low to moderate
Paliperidone	Low to moderate	Low	Low	Moderate	Low
Aripiprazole	Low to moderate	Low	Low	Mild reduction	Very low
Ziprasidone	None to low	Low	Low	Low	Moderate
Asenapine	Low to moderate	Low	Low	Low	Low to moderate
Iloperidone	Low to moderate	Low	Low	Low	Moderate
Lurasidone	Low	Low	Low	Low	0
Cariprazine	Low	Low	Low	Mild reduction	Low

The predictive confidence for asenapine, iloperidone, lurasidone, and cariprazine is restricted for these newer medicines because limited data are available for comparisons.

[a]Individual changes of < 30 ms unlikely to be of concern, and all these medications fall in a range below that value.

Assembled from data collected by Schumann and Ewigman (2008), Hasnain et al. (2010), Tschoner et al. (2007), Harrigan (2004, 2013), and Peuskens et al. (2014).

Clozapine (Clozaril)

Clozapine, a dibenzodiazepine, was approved by the FDA for marketing in the United States in late 1989. It differs from typical antipsychotic medications in its dopaminergic effects. It functions as a dopamine blocker at both D_1 and D_2 receptors, but does not induce catalepsy or inhibit apomorphine-induced stereotypy. Clozapine also appears to block limbic dopamine receptors more than striatal dopamine receptors. This may account for the fact that no confirmed cases of TD were reported in more than 20 years of worldwide experience in patients who received only clozapine (*PDR*, 2000) and even to this day the incidence remains very low.

Volavka (1999) suggested that clozapine's antiaggressive effect in patients diagnosed with schizophrenia may result from its unique pharmacologic properties of preferentially blocking the D_1-mediated function and its serotonergic actions.

Clozapine has significantly greater efficacy in treating the "negative" symptoms of schizophrenia and has shown a lower incidence of extrapyramidal symptoms (EPSs) than have traditional antipsychotics. There is also evidence that clozapine has a positive therapeutic effect on some patients with preexisting TD. As with traditional antipsychotic medications, clozapine initially suppresses the involuntary movements; but, unlike traditional antipsychotics, the abnormal movements do not worsen over time with clozapine, sometimes even with dose reduction. There is a suggestion that, although it may not be curative, clozapine may alleviate TD over time in some patients (Jann, 1991).

Because of the increased risk for serious and potentially life-threatening untoward effects that have been reported in patients receiving clozapine, its administration was previously deemed appropriate only for severely dysfunctional patients with schizophrenia who had not responded satisfactorily to adequate trials of at least two other antipsychotic medications or who could not tolerate the untoward effects present at therapeutic dose levels. Given the realization that neurodegeneration begins to occur with the first psychotic episode in the adolescent brain and continues each year, some clinicians now advocate the implementation of clozapine sooner than later. The logic of using clearly the most efficacious antipsychotic agent currently available is sound and acceptable to many clinicians given that the blood monitoring requirements have made the risk of serious injury or death exceedingly rare.

In their comparison of clozapine and olanzapine in the treatment of treatment-resistant schizophrenia with childhood onset, Kumra et al. (1998) reported that clozapine was superior to olanzapine and remains the "gold standard" treatment for schizophrenia. They also concluded that all children and adolescents with treatment-refractory schizophrenia should be given a trial of clozapine despite the increased risk of serious untoward effects (agranulocytosis/neutropenia and seizures) and the inconvenience of mandatory and necessary monitoring.

Pharmacokinetics of Clozapine

Peak plasma concentrations during steady-state maintenance at 100 mg twice daily occurred on an average of 2.5 hours (range, 1 to 6 hours) after dosing; mean peak plasma concentration was 319 ng/mL (range, 102 to 771 ng/mL). Clozapine is almost completely metabolized to demethylated, hydroxylated, and N-oxide derivatives, of which approximately 50% is secreted in the urine and 30% in the feces. Serum half-life after a single 75-mg dose averages 8 hours (range, 4 to 12 hours); at steady state on 100 mg twice daily, serum half-life averaged 12 hours (range, 4 to 66 hours). Food does not affect the absorption/bioavailability of clozapine; it may be taken with or without food.

Contraindications for Clozapine Administration

Hypersensitivity to clozapine is a contraindication. Also, patients with myeloproliferative disorders, uncontrolled epilepsy, or a history of clozapine-induced agranulocytosis or severe granulocytopenia should not take clozapine. Clozapine should not be administered together with another medication known to cause agranulocytosis or to suppress bone marrow function.

Tolerability and Adverse Effects of Clozapine

Agranulocytosis is reported to occur in association with administration of clozapine in 1% to 2% of patients. Because of this, weekly monitoring of white blood cell (WBC) counts is mandatory, with discontinuation of treatment if the WBC decreases significantly. It has been recommended that if the WBC falls below 3,500, monitoring should be increased to twice weekly, and if the WBC falls below 3,000, clozapine should be discontinued. Alvir et al. (1993) reported that 73 of 11,555 patients who received clozapine during a 15-month period developed agranulocytosis; of these, 2 died from complications of infection. The cumulative incidence of agranulocytosis was 0.80% after 1 year and 0.91% after 18 months. Agranulocytosis occurred during the first 3 months of treatment in the large majority of cases (61 [83.6%] of 73). In general, older patients and females appear to be at higher risk for developing agranulocytosis. An exception appeared to be that patients younger than 21 years of age were at somewhat higher risk than patients between 21 and 40 years of age. The authors also noted that subsequent to the period of their study, an additional five patients between 40 and 72 years of age died from complications resulting from agranulocytosis within 3 months of taking clozapine (Alvir et al., 1993).

Kumra et al. (1996) reported that 5 (24%) of 21 adolescent patients enrolled for up to 30 ± 15 months in their study had mild to moderate neutropenia, compared with an estimated cumulative risk of 1.5% to 2.0% in adults. They suggested that this might occur because, in metabolizing clozapine, children produce relatively higher concentrations of N-desmethyl-clozapine, which is associated with hematopoietic toxicity, than do adults.

Administration of clozapine is also associated with an increased incidence of seizures that is apparently dose dependent. At doses below 300 mg/day, approximately 1% to 2% of patients develop seizures; at moderate doses of 300 to 599 mg/day, approximately 3% to 4% develop seizures; and at high doses of 600 to 900 mg/day, approximately 5% of patients develop seizures. Baseline electroencephalogram (EEG) and periodic monitoring should be mandatory for children and adolescents receiving clozapine.

Gerbino-Rosen et al. (2005) reported a retrospective chart review of the hematologic adverse events (HAEs) in 172 children and adolescents admitted over a 12-year period to a long-term chronic care facility for treatment-resistant disorders, defined as having failed treatment (i.e., continued need for hospitalization secondary to potential for self-harm, harm to others, or inability to care for self) with at least two antipsychotics in at least two chemical classes in clinically appropriate doses; the large majority of patients were diagnosed with schizophrenia spectrum disorders ($N = 139$) or BPD ($N = 25$). Patients, none of whom had previously received clozapine, were administered clozapine (mean age at clozapine initiation was 15.03 ± 2.13 years) on an open-label basis following a standard medication-monitoring program, with weekly assessments of WBC counts with differential, including absolute neutrophil counts (ANCs). The median observation period was 8 months. Neutropenia (an ANC < 1,500/mm^3) occurred in 29 (16.9%) patients; 5 of these patients who continued clozapine as a repeated blood sample had a safe ANC and were not included among the patients who developed clozapine-induced HAE ($N = 24$). One of the 24 (0.4%) developed agranulocytosis (ANC < 500/mm^3). The cumulative probability of developing an HAE over a 1-year period was 16.1% (95% CI, 9.7% to 22.5%); for developing agranulocytosis, the cumulative probability over a 1-year period was 0.99% (95% CI, 0.98% to 1.0%). Twenty of the 24 patients with an HAE were rechallenged with clozapine; of these, 11 did not develop another episode of HAE and remained on clozapine. The nine patients who developed a second episode were administered a third trial of clozapine, with five being successfully maintained on clozapine without subsequent HAE, and four patients eventually stopping because of HAEs. Overall, only eight (5%) patients stopped clozapine because of HAEs. The authors noted that the risk for agranulocytosis in children and adolescents treated with clozapine is similar to that reported for adults; and that with careful monitoring and prompt discontinuation of clozapine at the first sign of an HAE, there were no long-term negative sequelae in these patients (Gerbino-Rosen et al., 2005).

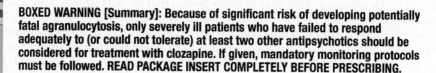

BOXED WARNING [Summary]: Because of significant risk of developing potentially fatal agranulocytosis, only severely ill patients who have failed to respond adequately to (or could not tolerate) at least two other antipsychotics should be considered for treatment with clozapine. If given, mandatory monitoring protocols must be followed. READ PACKAGE INSERT COMPLETELY BEFORE PRESCRIBING.

Indications for Clozapine in Child and Adolescent Psychiatry

Clozapine is indicated for the management of severely ill, treatment-resistant, schizophrenic patients, and to reduce the risk of recurrent suicidal behavior in patients with schizophrenia or schizoaffective disorder who are judged to be at risk of reexperiencing suicidal behavior. The manufacturer noted that safety and efficacy of clozapine have not been established in children younger than 16 years of age.

Clozapine Dosage Schedule

- *Adolescents 16 years of age and adults:* Initially, a dose of 12.5 mg once or twice daily is recommended. The dose can be increased daily by 25 to 50 mg, if tolerated, to reach a target dose of 300 to 450 mg by 2 weeks' time. Subsequent dose increases of a maximum of 100 mg may be made once or twice weekly. Total daily dosage should not exceed 900 mg.

Clozapine Dose Forms Available

- *Clozapine USP scored tablets:* 25, 50, 100, and 200 mg
- *Clozapine orally disintegrating (FazaClo ODT) orally disintegrating tablets:* 12.5, 25, 100, 150, and 200 mg for oral administration without water and may be chewed
- *Clozapine oral suspension (Versacloz):* 50 mg/mL

Mandatory Monitoring

Revisions to United States regulations in 2015 lowered certain ANC thresholds to ≥1,000/mm³, expanding the number of patients eligible to receive the medication, and permitted clinicians to override ANC-based treatment recommendations to continue or restart clozapine in patients for whom the benefits of clozapine clearly exceed the risk of agranulocytosis.

Baseline WBC count must be ≥3,500/mm³, with the differential having an ANC of ≥1,000/mm³. Weekly monitoring of these parameters is required during the first 6 months of treatment with WBC counts ≥3,000/mm³ and ANCs ≥1,000/mm³ necessary to continue on medication.

- Mild neutropenia (ANC 1,000 to 1,499/μL)—Continue treatment but increase monitoring frequency to three times per week.
- Moderate neutropenia (ANC 500 to 999/μL)—Interrupt *clozapine* treatment, increase monitoring to daily until ANC is 1,000/microL at which point clozapine can be reinstituted.
- Severe neutropenia/agranulocytosis (ANC < 500/μL)—Discontinue *clozapine*. Rechallenge should only occur if the benefits outweigh the risks, in consultation with hematology.

If ANC counts for the first 6 months are always within the acceptable range, biweekly monitoring may be initiated after 6 months. If ANC counts for the second 6 months are always within the acceptable range, monthly monitoring may be initiated after 12 months.

Benign ethnic neutropenia—Lower neutrophil thresholds were established for starting *clozapine* in patients with confirmed benign ethnic neutropenia, a cause of neutropenia often seen in patients of African descent. Treatment can be instituted and continued in patients with an ANC of at least 1,000/μL.

Read the complete monitoring instructions in package insert or *PDR* before prescribing.

Other untoward effects include adverse cardiovascular effects such as orthostatic hypotension, tachycardia, and ECG changes.

Reports of Interest

COS, defined as onset before age 13, is a rare but severe form of the disorder, which is often treatment refractory. Short-term studies have indicated superior efficacy of clozapine in controlled, comparative trials against haloperidol (Kumra et al., 1996), olanzapine (Shaw et al., 2006), and high-dose olanzapine (Kumra et al., 2008) in alleviating negative symptoms in patients with treatment-refractory COS compared with patients having adult-onset schizophrenia (AOS). However, there have been no data for patients with COS who have been maintained on clozapine for an extended period of time. To address this, Rapoport et al. (2016) conducted a study assessing functioning and compliance in patients on clozapine over a period of 2-plus years. In general, across various studies, clozapine generally appeared to be more efficacious in patients having COS than in populations with AOS (McGough & Faraone, 2009), especially in alleviating negative symptoms.

To conduct this long-term study, the Child Psychiatry Branch of the National Institutes of Health (NIH) in 1990 began to assemble a unique cohort of COS cases ($N = 131$) diagnosed with schizophrenia to enroll in several studies. Most of the patients had negative symptoms, and all had had clear deterioration of at least 6 months' duration. After the screening process to confirm COS, a 3-month inpatient observation period was initiated, including a 3-week, medication-free period for diagnostic and treatment purposes. Most patients with COS received either a double-blind or an open trial of clozapine before discharge. Two short-term, double-blind study cohorts and one open-label trial cohort were placed on clozapine during their inpatient stay. After dropout for various reasons, 99 patients who tolerated clozapine well in the NIH study were discharged on clozapine. Serious side effects, such as two patients experiencing clozapine-induced seizures and two patients developing neutropenia, resulted in their removal from the study. Four other patients who developed weight gain, palpitations, violence and aggression, and poor impulse control also had to leave the study. Two additional patients discontinued clozapine for unknown reasons. By the end of this process, 87 of the 120 reachable patients with COS, 72.5% were maintained on clozapine for more than 2 years. For patients meeting the criteria for clozapine maintenance, their dosage of clozapine at their most recent follow-up visit to the NIH ranged from 50 to 900 mg, with a median dosage of 500 mg. The lower quartile dosage was 275 mg, and the upper quartile dosage was 500 mg. At time of the last assessment, the average age of the study patients was 27.2 (SD 7.7) years within the COS cohort, and the study group have not found reduced compliance as the subjects become older. The high maintenance rate of COS, 72.5%, exceeds the limited evidence from randomized, double-blind controlled studies of treatment-refractory AOS by Juul Povlsen et al. (1985), Lindstrom (1988), Mattes (1989), Gaszner and Makkos (2004) in which the maintenance rates ranged from 32% to 57%. Despite the inconvenience of monthly hematologic monitoring and weekly, biweekly, and then monthly renewal of prescriptions, these patients made a concerted effort to remain on clozapine ranging from 2 to >20 years, with an average of 6.9 ± 4.98 years of maintenance. Compliance with treatment in the early months of clozapine therapy is important because approximately 30% of patients with treatment-resistant AOS require up to 6 months of treatment with clozapine before exhibiting a reduction in psychotic symptoms (Meltzer et al., 1989). The authors note that the rate of clozapine-related adverse effects in children exceeds those reported for adults (Frazier et al., 2003; Sporn et al., 2007). There is a greater toxicity and risk of agranulocytosis (6%) in younger subjects versus only 1% to 2% of adults experiencing neutropenia (Alvir et al., 1993). Children also have akathisia at a higher rate of 15% versus the 3% seen in adults (*PDR*, 2004). Also, undesirable side effects, such as sialorrhea, tachycardia, heart failure, seizures, weight gain, and metabolic changes may also warrant discontinuation of clozapine. Offsetting these issues of elevated side effects in youth populations that could potentially lead to higher rates of discontinuation of clozapine therapy may be the parental support that is available to these children and adolescents. Such family support is less consistently available for patients having AOS, who often lack insight into their illness. At the time of the last assessment, the average age of the study patients was 27.2 (SD 7.7) years within the COS cohort, and the study group have not found reduced compliance as the subjects become older, which is typically the trajectory.

Clozapine in the Treatment of Children and Adolescents Diagnosed with Schizophrenia

Siefen and Remschmidt (1986) administered clozapine to 21 inpatients, 12 of whom were younger than 18 years (average age, 18.1 years). Their patients had an average of 2.4 inpatient hospitalizations and had been tried on an average of 2.8 different antipsychotics without adequate therapeutic response or with severe extrapyramidal effects. In addition, the clinicians considered it a risk that their patients' psychotic symptoms would become chronic if clozapine was not administered.

Clozapine was administered over an average of 133 days. The average maximum dose was 415 mg/day (range, 225 to 800 mg/day) and the average maintenance dose was 363 mg/day (range, 150 to 800 mg/day). In addition, 11 of the 21 subjects were administered one or more other unidentified medications for about half of the time they were receiving clozapine.

Approximately 67% of symptoms that had been relatively resistant to previous treatment with antipsychotics disappeared or improved markedly in 11 (52%) of the patients, and an additional 6 (29%) patients showed at least slight improvement in the same number of symptoms. Four patients, however, had no changes or worsening of more than half of their psychopathologic symptoms during clozapine therapy. Positive symptoms of schizophrenia improved to a greater degree than did the negative symptoms. Specifically, improvements in incoherent/dissociative thinking, aggressiveness, hallucinations, agitation, ideas of reference, anxiety, inability to take decisions, psychomotor agitation, motivation toward achievement, impoverished and restricted thinking, and ambivalent behavior were reported. Symptoms such as lack of self-confidence, fear of failure, psychomotor retardation, irritability, slowed thinking, blunted affect, and unhappiness showed no improvement or deteriorated during treatment with clozapine (Siefen & Remschmidt, 1986). The most frequent untoward effects observed early in treatment with clozapine were daytime sedation, dizziness, tachycardia, orthostatic hypotension, sleepiness, and increased salivation. No patients developed agranulocytosis, and the hematologic changes that occurred in approximately 25% of patients were clinically insignificant and normalized during continued maintenance on clozapine (Siefen & Remschmidt, 1986).

Schmidt et al. (1990) reported a total of 57 cases of children and adolescents (age range, 9.8 to 21.3 years; mean, 16.8 years; 30 males and 27 females) who were treated with clozapine. Forty-eight patients were diagnosed with a schizophrenic disorder, five with schizoaffective disorder, two with bipolar manic disorder, and two with pervasive developmental disorders (PDDs). These patients had a mean duration of illness of 19.4 months (range, 0 to 74 months) before their hospitalization at the start of the study, which was the first hospitalization for 16 patients, the second for 16 patients, and the third or more for the remaining 25 patients. Clozapine was begun, on an average, approximately 3 months after hospitalization following treatment failures with other antipsychotic medications and concern about chronicity, intolerable untoward effects, or uncontrolled excitation. Average dose during the length of hospitalization was 318 mg/day (range, 50 to 800 mg/day); average dose at discharge was somewhat lower, 290 mg/day (range, 75 to 800 mg/day). Thirty-five patients received only clozapine. In 22 cases, one or more additional other neuroleptics, primarily phenothiazines, were administered simultaneously; but in about one-half of these cases, the additional medications were tapered off and discontinued so that eventually 80% of the patients were on clozapine only. Mean duration on clozapine during hospitalization was 78 days (range, 7 to 355 days).

Clozapine was discontinued in 15 (26%) of the patients between the 8th and 132nd days of treatment (average, 50th day) when they were taking a mean dose of 143 mg/day (range, 25 to 350 mg/day) for the following reasons: insufficient antipsychotic effect in 7 cases; poor compliance and a change to depot medication in 5 cases; and severe untoward effects in 3 cases (cholinergic delirium, seizure, and questionable clinically significant decrease of erythrocytes to 2.3 million).

The authors reported that two-thirds of the patients completing the study significantly improved in the whole range of symptoms. Paranoid-hallucinatory symptoms and excitation responded best, followed by a reduction in aggressivity. Clozapine was less effective in decreasing agitation and improving negative symptoms, and these symptoms sometimes worsened. Untoward effects were noted in all subjects. These included increased heart rate (during the first 8 weeks only) from 94 to 109 beats per minute in 37 (65%) patients, daytime sedation in 29 (51%) patients, hypersalivation in 20 (35%) patients, orthostatic hypotension in 20 (35%) patients, and an unspecified rise in temperature in 15 (26%) patients. Abnormal movements were observed in nine patients, including tremor (six cases), akathisia (one case), and unspecified EPSs in two cases. During the first 16 weeks of clozapine therapy, a significant decrease in various hematologic parameters, including number of erythrocytes, was observed, but did not reach pathologic values; a relative shift from lymphocytes to neutrophils was seen in the differential during the first 2 weeks. There was a reversible increase in liver enzymes, which peaked during the third and fourth weeks. On EEGs, there was evidence that clozapine induced increased neuronal disinhibition (e.g., spike discharges) and a shift in background activity to lower frequencies. Pathologic EEG changes were present in 30 (53%) patients on clozapine compared with 17 (30%) patients before its administration ($P < .01$). One patient developed a seizure (Schmidt et al., 1990). The authors later noted that they considered EEG monitoring before and during treatment with clozapine to be mandatory (Blanz & Schmidt, 1993).

Remschmidt et al. (1994) reported a retrospective study of 36 adolescent inpatients aged 14 to 22 years, diagnosed with schizophrenia, who were treated on an open basis with clozapine following treatment failures with at least two other antipsychotic medications. Doses ranged from 50 to 800 mg/day (mean, 330 mg/day), and the mean duration of clozapine administration was 154 ± 93 days. Twenty-seven patients (75%) had clinically significant improvement; four (11%) had complete remissions. Three patients (8%) showed no improvement. Six (17%) developed untoward effects, necessitating the discontinuation of clozapine: leukopenia without agranulocytosis (two patients); hypertension, tachycardia, and ECG abnormalities (two patients); elevations in liver transaminases to 10 times normal values without other signs of hepatitis (one patient); and worsening of symptoms and development of stupor when given in combination with carbamazepine 400 mg/day (one patient). Five patients developed EPSs over a period of several months: four (11%) developed akathisia and one developed a course tremor. Overall, positive symptoms improved significantly more than negative symptoms did. For example, delusions, hallucinations, and excitation improved in approximately 65% of patients. Some negative symptoms (e.g., flat affect and autistic behavior) showed little improvement, but other negative symptoms (e.g., anergy, muteness, bizarre behavior, and thought blocking) showed improvement in 11% to 22% of the patients. Nine of 10 (90%) patients who had predominantly negative symptoms did not improve clinically.

Levkovitch et al. (1994) treated 13 adolescents (7 males and 6 females; mean age, 16.6 years; range, 14 to 17 years) who were diagnosed with adolescent-onset schizophrenia with clozapine. All had experienced treatment failures, with an average of three traditional antipsychotics. Patients received an average daily dose of 240 mg of clozapine for a mean of 245 days. After 2 months, 10 patients (76.9%) showed significant improvement of at least a 50% decrease in scores on the Brief Psychiatric Rating Scale (BPRS); 2 patients showed more modest improvements. Clozapine was discontinued after 2 days in one patient because of significant orthostatic hypotension. Other untoward effects were tiredness in four (30.8%) patients, hypersalivation in one (7.7%), and temperature elevation in one (7.7%). No leukopenia occurred during weekly monitoring.

Frazier et al. (1994) treated 11 hospitalized adolescents (age range, 12 to 17 years; mean, 14.0 ± 1.5 years) diagnosed with COS with a 6-week open trial of clozapine. Subjects were chronically and severely ill and had received at least two previous neuroleptic medications without significant clinical benefit or experienced intolerable untoward effects. Following a 4-week washout/observation period, clozapine was begun at 12.5 or 25 mg/day. Dose was titrated individually depending on symptom response versus untoward effects and increased by one to two times the initial dose every 4 days to a potential maximum of 900 mg/day. The main untoward effects responsible for limiting dose increases were tachycardia (three patients) and sedation (seven patients). Other untoward effects reported included hypersalivation (eight patients), weight gain (seven patients), enuresis (four patients), constipation (four patients), orthostatic hypotension (two patients), nausea (one patient), and dizziness (one patient).

Extrapyramidal untoward effects also occurred: Four adolescents developed akathisia after several months and one developed a coarse tremor. The mean dose of clozapine at the end of the 6-week period was 370.5 mg/day (range, 125 to 825 mg/day). Six (55%) of the patients improved over 30% on the BPRS on optimal dose of clozapine, compared with admission ratings when nine of the patients were receiving other medications; nine (82%) of the patients improved on clozapine over 30% on the BPRS compared with ratings during the washout period. Nine of the 11 patients also received 6-week courses of haloperidol following 4-week washout/observation periods during their hospitalizations; of these, 5 (56%) showed more than a 30% improvement on the BPRS while on clozapine, compared with earlier ratings while on haloperidol. Both positive and negative symptoms of schizophrenia improved (Frazier et al., 1994).

Mozes et al. (1994) treated four children with clozapine; the three males and one female, 10 to 12 years of age, were diagnosed with schizophrenia and had not responded satisfactorily to other neuroleptics. Clozapine was begun in doses of 25 to 100 mg/day and titrated upward. Three patients had significantly reduced symptomatology in <2 weeks. Further decreases in both positive and negative symptoms occurred during the next 10 to 15 weeks of treatment. All four children improved significantly on the BPRS, with a mean reduction of 41 within 15 weeks. At the time of the report, patients had been in treatment between 23 and 70 weeks, and maintenance dosage ranged from 150 to 300 mg/day. The most frequent untoward effect was drooling, which spontaneously decreased over time; drowsiness, experienced by three patients, peaked during the first week and then gradually faded away. Excitatory EEG changes occurred in three patients, and dosage was not increased to decrease the likelihood of seizures. Of note, two cases of TD caused by previous neuroleptic medications disappeared on clozapine.

Kumra et al. (1996) reported a double-blind study comparing clozapine and haloperidol in 21 hospitalized patients (11 males and 10 females; mean age, 14.0 ± 2.3 years) who had been diagnosed with schizophrenia by DSM-III-R (American Psychiatric Association [APA], 1987) criteria by age 12 and who were treatment refractory. All patients had failed to respond to at least two standard neuroleptics, often at high doses, and augmented with mood stabilizers or antidepressants; most patients also had failed to respond to risperidone. Medications were discontinued over a 2-week period, which was followed by a 4-week washout before active medication whenever this could be tolerated. Patients were randomly assigned to a 6-week parallel treatment with clozapine ($N = 10$) or haloperidol ($N = 11$); the two groups did not differ significantly on any demographic variables. To maintain the blind and to minimize any extrapyramidal effects secondary to haloperidol, all patients receiving that medication were prescribed up to 6 mg/day of benztropine, whereas subjects on clozapine received identical placebo tablets. Initial doses were based on patients' weights and ranged from 6.25 to 25 mg/day for clozapine and from 0.25 to 1.0 mg/day for haloperidol. Increases in the dose by one or two times the initial dose were permitted every 3 to 4 days if clinically indicated. Three patients receiving clozapine and one patient on haloperidol were unable to complete the 6-week trial because of severe untoward effects and were dropped during the fourth and fifth weeks, and the ratings of the final week were carried forward in data analysis. The mean dose of haloperidol during the last treatment week was 16.0 ± 8 mg/day (range, 7 to 27 mg/day) or 0.29 ± 0.19 mg/kg/day (range, 0.08 to 0.69 mg/kg/day). The mean dose of clozapine during the last treatment week was 176 ± 149 mg/day (range, 25 to 525 mg/day) or 3.07 ± 2.59 mg/kg/day (range, 0.34 to 7.53 mg/kg/day); the mean dose of clozapine for the seven subjects who completed the entire 6-week trial was higher: 239 ± 134 mg/day. Clozapine was statistically superior to haloperidol on ratings at the 6-week endpoint on the BPRS ($P = .04$), the Bunney-Hamburg Psychosis Rating Scale ($P = .02$), the Scale for the Assessment of Positive Symptoms ($P = .01$), and the Scale for the Assessment of Negative Symptoms ($P = .002$). Clozapine was also superior to haloperidol on the depression ($P = .02$), thinking disturbance ($P = .05$), withdrawal ($P = .03$), and total ($P = .03$) rating scores on the BPRS. After the double-blind study was completed, the 11 patients who received haloperidol were administered clozapine openly for 6 weeks. The combined sample of 21 subjects was rated on the Clinical Global Impressions (CGI) Scale as follows: very much improved, 2 (9.5%); much improved, 11 (52.4%); minimally improved, 7 (33%); and worsened, 1 (4.8%). The authors also noted that for some patients, clinical improvement continued and peaked only after 6 to 9 months of treatment, as has been reported for adults.

Despite the superiority of clozapine over haloperidol, Kumra et al. (1996) noted serious untoward effects secondary to clozapine. Five of the 10 patients in the double-blind portion developed toxic hematopoietic effects with an ANC of <1,500. In three patients, the WBC normalized spontaneously and they were successfully restarted on clozapine; the other two patients, however, had recurrences of neutropenia when rechallenged with clozapine and were dropped from the study. One patient developed myoclonus and had a tonic-clonic seizure the next day; epileptiform spikes continued on the EEG despite lowering the dose of clozapine and antiepileptic medication, and clozapine was discontinued. Another patient who had bifrontal and posterior delta wave slowing during the study had tonic-clonic seizures as an outpatient on 275 mg/day of clozapine and continued to have petit mal seizures despite a reduction in dosage and treatment with valproate sodium, necessitating discontinuation of clozapine. Three of the 11 patients treated openly with clozapine also developed significant EEG changes associated with worsening behavior, such as increased aggression, psychosis, or irritability. Two of these individuals improved with a reduction of the dose of clozapine and addition of valproate sodium; however, the third experienced further clinical deterioration and facial myoclonus with associated EEG spikes, which required the discontinuation of clozapine. Children and adolescents appear to be at greater risk than are adults to develop clinically significant EEG changes. One patient on clozapine had clinically significant increases in liver enzymes and two had tachycardias of more than 100 beats per minute. The authors also felt that excessive weight gain occurred secondary to clozapine; the two best responders during the double-blind protocol gained the most weight. Only one patient was dropped from the haloperidol group, and that was for signs of incipient neuromalignant syndrome; the discontinuing of haloperidol and initiation of supportive measures resulted in normalization of laboratory abnormalities and vital signs within a few days. The extrapyramidal tract untoward effects expected from haloperidol were minimized by the prophylactic benztropine. This study provides significant support for the importance of clozapine in treatment-resistant schizophrenia in children and adolescents but underscores the importance of monitoring the WBC for untoward effects, such as neutropenia/agranulocytosis, and to monitor EEGs for epileptiform changes, to observe for myoclonic movements that may progress to tonic-clonic seizures, and for seizures as the pediatric age group may be at greater risk for all of these than are adults.

In a naturalistic treatment study, Kranzler et al. (2005) administered open-label clozapine, using a flexible titration schedule, to 20 treatment-refractory adolescents (14 males, 6 females; median age 14.19 years; age range 8.5 to 18 years) diagnosed with schizophrenia and hospitalized in a long-term treatment facility (Bronx Children's Psychiatric Center) to evaluate its effectiveness in the treatment of aggression. Subjects were judged to be acutely ill and required a change of medication because of the severity of their psychosis and aggression when clozapine was introduced. The current medication regime was continued and there was a slow cross-taper with clozapine. Using a mirror-image study design, effectiveness was measured by comparing the number of emergency oral and injected medications and frequency of seclusion or restraint events in the 12 weeks immediately preceding the trial of clozapine and during a similar period (from week 12 through 24 of clozapine treatment) when optimal clozapine levels had been reached. The mean dose at week 24 was 476 ± 119 mg/day, and 11 of the 20 subjects were on clozapine monotherapy. Comparison of preclozapine and optimal clozapine measures implemented for aggressive behavior showed significant decreases in emergency oral medication, injectable medication, and seclusion events. Another significant finding was that patients who had been hospitalized for a shorter length of time when started on clozapine showed a significantly greater reduction in seclusion events than did subjects who had been hospitalized for longer periods when the switch to clozapine was made ($P = .033$). These data suggested that, in such a patient population, clozapine reduces the incidence and severity of violence and aggression and may hasten discharge to a less restrictive setting. The authors think that clozapine treatment may be underutilized because of concerns about its untoward effects and the necessary frequent monitoring with blood tests.

Risperidone (Risperdal)

Risperidone belongs to the new chemical class of benzisoxazole derivatives. It was approved by the FDA for marketing in the United States in 1993. The manufacturer suggests that its antipsychotic properties may be mediated through its antagonism of dopamine type 2 (D_2) and serotonin type 2 ($5\text{-}HT_2$) receptors; it also has a high affinity for alpha-1 and alpha-2 adrenergic and H_1 histaminergic receptors (Risperdal [package insert], 2010).

Risperidone appears to have significantly greater efficacy in improving "negative" symptoms of schizophrenia than do the traditional antipsychotics (Chouinard et al., 1993).

Risperidone has significantly fewer EPSs than do typical antipsychotics. However, the appearance of EPSs is dose related and becomes increasingly greater than that for placebo in the upper approved dosage ranges.

Although the manufacturer notes that there have been isolated reports of TD associated with risperidone, it is likely that the incidence of TD occurring with risperidone only will be significantly less than that with typical antipsychotic agents. Nonetheless, TD has been reported with risperidone since soon after its adoption (Klykylo & Feeney, 1997), and clinicians using this and all antipsychotic agents must be alert for its occurrence.

Pharmacokinetics of Risperidone

Food does not affect the rate or extent of the absorption of risperidone. Peak serum levels of risperidone occur at a mean of 1 hour after ingestion. Risperidone is metabolized in the liver by cytochrome P450IID6 to 9-hydroxyrisperidone, which is the major active metabolite and similar to risperidone in its receptor binding activity. The 9-hydroxyrisperidone active metabolite, developed by Jansen Pharmaceuticals and marketed as Invega, is described later. Because of genetic polymorphism, approximately 7% of Caucasians and a very low percentage of Asians are slow metabolizers. Peak 9-hydroxyrisperidone levels occur in approximately 3 hours in extensive metabolizers and 17 hours in poor metabolizers. Half-life ($T_{1/2}$) of risperidone is approximately 3 hours in extensive metabolizers and 20 hours in poor metabolizers; $T_{1/2}$ of 9-hydroxyrisperidone is approximately 21 hours in extensive metabolizers and 30 hours in poor metabolizers.

Contraindications for Risperidone Administration

Risperidone is contraindicated in patients with a known hypersensitivity to it.

Risperidone should be administered with caution to patients with hepatic impairment, which may increase free risperidone by up to 35%, and/or renal impairment, which may decrease clearance of risperidone and its active metabolite by up to 60%.

Interactions of Risperidone with Other Medications

Carbamazepine

Plasma concentrations of risperidone and 9-hydroxyrisperidone were decreased by approximately 50% with coadministration of carbamazepine over a 3-week period. Plasma levels of carbamazepine did not appear to be affected.

Valproate

Oral doses (4 mg/day) of risperidone did not affect the predose or average plasma concentrations and exposure area under the curve (AUC) of valproate (a total of 1,000 mg administered in three divided doses), but there was a 20% increase in valproate peak plasma concentration after concomitant administration of risperidone.

Lithium

Risperidone (6 mg/day in two divided doses) did not affect the exposure (AUC) or lithium's peak plasma concentration.

Fluoxetine

Fluoxetine in doses of 20 mg/day increased risperidone's plasma concentration from 2.5 to 2.8 times, but did not affect the plasma concentration of 9-hydroxyrisperidone.

Paroxetine

Paroxetine in doses of 20 mg twice daily increased risperidone's plasma concentration by three to nine times and lowered the concentration of 9-hydroxyrisperidone by approximately 13%.

Tolerability and Adverse Effects of Risperidone

Extrapyramidal Symptoms

The incidence of EPSs in patients treated with risperidone appears to be dose related, and clinicians often opt to maintain the dosage below the 6 mg/day dosage.

Hepatotoxicity

Kumra et al. (1997) reviewed the medical records of the 13 children and adolescents (3 males and 10 females) diagnosed with schizophrenia who were admitted to the National Institute of Mental Health (NIMH) over a period of 28 months and treated with risperidone. Two of the three males, but none of the females, showed evidence of steatohepatitis with obesity, elevated liver enzyme values, and evidence of fatty liver on ultrasound, which was confirmed by biopsy in one case. Following discontinuation of risperidone, liver function tests returned to normal within 2 weeks to 3 months. The authors noted that two additional males who were subsequently admitted developed hepatotoxicity during long-term treatment with risperidone. The authors strongly recommended determining baseline liver function tests, obtaining liver aminotransferases, cholesterol, and triglycerides every 3 months, and monitoring weight frequently in pediatric patients who are being maintained on risperidone. Males in this age range may be particularly at risk for hepatotoxicity.

Szigethy et al. (1999) retrospectively reviewed the charts of 38 children and adolescents (32 males and 6 females; mean age, 10.6 ± 3.7; age range, 4 to 17 years) who had been treated with a mean dose of 2.5 mg/day (range, 0.5 to 10.0 mg/day) or 0.05 mg/kg/day (range, 0.01 to 0.11 mg/kg/day) of risperidone for a mean of 15.2 ± 10.0 months (range, 1 to 35 months) to assess hepatic function during risperidone treatment and to identify any clinical factors associated with hepatic dysfunction. Diagnoses of the subjects were autistic disorder ($N = 12$), other PDDs ($N = 8$), mood disorders ($N = 6$), disruptive behavior disorders (DBDs) ($N = 7$), and psychotic disorders ($N = 5$). Thirty-seven (97.4%) of the subjects had normal values for aspartate aminotransferase (AST), alanine aminotransferase (ALT), and total bilirubin after treatment with risperidone for a mean duration of 12.2 ± 9.8 months (range, 1 to 30 months). The 38th subject, who had received 24 months of risperidone and a peak dose of 4 mg/day, had an ALT of 46 U/L, 7 U/L above the upper limit of normal (ULN), which was not considered clinically significant. Baseline liver function tests were available for 14 subjects; comparison of these values with those obtained after an average of 5.47 ± 4.9 months (range, 1 to 19 months) showed no clinically meaningful increases. All subjects for whom baseline weights were available gained weight during treatment (see following text). The authors noted that obesity itself is associated with both steatohepatitis and elevated transaminases and that weight gain alone may have caused the elevated ALT in their patients. Overall, the authors concluded from their review that the risk for risperidone-induced hepatotoxicity is probably low in relatively short-term therapy in this age group.

Weight Gain

Weight gain is often a problem in patients treated with risperidone, usually secondary to a marked increase in appetite. Horrigan and Barnhill (1997) noted a positive correlation between the degree of clinical improvement, increased appetite, and weight gain. They noted that serotonin plays a role in signaling satiety and that, by blocking 5-HT$_2$ receptors, risperidone may cause dysregulation of the "satiety switch."

In their chart review of 38 patients who received risperidone, Szigethy et al. (1999) reported that weight gain occurred in all 23 subjects for whom baseline weights were available; mean baseline weight was 37.92 ± 16.0 kg (range, 15.0 to 73.6 kg), and mean end-of-study weight was 48.28 ± 18.97 kg (range, 19.10 to 82.95 kg). The mean weight gain was 1.01 ± 0.73 kg/month (range, 0.18 to 3.1 kg/month). The mean duration of risperidone therapy for all 38 subjects was 15.2 ± 10.0 months (range, 1 to 35 months), demonstrating that risk of weight gain with risperidone therapy is an important therapeutic issue.

Martin et al. (2000) conducted a retrospective chart review comparing 37 child and adolescent inpatients treated for a minimum of 6 continuous months with risperidone, with 33 inpatients having no exposure to atypical antipsychotics with regard to baseline weight, standardized z scores of weight for age and gender, and percentage of subjects whose weight increased ≥7% (chosen a priori as the standard cutoff for extreme weight gain in clinical trials). After 6 months of risperidone, significantly more subjects on risperidone (78%) versus 24% of controls gained ≥7% of their baseline weight ($P = .001$). A significant difference was evident within 2 months of treatment ($P = .001$). Risperidone-treated subjects gained an average of 1.2 kg/month over the 6-month study, and their weight gain showed no tendency to plateau during that period. There was no correlation between dose of risperidone and demographic or clinical characteristics such as discharge diagnosis or concomitant medication. Weight gain is an important consideration in the treatment of children and adolescents with risperidone and must be considered in the risks and benefits discussed as part of the informed consent process.

Hyperprolactinemia

Risperidone may cause elevations of prolactin that are significantly above normal values and may persist during chronic administration. This is discussed in detail and relevant literature reviewed under the section "Prolactin Levels" in Chapter 2.

Hyperglycemia and Type 2 Diabetes

Epidemiologic studies suggest an increased risk of treatment-emergent hyperglycemia-related adverse events (AEs) in patients treated with atypical antipsychotic medications, including risperidone (*PDR*, 2006).

Other Untoward Effects

Orthostatic hypotension, dizziness, tachycardia, increase of QTc interval on ECG to >450 ms, insomnia or somnolence, constipation, rhinitis, and many other untoward effects have been reported.

Indications for Risperidone in Child and Adolescent Psychiatry

Risperidone is indicated for the following:
- Treatment of schizophrenia in adolescents aged 13 to 17 years
- Treatment of acute manic or mixed episodes associated with bipolar I disorder in children and adolescents aged 10 to 17 years
- Treatment of irritability associated with autistic disorder in children and adolescents aged 5 to 16 years.

Risperidone Dosage Schedule for Schizophrenia

Adolescents 13 to 17 years of age: an initial dose of 0.5 mg once daily in AM or PM is recommended, with increases of 0.5 to 1.0 mg occurring in intervals of no less than 24 hours as tolerated to a recommended dose of 3 mg/day. It is recommended that any subsequent adjustments of dosage be made at weekly intervals to allow adequate time for steady-state serum levels to be achieved. The manufacturer indicates that although efficacy has been demonstrated in studies of adolescent patients with schizophrenia at doses between 1 and 6 mg/day, no additional benefit was seen above 3 mg/day, and higher doses were associated with more AEs. Doses higher than 6 mg/day have not been studied in adolescents. It is recommended that patients experiencing persistent somnolence may benefit from administering half the daily dose twice daily.

Risperidone Dosage Schedule for Bipolar Disorder

Children and adolescents aged 10 to 17 years of age: an initial dose of 0.5 mg once daily in AM or PM is recommended, with increases of 0.5 to 1.0 mg occurring in intervals of no less than 24 hours as tolerated to a recommended dose of 2.5 mg/day. The manufacturer indicates that although efficacy has been demonstrated in studies of adolescent patients with bipolar mania at doses between 0.5 and 6 mg/day, no additional benefit was seen above 2.5 mg/day, and higher doses were associated with more AEs. Doses higher than 6 mg/day have not been studied in children and adolescents.

Risperidone Dosage Schedule for Autism

Children and adolescents 5 to 16 years of age: Dosing should be initiated at 0.25 mg/day for patients <20 kg and 0.5 mg/day for patients ≥20 kg. After a minimum of 4 days from treatment initiation, the dose may be increased to the recommended dose of 0.5 mg/day for patients <20 kg and 1 mg/day for patients ≥20 kg. This dose should be maintained for a minimum of 14 days. In patients not achieving sufficient clinical response, dose increases may be considered at ≥2-week intervals in increments of 0.25 mg/day for patients <20 kg or 0.5 mg/day for patients ≥20 kg. Caution should be exercised with dosage for smaller children who weigh <15 kg. In clinical trials, 90% of patients who showed a response (based on at least 25% improvement

(continued)

Indications for Risperidone in Child and Adolescent Psychiatry (*continued*)

on Aberrant Behavior Checklist—Irritability subscale [ABC-I]), received dosages between 0.5 and 2.5 mg/day. The maximum daily dose of risperidone in one of the pivotal trials, when the therapeutic effect reached plateau, was 1 mg in patients <20 kg, 2.5 mg in patients ≥20 kg, or 3 mg in patients >45 kg. No dosing data are available for children who weighed <15 kg. The manufacturer recommends that consideration be given to gradually lowering the dose to achieve the optimal balance of efficacy and safety once sufficient clinical response has been achieved and maintained.

Risperidone Dose Forms Available

- *Tablets:* 0.25, 0.5, 1, 2, 3, and 4 mg
- *Orally disintegrating tablets (Risperdal M-TAB):* 0.5, 1, and 2 mg
- *Oral solution:* 1 mg/mL
- *Long-acting injection (Risperdal Consta):* 25, 37.5, and 50 mg vials. This dosage form is indicated for the treatment of schizophrenia and is designed to provide 2 weeks of medication coverage. Its use is not recommended in patients younger than 18 years of age because its safety and efficacy have not been studied in this age group.

Schizophrenia

U.S. Food and Drug Administration Registry Trials

The efficacy and safety of risperidone in the short-term treatment of schizophrenia in adolescents aged 13 to 17 years was demonstrated in two short-term (6 and 8 weeks), double-blind controlled trials. All patients met DSM-IV diagnostic criteria for schizophrenia and were experiencing an acute episode at time of enrollment.

In the first trial (study 1), patients were randomized into one of three treatment groups: risperidone 1 to 3 mg/day ($N = 55$, mean modal dose = 2.6 mg), risperidone 4 to 6 mg/day ($N = 51$, mean modal dose = 5.3 mg), or placebo ($N = 54$). In the second trial (study 2), patients were randomized to either risperidone 0.15 to 0.6 mg/day ($N = 132$, mean modal dose = 0.5 mg) or risperidone 1.5 to 6 mg/day ($N = 125$, mean modal dose = 4 mg).

In all cases, study medication was initiated at 0.5 mg/day (with the exception of the 0.15 to 0.6 mg/day group in study 2, where the initial dose was 0.05 mg/day) and titrated to the target dosage range by approximately day 7. Subsequently, dosage was increased to the maximum tolerated dose within the target dose range by day 14. The primary efficacy variable in all studies was the mean change from baseline in total Positive and Negative Syndrome Scale (PANSS) score. Results of the studies demonstrated efficacy of risperidone in all dose groups from 1 to 6 mg/day compared with placebo, as measured by significant reduction of total PANSS score. The efficacy on the primary parameter in the 1- to 3-mg/day group was comparable to the 4- to 6-mg/day group in study 1, and similar to the efficacy demonstrated in the 1.5- to 6-mg/day group in study 2. In study 2, the efficacy in the 1.5- to 6-mg/day group was statistically significantly greater than that in the 0.15- to 0.6-mg/day group.

Doses higher than 3 mg/day did not reveal any trend toward greater efficacy (Risperdal [package insert], 2010).

Autism

U.S. Food and Drug Administration Registry Trials

The efficacy and safety of risperidone in the treatment of irritability associated with autistic disorder were established in two 8-week, double-blind, placebo-controlled trials in 156 children and adolescents (aged 5 to 16 years) who met the DSM-IV criteria for autistic disorder. The Research Units on Pediatric Psychopharmacology (RUPP) Autism Network Study Part 1 was a randomized 8-week, multisite, randomized, double-blind, placebo-controlled, parallel-group, flexible-dose study.

This study was to compare the safety and efficacy of risperidone and placebo in the treatment of severe tantrums, aggression, and/or self-injurious behavior (SIB) in 101 children (82 males and 19 females; age range 5 to 17 years, mean age 8.8 + 2.7 years) who were diagnosed with autistic disorder by DSM-IV (APA, 1994) criteria. The primary outcome measures were the Irritability subscale of the Aberrant Behavior Checklist (ABC) and the Clinical Global Impressions–Improvement (CGI-I) Scale; a positive response required a minimum 25% reduction on the Irritability score and a rating of 1 or 2 (much improved or very much improved) on the CGI-I Scale at time 8 weeks. Forty-nine subjects were assigned to risperidone and 52 to placebo.

The initial dose of risperidone was determined by subjects' weight. More than 90% of these subjects were below 12 years of age and most weighed more than 20 kg (16 to 104.3 kg). Children weighing ≤20 kg received 0.25 mg daily; those weighing 20 to 45 kg received 0.5 mg daily at bedtime for the first 3 days and then increased to 0.5 mg twice daily on day 4 followed by titration in 0.5-mg increments to a maximum of 1 mg in the morning and 1.5 mg at bedtime by day 29. Children weighing ≥45 kg were prescribed medication at a somewhat accelerated rate to achieve a maximum permitted dose of 1.5 mg in the morning and 2.0 mg at bedtime. The final mean dose of risperidone was 1.8 + 0.7 mg/day, with a range of 0.5 to 3.5 mg.

At 8 weeks, subjects on risperidone had a 56.9% decrease on the Irritability subscale of the ABC versus 14.1% decrease for subjects receiving placebo ($P < .001$). On the CBI-I Scale, 75.5% of subjects on risperidone were rated 1 or 2 (very much improved or much improved) versus only 11.5% of subjects on placebo. Positive responders included 69% of the risperidone group versus only 12% of the group on placebo ($P < .001$). The authors also noted that, compared with the group receiving placebo, the risperidone group improved significantly on the Stereotypy and Hyperactivity Scales, but there were no significant differences on the Social Withdrawal and Inappropriate Speech Scales of the ABC. The authors also noted that 23 of the 34 subjects who were "responders" continued to show benefit after 6 months on medication.

No child dropped out of the study because of AEs; no serious AEs occurred in the risperidone group and most were mild and self-limited (e.g., fatigue/drowsiness subsided in most subjects within 4 to 6 weeks). Increased appetite ("mild" 49% vs. 25%, $P = .03$; "moderate" 24% vs. 4%, $P = .01$), fatigue 59% versus 27%, drowsiness 49% versus 12% ($P < .001$), dizziness 16% versus 4% ($P = .05$), and drooling 27% versus 6% ($P = .02$) were each significantly more frequent in the risperidone group than in the placebo group. Over the 8-week study, subjects on risperidone gained significantly more weight—an average of 2.7 + 2.9 kg versus 0.8 + 2.2 kg for subjects in the placebo group ($P < .001$). Three (6%) of the subjects in the risperidone group withdrew from the study because of lack of clinical efficacy versus 18 (35%) of the subjects in the placebo group, of whom 12 withdrew because of lack of clinical efficacy ($P = .001$).

The authors concluded that risperidone was safe and effective, with a favorable risk–benefit ratio in the short-term treatment of children diagnosed with autistic disorder. Significant improvements were noted in tantrums, aggression, SIB, stereotypic behavior, and hyperactivity.

Long-term Trials

Additional safety information was also assessed in a long-term study in patients with autistic disorder, or in short- and long-term studies involving 1,885 pediatric patients with psychiatric disorders other than autistic disorder, schizophrenia, or bipolar mania who were of similar age and weight and who received similar dosages of risperidone as patients treated for irritability associated with autistic disorder (Risperdal [prescribing information], 2007).

Weight Changes

In longer term pediatric studies, the majority of weight gain occurred during the first 6 months. At 12 months, expected normal growth (7 to 8 lb) accounted for approximately half of the 17-lb weight gain observed with risperidone.

Tardive Dyskinesia

Of the 1,885 patients with autistic disorder and other psychiatric disorders, two patients were reported to have TD (0.1%). In both cases, TD resolved upon discontinuation.

Reports of Interest

Horrigan and Barnhill (1997) reported treating 11 males ranging from children to adults with risperidone (mean age, 18.3 years; age range, 6 to 34 years); 10 of these subjects were diagnosed with autistic disorder with comorbid moderate to severe mental retardation. All 11 exhibited explosive aggressive behavior, including SIBs of such a magnitude that their present caretakers were considering placing them elsewhere; 8 of them had poor sleep patterns, which additionally aggravated the situation. On average, the 11 patients had prior trials on 5.45 psychotropic medications with no, or only partial, improvement. After appropriate washout, five subjects were begun on risperidone only and six had risperidone added to partially efficacious medications, which were continued. Risperidone was initiated with a bedtime dose of 0.5 mg daily and titrated upward in 0.25- to 0.5-mg increments every 5 to 7 days. All patients improved, with the most significant clinical gains apparent within 24 hours. Aggression, self-injury, explosivity, overactivity, and poor sleep patterns improved the most, and caregivers reported that many of the patients tolerated frustration and transitions better and appeared calmer and focused. Optimal daily dose after 4 weeks ranged from 0.5 to 2.0 mg, with a modal dose of 0.5 mg bid ($N = 10$); after 4 months, the modal dose remained unchanged for the eight patients who continued on the study. Untoward effects reported included three patients with initial mild sedation that ceased by the third week. One patient developed possible chemical hepatitis, with gamma-glutamyltranspeptidase increasing from a baseline of 32 to 295 at week 10, necessitating discontinuation. Possible precipitation of a new complex partial seizure disorder and a weight loss of 3.5 kg occurred in one patient, and significant weight gain was reported in eight patients, with gains of 1.6 to 3.6 kg within 4 weeks. None of the patients developed any extrapyramidal tract symptoms or significant changes in blood pressure or heart rate.

Bipolar Disorder

U.S. Food and Drug Administration Registry Trials

The efficacy and safety of risperidone in the short-term treatment of acute manic or mixed episodes associated with bipolar I disorder (BP-I) in 169 children and adolescent patients, aged 10 to 17 years, were demonstrated in one double-blind, placebo-controlled, 3-week trial.

Reports of Interest

Risperidone in the Treatment of Children and Adolescents Diagnosed with Bipolar Disorder

Frazier et al. (1999) conducted a retrospective chart review of outpatients at a university center who were diagnosed by DSM-IV criteria (APA, 1994) with BPD and treated with risperidone. Twenty-eight such subjects, mean age 10.4 ± 3.8 (range, 4 to 17 years; 27 males, 1 female), were identified. Twenty-five subjects were diagnosed with BP-I, most recent episode mixed, and three with BP-I, most recent episode hypomanic. In addition, there was an average of 2.6 ± 0.8 comorbid diagnoses, including attention-deficit/hyperactivity disorder (ADHD) in 25 (89%) and PDD in 8 (29%), and 13 subjects had psychotic symptoms. Subjects had been previously medicated with an average of 3.6 ± 1.7 medications. Outcome was measured using the NIMH CGI Scale, including CGI-S (illness severity) and CGI-I (global improvement).

Risperidone was begun at a low dose and titrated to reach the lowest dose, achieving acceptable clinical improvement. Mean optimal daily dose of risperidone was 1.7 ± 1.3 mg. Mean length of treatment was 6.1 ± 8.5 months (range, 1 week to 34 months). A mean of 1.8 ± 1.1 medications was administered concurrently to 27 (96%) of the subjects. Optimal clinical response to risperidone was 1.9 ± 1.0 months; 16 (57%) responded within the first month. CGI-S scores stratified for syndromes of mania, psychosis, and aggression all showed significant improvement, with decreases from marked severity to within the mild severity range. Such scores for ADHD declined significantly, but still remained in the moderately severe range. Using a CGI-I rating of 2 or less ("much" or "very much improved") to define robust improvement, 82% of subjects improved for mania, 82% for aggression, 69% for psychosis, and 8% for ADHD. No serious untoward effects were reported; common untoward effects were weight gain (18%), mild sedation (18%), and drooling (7%). There were no cases of extrapyramidal side effects. Prolactin levels were available for 11 subjects; mean prolactin level was 32.8 ± 12.05 ng/mL (normal range, 0 to 15 ng/mL) and was above normal in 9 (82%) of these subjects.

The authors concluded that risperidone treatment resulted in rapid and sustained improvement of manic, psychotic, and aggressive symptoms in these 28 children diagnosed with BP-I, all but 1 of whom had been previously medicated with limited success. They noted that the efficacy of risperidone was in contrast to similar subjects treated with mood stabilizers, which, although efficacious, took many months to reach maximum clinical improvement and were associated with a high percentage of relapse.

Risperidone in the Treatment of Children and Adolescents Diagnosed with Conduct Disorder (and Various Intelligence Quotients)

Findling et al. (2000) conducted a small 10-week, randomized, double-blind, placebo-controlled study at an inner-city, academic medical center to address whether risperidone was superior to placebo in ameliorating aggression in children and adolescents. More specifically, the study attempted to examine the safety, tolerability, and efficacy of risperidone in children and adolescents suffering from a primary diagnosis conduct disorder (CD) with prominent aggressive behavior. Notably, exclusion criteria included moderate or severe ADHD and significant psychiatric comorbidity including mood disorders.

Twenty youths (19 males and 1 female) were selected as subjects. Ten were randomly assigned to receive placebo and 10 youths were randomly assigned to receive risperidone. Half of the youths assigned to each treatment arm were White. The ages of the patients ranged from 6 to 14 years. Nine of the youths (six in the risperidone group and three in the placebo group) had not improved with community-based treatments with other psychotropic medications. These nine youths had all previously received methylphenidate. Other medications that had been previously prescribed to these youths included dextroamphetamine ($N = 4$), clonidine ($N = 3$), an antidepressant ($N = 5$), divalproex sodium ($N = 2$), and thioridazine ($N = 1$).

Patients were seen weekly throughout the trial. The starting dose of medication was one 0.25 or 0.50 mg tablet per day, depending on patient weight, given in the morning. Medications could be increased at weekly intervals during the first 6 weeks of the study. Patients weighing <50 kg had a maximum total daily dose of risperidone of 1.5 mg. Patients weighing 50 kg or greater had a maximum total daily dose of risperidone of 3.0 mg.

Of the 10 youths assigned to risperidone, 6 completed the entire study. Only three youths who received placebo finished the trial. The average estimated end-of-study dose for those youths assigned to risperidone was 0.028 ± 0.004 mg/kg/day (range, 0.75 to 1.50 mg/day). Although investigators were permitted to use their discretion to alter dosing to bedtime or in divided dosages, all but one subject received their medication as a once-daily dose in the morning.

The primary outcome measure was the Rating of Aggression Against People and/or Property Scale (RAAPPS). The authors concluded that risperidone was clearly superior to placebo in ameliorating aggression on this primary outcome measure during the last 4 weeks of the study. Statistically significant differences were not found for all measures of aggression in the secondary outcome measures, but there were positive trends on many measures and this finding may have been the result of the small sample size. The once-a-day dosages used in this study were fairly modest, and larger dosages or the utilization of multiple dosages over the course of a day may have been more beneficial for some patients. Risperidone was reasonably well tolerated, with none of the risperidone-treated patients developing extrapyramidal side effects or requiring treatment with oral benztropine, which the study allowed. There were no clinically significant changes in any laboratory values such as elevations of serum transaminases or electrocardiogram (ECG) findings. The predicted weight gain for the risperidone group was 4.2 ± 0.7 kg and for the placebo group 0.74 ± 0.9 kg, suggesting that treatment with risperidone was associated with weight gain. The modest side-effect rates found in the study were likely due to the low dosing ranges and slow titration utilized in the study as well as the short duration of the study. The authors concluded that these data provide preliminary evidence that risperidone may have efficacy in the treatment of youths with CD. Because of the small sample size and the brief length of this study, further research is necessary to confirm these findings.

Findling et al. (2000) noted that, despite the small sample size, clinical improvement on almost all measures of aggressive behavior were highly significant in patients receiving risperidone compared with those on placebo. Risperidone, in low daily doses, appears to be a promising short-term treatment for at least some youngsters diagnosed with CD and exhibiting prominent aggressive behavior (Findling et al., 2000).

Aman et al. (2000) conducted a 6-week, randomized, double-blind, placebo-controlled study of risperidone in the treatment of 118 children (age range, 5 to 12 years) exhibiting severe conduct problems and who had intelligence quotients (IQs) ranging from 35 (moderate retardation) to 84 (borderline intelligence). Efficacy was determined by ratings on the Nisonger Child Behavior Rating Form (N-CBRF), the ABC, the Behavior Problems Inventory, and the CGI Scale. Risperidone dosage was titrated to be within a range of 0.02 to 0.06 mg/kg/day. The mean treatment dose was 1.23 mg/day. Patients on risperidone improved significantly more on the N-CBRF than did patients on placebo, beginning within the first week and continuing for the duration of the study. At endpoint, risperidone was also significantly better than placebo, as evidenced by ratings on the other scales. No serious untoward effects were reported.

Snyder et al. (2002) conducted a double-blind, placebo-controlled 6-week study of 110 children (age range, 5 to 12 years) with subaverage IQs (15 were moderately retarded [IQ = 35 to 49], 42 were mildly retarded [IQ = 50 to 69], and 53 had borderline IQs [IQ = 70 to 85]) to determine the efficacy of risperidone in reducing the severe disruptive behaviors they exhibited, including aggression, destruction of property, impulsivity, and defiance of authority. The children were diagnosed with CD, oppositional defiant disorder, or DBD NOS; 80% of subjects were also diagnosed with ADHD, and 45 of these continued treatment with the stimulant medication they were already receiving at time of entry to this study. Subjects had to have a score of 24 or greater on Conduct Problem subtest of the N-CBRF at baseline and at the end of a weeklong single-blind placebo run-in period that preceded the 6-week study to enter the double-blind phase. Of the 133 children beginning the study, 23 (17.3%) were placebo responders who dropped out of the study before the double-blind phase.

Subjects were randomly assigned to placebo ($N = 57$) or risperidone ($N = 53$). Twenty-five subjects dropped out of the double-blind portion; the most common reason being insufficient response. All 19 dropouts from the placebo group were for insufficient response, whereas only 2 of the 6 dropouts from the risperidone group were for this reason ($P < .001$).

Risperidone or placebo was administered as an oral solution, beginning at 0.01 mg/kg/day and titrated upward with a maximum permitted weekly increase of 0.02 mg/kg to a total maximum dose of 0.06 mg/kg/day. The mean dose of risperidone at the endpoint was 0.98 ± 0.06 mg/day (range 0.40 to 3.80 mg/day) or 0.033 ± 0.001 mg/kg/day. The risperidone group showed a significantly greater reduction in ratings on the primary outcome variable, the N-CBRF Conduct Problem subtest, than the placebo group (47.3% vs. 20.9% reduction, $P < .001$). In addition, significant improvements for subjects on risperidone were reported on several other subscales of the N-CBRF (Conduct Problem scale) and on various subscales of the Behavior Problems Inventory (aggressive behavior), the ABC (Irritability), and the Visual Analog Scale (VAS) (symptom) compared with the placebo group. Ratings on the CGI-I Scale for subjects who completed the 6-week double-blind phase were significantly better for the risperidone group ($N = 42$), which improved significantly more than those in the placebo group ($N = 37$). No clinically significant ECG changes occurred. There were no significant cognitive changes on the Continuous Performance Test (CPT) or on the modified children's version of the California Verbal Learning Test (MCVLT-CV).

The most common adverse effects reported in the risperidone group were somnolence (41.5%), headache (17%), appetite increase (15.1%), and dyspepsia (15.1%). At endpoint, the risperidone group gained significantly more weight than did the placebo group, 2.2 versus 0.2 kg ($P < .001$). Prolactin levels increased significantly in both males (from 6.96 at baseline to 27.08 at endpoint) and females (from 11.30 at baseline to 30.38 at endpoint) taking risperidone; the authors attributed this increase in the group to a minority of subjects whose increased prolactin levels fell within the 35 to 105 ng/mL range (normal range is 2 to 18 ng/mL for males and 3 to 30 ng/mL for females).

The authors concluded that risperidone was effective in reducing aggression, hyperactivity, and self-injury associated with DBDs and that it was adequately tolerated.

Risperidone in the Treatment of an Adolescent Diagnosed with Obsessive-Compulsive Disorder

Simeon et al. (1995) reported that a 16-year-old male diagnosed with severe obsessive-compulsive disorder, symptoms of anxiety, and aggressive and oppositional behavior and who had failed prior trials of clomipramine alone and in combination with standard neuroleptics and fluvoxamine showed minimal improvement and remained severely dysfunctional when risperidone was used in combination with clomipramine and fluvoxamine.

Risperidone in the Treatment of Children and Adolescents Diagnosed with Tic Disorders

Gilbert et al. (2004) conducted a randomized, double-blind crossover trial comparing risperidone and pimozide in 19 children and adolescents (15 males and 4 females; age range, 7 to 17 years, mean 11 ± 2.5 years) who were diagnosed with Tourette disorder ($N = 16$) or chronic motor tic disorder ($N = 3$). Subjects were randomized to active treatment for a 4-week period; this was followed by a 2-week washout and administration of the other medication for an additional 4 weeks. All subjects received placebo for an initial 2-week period, at the completion of which baseline tic severity was determined. The active medications were titrated for the first 2 weeks and then held constant for the final 2 weeks of each period. Doses were increased if there was minimal or no improvement and held constant if untoward effects developed. Both treatments were administered twice daily; however, the morning dose of pimozide was a placebo. Pimozide was begun at a dose of 1 mg at bedtime and could be titrated up to a maximum of 4 mg/day. Risperidone was begun at a dose of 0.5 mg twice daily (morning and bedtime) and could be titrated up to a maximum of

2 mg twice daily. Two subjects taking risperidone and one subject taking pimozide discontinued the study because of worsening tics. Thirteen subjects completed the study. The final daily doses of risperidone ranged from 1 to 4 mg (mean 2.5 mg/day); final daily doses of pimozide ranged from 1 to 4 mg (mean 2.4 mg/day). Changes in tic severity were rated on the Yale Global Tic Severity Scale (YGTSS; baseline rating = 43.3 ± 17.5). For the first 4-week period, subjects on risperidone had significantly lower tic severity scores on the YGTSS than did subjects on pimozide (25.2 ± 13.6 vs. 34.2 ± 14.2; $P = .05$). The mean 18-point (42%) decrease on the YGTSS in the subjects receiving risperidone is clinically meaningful. Subjects on both medications experienced weight gain; during the 4-week treatment periods, subjects on risperidone gained a mean of 1.9 kg, whereas those on pimozide gained about half as much, 1.0 kg. Untoward effects were rated as mild. The authors conclude that their study supports the idea that risperidone and other atypical dopamine blocking agents are effective in treating Tourette disorder, but caution that excessive weight gain and high dropout rates in this and other studies suggest that, when such medications are used as monotherapy, the efficacy–to–adverse-effect ratio is unfavorable for some patients.

Olanzapine (Zyprexa)

Olanzapine belongs to the thienobenzodiazepine class. It was approved by the FDA for marketing in the United States in 1997. The manufacturer suggests that its antipsychotic properties may be mediated through a combination of dopamine and serotonin type 2 ($5\text{-}HT_2$) antagonism. Olanzapine also antagonizes muscarinic M_{1-5} receptors, which may explain its anticholinergic effects; histamine H_1 receptors, which may explain the somnolence that may occur; and adrenergic alpha-1 receptors, which may explain the orthostatic hypotension sometimes observed.

Pharmacokinetics of Olanzapine

Food does not affect the rate or extent of absorption of olanzapine. Peak serum concentrations occur approximately 6 hours after oral administration. The half-life of olanzapine ranges from 21 to 54 hours in 90% of the population, with a mean half-life of 30 hours. With once-daily dosing, steady-state serum concentrations occur in approximately 7 days.

Olanzapine is metabolized primarily by direct glucuronidation and cytochrome P450 (CYP)-mediated oxidation. The major circulating metabolites during steady-state, 10-N-glucuronide and 4-N-desmethyl olanzapine are clinically inactive at usual doses. The medication is highly metabolized, with only approximately 7% being recovered unchanged in the urine. Approximately 60% of the medication is excreted through the kidneys, and approximately 30% is recovered in the feces.

Tobacco smoking induces cytochrome CYP1A2, a principal enzyme mediating the metabolism of olanzapine; hence, adult smokers have lower plasma olanzapine levels than do nonsmokers.

It is noted that olanzapine clearance is approximately 30% greater in males than in females and approximately 40% greater in smokers than in nonsmokers; however, dosage modifications are not usually necessary.

Grothe et al. (2000) studied the pharmacokinetics (PK) of olanzapine in an 8-week, open-label treatment of eight inpatients (4 males and 4 females; age range, 10 to 18 years) diagnosed with schizophrenia who were subjects in the NIMH study investigating the efficacy and safety of atypical antipsychotic medications in treatment-refractory schizophrenia with childhood onset. Because all eight were nonsmokers, their olanzapine PK were compared with those reported for adult nonsmokers. Olanzapine was begun at a dose of 2.5 mg/day, with an increase to 5.0 mg/day on day 3. Subsequently, olanzapine was titrated upward in 2.5- to 5.0-mg increments every 5 to 9 days on the basis of the clinical response up to a maximum of 20 mg/day. Blood samples were drawn weekly; at the end of treatment, plasma level determinations were made for 0, 1, 2, 4, 8, 12, 24, and 36 hours after the final dose. At the end of the 8-week study, seven subjects were receiving olanzapine 20 mg/day and one was receiving 15 mg/day. Plasma olanzapine levels increased linearly in this dose range, making dose adjustments relatively predictable. At a fixed-dose, steady-state levels developed in approximately 7 days, with olanzapine's concentration approximately doubling over that period. The seven subjects receiving 20 mg/day had an average steady-state plasma olanzapine concentration of 92.6 ± 27.0 ng/mL; average trough concentration (measured 24 hours after the last dose) was 75.6 ± 27.2 ng/mL. The seven subjects' mean maximum plasma concentration (C_{max}) was 115.6 ± 26.7 ng/mL, which occurred at a mean time (T_{max}) of 4.7 ± 3.7 hours after the dose was given. Mean elimination half-life ($T_{1/2}$) was 37.2 ± 5.1 hours. Olanzapine plasma levels of these seven mostly adolescent subjects were comparable to those reported for adult nonsmokers.

Interactions of Olanzapine with Other Medications

Of particular note, carbamazepine, a potent inducer of CYP1A2 activity, in doses of 200 mg bid causes an increase of approximately 50% in the clearance of olanzapine; higher doses may cause an even greater increase, necessitating upward adjustment of the dose of olanzapine.

Contraindications for Olanzapine Administration

Olanzapine is contraindicated in patients with known hypersensitivity to the medication.

Tolerability and Adverse Effects of Olanzapine

Extrapyramidal Symptoms

At doses up to 15 ± 2.5 mg, there were no statistically significant differences in treatment-emergent EPSs assessed by rating scales between placebo and olanzapine. This was also true for adverse effects spontaneously reported by patients, except that akathisia was reported significantly more frequently at doses of 10 ± 2.5 mg or more for olanzapine than for placebo.

Other Adverse Effects

Orthostatic hypotension, tachycardia, weight gain, liver transaminase elevations, somnolence, insomnia, constipation, dizziness, agitation, and dry mouth have been reported to occur in patients treated with olanzapine.

Indications for Olanzapine in Child and Adolescent Psychiatry

- Olanzapine is indicated in adolescents 13 to 17 years of age for the treatment of schizophrenia.
- Olanzapine is indicated in adolescents 13 to 17 years of age for and the treatment of acute mixed or manic episodes associated with bipolar I disorder.
- Olanzapine is also indicated for the treatment of depressive episodes associated with n bipolar I disorder in children and adolescents 10 to 17 years of age.

Olanzapine Dosage Schedule

- *Children and adolescents 12 years of age and less:* not recommended. The safety and effectiveness of olanzapine have not been established for pediatric populations <13 years of age.

Treatment of Schizophrenia

Adolescents 13 to 17 years of age: An initial dose of 2.5 to 5 mg without regard to meals is recommended, with dose increases in increments of 2.5 to 5.0 mg over several days as tolerated to a target dose of 10 mg/day.

(continued)

Indications for Olanzapine in Child and Adolescent Psychiatry (*continued*)

Although a flexible-dose range of 2.5 to 20 mg was used in clinical trials and was shown to be efficacious, doses above 10 mg/day have not been demonstrated to clearly increase efficacy. The safety of doses above 20 mg/day has not been evaluated in clinical trials.

Treatment of Acute Mixed or Manic Episodes Associated with Bipolar I Disorder

Adolescents 13 to 17 years of age: An initial dose of 2.5 to 5 mg without regard to meals is recommended, with dose increases in increments of 2.5 to 5.0 mg over several days as tolerated to the dose range of 2.5 to 20 mg/day which demonstrated efficacy in clinical trials. The safety of doses above 20 mg/day has not been evaluated in clinical trials.

   Treatment of depressive episodes associated with bipolar I disorder in children and adolescents 10 to 17 years of age: Oral olanzapine should be administered in combination with fluoxetine once daily in the evening, without regard to meals, beginning with 2.5 mg of oral olanzapine and 20 mg of fluoxetine. Dosage adjustments, if indicated, can be made according to efficacy and tolerability. Safety of coadministration of doses above 12 mg olanzapine with 50 mg fluoxetine has not been evaluated in pediatric clinical studies.

Olanzapine Dose Forms Available

Tablets: 2.5, 5, 7.5, 10, 15, and 20 mg
Orally disintegrating tablets (Zyprexa Zydis): 5, 10, 15, and 20 mg
Injection, intramuscular: 10 mg vial

Olanzapine/Fluoxetine (Symbyax) Dose Forms Available

Symbyax (olanzapine/fluoxetine HCl) is a fixed-dose combination
- 3 mg olanzapine/25 mg fluoxetine
- 6 mg olanzapine/25 mg fluoxetine
- 12 mg olanzapine/25 mg fluoxetine
- 6 mg olanzapine/50 mg fluoxetine
- 12 mg olanzapine/50 mg fluoxetine

The PI sheet states that the increased potential (in adolescents compared with adults) for weight gain and hyperlipidemia may lead clinicians to consider prescribing other medications first in adolescents.

Schizophrenia

U.S. Food and Drug Administration Registry Trials

Adolescents (ages 13 to 17): Efficacy was established in one 6-week trial in patients with schizophrenia. Prescribing Information (PI) indicates the increased potential (in adolescents compared with that in adults) for weight gain, and hyperlipidemia may lead clinicians to consider prescribing other medications first in adolescents. Compared with patients from adult clinical trials, adolescents were likely to gain more weight, experience increased sedation, and have greater increases in total cholesterol, triglycerides, low-density lipoprotein (LDL) cholesterol, prolactin, and hepatic aminotransferase levels.

Commonly Observed Adverse Reactions

Commonly observed treatment-emergent adverse reactions of ≥5% incidence among adolescents (13 to 17 years old; combined incidence from short-term, placebo-controlled clinical trials of schizophrenia or BP-I manic or mixed episodes) were sedation, weight increase, increased appetite, headache, fatigue, dizziness, and dry mouth in decreasing order of incidence (Zyprexa [package insert], 2011).

Reports of Interest

Olanzapine in the Treatment of Children and Adolescents Diagnosed with Schizophrenia

Sholevar et al. (2000) treated with olanzapine 15 hospitalized subjects (9 males and 6 females; age range, 6 to 13 years; mean age, 9.4 ± 1.99 years) who were diagnosed with childhood-onset acute schizophrenia by DSM-IV criteria before age 12. Medication was begun between 24 and 48 hours after admission. Because the first three subjects experienced morning sedation and lethargy on initial doses of 5 mg of olanzapine daily, the subsequent 12 patients were begun on 2.5 mg daily. Medication was increased to 5 mg daily after 5 days if no untoward effects were apparent. Average hospitalization during which this study took place was 11.3 days. At the end of hospitalization, 14 (93%) of the subjects were maintained on 5-mg olanzapine daily. Psychiatric improvement was rated on a 4-point scale: 0 = no improvement, 1 = slight improvement, 2 = moderate improvement, and 3 = great improvement. Five subjects (33.3%) were greatly improved, five (33.3%) were moderately improved, three (20%) were slightly improved, and two (13.3%) showed no improvement. Sedation was the most common untoward effect and lasted from 0 to 4 days. There were no clinically significant changes in laboratory values or vital signs. The authors reported that longer duration of initial sedation was significantly positively correlated with increased clinical improvement ($P = .004$). Younger age was significantly correlated with increased clinical improvement ($P < .05$). The 11 subjects who were being treated for the first time with an antipsychotic showed greater clinical improvement than did the 4 who had failed prior treatments with antipsychotics.

Head-to-Head Trial of Olanzapine Versus Clozapine

Kumra et al. (1998) compared the efficacy of olanzapine in an 8-week, open-label trial in 8 patients (mean age, 15.3 ± 2.3 years) with that of clozapine in a 6-week, open-label trial in 15 patients (mean age, 13.6 ± 1.5 years) in the treatment of subjects diagnosed with schizophrenia by DSM-III-R (APA, 1987) criteria. Subjects receiving olanzapine in this study had treatment-resistant schizophrenia (all had failed prior treatment with at least two other neuroleptics) with childhood onset, which comprises an even rarer subgroup than schizophrenia with childhood onset. In addition, four of the subjects on olanzapine had experienced good clinical response to clozapine but developed significant untoward effects requiring its discontinuation. In addition, most clinicians would now administer a trial of an atypical antipsychotic rather than a standard neuroleptic as a first-line medication.

Mean dose of olanzapine at the sixth week of treatment was 17.5 ± 2.3 mg/day (range, 12.5 to 20 mg/day) or 0.27 ± 0.11 mg/kg/day (range, 0.15 to 0.41 mg/kg/day). The mean dose of clozapine at the sixth week of treatment was 317 ± 147mg/day (range, 100 to 600 mg/day) or 5.42 ± 2.84 mg/kg/day (range, 1.28 to 8.88 mg/kg/day). Efficacy was rated using scores of the BPRS and the CGI Scale.

The most clinically important findings of this study were that 8 (53%) of the 15 subjects on clozapine and none of the 8 subjects on olanzapine met "responder" criteria by week 6. At week 8, two (25%) of the subjects receiving olanzapine met "responder" criteria and one (12.5%) was a partial responder. Clinical improvement of subjects on clozapine at 6 weeks was rated better than that of subjects on olanzapine at 8 weeks for all clinical ratings. Even the four subjects who could not tolerate clozapine because of untoward effects had shown greater clinical improvement on clozapine than on olanzapine. Of the eight patients on olanzapine, three were rated "much improved"; two, "minimally improved"; one, "no change"; one, "minimally worse"; one, "much worse." Four subjects, who improved on olanzapine at 8 weeks and continued to take the medication, showed further clinical improvement. Untoward effects of olanzapine were moderate but frequent; the most common were insomnia (seven, 87.5%), transient liver transaminase elevation (seven, 87.5%), increased appetite (six, 75%), nausea/vomiting (six, 75%), headache (six, 75%), sustained tachycardia (six, 75%), increased agitation (six, 75%), difficulty concentrating (five, 62.5%), and constipation (five, 62.5%). During the 8-week trial, seven (87.5%) of the patients on olanzapine were treated with lorazepam, 2 to 8 mg/day, for agitation or insomnia. No patient on olanzapine required prophylactic anticonvulsant treatment for developing an abnormal EEG or convulsions, but four of the patients on clozapine required such medication. The authors concluded that clozapine remains the "gold standard" for the treatment of schizophrenia; but that because of olanzapine's much more favorable untoward-effect profile and indication of therapeutic efficacy in some of their subjects, it is a good first-line choice for treating schizophrenia with childhood onset.

Olanzapine in the Treatment of Children and Adolescents Diagnosed with Pervasive Developmental Disorders

Potenza et al. (1999) reported a 12-week, open-label, pilot study in which olanzapine monotherapy was prescribed to eight patients (mean age, 20.9 ± 11.7 years; range, 5 to 42 years), of whom four were children or adolescents, diagnosed by DSM-IV (APA, 1994) criteria with autistic disorder ($N = 5$) or with PDD not otherwise specified (PDD NOS) of at least moderate severity. Four subjects had full-scale intelligence quotients (FSIQs) in the mildly retarded range, and three subjects had FSIQs in the moderately retarded range. Seven of the subjects had prior medication trials, including at least one typical antipsychotic that was clinically ineffective or produced unacceptable untoward effects. Efficacy was assessed using the Yale-Brown Obsessive-Compulsive Scale Compulsion Subscale (Y-BOCS-CS), the Self-Injurious Behavior Questionnaire (SIB-Q), the Vineland Adaptive Behavior Scale Maladaptive Behavior subscales, the Ritvo-Freeman Real-Life Rating Scale (RFRLRS), the CGI-I Scale, and the clinician-rated VAS.

All subjects had a 4-week, medication-free period before beginning the 12-week protocol. An initial daily dose of 2.5 mg of olanzapine was prescribed for the first 2 weeks. Olanzapine was then titrated upward in 2.5- to 5.0-mg increments to a maximum of 20 mg/day, usually given at bedtime. Seven subjects completed the study and the eighth dropped out after 9 weeks because of failure to improve, the last observation of that case was carried forward, intent-to-treat methodology was used in the data analysis. The mean dose of olanzapine at week 12 was 7.8 ± 4.7 mg/day (range, 5 to 20 mg/day). Six patients were considered responders, and the response was not correlated with dose, age, IQ, SIBs or repetitive behaviors, or baseline severity of illness. By the end of week 4, subjects showed a significant mean improvement over baseline on the CGI-I ($P = .015$) with further improvement at the end of the 8th and 12th weeks ($P < .001$). There was also significant improvement on items of the VAS, such as temper tantrums, impulsivity, anxiety, social withdrawal, rocking, destruction of property, and inappropriate sexual behavior; and the RFRLRS behavioral constellations for sensory motor behaviors, social relationship to people, affectual reactions, sensory responses, and language use and response, and the SIB-Q showed a significant reduction in aggressive behavior over time. Repetitive behaviors rated on the Y-BOCS-CS showed no significant improvement. The most clinically significant untoward effects were sedation in three subjects and significant weight gain in six subjects. The group mean weight at the end of the 12-week period was 70.88 ± 25.06 kg, compared with 62.50 ± 25.37 kg at baseline ($P = .008$). The guardians of two children who were responders discontinued their olanzapine 2 and 8 weeks after the initial period because they felt the clinical benefit was not sufficient to tolerate the significant weight gain.

Bipolar Disorder

U.S. Food and Drug Administration Registry Trials

Adolescents (ages 13 to 17): Efficacy was established in one 3-week trial in patients with manic or mixed episodes associated with BP-I. The increased potential (in adolescents compared with that in adults) for weight gain and hyperlipidemia may lead clinicians to consider prescribing other medications first in adolescents. Compared with patients from adult clinical trials, adolescents were likely to gain more weight, experience increased sedation, and have greater increases in total cholesterol, triglycerides, LDL cholesterol, prolactin, and hepatic aminotransferase levels.

Children and adolescents (ages 10 to 17): Efficacy was established in one 8-week trial in patients currently in a depressed episode associated with BP-I.

Detke et al. (2015) conducted a randomized, double-blind, placebo-controlled study to assess the efficacy and safety of olanzapine/fluoxetine combination (OFC) for the acute treatment of bipolar I depression in children and adolescents.

Patients 10 to 17 years of age with BP-I, currently in a depressed episode, with a baseline Children's Depression Rating Scale—Revised (CDRS-R) total score ≥ 40, a Young Mania Rating Scale (YMRS) total score ≤ 15, and a YMRS-item 1 ≤ 2 were accepted into the study. A total of 170 patients were randomized to OFC (6/25 to 12/50 mg/day and 85 patients were placed on placebo for up to 8 weeks of double-blind treatment. The primary efficacy measure was mean change in CDRS-R using mixed-model repeated-measures methodology.

The results evidenced that from baseline to week 8, the least-squares mean change in CDRS-R total score was greater for OFC-treated patients than for placebo-treated patients (-28.4 versus -23.4, $P = .003$; effect size $= 0.46$), with between-group differences statistically significant at week 1 ($P = .02$) and all subsequent visits (all $P < .01$). Rates of and times to response and remission were statistically significantly greater for OFC- than for placebo-treated patients. The most frequent treatment-emergent AEs in the OFC group were weight gain, increased appetite, and somnolence. Mean weight gain at patient's endpoint was significantly greater for OFC- than for placebo-treated patients (4.4 kg vs. 0.5 kg, $P < .001$). Treatment-emergent hyperlipidemia was very common among OFC-treated patients. Abnormal increases in hepatic analytes, prolactin, and corrected QT interval (QTc) were also common or very common but generally not clinically significant.

The authors concluded that OFC was superior to placebo in this study, which led to OFC being approved by the FDA for the acute treatment of bipolar I depression in patients 10 to 17 years of age. The authors instructed that the benefits of OFC should be weighed against the risk of AEs, particularly weight gain and hyperlipidemia with the olanzapine component.

Olanzapine in the Treatment of Children and Adolescents Diagnosed with Bipolar Disorder

Frazier et al. (2000) treated 23 subjects (age range, 5 to 14 years), diagnosed with BPD and currently manic or mixed, with olanzapine on an open-label basis for up to 8 weeks. The dose ranged from 2.5 to 20 mg/day. Efficacy was evaluated by ratings on the YMRS with responders defined a priori as having $\geq 30\%$ improvement in total score from baseline to endpoint and by ratings of ≤ 3 ("very much improved," "much improved," or "improved") on the Clinical Global Impressions–Bipolar Mania (CGI-BP) Improvement Scale. Twenty-two (95.7%) completed the study; the 23rd developed depressive symptoms and dropped out. Mean ratings on the YMRS decreased by 19.04 ± 9.21 ($P < .001$), and 60.9% were rated as responders. No significant EPSs were noted; however, subjects' weight increased significantly (4.98 ± 2.32 kg over the course of the treatment).

Quetiapine Fumarate (Seroquel)

Quetiapine fumarate (Seroquel) belongs to a new chemical class, the dibenzothiazepine derivatives. The medication antagonizes 5-HT_{1a}, 5-HT_3, dopamine D_1, dopamine D_2, histamine H_1, adrenergic alpha-1, and adrenergic alpha-2 neurotransmitter receptors in the brain. It has no appreciable affinity at cholinergic-muscarinic and benzodiazepine receptors. It is suggested that its antipsychotic properties may be mediated through its antagonism of dopamine type 2 (D_2) and serotonin type 2 (5-HT_2) receptors. Quetiapine's antagonism of H_1 and adrenergic alpha-1 receptors may explain the sedation and hypotension, respectively, sometimes observed with the medication. It was approved by the FDA in 1997 for adult patients.

Pharmacokinetics of Quetiapine Fumarate

Food affects the bioavailability of quetiapine fumarate only marginally. Peak serum levels occur at a mean of 1.5 hours after ingestion. Quetiapine fumarate is extensively metabolized, primarily in the liver, by sulfoxidation by cytochrome P450 3A4 (CYP3A4) isoenzyme, to its major, sulfoxide metabolite, and by oxidation; both metabolites are pharmacologically inactive.

Steady-state serum concentrations occur after approximately 2 days on a given dose regimen. Terminal serum half-life is approximately 6 hours.

Gender, race, and smoking have no clinically significant effects on the metabolism of quetiapine fumarate.

Contraindications for Quetiapine Fumarate Administration

Quetiapine fumarate is contraindicated in patients with a known hypersensitivity to it. Quetiapine fumarate should be administered with caution to patients with hepatic impairment, which may increase plasma levels.

Advantages of Quetiapine Fumarate

Quetiapine fumarate does not cause statistically significant changes in the QT, QTc, and PR intervals of the ECG.

Tolerability and Adverse Effects of Quetiapine Fumarate

Extrapyramidal Symptoms

The incidence of treatment-emergent EPSs in patients treated with quetiapine fumarate is not significantly different from that in patients treated with placebo over a daily dose range of 75 to 750 mg.

Other Adverse Effects

Orthostatic hypotension, dizziness, tachycardia, weight gain, somnolence, constipation, dry mouth, dyspepsia, and many other untoward effects have been reported in patients taking quetiapine.

Indications for Quetiapine Fumarate in Child and Adolescent Psychiatry

The PI states that because of the increased potential (in adolescents compared with adults) for weight gain and hyperlipidemia may lead clinicians to consider prescribing other medications first in adolescents.

Quetiapine is indicated in adolescents 13 to 17 years of age for the treatment of schizophrenia and in children and adolescents 10 to 17 years of age for the treatment of manic episodes associated with bipolar I disorder.

Quetiapine Dosage Schedule

Quetiapine can be taken without regard to food.

Clinical Pearl: Because of quetiapine's common side effect of sedation, it is often administered with the largest dose before bedtime to aid sleep onset as well.

Treatment of Schizophrenia

Adolescents 13 to 17 years of age: Day 1: 25 mg twice daily. Day 2: twice-daily dosing totaling 100 mg. Day 3: twice-daily dosing totaling 200 mg. Day 4: twice-daily dosing totaling 300 mg. Day 5: twice-daily dosing totaling 400 mg. A flexible-dose range of 400 to 800 mg was used in clinical trials based on response and tolerability and shown to be efficacious. However, no additional benefit was seen in the 800-mg group. The safety of doses over 800 mg/day has not been evaluated in clinical trials. On the basis of tolerability issues, quetiapine may be administered three times daily when indicated.

Treatment of Acute Manic Episodes Associated with Bipolar I Disorder

Children and adolescents 10 to 17 years of age: Day 1: 25 mg twice daily. Day 2: twice-daily dosing totaling 100 mg. Day 3: twice-daily dosing totaling 200 mg. Day 4: twice-daily dosing totaling 300 mg. Day 5: twice-daily dosing totaling 400 mg. Dosage adjustments should be in increments of no greater than 100 mg/day. A flexible-dose range of 400 to 600 mg was used in clinical trials depending on response and tolerability and shown to be efficacious. However, no additional benefit was seen in the 600-mg group. The safety of doses

(continued)

Indications for Quetiapine Fumarate in Child and Adolescent Psychiatry (*continued*)

over 600 mg/day has not been evaluated in clinical trials. On the basis of tolerability issues, quetiapine may be administered three times daily when indicated.

Quetiapine Fumarate Dose Forms Available

- *Tablets:* 25, 50, 100, 200, 300, and 400 mg

Quetiapine Fumarate XR (Extended-Release) Dose Forms Available

- *Tablets:* 50, 150, 200, 300, and 400 mg.
- *Clinical Pearl:* Note that the XR formulation is less sedating versus IR quetiapine, often allowing daytime dosing with less sedation. Some clinicians prefer to use Quetiapine XR up to twice a day during the daytime to reduce the SE of sedation and use the more sedating IR quetiapine before bedtime to aid sleep onset.

Schizophrenia

U.S. Food and Drug Administration Registry Trials

Adolescents (ages 10 to 17): Efficacy was established in one 3-week, double-blind, placebo-controlled trial in patients with schizophrenia.

Bipolar Disorder

U.S. Food and Drug Administration Registry Trials

Adolescents (ages 13 to 17): Efficacy was established in one 3-week double-blind, placebo-controlled, multicenter trial in patients with manic episodes associated with BP-I.

The increased potential (in adolescents compared with adults) for weight gain and hyperlipidemia may lead clinicians to consider prescribing other medications first in adolescents. Compared with patients from adult clinical trials, adolescents were likely to gain more weight, experience increased sedation, and have greater increases in total cholesterol, triglycerides, LDL cholesterol, prolactin, and hepatic aminotransferase levels.

Reports of Interest—Failed Trials

Beginning in 2009, two double-blind, placebo-controlled, monotherapy studies of quetiapine in pediatric bipolar depression (utilizing extended [ER]- and immediate-release [IR] formulations) *failed* to demonstrate significant antidepressant efficacy (DelBello et al., 2009; Findling et al., 2014).

Reports of Interest

Quetiapine Fumarate in the Treatment of Children and Adolescents Diagnosed with Autistic Disorder

Martin et al. (1999) treated six male outpatients (mean age, 10.9 ± 3.3 years; age range, 6.2 to 15.3 years) diagnosed with autistic disorder by DSM-IV (APA, 1994) criteria with quetiapine in a 16-week, open-label study. All were mentally retarded (two mild, three moderate, one severe). Target symptoms for five patients were aggression, self-injury, and poor impulse control, and for the sixth interfering stereotypies and repetitive behaviors. Quetiapine was begun with a nighttime dose of 25 mg and titrated on the basis of clinical response, with increases up to 100 mg/week permitted. Efficacy was assessed by ratings on the ABC, the CGI-I Scale, with subjects rated "much improved" or "very much improved" considered responders, the RFRLRS, and the Children's Yale-Brown Obsessive-Compulsive Scale. Only two subjects completed the 16-week study. Three (50%) dropped out (two after 4 weeks and one after 8 weeks) because sedation and the lack of clinical improvement were so problematic that the dose of quetiapine could not be increased (one of the three also had an apparent seizure), and the fourth dropped out after 4 weeks because of behavioral activation and apparent akathisia. Mean dose of quetiapine at endpoint or at dropout was 225 ± 108 mg/day (range, 100 to 350 mg/day). On the basis of the CGI-I, only the two subjects who completed the 16 weeks were responders, one "very much improved" and the other "much improved"; of the four nonresponders, one was "much worse," two were "minimally worse," and one was "no change." Four subjects experienced increased appetite and a mean weight gain of 2.9 ± 3.6 kg. Overall, quetiapine was poorly tolerated and/or ineffective for two-thirds of the subjects, and only one of the two responders continued to benefit from long-term treatment with quetiapine.

Findling et al. (2004) reported a 12-week, open-label study in nine subjects (age range 12.0 to 17.3 years; eight males, one female) diagnosed with autistic disorder and having a score of >30 on the Childhood Autism Rating Scale, and a rating on the CGI-S of at least moderately ill. Target symptoms included aggression, SIBs, tantrums, irritability, overactivity, and social withdrawal. Quetiapine was begun at 25 mg twice daily for 3 days and then increased to 50 mg twice daily for the next 11 days. At the beginning of week 3, the dose was increased by 50 mg twice daily every other week to reach a target dose of 150 mg twice daily (300 mg/day). Following this, the dose could be increased by a total of 25 to 75 mg/week, depending on tolerability and clinical response, to a maximum of 750 mg/day.

Mean total quetiapine daily dose was 291.7, dose range 100 to 450 mg. Responders were defined as having ratings of 1 (very much improved) or 2 (much improved) on the CGI-I rating at endpoint. Six patients completed the study; one dropped out because of increased aggression/agitation and one dropped out because of drowsiness, whereas the final patient was lost to follow-up after 1 week. Only two of the eight patients (25%) who received medication were responders. The most frequent side effects reported by parents were sedation ($N = 7$), weight gain ($N = 5$), agitation ($N = 4$), and aggression ($N = 2$). The authors noted that quetiapine was not particularly effective clinically in these treatment-resistant adolescents with autistic disorder (Findling et al., 2004).

Quetiapine in Children and Adolescents with Conduct Disorder

Findling et al. (2006b) conducted an 8-week, open-label outpatient trial of quetiapine in patients aged 6 to 12 years with a primary diagnosis of CD to address whether quetiapine was superior to placebo in ameliorating aggression in children. Study patients could have comorbid ADHD, but were excluded if an organic mental syndrome including mental retardation was present. Of the 17 subjects enrolled, 16 were boys with a mean age of 8.9 years and all subjects met diagnostic symptom criteria for comorbid ADHD/combined type.

During the acute trial phase, patients were dosed depending on weight, with patients weighing <35 kg administered a single morning dose of 25 mg quetiapine. Patients weighing >35 kg began treatment with 25-mg quetiapine in the morning and 25-mg quetiapine 1 hour before bedtime. Each subject's study medication was increased in a twice-daily manner until a total daily dose of approximately 3 mg/kg/day was reached by the end of week 1. Beginning week 2 and up to the end of week 7, patients could then have their medication increased at the discretion of the treating psychiatrist to either a total daily dose of 6 mg/kg/day or 750 mg/day (whichever was lower). Dose decreases were also permitted.

The primary outcome measure was the RAAPPS score (Kemph et al., 1993). The clinician-rated RAAPPS records severity of aggressive behaviors, with lower scores representing more modest degrees of aggressive behavior. This single-item scale has a possible score ranging from 1 (no aggression) to 5 (intolerable). Multiple secondary measures were utilized to assess various behaviors and emotions, overall psychosocial functioning, and the severity of a patient's psychiatric condition.

At the patient's final study visit, those attaining a CGI-I Scale score of 1 or 2, indicative of being "very much" or "much improved," respectively, were considered responders.

Twelve of the 17 patients enrolled completed all 8 weeks of the study. The median study dose of quetiapine at week 8 was 150 mg (range 75 to 300 mg) with a mean dose of 4.4 mg/kg. RAAPPS and CGI-S scores at weeks 4 and 8 evidenced significant differences reflecting improvement for several domains, including aggression and conduct problems. At week 8, 6 of the 12 patients who completed treatment were given CGI-I scores of 1 or 2 and were considered responders.

Regarding AEs, 15 (88.2%) of the 17 dosed patients experienced an AE during the course of the study. The most frequently reported side effects included the following in decreasing order: fatigue, nasal congestion, headache, nausea, sedation, increased appetite, vomiting, stomach pain, irritability, and fever. No patient withdrew from the study because of an AE. However, over the course of the study there was a median increase in weight of 2.3 kg ($P < .001$) in the 12 patients who completed the study. Fasting morning blood chemistry evaluations showed no clinically significant changes between baseline and week 8 last observation carried forward (LOCF) visits. Prolactin levels were obtained in 16 patients at the screening visit and in 10 patients at week 8. No elevation of prolactin levels was found. No neurologic symptoms were observed during the course of the study as measured by the Neurological Rating Scale, Barnes Akathisia Scale, and the Abnormal Involuntary Movement Scale. In addition, no significant changes on physical examination were noted during the course of this study.

A statistical analysis of quetiapine PK data was conducted via blood sampling for those patients in the study at study week 2 and study week 8. Calculated quetiapine PK parameter estimates for both study periods indicate that the medication was rapidly absorbed from the intestinal tract, reflected by the average T_{max} of 1.2 and 1 hour at study weeks 2 and 8, respectively. Quetiapine $T_{1/2}$ averaged 3.9 and 2.9 hours and total body clearance (Cl) averaged 3.5 and 3.0 L/hour/kg at weeks 2 and 8, respectively. Furthermore, the disposition of quetiapine was linear over the dose range studied. No statistically significant relationships or differences were observed for quetiapine C_{max}, T_{max}, or Cl relative to age, study period, or dose. In general, it appears that the PK profile of quetiapine, including the critical assessment of medication body elimination, is similar across studies of adults (DeVane & Nemeroff, 2001), adolescents (McConville et al., 2000), and children based on this study. Week 8 concentration data were used to examine graphically the possibility that overall concentrations, or concentration at a single time point could differentiate between responder and nonresponder status. No relationships were observed. In contrast, for the 10 patients with plasma quetiapine concentration determinations at week 8, statistical analysis revealed patients with 1-hour postdose quetiapine plasma concentrations >300 ng/mL were significantly more likely to be considered responders than were those patients with plasma quetiapine concentrations <300 ng/mL (Fisher exact test, $P = .048$). Despite these observed trends, caution should be used in considering this preliminary finding because of the small number of patients that were studied and the limited age range (6 to 12 years) of these patients.

Because approximately 99% of quetiapine is metabolized in the liver predominantly via CYP3A4 and a small contribution by CYP2D6 (DeVane & Nemeroff, 2001), concurrent medication administration and/or hepatic dysfunction affecting these pathways may markedly affect PK parameters.

Given the limitations of a short, open-label design study with a small sample size, the authors proposed that quetiapine was found to be beneficial and generally well tolerated in the acute treatment of aggressive behavior in a small number of children with CD. Quetiapine continues to be considered an agent with a mild risk of EPSs or other neurologic side effects, but its potential for significant weight gain and metabolic syndrome long term are clearly relative to a risk–benefit analysis when considering quetiapine in this pediatric population.

Quetiapine Fumarate in the Treatment of Adolescents Diagnosed with Conduct Disorder

Connor et al. (2008) in a small 7-week, randomized, double-blind, placebo-controlled pilot study with two parallel arms of 19 patients found that for adolescents with CD, quetiapine dosed in a twice-a-day manner at 200 to 600 mg/day was effective in decreasing overt aggression. The primary outcome measures were the clinician-assessed secondary outcome measures and included parent-assessed quality of life, the overt aggression scale (OAS), and the Conduct Problems subscale of the Conners' Parent Rating Scale (CPRS-CP). The final mean dose of quetiapine was 294 ± 78 mg/day (range 200 to 600 mg/day). Quetiapine was superior to placebo on the clinician-assessed measures utilized, which were the CGI-S and the CGI-I scales. No differences were found on the parent-completed OAS and CPRS-CP. Quetiapine was well tolerated. One patient randomized to quetiapine developed akathisia, requiring medication discontinuation. No other extrapyramidal side effects occurred in patients receiving active medication. The average weight gain in the quetiapine group was 2.3 kg compared to an average weight gain in the placebo group of 1.1 kg, comparing weights at the initial and final visits. This was reported as a nonsignificant difference. The authors concluded the study results suggest that quetiapine may be broadly beneficial in adolescents meeting diagnostic criteria for CD.

Aripiprazole (Abilify)

Aripiprazole belongs to the chemical class of quinolinone derivatives. The FDA approved it for marketing in the United States in 2002 for adults. The manufacturer suggests that its antipsychotic properties may be mediated through its partial agonism of dopamine type 2 (D_2) and serotonin type 1 ($5-HT_{1A}$) receptors and antagonism of serotonin type 2 ($5-HT_{2A}$) receptors.

Pharmacokinetics of Aripiprazole

Taken orally, aripiprazole is well absorbed, and peak plasma concentrations occur within 3 to 5 hours. Taking it with food does not significantly alter peak plasma concentrations; however, it may delay them for several hours. Activity is due to aripiprazole (approximately 60%) and its major metabolite dehydro-aripiprazole (approximately 40%) at steady-state plasma levels, which are achieved for both within 14 days. Mean elimination half-lives are approximately 75 hours for aripiprazole and approximately 94 hours for dehydro-aripiprazole. The major metabolism is through the hepatic P450 isomers CYP2D6 and CYP3A4. Most of the metabolites and some unchanged medication are excreted in the feces; a lesser but significant amount is excreted by the kidneys.

Approximately 8% of Caucasians are poor metabolizers of aripiprazole because they have decreased ability to metabolize CYP2D6 substrates. Such individuals have a net increase of approximately 60% on exposure to the medication, compared with extensive (normal) metabolizers of the medication. The elimination half-life of aripiprazole for poor metabolizers is approximately 146 hours, nearly twice that of extensive metabolizers.

Interactions of Aripiprazole with Other Medications

Medications such as quinine, which inhibit CYP2D6, can result in more than a doubling of the plasma levels and require downward adjustment of the dose of aripiprazole. If fluoxetine or paroxetine, both potential CYP2D6 inhibitors, is given concomitantly, the aripiprazole dose should be reduced by at least one-half of the usual dose.

Contraindications for Aripiprazole Administration

Aripiprazole is contraindicated in patients with known hypersensitivity to the medication.

Tolerability and Adverse Effects of Aripiprazole

Commonly observed adverse reactions (>5% incidence and at least twice the rate of placebo for aripiprazole vs. placebo, respectively):

- Pediatric patients (13 to 17 years) with schizophrenia: extrapyramidal disorder (17% vs. 5%), somnolence (16% vs. 6%), and tremor (7% vs. 2%)
- Pediatric patients (10 to 17 years) with bipolar mania: somnolence (23% vs. 3%), extrapyramidal disorder (20% vs. 3%), fatigue (11% vs. 4%), nausea (11% vs. 4%), akathisia (10% vs. 2%), blurred vision (8% vs. 0%), salivary hypersecretion (6% vs. 0%), and dizziness (5% vs. 1%)

Electrocardiographic Changes

No significant ECG differences were found between subjects administered placebo and aripiprazole in the pooled data of the premarketing trials; within the dose range of 10 to 30 mg, aripiprazole tended to slightly shorten the QTc interval. There was a median increase in heart rate of 4 beats per minute in subjects treated with aripiprazole.

Weight

In premarketing studies of 4 to 6 weeks' duration, subjects receiving aripiprazole gained a mean of 0.7 kg compared with subjects on placebo who lost a mean of 0.05 kg. In a 52-week study, weight gain or loss was related to initial BMI. Subjects with a BMI of <23 gained a mean of 2.6 kg, and 30% had an increase in weight of >7% over baseline measures. The data for subjects with baseline BMIs of 23 to 27 were a mean weight gain of 1.4 kg with 19% experiencing a weight gain of >7%. Subjects with a BMI >27 lost a mean weight of 1.2 kg, but 8% of them still gained >7% of their baseline body weight.

Indications for Aripiprazole in Child and Adolescent Psychiatry

- Adolescents 13 to 17 years of age for the treatment of schizophrenia
- Children and adolescents 10 to 17 years of age for the treatment of manic or mixed episodes associated with bipolar I disorder, both as monotherapy, and as an adjunct to lithium or valproate
- Children and adolescents 10 to 17 years of age for the treatment of irritability associated with autistic disorder
- Children and adolescents 6 to 18 years of age for treatment of Tourette disorder

Aripiprazole Dosage Schedule

- *Children 9 years of age and less:* not recommended. The safety and effectiveness of olanzapine have not been established for pediatric populations <12 years of age.

Treatment of Schizophrenia

Adolescents 13 to 17 years of age: The recommended starting daily dose of the tablet formulation is 2 mg, which in the studies was titrated to 5 mg after 2 days and to the target dose of 10 mg after 2 additional days. Subsequent dose increases should be administered in 5 mg increments. The 30-mg/day dose was not shown to be more efficacious than the 10-mg/day dose. Aripiprazole can be administered without regard to meals. Maintenance efficacy was demonstrated in one trial in adults and can be extrapolated to adolescents.

Treatment of Acute Manic Episodes Associated with Bipolar I Disorder

Children and adolescents 10 to 17 years of age: The recommended starting dose as monotherapy is 2 mg/day, with titration to 5 mg/day after 2 days, and a target dose of 10 mg/day after 2 additional days. Recommended

(continued)

Indications for Aripiprazole in Child and Adolescent Psychiatry (*continued*)

dosing as adjunctive therapy to lithium or valproate is the same. Subsequent dose increases, if needed, should be administered in 5-mg/day increments. Aripiprazole can be given without regard to meals. The recommended dose for maintenance treatment, whether as monotherapy or as adjunctive therapy, is the same dose needed to stabilize patients during acute treatment, both for adult and pediatric patients. Patients should be periodically reassessed to determine the continued need for maintenance treatment.

Treatment of Irritability Associated with Autistic Disorder

Children and adolescents 6 to 17 years of age: The recommended starting dose is 2 mg/day. The dose should be increased to 5 mg/day, with subsequent increases to 10 or 15 mg/day if needed. Dose adjustments of up to 5 mg/day should occur gradually, at intervals of no less than 1 week. The efficacy of aripiprazole for the maintenance treatment of irritability associated with autistic disorder has not been evaluated. Although there is no body of evidence available to answer the question of how long the patient treated with aripiprazole should be maintained, patients should be periodically reassessed to determine the continued need for maintenance treatment.

Treatment of Tourette Disorder

Children and adolescents 6 to 18 years of age: The recommended dosage range for Tourette disorder is 5 to 20 mg/day. For patients weighing less than 50 kg, dosing should be initiated at 2 mg/day with a target dose of 5 mg/day after 2 days. The dose can be increased to 10 mg/day in patients who do not achieve optimal control of tics. Dosage adjustments should occur gradually at intervals of no less than 1 week. For patients weighing 50 kg or more, dosing should be initiated at 2 mg/day for 2 days, and then increased to 5 mg/day for 5 days, with a target dose of 10 mg/day on day 8. The dose can be increased up to 20 mg/day for patients who do not achieve optimal control of tics. Dosage adjustments should occur gradually in increments of 5 mg/day at intervals of no less than 1 week. Patients should be periodically reassessed to determine the continued need for maintenance treatment.

  Clinical Pearl: Note that for many individuals, tics may not begin to decrease in intensity or frequency until late teens/early 20s and that treatment does not abbreviate the natural course of the disorder. Some individuals will have a degree of residual tics the entirety of their lives.

Aripiprazole Dose Forms Available

- *Tablets:* 2, 5, 10, 15, 20, and 30 mg
- *DISCMELT orally disintegrating tablets:* 10 and 15 mg
- *Oral solution:* 1 mg/mg
- Injection for intramuscular use is a clear, colorless solution available as a ready-to-use, 9.75 mg/1.3 mL (7.5 mg/mL)
- Abilify MyCite: 2-, 5-, 10-, 15-, 20-, and 30-mg strength tablets with sensors in 30-count bottles copackaged with seven patches.

Schizophrenia

U.S. Food and Drug Administration Registry Trials

Adolescents (ages 13 to 17): The efficacy of aripiprazole (aripiprazole) in the treatment of schizophrenia in pediatric patients (13 to 17 years of age) was evaluated in one 6-week, placebo-controlled trial of outpatients who met DSM-IV criteria for schizophrenia and had a PANSS score ≥70 at baseline. In this trial ($N = 302$) comparing two fixed doses of aripiprazole (10 or 30 mg/day) to placebo, aripiprazole was titrated starting from 2 mg/day to the target dose in 5 days in the 10-mg/day treatment arm and in 11 days in the 30-mg/day treatment arm. Both doses of aripiprazole were superior to placebo in the PANSS total score, the primary outcome measure of the study. The 30-mg/day dosage was not shown to be more efficacious than the 10-mg/day dose.

Commonly Observed Adverse Reactions

Commonly observed adverse reactions associated with the use of aripiprazole in adolescent patients with schizophrenia (incidence of 5% or greater and aripiprazole incidence at least twice that for placebo) were extrapyramidal disorder, somnolence, and tremor.

Bipolar Disorder

U.S. Food and Drug Administration Registry Trials

Children and adolescents (ages 10 to 17): The efficacy of aripiprazole in the treatment of BP-I in pediatric patients (10 to 17 years of age) was evaluated in one 4-week, placebo-controlled trial ($N = 296$) of outpatients who met DSM-IV criteria for BP-I manic or mixed episodes with or without psychotic features and had a YMRS score ≥20 at baseline. This double-blind, placebo-controlled trial compared two fixed doses of aripiprazole (10 or 30 mg/day) with placebo. The aripiprazole dose was started at 2 mg/day, which was titrated to 5 mg/day after 2 days, and to the target dose in 5 days in the 10-mg/day treatment arm and in 13 days in the 30-mg/day treatment arm. Both doses of aripiprazole were superior to placebo in change from baseline to week 4 on the YMRS total score.

Tolerability and Adverse Effects of Aripiprazole

Commonly observed adverse reactions associated with the use of aripiprazole in adolescent patients with schizophrenia (incidence of 5% or greater and aripiprazole incidence at least twice that for placebo) were somnolence, extrapyramidal disorder, fatigue, and nausea.

Autistic Disorder

U.S. Food and Drug Administration Registry Trials

Children and adolescents (ages 6 to 17): The efficacy of aripiprazole in the treatment of irritability associated with autistic disorder was established in two 8-week, placebo-controlled trials in pediatric patients (6 to 17 years of age) who met the DSM-IV criteria for autistic disorder and demonstrated behaviors such as tantrums, aggression, SIB, or a combination of these problems. More than 75% of these subjects were below 13 years of age.

Efficacy was evaluated using two assessment scales: the ABC and the CGI-I Scale. The primary outcome measure in both trials was the change from baseline to endpoint in the Irritability subscale of the ABC (ABC-I). The ABC-I subscale measured the emotional and behavioral symptoms of irritability in autistic disorder, including aggression toward others, deliberate self-injuriousness, temper tantrums, and quickly changing moods. The results of these trials are as follows:

In one of the 8-week, placebo-controlled trials, children and adolescents with autistic disorder ($N = 98$), aged 6 to 17 years, received daily doses of placebo or aripiprazole 2 to 15 mg/day. Aripiprazole, starting at 2 mg/day with increases allowed up to 15 mg/day depending on clinical response, significantly improved scores on the ABC-I subscale and on the CGI-I Scale compared with placebo. The mean daily dose of aripiprazole at the end of 8-week treatment was 8.6 mg/day.

In the other 8-week, placebo-controlled trial in children and adolescents with autistic disorder ($N = 218$), aged 6 to 17 years, three fixed doses of aripiprazole (5, 10, or 15 mg/day) were compared with placebo. Aripiprazole dosing started at 2 mg/day and was increased to 5 mg/day after 1 week. After the second week, it was increased to 10 mg/day for patients in the 10- and 15-mg dose arms, and after the third week, it was increased to 15 mg/day in the 15-mg/day treatment arm. All three doses of aripiprazole significantly improved scores on the ABC-I subscale compared with placebo (Aripiprazole [package insert], 2012).

Commonly Observed Adverse Reactions

Commonly observed adverse reactions associated with the use of aripiprazole in adolescent patients with autism in decreasing order (incidence of 5% or greater and aripiprazole incidence at least twice that for placebo) were sedation, fatigue, vomiting, somnolence, tremor, pyrexia, drooling, decreased appetite, salivary hypersecretion, extrapyramidal disorder, and lethargy.

Tourette Disorder—Pediatric

U.S. Food and Drug Administration Registry Trials

Children and adolescents (ages 6 to 18): The efficacy of aripiprazole in the treatment of Tourette disorder was established in one 8-week (7 to 17 years of age) and one 10-week (6 to 18 years of age), placebo-controlled trials in pediatric patients (6 to 18 years of age) who met the DSM-IV criteria for Tourette disorder and had a Total Tic Score (TTS) $\geq$20 to 22 on the YGTSS. The YGTSS is a fully validated scale designed to measure current tic severity. Efficacy was evaluated using two assessment scales: the TTS of the YGTSS and the Clinical Global Impressions Scale for Tourette Syndrome (CGI-TS), a clinician-determined summary measure that takes into account all available patient information. Over 65% of these patients were under 13 years of age

In the 8-week, placebo-controlled, fixed-dose trial, children and adolescents with Tourette disorder (N = 133), aged 7 to 17 years, were randomized 1:1:1 to low-dose aripiprazole, high-dose aripiprazole, or placebo. The target doses for the low- and high-dose aripiprazole groups were based on weight. Patients <50 kg in the low-dose aripiprazole group started at 2 mg/day with a target dose of 5 mg/day after 2 days. Patients $\geq$50 kg in the low-dose aripiprazole group started at 2 mg/day and increased to 5 mg/day after 2 days, with a subsequent increase to a target dose of 10 mg/day at day 7. Patients <50 kg in the high-dose aripiprazole group started at 2 mg/day and increased to 5 mg/day after 2 days, with a subsequent increase to a target dose of 10 mg/day at day 7. Patients $\geq$50 kg in the high-dose aripiprazole group started at 2 mg/day and increased to 5 mg/day after 2 days, with a subsequent increase to a dose of 10 mg/day at day 7 and were allowed weekly increases of 5 mg/day up to a target dose 20 mg/day at day 21. Aripiprazole (both high- and low-dose groups) demonstrated statistically and significantly improved scores on the YGTSS TTS and on the CGI-TS scale compared with placebo. Improvement measured by reduction in the YGTSS TTS was evident by week 1 to 2 with increasing decline in tics by weeks 4 to 6 when maximal effect began to plateau at a 13.4-point reduction compared to placebo for the low-dosage group and a 16.9-point reduction compared to placebo for the high-dose group as measured by the YGTSS TTS.

In the 10-week, placebo-controlled, flexible-dose trial in children and adolescents with Tourette disorder (N = 61), aged 6 to 18 years, patients received daily doses of placebo or aripiprazole, starting at 2 mg/day, with increases allowed up to 20 mg/day depending on clinical response. Aripiprazole demonstrated statistically and significantly improved scores of a 15-point reduction on the YGTSS TTS Scale compared with placebo. The mean daily dose of aripiprazole at the end of 10-week treatment was 6.54 mg/day.

The most commonly observed adverse reactions in short-term, placebo-controlled trials of pediatric patients (6 to 18 years) with Tourette disorder treated with oral aripiprazole versus placebo were sedation (13% vs. 6 %); somnolence (13% vs. 1%); nausea (11% vs. 4%); headache (10% vs. 3%); nasopharyngitis (9% vs. 0%); fatigue (8% vs. 0%); and increased appetite (7% vs. 1%).

In two short-term, placebo-controlled trials in patients (6 to 18 years) with Tourette disorder with median exposure of 57 days, the mean change in body weight in aripiprazole-treated patients was +1.5 kg (N = 105) compared with +0.4 kg (N = 66) in placebo-treated patients. The incidence of reported EPS-related events, excluding events related to akathisia. In the pediatric (6 to 18 years) short-term Tourette disorder trials, changes in the Simpson Angus Rating Scale, Barnes Akathisia Scale, and Assessments of Involuntary Movement Scale were not clinically meaningfully different for aripiprazole and placebo.

In the study of pediatric patients (7 to 17 years of age) with Tourette disorder, no common adverse reaction(s) had a dose–response relationship (Abilify [package insert], 2017).

Reports of Interest

Aripiprazole in Children and Adolescents with Conduct Disorder

Findling et al. (2009) conducted an open-label, 15-day, three-center study with an optional 36-month extension that enrolled a total of 23 patients: 12 children (6 to 12 years) and 11 adolescents (13 to 17 years) with CD and a score of 2 to 3 on the RAAPP. This study consisted of an initial 15-day, outpatient PK study (phase A) at the end of which subjects were permitted to enter the open-label extension treatment period (phase B) of 36 months, during which frequent reassessment for safety and efficacy occurred. Throughout phase B, the dose could be adjusted at the discretion of the investigator up to a maximum of 15 mg/day. Notably, stimulants were allowed from months 2 through 36. All 23 subjects completed the initial 14 days of treatment (phase A) and continued into the 36-month continuation phase (phase B). Of these, only five patients (21.7%, two children and three adolescents) completed 36 months of treatment and 18 (78.3%) discontinued before the 36-month time point. The aripiprazole dose was adjusted upward in phase B for most patients ($N = 14/23$, 60.9%), with 6 of these 14 patients eventually receiving the maximum dose. Overall, RAAPP scores improved during the course of the study. Treatment effects appeared early because both children and adolescents showed a median score of 2 at day 14 and remained at this level at month 36. By day 14, 63.6% of children and 45.5% of adolescents were rated as much or very much improved on the CGI-I score. At month 36, 66.7% of children and 100% of adolescents showed this level of CGI-I score (much or very much improved) (observed cases). A neuropsychologic battery consisting of the Wisconsin Card Sort Test, pediatric version (WCST), Conners' CPT II, and the Verbal Fluency Test showed, on average, minor improvements per the authors.

Treatment with aripiprazole was generally well tolerated after the initial dose adjustment was revised following vomiting in four and somnolence in three children. Throughout the study, there were five reports of EPSs, three of them being in phase A. All EPS reports were considered to be of mild intensity by the investigator and did not lead to discontinuation. There were no serious AEs and no subjects discontinued because of AEs. Only two laboratory findings of potential clinical significance were observed; an elevated creatine phosphokinase of 737 that lasted for 3 days in one subject and a mild elevation of hepatic enzymes on day 169 that lasted for 15 days in another subject. Both investigators considered these to be not clinically significant and it was not reported as an AE. An elevated prolactin level was not reported for any subject. No subjects were discontinued from the study because of vital-sign abnormalities.

Mean weight change (LOCF) in patients ≤12 years old from baseline to week 72 was 9.0 ± 11.0 kg. In patients ≤13 years old, the mean change in weight was 3.3 ± 15.5 kg. Mean BMI change in patients ≤12 years old from baseline to week 72 was 1.8 kg/m². In patients ≤13 years old, the mean change in BMI from baseline was 3.4 kg/m². The authors proposed that although weight and BMI increased in children and adolescents over the study duration, weight gain in this population was normal and the findings were therefore not unexpected. No patients discontinued because of weight gain. Total cholesterol and glucose levels did not appear to be affected negatively by treatment.

In regard to the PK studies, it appears the steady state was attained within 14 days of once-daily aripiprazole dosing. The authors concluded that the mean apparent oral clearance of aripiprazole, when normalized for body weight, was similar across age groups.

The authors proposed that the preliminary data from this study (which was done before aripiprazole was FDA approved for treatment of schizophrenia and BPD in adolescent patients) suggest that aripiprazole may improve symptoms of CD with modest impact on cognitive function in both children and adolescents; however, the sample size was too small to draw any firm conclusions. It also supported the learned clinical practice enacted by early clinicians of starting aripiprazole at low doses initially and titrating gradually over the first 10 to 14 days to reduce the incidence of nausea and vomiting, which was unfortunately too frequent when more aggressive dosing was utilized.

Ziprasidone Hydrochloride (Geodon)

The manufacturer suggests that ziprasidone's antipsychotic properties may be mediated through its antagonism of dopamine type 2 (D_2) and serotonin type 2 (5-HT_{2A}) receptors.

It was approved by the FDA for marketing in the United States in 2001.

Pharmacokinetics of Ziprasidone Hydrochloride

Taken orally, ziprasidone is well absorbed and peak plasma concentrations occur within 6 to 8 hours. Absorption is increased up to twofold when taken with food. Elimination is mainly through hepatic metabolism; about one-third of the excretory metabolites are oxidized by CYP3A4, and about two-thirds result from reduction by aldehyde oxidase. Approximately 20% is excreted in the urine and 66% in the feces. Mean terminal half-life is approximately 7 hours for doses in the recommended clinical range. Steady-state plasma levels are achieved within 1 to 3 days at a constant dose.

Interactions of Ziprasidone with Other Medications

Carbamazepine, an inducer of CYP3A4, resulted in a decrease of approximately 35% in ziprasidone AUC (the total amount of medication absorbed into the systemic circulation and available for distribution to the target organ and site of action).

Contraindications for Ziprasidone Administration

Ziprasidone is contraindicated in patients with known hypersensitivity to the medication or in patients who have familial long QT syndrome or a history of cardiac arrhythmias or other significant cardiovascular illnesses.

Ziprasidone should not be prescribed concomitantly with other medications that are known to prolong the QTc interval.

Tolerability and Adverse Effects of Ziprasidone

ECG changes: Ziprasidone is associated with increases in the QTc interval. In placebo-controlled trials, ziprasidone increased the QTc interval by approximately 10 ms at a dose of 160 mg/day compared with that in placebo. In direct comparisons with five other antipsychotic medications, the mean increase in QTc over baseline in subjects receiving ziprasidone ranged from 9 to 14 ms greater than that for subjects receiving risperidone, olanzapine, quetiapine, and haloperidol; but was approximately 14 ms less than that for subjects receiving thioridazine.

Indications for Ziprasidone Hydrochloride in Child and Adolescent Psychiatry

Ziprasidone does *not* have FDA approval for any condition in child and adolescent psychiatry.

Ziprasidone is indicated only for adults for the treatment of schizophrenia and the treatment of acute mania episodes or mixed episodes associated with bipolar disorder. Ziprasidone intramuscular is indicated for the treatment of acute agitation in adult patients with schizophrenia and adult patients who need intramuscular antipsychotic medication for rapid control of the agitation.

Because of ziprasidone's greater capacity to increase the QT/QTc interval compared with several other antipsychotics, careful clinical consideration should be given to prescribing one or more trials of such alternative antipsychotics before undertaking a trial with ziprasidone.

(continued)

Indications for Ziprasidone Hydrochloride in Child and Adolescent Psychiatry (*continued*)

There is an interesting history behind ziprasidone in child and adolescent psychiatry. Ziprasidone was initially voted to be "acceptably safe" and effective for the treatment of bipolar disorder in teenagers and children by an FDA panel of outside medical experts that reviewed trial data for the FDA in 2009. However, there were comparatively more concerns about its efficacy compared with the other agents in the subgroups of younger patients aged 10 to 14 and patients weighing <45 kg, where ziprasidone did not achieve statistically significant difference versus placebo. It appears the small numbers of patients in these younger subgroups precluded any meaningful conclusions. Possibly because of these clinical efficacy issues, other safety issues, and concerns about data collection at certain sites, ziprasidone's final formal FDA approval never materialized.

Ziprasidone Dosage Schedule

- *Children and adolescents 17 years of age and less:* not recommended. The safety and efficacy of ziprasidone have not been established for pediatric populations.
- *Adolescents 18 years of age and older and adults:* an initial dose of 20 mg twice daily is recommended. Maximum total daily doses over 160 mg are not usually recommended. As it takes 1 to 3 days to achieve steady-state plasma levels, adjustments in dose should not be made at intervals of <2 days. In long-term studies (52 weeks) of subjects maintained on ziprasidone doses ranging from 20 to 80 mg twice a day, no clinical advantage was demonstrated for doses over 20 mg twice a day.

Ziprasidone Hydrochloride Dose Forms Available

- *Capsules:* 20, 40, 60, and 80 mg
- *Injection:* (ziprasidone mesylate) single-use vials 20 mg/mL for intramuscular injection. Doses are different from the oral doses; read package insert before use.

Per the ziprasidone PI, patients should be instructed to take ziprasidone capsules with food for optimal absorption. The absorption of ziprasidone is increased up to twofold in the presence of food (Geodon [package insert], 2015).

Reports of Interest

Ziprasidone in the Treatment of Children and Adolescents Diagnosed with Autistic Disorder

McDougle et al. (2002) conducted an open-label trial to evaluate the safety and effectiveness of ziprasidone in treating 12 subjects (mean age 11.62 ± 4.38 years; age range 8 to 20 years) who were diagnosed with autistic disorder ($N = 9$) or PDD not otherwise specified (PDD NOS); ($N = 3$) by DSM-IV criteria; 11 subjects had co-diagnoses of mental retardation (mild $= 4$, moderate $= 6$, and severe $= 1$). Target symptoms were aggression, self-injury, property destruction, agitation, irritability, and mood instability. Most subjects were treatment resistant, and 11 were previously treated with one or more other atypical antipsychotic medications, with significant weight gain often causing their discontinuation. At the beginning of the study, five subjects were receiving an atypical antipsychotic, which was discontinued over a 4-week taper. Four subjects were permitted to continue on their usual dose of other medications during the study.

The initial dose of ziprasidone was 20 mg at bedtime and titrated upward according to clinical response and AEs, in increments of 10 to 20 mg/week, and divided into two daily doses. All subjects completed a minimum of 6 weeks of the study; mean duration was 14.15 ± 8.29 weeks, range 6 to 30 weeks. The final mean ziprasidone dose was 59.23 ± 34.76 mg/day, dose range 20 to 120 mg/day. Responders were defined as subjects with a CGI-I rating of 1 (very much improved) or 2 (much improved). Six (50%) subjects were responders; two subjects with comorbid BPD were rated much worse. AEs were evaluated using a checklist used by the RUPP Autism Network. Four subjects reported no AEs. Sedation ($N = 5$), usually transient, was the most frequent AE, three experienced increased appetite and two had insomnia. Both the subjects with comorbid BPD experienced agitation and insomnia. One subject who had a history of TD of the hands developed an oral dyskinesia that resolved when ziprasidone was discontinued. The mean weight change was -5.83 ± 12.52 lb, range -35 to $+6$ lb. No cardiovascular AEs were reported; however, only a baseline ECG was performed. The authors suggested that ziprasidone is a potentially useful treatment for aggression, agitation, and irritability in children, adolescents, and young adults diagnosed with autistic disorder or PDDNOS and that further studies should be undertaken (McDougle et al., 2002).

Ziprasidone (Intramuscular) in the Treatment of Children and Adolescents Exhibiting Acute Agitation, Aggression, or Anxiety

Staller (2004) conducted a retrospective chart review of 49 children and adolescents (17 males and 32 females; age range 8 to 16 years), who were administered intramuscular ziprasidone for acute agitation and agitation/anxiety/threat ($N = 47$) or psychosis ($N = 2$) during hospitalization in an acute care private psychiatric hospital in central upstate New York. Most subjects (87%) were administered 20-mg injections; however, six subjects (two males and four females), all 13 years of age or younger, received 10-mg injections. Nursing notes indicated that only two patients continued to exhibit agitation and aggression during the subsequent shift and that only one of these was given a repeat 20-mg dose. There were no adverse reactions reported.

Ziprasidone Treatment of Children and Adolescents with Tourette Syndrome: A Pilot Study

Sallee et al. (2000a) conducted a study to evaluate the efficacy and tolerability of ziprasidone in children and adolescents with Tourette syndrome and chronic tic disorders. Twenty-eight patients aged 7 to 17 years were randomly assigned to ziprasidone or placebo for 56 days. Ziprasidone was initiated at a dose of 5 mg/day and flexibly titrated to a maximum of 40 mg/day. Ziprasidone was significantly more effective than placebo in reducing the Global Severity ($P = .016$) and TTSs ($P = .008$) on the YGTSS. Compared with placebo, ziprasidone significantly reduced tic frequencies as determined by blind videotape tic counts ($P = .039$). The mean ($\pm$SD) daily dose of ziprasidone during the last 4 weeks of the trial was 28.2 $\pm$ 9.6 mg. Ziprasidone in a dosage from 5 to 40 mg/day appeared to be effective in the treatment of Tourette syndrome and was well tolerated with mild transient somnolence as the most common AE. No clinically significant effects were observed on specific ratings of EPS, akathisia, or TD.

Paliperidone Extended-Release Tablets (Invega)

Similar to risperidone, paliperidone is a psychotropic agent belonging to the chemical class of benzisoxazole derivatives. In fact, paliperidone 9-hydroxyrisperidone is the chief active metabolite of risperidone, an established antipsychotic agent. Paliperidone, which is available in ER tablets (paliperidone ER; Invega), is an oral atypical antipsychotic medication. Paliperidone demonstrates high affinity for central dopamine 2 and serotonin 2a receptors. In addition, it has affinity for both alpha-adrenergic 1 and 2 and histaminic 1 receptors. Paliperidone does not possess affinity for muscarinic-cholinergic and beta-adrenergic receptors.

Paliperidone was first approved in December 2006 for the acute and maintenance treatment of schizophrenia in adults. It was the seventh SGA to be introduced to the U.S. market. In April 2011, the FDA approved Invega (paliperidone) ER tablets for the treatment of schizophrenia in children and adolescents 12 to 17 years of age.

Pharmacokinetics of Paliperidone

Paliperidone ER utilizes the Osmotic-Controlled Release Oral Delivery System (OROS), which allows for once-daily dosing and a resulting PK profile, which exhibits a more stable serum concentration. OROS formulation delivers paliperidone at a controlled rate over a 24-hour period. This is the same delivery system that was originally developed for the long-acting stimulant methylphenidate ER (OROS). Rossenu et al. (2007) found that the OROS technology results in reduced fluctuations between medication peak and trough serum concentrations (e.g., 38% paliperidone ER vs. 125% risperidone IR). To preserve the integrity of the OROS delivery system, the tablet should be swallowed whole and not chewed, split, or crushed (Invega [package insert], 2012). Because the shell of the tablet is nonabsorbable, prescribers should inform patients that the undissolved residue may be observed in their stool.

Administration of this agent after a high-fat or high-calorie meal increased the maximum serum concentration and AUC values by 60% and 54%, respectively. Although paliperidone ER can be taken without regard to meals, the presence of food may increase its exposure. Patients in the clinical efficacy trials, however, were dosed without regard to meal timing. The terminal half-life of paliperidone ER is about 23 hours in extensive metabolizers and 30 hours in poor metabolizers with steady-state concentration attained in 4 to 5 days.

Metabolism and Absorption

In vivo studies suggest that the CYP enzyme system plays a minimal role in paliperidone metabolism, with none of the metabolites accounting for >10% of a dose. Because of this limited hepatic metabolism, paliperidone should have minimal risks for hepatic medication–medication and medication–disease interactions. The majority (59%) of paliperidone is eliminated through the kidneys as unchanged medication.

Vermeir et al. (2005) reported that paliperidone ER undergoes very limited hepatic metabolism, with approximately 60% of the unchanged medication eliminated renally and 11% eliminated unchanged in the feces. Paliperidone is not expected to cause clinically important PK interactions with medications that are metabolized by CYP isozymes. In vitro studies in human liver microsomes showed that paliperidone does not substantially inhibit the metabolism of medications metabolized by CYP isozymes, including CYP1A2, CYP2A6, CYP2C8/9/10, CYP2D6, CYP2E1, CYP3A4, and CYP3A5 (Invega [package insert], 2012), which should translate into less hepatic medication–medication or medication–disease interactions. Rossenu et al. (2006) ascertained that, in general, the paliperidone ER PK profile demonstrates dose proportionality within the recommended clinical range of 3 to 12 mg/day.

Contraindications for Paliperidone Administration

Paliperidone is contraindicated in patients with a known hypersensitivity to it.

Interactions of Paliperidone with Other Medications

Carbamazepine. Plasma concentrations of 9-hydroxyrisperidone were decreased by approximately 37% with coadministration of carbamazepine, although plasma levels of carbamazepine did not appear to be affected.

Divalproex Sodium. Plasma concentrations (C_{max}) and AUC of 9-hydroxyrisperidone were increased by approximately 50% with coadministration of divalproex sodium. In a clinical study, subjects on stable doses of valproate had comparable valproate average plasma concentrations when paliperidone ER 3 to 15 mg/day was added to their existing valproate treatment (Invega [package insert], 2012).

PK interaction between lithium and paliperidone ER is unlikely.

In an interaction study in healthy subjects in which a single 3-mg dose of paliperidone ER was administered concomitantly with 20 mg/day of paroxetine (a potent CYP2D6 inhibitor), paliperidone exposures were on average 16% higher in CYP2D6 extensive metabolizers.

Extrapyramidal Symptoms. In the adolescents with schizophrenia trial akathisia, tremor, dystonia, and cogwheel rigidity were observed adverse reactions with an incidence ≥5% and at least twice that for placebo.

Hepatotoxicity. Paliperidone should have less hepatic issues than risperidone does.

Weight Gain. Weight gain in adolescent subjects (12 to 17 years of age) with schizophrenia was assessed in a 6-week, double-blind, placebo-controlled study and an open-label extension with a median duration of exposure to paliperidone ER of 182 days.

In the open-label long-term study, the proportion of total subjects treated with paliperidone ER with an increase in body weight of ≥7% from baseline was 33%. However, this weight gain should be assessed against that expected increase in weight that occurs with normal growth over the 182-day length of the study to achieve a more clinically relevant measure of changes in weight. The mean change from open-label baseline to endpoint in standardized score for weight was 0.1 (4% above the median for normative data). On the basis of the comparison with the normative data, these changes are not considered to be clinically significant. Although paliperidone ER appears to be well tolerated in short-term studies, long-term follow-up investigations of 1 to 2 years with ongoing clinical monitoring are necessary to confirm their safety in this age group.

Hyperprolactinemia. Paliperidone has a prolactin-elevating effect similar to that seen with risperidone, a medication that is associated with higher levels of prolactin than other antipsychotic medications.

Hyperglycemia and Dyslipidemia. Previous epidemiologic studies suggested an increased risk of treatment-emergent hyperglycemia-related AEs in patients treated with atypical antipsychotic medications, including risperidone (PDR, 2006). Also, undesirable alterations in lipids have been observed in patients treated with atypical antipsychotics; but because paliperidone was not marketed at the time these studies were performed, it is not known whether paliperidone is associated with these increased risks. There were only limited changes in these parameters in the adolescent schizophrenia studies, but these trials were only 6 weeks in duration and of limited benefit in determining the true metabolic risk of paliperidone.

Other Untoward Effects. Paliperidone can induce orthostatic hypotension, tachycardia, dizziness, and syncope in some patients because of its alpha-blocking activity; thus, titration of dosages is indicated. Paliperidone causes a modest increase in the QTc interval. The use of paliperidone should be avoided in combination with other medications that are known to prolong QTc. In an adult QTc study, a 4-mg dose of the IR oral formulation of paliperidone showed an increased placebo-subtracted QTcLD of 6.8 ms on day 2 at 1.5 hours post dose. None of the subjects had a change exceeding 60 ms or a QTcLD exceeding 500 ms at any time during this study (Invega [package insert], 2012).

Indications for Paliperidone in Child and Adolescent Psychiatry

Paliperidone is indicated for the management of the manifestations of schizophrenia in adolescents aged 12 to 17 years.

Paliperidone ER Dosage Schedule for Schizophrenia

- *Children 11 years of age or less:* not recommended. The safety and effectiveness of paliperidone in this young pediatric age group have not been established.
- *Adolescents <51 kg:* an initial dose of 3 mg once daily, with a recommended dosing range of 3 to 6 mg and a maximum dosage of 6 mg.

(continued)

Indications for Paliperidone in Child and Adolescent Psychiatry (*continued*)

- *Adolescents >51 kg:* an initial dose of 3 mg once daily, with a recommended dosing range of 3 to 12 mg and a maximum dosage of 12 mg.

Initial dose titration is not required. Dose increases, if considered necessary, should be made only after clinical reassessment and should occur at increments of 3 mg/day at intervals of more than 5 days. The manufacturer indicates that there was no clear enhancement to efficacy at the higher doses, that is, 6 mg for subjects weighing <51 and 12 mg for subjects weighing ≥51 kg, whereas AEs were dose related.

Clinical Pearl: To compare dosages of paliperidone to risperidone, a virtual comparison of the two medications was conducted by Schooler et al. (2006). The authors combined data from all available randomized placebo-controlled studies of risperidone and paliperidone in adults with schizophrenia. Paliperidone 6 to 12 mg/day was found to be similarly efficacious to risperidone 4 to 6 mg/day, with some tolerability benefits. In addition, paliperidone 6 to 12 mg/day was found to be more efficacious than risperidone 2 to 4 mg/day, but was associated with increased tachycardia.

Paliperidone ER Dose Forms Available

- *Tablets:* 1.5, 3, 6, and 9 mg

Paliperidone Dosage Schedule for Bipolar Disorder

Paliperidone is not approved for bipolar disorder in children, adolescents, or adults.

Schizophrenia

U.S. Food and Drug Administration Registry Trials

The efficacy of paliperidone ER in adolescents with schizophrenia was established in a single, 6-week randomized, double-blind, placebo-controlled study using a fixed-dose weight-based treatment group design over a dose range of 1.5 to 12 mg/day.

The study was conducted in several countries, including in the United States, and involved adolescents ranging in age from 12 to 17 years, all of whom met DSM-IV criteria for schizophrenia, with diagnosis confirmation using the Kiddie Schedule for Affective Disorders and Schizophrenia–Present and Lifetime Version. Efficacy was evaluated using the PANSS, a validated multi-item inventory composed of 30 individual items to evaluate positive symptoms, negative symptoms, disorganized thoughts, uncontrolled hostility/excitement, and anxiety/depression.

The study used a weight-based dosing regimen with a low (1.5 mg), medium (3 mg), and high (9 mg) dose groups. Dosing was in the morning without regard to meals. Overall, this study demonstrated efficacy of paliperidone ER in adolescents within the dose range of 3 to 12 mg a day; however, there was no clear indication of enhanced efficacy at the higher doses, and AEs were dose related.

In the treatment group, the most commonly reported AEs in this study were somnolence (13%), akathisia (9%), headache (9%), and insomnia (9%). As with most atypical antipsychotic medications, significant weight gain can be a side effect as well.

Reports of Interest

Paliperidone Extended Release for Irritability in Autistic Disorder

Stigler et al. (2010) reported on two case reports of patients with autism who manifested treatment-resistant aggression that benefited markedly when treated with paliperidone ER. The authors noted that, given the efficacy of risperidone in youths and adults with autism, paliperidone ER may be of benefit as well and have the advantages of once-daily dosing, much less PK interactions, and a lower incidence of EPSs and weight gain because the latter was of considerable concern in the risperidone Registry Trials. During the trial, the two patients received repeated health assessment via ECGs, vitals (including height and weight), and lab work (complete blood count [CBC], liver function tests, fasting glucose, and fasting lipid panel). Symptom improvement with the focus on the target symptom domain of irritability (aggression, SIBs, tantrums) was measured by utilizing the CGI-I Scale (Guy, 1976b) and rated 1 to 7 (1 = very much improved; 2 = much improved; 3 = minimally improved; 4 = no change; 5 = minimally worse; 6 = much worse; 7 = very much worse). In this report, patients were judged treatment responders if assigned a posttrial CGI-I rating of 1 (very much improved) or 2 (much improved).

One patient was female and 16 years of age with verbal autism, comorbid mild mental retardation, and intermittent explosive disorder, which was representative of her severe irritability, impulsive aggression toward others, as well as SIB. The patient also had a seizure disorder that was diagnosed in early childhood. Owing to the severity of her irritability, physical aggression, SIB, and tantrums, she had received several prior adequate medication trials that were reported as ineffective. These trials included quetiapine, risperidone, aripiprazole, and valproic acid.

At the time of initial assessment, the patient was taking a medication regimen of ziprasidone 80 mg twice daily, naltrexone 75 mg daily, diazepam 10 mg three times daily, and oxcarbazepine 300 mg daily for her seizure disorder, which was well controlled. Her baseline lab work was notable for elevated liver function tests (AST, 74 [reference range, 15 to 41] and ALT, 108 [reference range, 0 to 45]). Fasting lipid panel revealed an elevated total cholesterol of 268 (reference range, <200) and LDL of 191 (reference range, 118 to 142). The investigators tapered off the ziprasidone over a period of 1 month. Paliperidone ER was subsequently initiated at a dosage of 3 mg daily. When the patient was continued at this dosage for 4 weeks with only modest improvement in her symptoms, overall it was elected to increase her dosage to 6 mg daily to target her residual symptoms. The patient responded to such a degree that she was judged to be "very much improved," in relation to her target symptoms of irritability (aggression, SIB, and tantrums). Owing to her markedly improved functioning, naltrexone and diazepam were successfully tapered and discontinued over a period of 2 and 4 months, respectively. Repeat lab work obtained at 44 weeks continued to demonstrate a normal CBC and fasting glucose level with a normalizing of her liver function tests. Her fasting lipid panel measures improved as well, with a decrease in total cholesterol to 230 and LDL of 160. An ECG recording was normal. The investigators reported the patient was maintained at this 6-mg dosage of paliperidone for 50 weeks. No additional adverse effects were observed or recorded including EPSs or changes in vital signs. Over the 50 weeks of treatment, the patient recorded a loss of 10 lb (from 162 to 152 lb).

The second patient was a 20-year-old male with minimal language classic autism and moderate mental retardation. He had a history of severe irritability that included multiple daily episodes of aggression, SIB (head banging), and tantrums. Prior adequate medication trials included fluvoxamine, mirtazapine, olanzapine, chlorpromazine, haloperidol, quetiapine, and lithium. At the time of assessment, the patient had been on an ineffective 7-month trial of risperidone 4 mg twice daily, guanfacine 1 mg twice daily, and valproic acid ER 1,500 mg nightly. His baseline blood work was notable for an elevated total cholesterol of 232 (reference range, <200); triglycerides of 317 (reference range, <150); and a low high-density lipoprotein (HDL) of 35 (reference range, >40). Owing to the health risk of his SIB, it was elected to replace the risperidone with paliperidone ER without a taper period, which he tolerated without incident. The patient was reported to have had a marked reduction in his irritability, aggression, SIB, and tantrums across multiple settings, which warranted a classification of "much improved," with a CGI-I score of 2. The baseline fasting lipid panel measures that were out of normal range improved with a total cholesterol of 212, triglycerides of 192, and HDL of 42. An ECG recording was normal. He maintained satisfactorily on this dosage of paliperidone ER for 42 weeks. Over this treatment duration, his weight decreased by 2 lb (from 204 to 202 lb).

Albeit a small case study series, the authors proposed that their preliminary experience suggested that paliperidone may be an effective and well-tolerated treatment for severe irritability in adolescent and adult patients with autism and worthy of future study.

The Origins of U.S. Food and Drug Administration–Approved Second-Generation Antipsychotics as Mood Stabilizers in Pediatrics

Lithium was the first medication to be approved for pediatric BPD for 12- to 17-year-olds in the early 1970s. Beginning in late 2009, several of the atypical antipsychotic agents (olanzapine, risperidone, paliperidone, and quetiapine) received FDA approval for the treatment of BPD in youth. Although FDA approval was given to these aforementioned four atypical antipsychotic/mood stabilizers for the treatment of pediatric BPD, the FDA panel expressed concerns about the side effects of these medications, especially the propensity for weight gain and metabolic issues such as diabetes or lipid disorders. A study by Correll et al. (2009) found that teens are more prone to weight gain when taking atypical antipsychotic medications than are adults. Some have speculated that the higher density of histamine receptors in the pediatric versus adult brain may account for this greater propensity for weight gain. The study found children and teens can gain nearly 20 lb and become obese within just 11 weeks. Reviewing the weight gain reported in the randomized controlled trials (RCTs) of the currently available second- and third-generation mood stabilizers, one could rank the weight gain from most to least as olanzapine > quetiapine > risperidone > paliperidone ER > aripiprazole > iloperidone > asenapine > cariprazine/lurasidone > ziprasidone.

Newer U.S. Food and Drug Administration–Approved and Non-Approved Pediatric Antipsychotic/Mood Stabilizer Medications of Interest

In 2010, three new antipsychotics, namely, lurasidone (Latuda), iloperidone (Fanapt), and asenapine (Saphris), were approved for adult schizophrenia. Subsequently asenapine was approved for pediatric BPD and lurasidone was approved for pediatric schizophrenia and BPD as well. Iloperidone has no FDA approval for any conditions in children and adolescents at the time of this printing and it is unlikely that it ever will as no pediatric clinical trials are under way. Some of these newly released antipsychotic/mood stabilizer medications may never receive FDA approval for various pediatric psychiatric conditions; but because of their preferable side-effect profile with regard to extrapyramidal issues, TD risks, potential for neuroleptic malignant syndrome, and concerning degenerative brain issues, they are of interest to pediatric clinicians, given the current medication options available to them. As such, those second- and third-generation agents currently lacking FDA approval for pediatric indications are discussed at the end of the chapter in the section "Non-FDA-Approved Pediatric Antipsychotic/Mood Stabilizer Medications of Clinical Interest."

As of 2018, clinicians have several additional FDA-approved medications for pediatric BPD, and utilizing one of these agents as a first-line treatment is appropriate given their efficacy in RCTs. The studies on the originally approved agents indicated some variance in the number needed to treat (NNT), which is the number of how many patients need to be treated for one to benefit. The NNTs were predominantly in the 3 to 4 range, which indicates a clinically significant treatment effect. It is not always possible to accurately compare efficacy data across different studies, and as such many clinicians are apt to select an initial medication based on its side-effect profile and how that relates to the patient or their family medical history. These patient variables considered could entail current issues such as BMI, health history, and family history because it relates to obesity, diabetes, lipidemias, or cholesterol problems (Bowers et al., 2012).

For children <10 years old requiring treatment for BPD, there is very limited data to guide a clinician. Biederman et al. (2005a) evaluated short-term safety and efficacy in 31 preschoolers (4 to 6 years) in an open-label prospective study and found that both risperidone (at 1 week) and olanzapine (at 2 weeks) resulted in a rapid reduction of symptoms of mania in children with BPD; however, there were substantial adverse effects and the benefit may not outweigh the substantial risks in this population.

These agents are discussed in this section focusing on clinical relevance.

Lurasidone (Latuda)

Indications for Lurasidone in Child and Adolescent Psychiatry

Lurasidone is an atypical antipsychotic agent initially approved in 2010 in the United States for the treatment of schizophrenia in adults and in 2013 for bipolar depression in adults as monotherapy and as adjunctive therapy with lithium or valproate. In January 2017, lurasidone was approved to treat schizophrenia in adolescents aged 13 to 17 years. Lurasidone was approved in March 2018 for the acute treatment of depression in pediatric BPD as well. The efficacy of lurasidone in the treatment of mania associated with BPD has not been established.

Similar to most other atypical antipsychotics, lurasidone has high binding affinity and antagonism at serotonin 2A (5-HT_{2A}) and dopamine D_2 receptors. High binding affinity at 5-HT_7, as well as moderate binding affinity at 5-HT_{1A}, and alpha-2C adrenergic receptors is believed to possibly enhance cognition, and 5-HT_7 is being studied for a potential role in mood regulation and sensory processing. Lurasidone's low activity on alpha-1, H_1, and M_1 receptors suggests a low risk of orthostatic hypotension, H_1-mediated sedation and weight gain, and H_1- and M_1-mediated cognitive blunting. In 2010, the FDA approved lurasidone for the acute treatment of schizophrenia at a dose of 40 or 80 mg, administered once daily with food. Subsequent dosing revisions now support an upper dosing range of 160 mg/day. In 2017, the FDA approved lurasidone for the treatment of adolescent patients aged 13 to 17 years with schizophrenia.

Pharmacokinetics of Lurasidone

The activity of lurasidone is primarily due to the parent medication. The PK of lurasidone is dose-proportional within a total daily dose range of 20 mg to 160 mg. Lurasidone is absorbed in the gastrointestinal tract, but its concentration (C_{max}) doubles when lurasidone is administered with food (≥ 350 cal). Absorption, however, is independent of the meal's fat content. The elimination half-life is approximately 18 hours, and steady-state concentration is reached within 7 days.

Metabolism and Absorption

Lurasidone is eliminated predominantly through CYP3A4 metabolism in the liver. The PI indicates that the starting and maintenance does of lurasidone should be reduced by 50% for patients who are taking moderate CYP3A4 inhibitors such as diltiazem. Lurasidone should be avoided if used in combination with a strong CYP3A4 inhibitor (e.g., ketoconazole) or a strong CYP3A4 inducer (e.g., rifampin).

Tolerability and Adverse Effects of Lurasidone

Most of the safety data comes from clinical studies in adults and is reported here with additional relevant side-effect data for children and adolescents discussed in the pediatric Schizophrenia FDA registry trial that follows. Tolerability was quite good, and the rate of discontinuation from clinical trials because of adverse effects was 9.4% for lurasidone versus 5.9% for placebo. Somnolence, akathisia, nausea, parkinsonism, and agitation were the most commonly reported adverse reactions; somnolence and akathisia appear dose related. Of note, orthostatic hypotension associated with dizziness, tachycardia or bradycardia, and syncope may occur, especially early in treatment. Other adverse effects associated with lurasidone were nausea, vomiting, dyspepsia, dystonia, dizziness, insomnia, agitation, and anxiety.

Metabolic changes (hyperlipidemia, hyperglycemia, and increased body weight) were quite favorable, and lurasidone is considered to have insignificant effects on serum lipids or glucose while being weight-neutral in 52-week open-label extension studies in adults.

As is the case with other D_2 antagonists, lurasidone is associated with increased prolactin in a small subset of patients, which appears to be greater in females and is dose dependent. However, in the longer term studies, there was no signal of any prolactin increase, suggesting that much as with olanzapine and others, and unlike risperidone, any significant elevation in prolactin levels is not sustained.

Lurasidone is not associated with significant QTc prolongation, seizures, transaminases increase, or changes in serum chemistry, hematology, or urinalysis.

Lurasidone does not require initial dose titration in adults and should be given with food that provides ≥350 cal to improve medication absorption. Lurasidone is manufactured as 20-, 40-, 80-, and 120-mg tablets. The tablets are not a long-acting formulation.

The recommended starting dose in adults is 40 mg/day, and the maximum recommended dose is 160 mg/day (a starting dose of 20 mg and a maximum dose of 80 mg is recommended in those on a moderate CYP3A4 inhibitor such as diltiazem) (Latuda [package insert], 2012).

Indications for Lurasidone in Child and Adolescent Psychiatry

Lurasidone Dosage Schedule for Schizophrenia and Bipolar Depression

Lurasidone should be taken with food (at least 350 cal). Administration with food substantially increases the absorption of lurasidone twofold. Grapefruit and grapefruit juice should be avoided in patients taking lurasidone, because these may inhibit CYP3A4 and alter lurasidone concentrations.

Treatment of Schizophrenia

Adolescent patients aged 13 to 17 years: The recommended starting dose of the tablet formulation is 40 mg once daily. Initial dose titration is not required. Lurasidone has been shown to be effective in a dose range of 40 to 80 mg/day. The maximum recommended dose is 80 mg/day.

Moderate and severe renal impairment: Recommended starting dose is 20 mg/day, and the maximum recommended dose is 80 mg/day.

Moderate and severe hepatic impairment: Recommended starting dose is 20 mg/day. The maximum recommended dose is 80 mg/day in moderate hepatic impairment and 40 mg/day in severe hepatic impairment.

Concomitant use of a moderate CYP3A4 inhibitor (e.g., diltiazem): Lurasidone dose should be reduced to half of the original dose level.

Treatment of Depressive Episode Associated with Bipolar I Disorder (Bipolar Depression)

Children and adolescents aged 10 to 17 years (monotherapy): The recommended starting dose as monotherapy is 20 mg/day. Initial dose titration is not required. The dose may be increased after 1 week based on clinical response. Lurasidone has been shown to be effective in a dose range of 20 to 80 mg per day as monotherapy. At the end of the clinical study, most of the patients (67%) received 20 or 40 mg once daily. The maximum recommended dose is 80 mg per day.

Lurasidone Dose Forms Available

* Tablets: 20, 40, 60, 80, and 120 mg

Schizophrenia

U.S. Food and Drug Administration Registry Trials

The efficacy of lurasidone was established in a 6-week, multicenter, randomized, double-blind, placebo-controlled study of adolescents (13 to 17 years) who met DSM-IV-TR criteria for schizophrenia ($N = 326$). Patients were randomized to one of two fixed doses of lurasidone (40 or 80 mg/day) or placebo. The primary rating instrument used to assess psychiatric signs and symptoms was the PANSS. The key secondary instrument was the CGI-S. For both dose groups, lurasidone was superior to placebo in reduction of PANSS and CGI-S scores at week 6. On average, the 80-mg/day dose did not provide additional benefit compared to the 40-mg/day dose as in both groups the PANSS dropped about 18 points from the baseline score, approximating 94 in both groups.

Tolerability and Adverse Effects

In studies of adolescents and adults with schizophrenia, changes in fasting glucose levels were similar. In the short-term, placebo-controlled study of adolescents, fasting serum glucose mean values were -1.3 for placebo ($N = 95$), $+0.1$ for 40 mg ($N = 90$), and $+1.8$ for 80 mg ($N = 92$).

The mean weight gain was $+0.5$ kg for lurasidone-treated patients compared to $+0.2$ kg for placebo-treated patients. The proportion of patients with a $\geq 7\%$ increase in body weight (at endpoint) was 3.3% for lurasidone-treated patients versus 4.5% for placebo-treated patients.

Regarding prolactin levels, the median change from baseline to endpoint in prolactin levels for lurasidone-treated patients was $+1.1$ ng/mL versus $+0.1$ ng/mL for placebo-treated patients. For lurasidone-treated patients, the median change from baseline to endpoint for males was $+1.0$ ng/mL and for females was $+2.6$ ng/mL. Although there was a dose-proportional increase in prolactin for males and females, the prolactin elevations were very mild on average; but the proportion of patients on lurasidone with prolactin elevations $\geq 5\times$ the ULN was 0.6% for females and 0% for male patients versus 0% for placebo-treated female and male patients.

Bipolar Disorder

FDA Registry Trials

A Supplemental New Drug Application was accepted for review on June 30, 2017, by the FDA for the use of lurasidone in children and adolescents with bipolar depression. In March 2018, lurasidone was FDA approved for the acute treatment of bipolar depression in children and adolescents 10 to 17 years of age.

In October 2017, DelBello et al. published announced post hoc analysis results of a positive phase 3 placebo-controlled clinical study, and interim data from a long-term open-label extension study, evaluating lurasidone in children and adolescents with major depressive episodes associated with BP-I with or without rapid cycling, and without psychotic features.

The trial studied 343 children and adolescents 10 to 17 years of age with bipolar depression. Participants received once-daily lurasidone, flexibly dosed 20 to 80 mg/day, or placebo. Treatment with lurasidone was initiated at a daily dose of lurasidone 20 mg for 7 days, with flexible dosing, in the range of 20 to 80 mg/day permitted after 7 days.

Study results at the 6-week endpoint of treatment with lurasidone was associated with statistically significant and clinically meaningful improvement in a wide range of depressive symptoms measured by the CDRS-R (total score -21.0 vs. -15.3; $P < .0001$; effect size, 0.45), compared to the placebo. More specifically, patients randomized to lurasidone demonstrated greater improvement on 13 of the 17 CDRS-R items including social withdrawal, sleep disturbance, listless speech, depressed facial effect, excessive guilt, difficult having fun, depressed feelings, low self-esteem, excessive weeping, hypoactivity, impaired schoolwork, irritability, and appetite disturbance.

Lurasidone was also associated with statistically significant improvement in the Clinical Global Impression–Bipolar Severity (key secondary measure), and measures of anxiety, quality of life, and global functioning.

The percentage of participants meeting a priori response criteria was significantly greater in the lurasidone group compared with the placebo group at week 6 (59.5% vs. 36.5%; $P < .0001$; NNT = 5; LOCF). However, when evaluating the percentage of patients achieving remission, on the basis of a priori composite criteria, this was not significantly different between the lurasidone and placebo groups at week 6 (26.0% vs. 18.8%; $P = .082$; NNT = 14; LOCF). The authors commented that there was greater mean improvement in the CDRS-R total at week 6 in the placebo group for the younger age group (−17.3 [1.5] vs. −14.7 [1.6]) versus the older group, resulting in a smaller and nonsignificant week 6 lurasidone effect size (0.29 vs. 0.61) on the CDRS-R total score. This latter anomaly was also felt to contribute to the finding of a significant treatment-by-age stratum interaction (10 to 14 vs. 15 to 17 years), whereby the younger age group had a nonsignificant effect size on the CDRS-R total score at week 6 endpoint. This finding is consistent with previous reports (Wagner et al., 2003, 2006) of higher placebo response rates among younger patients in pediatric trials of standard antidepressants.

There were low discontinuation rates of 1.7% due to AEs in both groups, with the two most common AEs on lurasidone being nausea and somnolence. The most common side effects with an incidence greater than 5% of lurasidone-treated patients included nausea, somnolence, weight increase, vomiting, dizziness, and insomnia. Treatment with lurasidone was associated with few effects on weight and metabolic parameters. The mean daily dose of lurasidone during the study was 31.5 mg/day in the 10- to 14-year-old age group, and 33.8 mg/day in the 15- to 17-year-old age group, and 32.5 mg/day in the combined age groups. The modal daily dose of lurasidone (combined age groups) was 20 mg in 52.3% of patients, 40 mg in 26.2% of patients, 60 mg in 12.8% of patients, and 80 mg in 8.7% of patients.

Treatment with lurasidone in the study was associated with low rates of akathisia and extrapyramidal symptoms, with only a small percentage of patients receiving anticholinergic medications for acute EPSs (1.2% vs. 0.6%). Small increases in prolactin were observed, but prolactin-related AEs were not observed. No changes in QTc interval were observed in association with lurasidone treatment in this study.

When compared with placebo, treatment with lurasidone was not associated with treatment-emergent suicidal ideation or behavior, or treatment-emergent mania. Suicidal ideation, as an AE, was reported by none of the patients in the lurasidone group, and by one patient in the placebo group. One component of this study that represented a real-world scenario was the inclusion of patients with ADHD and their ongoing stimulant treatment. There were no statistically significant treatment interactions for those patients on stimulant use for ADHD as observed for either the CDRS-R total or Clinical Global Impression–Bipolar Version, Severity of Illness (CGI-BP-S) depression scores based on ANCOVA analyses.

The long-term open-label extension study focused on 223 participants who completed the 6-week trial. The 2-year, open-label, flexible-dose, extension study showed that among the 155 people who completed 28 weeks of treatment, lurasidone-treated patients continued to improve in depressive symptoms on the CDRS-R total score. There was also continued improvement in the CGI-BP-S depression score.

During the extension phase, there was minimal effect noted on weight and metabolic parameters. In fact, the AEs were similar to those reported in the 6-week pivotal trial. The most common adverse effects greater than 10% were headache, 19.7%; somnolence 18.5%; and nausea, 14.3%.

The findings that lurasidone was effective for depression in bipolar depression, is well tolerated, and has a favorable side-effect profile including weight metabolic issues is promising because additional treatment options are clearly needed for those children and adolescents who suffer from bipolar depression given it is the most dominant phase in their lives.

Reports of Interest

Lurasidone Treatment in a Child with Autism Spectrum Disorder with Irritability and Aggression

Millard et al. (2014) reported a case report of using lurasidone for treating a 13-year-old boy with intellectual disability, autism spectrum disorder (ASD), and ADHD referred for evaluation of irritability and aggressive behavior. The patient exhibited classic autism with hand flapping, very limited language development, no reciprocal speech, and perseveration on special interests which when interrupted resulted in loss of temper and repeated aggressive behavior such as hitting himself, hitting objects, lashing out at his mother, and physically injuring her at times. The patient had received extensive special education and speech, occupational, and physical therapy services starting at 3 years of age, and was in a classroom dedicated to education of children with ASD.

He was first started on medications at the age of 10 years. By age 12, his temper and aggression had escalated to the degree that he required constant redirection. Initial treatment was with clonidine for insomnia and hyperactivity, which was ineffective. Later trials of risperidone, citalopram, long-acting guanfacine ER, quetiapine, lorazepam, and aripiprazole were enacted at the parents' request. These various agents used in combination were initiated to address very problematic behaviors such head banging, irritability, and aggressive behaviors or side effects such as extreme appetite with problematic weight gain and vomiting. After two separate trials of aripiprazole failed, it was discontinued to initiate a trial of lurasidone 10 mg/day that when titrated to 20 mg/day improved his irritability and aggressive behaviors. Because there were no significant adverse effects, the dose was increased to 30 mg/day, and trazodone was initiated for insomnia. Two months later, he was noted to be significantly less irritable, aggressive, and impulsive on this combination. He remained on lurasidone 30 mg daily, citalopram 30 mg daily, clonidine 0.2 mg qhs, and trazodone 75 mg qhs.

The authors utilized the first-line FDA-approved pharmacotherapies of risperidone and aripiprazole, which are the only two agents approved for irritability in autism, but they were ineffective and intolerable because of side effects in this adolescent with ASD. The authors propose that lurasidone may be a reasonable alternative, especially if the patient has a history of metabolic adverse effects. They further elaborated that given the risk of long-term metabolic adverse effects of most atypical antipsychotics, lurasidone may serve as an alternative, because it has shown to have fewer effects on weight gain, hyperlipidemia, elevated blood sugar, and insulin resistance in adults. In addition to the favorable metabolic profile, lurasidone has been shown to have antidepressant effects in studies with adults. Mood benefits and decrease in depression and irritability are thought to be associated with 5-HT_7 and alpha-2 receptor antagonism and partial 5-HT_{1A} agonist properties. In addition to lurasidone's potential benefits for treatment of irritability in children with ASD, there may also be a potential antidepressant effect, which may influence the overall symptom profile.

Asenapine (Saphris)

In 2009, the FDA approved asenapine for the treatment of schizophrenia and BPD in adults. In early 2017 *asenapine* was approved as monotherapy for the acute treatment of manic or mixed episodes associated with BP-I in children and adolescents 10 to 17 years of age.

Pharmacodynamics of Asenapine

Asenapine is an oral atypical antipsychotic agent that belongs to the class dibenzo-oxepino pyrroles. Asenapine exhibits high affinity for serotonin 5-HT_{1A}, 5-HT_{1B}, 5-HT_{2A}, 5-HT_{2B}, 5-HT_{2C}, 5-HT_5, 5-HT_6, and 5-HT_7 receptors, dopamine D_2, D_3, D_4, and D_1 receptors, alpha-1- and alpha-2-adrenergic receptors, and histamine H_1 receptors.

Asenapine has moderate affinity for H_2 receptors and has no appreciable affinity for muscarinic-cholinergic receptors.

Pharmacokinetics of Asenapine

Following a single 5-mg dose of asenapine, the mean T_{max} was observed at 1 hour. Following an initial more rapid distribution phase, the mean terminal half-life is approximately 24 hours. With multiple-dose twice-daily dosing, steady state is attained within 3 days. Overall, steady-state asenapine PK are similar to single-dose PK. This long terminal half-life gives some clinicians the confidence to prescribe asenapine in once-a-day dosing, usually in the evening, after the patient has reached a steady state. Reduced exposure to asenapine was observed following consumption of water at 2 minutes (19% decrease) and at 5 minutes (10% decrease).

Metabolism and Elimination

Elimination of asenapine is primarily through direct glucuronidation by UGT1A4 and oxidative metabolism by CYP isoenzymes (predominantly CYP1A2). To assess the potential for other medications to affect asenapine, the potential effects of inhibitors of several of these enzyme pathways on asenapine clearance were studied. The only notable finding was that fluvoxamine (a CYP1A2 inhibitor), even at a subtherapeutic dose of 25 mg bid, elevated the C_{max} by 13% and AUC by 29% for asenapine, and thus caution is advised when coadministering. In vitro studies indicate that asenapine weakly inhibits CYP2D6, and thus the potential for asenapine to affect other CYP2D6 substrate medications was conducted. Coadministration of a single 20-mg dose of paroxetine (a CYP2D6 substrate and inhibitor) during treatment with 5-mg asenapine twice daily in 15 healthy adult male subjects resulted in an almost twofold increase in paroxetine exposure. Asenapine should be coadministered cautiously with medications that are both substrates and inhibitors for CYP2D6. Dextromethorphan, valproic acid, and lithium predose serum concentrations collected from an adjunctive therapy study were comparable between asenapine-treated patients and placebo-treated patients, indicating a lack of effect of asenapine on valproic and lithium plasma levels. Food does have an impact on absorption. A crossover study in 26 healthy adult male subjects was performed to evaluate the effect of food on the PK of a single 5-mg dose of asenapine. Consumption of food immediately before sublingual administration decreased asenapine exposure by 20%; consumption of food 4 hours after sublingual administration decreased asenapine exposure by about 10%. These effects are probably due to increased hepatic blood flow.

Adverse Effects of Asenapine in Pediatric Trials

The most common side effects in children (ages 10 to 17) were sleepiness, dizziness, strange sense of taste, numbing of the mouth, nausea, increased appetite, feeling tired, weight gain, and extrapyramidal effects. In postmarketing experience, patients taking asenapine have reported reactions under the tongue (where you place asenapine), such as sores, oral blisters, peeling/sloughing, or inflammation. Patients have reported choking; some may have also experienced oropharyngeal muscular dysfunction or hypoesthesia.

In summary, compared to patients from adult clinical trials, adolescents were likely to gain more weight, experience increased sedation, and have greater increases in total cholesterol, triglycerides, LDL cholesterol, prolactin, and hepatic aminotransferase levels. In adult studies, asenapine was associated with increases in prolactin during the early phases of treatment. However, in a longer term 52-week study, there was no signal of any prolactin increase but rather a decrease, suggesting any significant elevation in prolactin levels may not be sustained although this is has not been studied in adolescents long term. Asenapine is pregnancy category C.

Refer to the pediatric Bipolar I FDA Registry Trials section on *Tolerability and Adverse Effects* later in the chapter for a more detailed discussion of side effects in the short 3-week pediatric study. Owing to the short 3-week duration of the pediatric trial, select data from the adult trials is discussed later because it is much more informative, especially in the area of cardiac function and long-term side effect data.

Tolerability and Adverse Effects of Asenapine in Adult Studies

In the adult schizophrenia clinical studies, tolerability was quite good; and the rate of discontinuation because of adverse effects was approximately 9% in asenapine-treated patients compared with about 10% of placebo-treated patients. The most common adverse reactions ($\geq 5\%$ and at least twice the rate of placebo) reported with acute treatment in schizophrenia were akathisia, oral hypoesthesia, and somnolence.

The most common adverse reactions ($\geq 5\%$ and at least twice the rate of placebo) reported with acute monotherapy treatment of manic or mixed episodes associated with BP-I were somnolence, dizziness, EPSs other than akathisia, and weight increase. In short-term, placebo-controlled schizophrenia trials, the mean weight gain was 1.1 kg for asenapine-treated patients compared with 0.1 kg for placebo-treated patients. In a 52-week, double-blind, comparator-controlled trial of patients with schizophrenia or schizoaffective disorder, the mean weight gain from baseline was 0.9 kg.

To assess EPSs in the short-term, placebo-controlled schizophrenia and bipolar mania trials, data were objectively collected on the Simpson Angus Rating Scale for EPS, the Barnes Akathisia Scale (for akathisia), and the Assessments of Involuntary Movement Scales (for dyskinesias). The mean change from baseline for the all-asenapine 5- or 10-mg twice-daily-treated group was comparable to placebo in each of the rating scale scores.

The effects on fasting serum glucose levels as well as the total cholesterol and fasting triglycerides in the short-term schizophrenia and bipolar mania trials revealed no clinically relevant mean changes. In a 52-week, double-blind, comparator-controlled trial of patients with schizophrenia and schizoaffective disorder, the mean increase from baseline of fasting glucose was 2.4 mg/dL. The mean decrease from baseline of total cholesterol was 6 mg/dL and the mean decrease from baseline of fasting triglycerides was 9.8 mg/dL. As is the case with other D_2 antagonists, asenapine is associated with increases in prolactin during the early phases of treatment; however, in the longer term 52-week study, there was no signal of any prolactin increase but rather a decrease, suggesting any significant elevation in prolactin levels is not sustained. Asenapine is pregnancy category C.

Although rare, asenapine may induce orthostatic hypotension and syncope in some patients, especially early in treatment, because of its alpha-1-adrenergic antagonist activity. The effects of asenapine on the QT/QTc interval were evaluated in a dedicated QT study. This trial involved asenapine doses of 5, 10, 15, and 20 mg twice daily, and placebo, and was conducted in 151 clinically stable patients with schizophrenia, with ECG assessments throughout the dosing interval at baseline and steady state. At these doses, asenapine was associated with increases in QTc interval ranging from 2 to 5 ms compared with placebo. No patients treated with asenapine experienced QTc increases ≥ 60 ms from baseline measurements, nor did any patient experience a QTc of ≥ 500 ms. Despite these small increases of 2 to 5 ms in QTc, the PI indicates that the use of asenapine should be avoided in combination with other medications known to prolong QTc including class 1A antiarrhythmics (e.g., quinidine, procainamide) or class 3 antiarrhythmics (e.g., amiodarone, sotalol), antipsychotic medications (e.g., ziprasidone, chlorpromazine, thioridazine), and antibiotics (e.g., gatifloxacin, oxifloxacin). It is also recommended to avoid asenapine in patients with congenital prolongation of QT interval or a history of cardiac arrhythmias, and in circumstances that may increase occurrence of torsades de pointes and/or sudden death in association with the use of medications that prolong QTc interval (Saphris [package insert], 2017).

Indications for Asenapine in Child and Adolescent Psychiatry

Asenapine is indicated as monotherapy for the acute treatment of manic or mixed episodes associated with BP-I in children and adolescents 10 to 17 years of age.

Asenapine Dosage Schedule for Bipolar Disorder

Children and Adolescents 10 to 17 years of age: The recommended starting daily dose is 2.5 mg sublingually (SL) q12hr initially; may increase to 5 mg SL q12hr after 3 days and to 10 mg SL q12hr after 3 additional days. Asenapine is a sublingual tablet. To ensure optimal absorption, patients should be instructed to place the tablet under the tongue and allow it to dissolve completely. The tablet will dissolve in saliva within seconds. Asenapine sublingual tablets should not be split, crushed, chewed, or swallowed. Patients should be instructed to not eat or drink for 10 minutes after administration to ensure proper absorption. Oral hypoesthesia and/or oral paresthesia may occur directly after administration of asenapine and usually resolves within 1 hour.

Asenapine Dose Forms Available

Sublingual tablets: 2.5, 5, and 10 mg. Sublingual tablets are black-cherry flavored.

Bipolar I Disorder

U.S. Food and Drug Administration Registry Trial

The efficacy of asenapine in the treatment of acute mania in children and adolescents 10 to 17 years of age was established in a single, 3-week, placebo-controlled, double-blind trial of 403 pediatric patients 10 to 17 years of age. In the study, 302 of the 403 pediatric patients received asenapine at fixed doses of 2.5, 5, and 10 mg twice daily. All patients were started on 2.5 mg twice daily. For those assigned to 5 mg twice daily, the dose was increased to 5 mg twice daily after 3 days. For those assigned to 10 mg twice daily, the dose was increased from 2.5 to 5 mg twice daily after 3 days, and then to 10 mg twice daily after 3 additional days. Asenapine was statistically superior to placebo in improving the YMRS total score and the CGI-BP-S overall score as measured by the change from baseline to week 3. An examination of subgroups did not reveal any clear evidence of differential responsiveness on the basis of age, sex, and race.

Tolerability and Adverse Effects of Asenapine

The incidences of EPS-related events, excluding events related to akathisia, were 4%, 3%, and 5% for patients treated with asenapine 2.5, 5, and 10 mg twice daily, respectively, as compared to 3% for placebo-treated patients. For events of akathisia, incidences were 2%, 2%, and 1% for pediatric patients treated with asenapine 2.5, 5, and 10 mg twice daily, respectively, as compared to 0% for placebo-treated patients.

Overall, there were dose-proportional elevations in fasting serum glucose, total cholesterol, and triglycerides levels found in the study; but overall these were quite modest and revealed no clinically relevant mean changes, which is in line with data from the longer adult trials. The proportion of subjects with a ≥7% increase in body weight was placebo—1.1% versus asenapine 2.5 mg bid—12.0%, 5 mg bid—8.9%, and 10 mg bid—8.0%. The incidence of AEs related to abnormal prolactin levels were 0% in the asenapine 2.5-mg twice-daily treatment group, 2% in the asenapine 5-mg twice-daily treatment group, and 1% in the asenapine 10-mg twice-daily treatment group versus 1% for patients treated with placebo. The mean increases (at endpoint) in prolactin levels were 3.2 ng/mL for patients treated with asenapine 2.5 mg twice daily, 2.1 ng/mL for patients treated with asenapine 5 mg twice daily, and 6.4 ng/mL for patients treated with asenapine 10 mg twice daily compared to an increase of 2.5 ng/mL for placebo-treated patients. Galactorrhea or dysmenorrhea were reported in 0% of patients treated with asenapine 2.5 mg twice daily, 2% of patients treated with asenapine 5 mg twice daily, and 1% of patients treated with asenapine 10 mg twice daily compared to 1% of placebo-treated patients. There were no reports of gynecomastia in this trial. Note that incidence of fatigue appeared to be dose related.

Asenapine in the Treatment of Children and Adolescents Diagnosed with Schizophrenia

Asenapine is not approved for schizophrenia in children or adolescents.

Failed Registry Trial: The efficacy of asenapine was *not* demonstrated in an 8-week, placebo-controlled, double-blind trial, in 306 adolescent patients aged 12 to 17 years with schizophrenia at doses of 2.5 and 5 mg twice daily. Note that the maximal dosing of asenapine in the successful registry trial for the treatment of children and adolescents diagnosed with BPD was 10 mg SL q12hr or twice the dosage used in the failed schizophrenia trial. Although one may suspect that this lower dosage range in the schizophrenia trial contributed to the failed study, no further trials were conducted to study a higher dosing paradigm.

In this failed schizophrenia trial, the PI indicates the most common adverse reactions (proportion of patients equal or greater than 5% and at least twice placebo) reported were somnolence, akathisia, dizziness, and oral hypoesthesia or paresthesia. The proportion of patients with an equal or greater than 7% increase in body weight at endpoint compared to baseline for placebo, asenapine 2.5 mg twice daily, and asenapine 5 mg twice daily was 3%, 10%, and 10%, respectively. The clinically relevant adverse reactions identified in the pediatric schizophrenia trial were generally similar to those observed in the pediatric bipolar I and adult bipolar I and schizophrenia trials. No new major safety findings were reported from a 26-week, open-label, uncontrolled safety trial in pediatric patients with schizophrenia treated with asenapine monotherapy (Saphris [package insert], 2017).

TABLE 7.1 » FDA-Approved Mood Stabilizers in Pediatrics

Agent	Pediatric Indication	Dosage
Risperidone	Acute treatment of manic and mixed episodes associated with bipolar I disorder in children and adolescents (10–17 y of age)	0.5–6.0 mg/d
Aripiprazole	Acute and maintenance treatment of manic or mixed episodes associated with bipolar I disorder in children and adolescents (10–17 y of age), both as monotherapy and as an adjunct to lithium or divalproex	10–30 mg/d
Quetiapine	Acute treatment of manic episodes associated with bipolar I disorder in children and adolescents (10–17 y of age),	400–600 mg/d
Quetiapine XR	Acute treatment of manic episodes associated with bipolar I disorder in children and adolescents (10–17 y of age),	400–600 mg/d
Olanzapine	Acute treatment of manic and mixed episodes associated with bipolar I disorder in adolescents (13–17 y of age)	2.5–20 mg/d
Olanzapine/fluoxetine	Acute treatment of bipolar I depression in patients 10–17 y of age	6/25; 6/50; 12/25; 12/50 mg/d
Lithium	Acute treatment of bipolar disorder in adolescents aged 12 y and above	Therapeutic levels 0.8–1.2 mEq/L
Asenapine	Acute treatment of manic or mixed episodes associated with bipolar I disorder in children and adolescents 10–17 y of age	2.5mg SL q12h–10 mg SL q12h
Lurasidone	Acute treatment of bipolar depression in children and adolescents 10–17 y of age	20–80 mg/d

Pending Pediatric Clinical Trials (clinicaltrials.gov)
None.

It is notable that lurasidone is only the second agent (olanzapine/fluoxetine being the first dual-agent) in children and adolescents that is approved for bipolar depression. Treatment of bipolar depression in children and adolescents remains a major unmet medical need because all of the initial FDA approvals were agents that demonstrated efficacy for the treatment of manic or mixed episodes in BPD. This deficit in research exists despite the fact that depressive episodes in BPD are more frequent and of longer duration than manic episodes. In addition, most of the disease burden and suicidality is associated with the depressive phases of BPD. Only in the past decade have prospective studies in children and adolescents with acute bipolar depression been conducted. Findling et al. (2014) and DelBello et al. (2009) conducted two double-blind, placebo-controlled, monotherapy studies of quetiapine in pediatric bipolar depression (utilizing ER and IR formulations) that failed to demonstrate significant antidepressant efficacy. In contrast, Detke et al. (2015) utilizing (OFC) therapy demonstrated significant efficacy in an 8-week bipolar depression trial in children and adolescents. The antidepressant effect of lurasidone in the Debello et al. (2017) study was comparable to results reported in the 8-week OFC trial, both in terms of CDRS-R improvement (effect size 0.45 vs. 0.46), and responder rates (NNT, 5 vs. 6). However, treatment with OFC was associated with relatively high discontinuation rates, both overall (31.8%) and due to AEs (14.1%). Treatment with OFC was also associated with a mean weight gain of 4.4 kg (vs. 0.5 kg on placebo), and a high proportion of patients (52%) experienced clinically significant ($\geq$7%) weight gain on OFC compared with placebo (4%).

Non-FDA-Approved Pediatric Antipsychotic/Mood Stabilizer Medications of Clinical Interest.

Brexpiprazole (Rexulti)

Brexpiprazole is *not* FDA indicated for any psychiatric condition in children and adolescents. Brexpiprazole is an atypical antipsychotic, and specifically a dopamine D_2 receptor partial agonist, placing it in the category of a TGA. In July 2015, the FDA approved brexpiprazole to treat schizophrenia and as an adjunct for major depressive disorder (MDD). For both adult indications, brexpiprazole demonstrated positive results compared with placebo in phase III trials. Brexpiprazole is not an isomer aripiprazole but rather a distinct novel compound from aripiprazole, although both agents share properties of being dopamine D_2 receptor partial agonists. It is the clinical impression of some pediatric prescribers using this agent off-label that brexpiprazole may have less weight gain than aripiprazole, but this clinical impression has not been confirmed in any studies to this point in time. Thus, it has been the practice of some clinicians treating patients who have experienced good efficacy with aripiprazole, but excessive weight gain, to trial brexpiprazole in an attempt to address this side-effect issue. Brexpiprazole will be discussed in a brief manner until the current pending registry trial utilizing brexpiprazole as Monotherapy for the Treatment in Adolescents (13–17 Years Old) with Schizophrenia is completed in 2020 (estimated). This trial should address many of the issues of safety, efficacy, and tolerability regarding its use in the pediatric population.

Pharmacodynamics of Brexpiprazole

Similar to aripiprazole, brexpiprazole is a dopamine D_2 partial agonist, but differs from aripiprazole because it is more potent at serotonin 5-HT_{1A} and 5-HT_{2A} receptors. It also has more noradrenergic effects that reportedly could aid cognition in a general sense and less activity at D_2 receptors, which could lead to better tolerability.

Pharmacokinetics of Brexpiprazole

Brexpiprazole has a long half-life of 91 hours, allowing a steady-state concentration to be obtained in approximately 2 weeks. Metabolism of brexpiprazole is mediated principally by CYP3A4 and CYP2D6. On the basis of *in vitro* data, brexpiprazole shows little or no inhibition of CYP450 isozymes.

Contraindications for Brexpiprazole Administration

The only absolute contraindication for brexpiprazole is known hypersensitivity to brexpiprazole or any of its components. Reactions have included rash, facial swelling, urticaria, and anaphylaxis.

As with all antipsychotics and agents with an indication for a depressive disorder, there is a bolded boxed warning in the product label that antidepressants increase the risk of suicidal thoughts and behaviors in patients aged 24 years and younger. Monitor for clinical worsening and emergence of suicidal thoughts and behaviors. The safety and efficacy of brexpiprazole has *not* been established in pediatric patients.

Interactions of Brexpiprazole with Other Medications

In patients with moderate to severe hepatic impairment, or moderate, severe, or end-stage renal impairment, the maximum recommended dosage is 3 mg/day for patients with schizophrenia, and 2 mg/day for patients with MDD.

In general, the PI recommends dosage adjustments in patients with various CYP considerations:

- For strong CYP2D6 or CYP3A4 inhibitors, administer one-half the usual dosage.
- For strong/moderate CYP2D6 with strong/moderate CYP3A4 inhibitors, administer a one-quarter of the usual dosage.
- For known CYP2D6 poor metabolizers taking strong/moderate CYP3A4 inhibitors, also administer a one-quarter of the usual dosage.
- For strong CYP3A4 inducers, double the usual dosage and further adjust depending on clinical response.

Tolerability and Adverse Effects of Brexpiprazole

The most commonly encountered AEs for MDD in the adult studies (incidence ≥5% and at least twice the rate for placebo (PBO)) were akathisia (8.6% vs. 1.7% PBO) and dose-related weight gain (6.7% vs. 1.9% PBO). The most commonly encountered AE in schizophrenia studies (incidence ≥4% and at least twice the rate for placebo) was weight gain (4% vs. 2% PBO). Akathisia in the schizophrenia trials were 5.5% for brexpiprazole and 4.6% for placebo, yielding a non-statistically significant value.

Short-term weight gain appears modest in adults; but as usual there were outliers with an increase of ≥7% of body weight in open-label long-term safety studies. This is of larger significance for pediatric patients because they consistently gain weight at levels than found in adult studies. Effects on glucose and lipids were small; but because these issues are often related to weight gain, they may be more of a concern for pediatric patients as well considering long-term risks. As to be expected with a partial dopamine agonist, minimal effects on prolactin were observed. Brexpiprazole is associated with small increases in the hormone prolactin, as opposed to the small decreases in prolactin seen with aripiprazole.

In the adult studies, no clinically relevant effects on the QT interval were evident.

Indications for Brexpiprazole in Child and Adolescent Psychiatry

Brexpiprazole is *not* FDA indicated for any psychiatric condition in children and adolescents.

Brexpiprazole Dosage Schedule in Adults

Brexpiprazole can be taken without regard to food.

Schizophrenia. The recommended starting dosage for brexpiprazole for schizophrenia is 1 mg/day on days 1 to 4. Brexpiprazole can be titrated to 2 mg/day on day 5 through 7, then to 4 mg/day on day 8 depending on the patient's response and ability to tolerate the medication. The recommended target dosage is 2 to 4 mg/day with a maximum recommended daily dosage of 4 mg.

Major Depressive Disorder. The recommended starting dosage for brexpiprazole as adjunctive treatment for MDD is 0.5 mg or 1 mg/day. Brexpiprazole can be titrated to 1 mg/day, then up to the target dosage of 2 mg/day, with dosage increases occurring at weekly intervals depending on the patient's clinical response and ability to tolerate the agent, with a maximum recommended dosage of 3 mg/day.

Brexpiprazole Dose Forms Available

Tablets: 0.25, 0.5, 1, 2, 3, and 4 mg
   Rexulti [package insert] (2017).

Schizophrenia

Reports of Interest. Pending pediatric clinical trials (clinical trials.gov).
   Description: This is a multicenter, randomized, double-blind, placebo- and active-controlled trial to evaluate the safety and efficacy of brexpiprazole monotherapy compared to placebo in adolescent subjects (13 to 17 years old) with a DSM-5 diagnosis of schizophrenia.
   Dosing Regimens:
   Study agent brexpiprazole: Dosing range = 2 to 4 mg/day. Initiation at 0.5 mg/day, then titrate to a maximum of 4 mg/day
   Active Comparator: Aripiprazole dosing range = 10 to 20 mg/day. Initiation at 2 mg/day, then titrate up to a maximum of 20 mg/day
   Placebo Comparator: Placebo matching placebo taken daily

Estimated enrollment:	387 subjects
Actual study start date:	June 30, 2017
Estimated study completion date:	April 2020
Estimated primary completion date:	April 2020 (final data collection date for primary outcome measure)

Cariprazine (Vraylar)

Cariprazine is *not* FDA indicated for any psychiatric condition in children and adolescents. Cariprazine is an atypical antipsychotic, and specifically a dopamine D_2 and D_3 receptor partial agonist, placing it in the category of a TGA. However, cariprazine differs from the other dopamine D_2 receptor partial agonists and other antipsychotic/mood stabilizers currently available in that it is more potent at dopamine D_3 receptors than at D_2 receptors. It is thought that effects on D_3 receptors may provide better antidepressant effects, but this proposition has not yet been tested. In September 2015, the FDA approved cariprazine to treat schizophrenia, and in 2017 cariprazine was approved for maintenance treatment of adults with schizophrenia. It is also approved for the treatment of bipolar mania and depression, and as an add-on treatment to antidepressants in unipolar depression.
   Cariprazine is *not* FDA indicated for any psychiatric condition in children and adolescents and currently has no pediatric Registry Trials under way. Thus, it is discussed in limited manner referencing dosing, efficacy, issues of safety, and tolerability data in adult studies thus far.

Cariprazine acts as a partial agonist at the dopamine D_3 and D_2 receptors with high binding affinity that is preferential for dopamine D_3 receptors. It also has high binding affinity partial agonist activity at the serotonin 5-HT_{1A} receptors. Cariprazine acts as an antagonist at 5-HT_{2B} and 5-HT_{2A} receptors with high and moderate binding affinity, respectively, and lower binding affinities for histamine H_1 receptors. Cariprazine has little or no affinity for adrenergic or cholinergic receptors.

The relative contribution of D_3 partial agonism is an area of ongoing scientific inquiry with no definite conclusions yet. Veselinovic et al. (2013) and Cutler et al. (2013) have contributed to the clinical understanding of the D_3 receptor by noting that D_3 is an autoreceptor that in animal studies (1) controls phasic, but not tonic, activity of dopamine nerve cells and (2) mediates behavioral abnormalities induced by glutamate and NMDA receptor antagonists. In these animal studies, D_3-preferring agents have been shown to exert pro-cognitive effects and improve anhedonic symptoms. Nemeth et al. (2017) conducted a European study utilizing cariprazine and risperidone in patients with schizophrenic aged 18 to 65 years suffering from predominantly negative symptoms for at least 6 months. The participants were randomly allocated to groups of 230 patients each for treatment either with cariprazine at a dose of 3 mg, 4.5 mg (target dose), or 6 mg/day or risperidone at a dose of 3 mg, 4 mg (target dose), or 6 mg/day. More patients in the cariprazine group had a response to treatment, defined as a decrease in the Positive and Negative Syndrome Scale factor score for negative symptoms (PANSS-FSNS) scores of 20% or more, by 26 weeks than in the risperidone group, with an NNT of 9. The fact that this study targeted patients specifically with negative symptoms is significant because they are often treatment resistant with medication therapies. The effect size of 0.31 indicates a modest improvement, but it was deemed clinically meaningful by patients. The study authors proposed that the results support the efficacy of cariprazine in the treatment of predominant negative symptoms of schizophrenia.

Cariprazine has a long half-life of 2 to 5 days in the prescribed dosing range, which allows once-a-day dosing. Because of the long half-life of cariprazine and its active metabolites, changes in dose will not be fully reflected in the plasma for several weeks. Prescribers should monitor patients for adverse reactions and treatment response for several weeks after starting cariprazine and after each dosage change.

Cariprazine is extensively metabolized by hepatic metabolism via CYP3A4 and, to a lesser extent, by CYP2D6 to two active metabolites: desmethyl-cariprazine (DCAR) and didesmethyl-cariprazine (DDCAR), both of which are equipotent to cariprazine. DCAR is further metabolized into DDCAR by CYP3A4 and CYP2D6. DDCAR is then metabolized by CYP3A4 to a hydroxylated metabolite. After multiple-dose administration, mean cariprazine and DCAR levels reach steady state in 1 to 2 weeks; DDCAR, in 4 to 8 weeks. The systemic exposure and serum levels of DDCAR are roughly threefold greater than cariprazine because of the longer elimination half-life of DDCAR.

As with all antipsychotics and other agents with an indication for a depressive disorder, there is a bolded boxed warning in the product label that antidepressants increase the risk of suicidal thoughts and behaviors in patients aged 24 years and younger. Clinicians are advised to monitor for clinical worsening and emergence of suicidal thoughts and behaviors.

Cariprazine is contraindicated in patients with a history of a hypersensitivity reaction to cariprazine. Reactions have ranged from rash, pruritus, urticaria, and events suggestive of angioedema (e.g., swollen tongue, lip swelling, face edema, pharyngeal edema, and swelling face). The safety and efficacy of cariprazine has *not* been established in pediatric patients.

Interactions of Cariprazine with Other Medications

Because the medication is metabolized primarily by CYP3A4, a 50% reduction in the cariprazine dosage is required in the presence of a CYP3A4 inhibitor such as ketoconazole. This would require dosing cariprazine every other day if taking the 1.5-mg daily dose. For patients initiating cariprazine therapy while already on a strong CYP3A4 inhibitor, patients should be administered 1.5 mg of cariprazine on day 1 and on day 3, with no dose administered on day 2. From day 4 onward, the dose should be administered at 1.5 mg daily, and then increased to a maximum dose of 3 mg daily. When the CYP3A4 inhibitor is withdrawn, cariprazine dosage may need to be increased. Because data are not available regarding concomitant use of cariprazine with a strong CYP3A4 inducer such as carbamazepine, this practice is not recommended.

Treatment discontinuation following discontinuation of cariprazine has clinical implications because the slow decline in plasma concentrations due to the long half-life of the active medication and its active metabolites may not be immediately reflected in patients' clinical symptoms; the plasma concentration of cariprazine and its active metabolites will decline by 50% in approximately 1 week.

Tolerability and Adverse Effects of Cariprazine

AEs may first appear several weeks after the initiation of cariprazine treatment, probably because plasma levels of cariprazine and its major metabolites accumulate over time.

Cariprazine generally was well tolerated in short-term trials for schizophrenia and Bipolar I (BP-I). The major tolerability issue in the short-term studies and open-label extensions for schizophrenia and BP-I was akathisia. In the BP-I extension, this side effect developed in 37% of patients and led to a 5% withdrawal rate, which would seem to indicate that it was usually mild in nature.

Patients with schizophrenia received open-label cariprazine for as long as 48 weeks. Treatment-emergent AEs reported in at least 10% of patients included akathisia (14.0%), insomnia (14.0%), and weight gain (11.8%). The mean change in laboratory values, blood pressure, pulse rate, and ECG parameters was clinically insignificant.

In short- and long-term studies for either indication, the effect of the medication on metabolic parameters appears to be small. In the long term, uncontrolled trials with cariprazine in schizophrenia, the mean changes from baseline in weight at 12, 24, and 48 weeks were 1.2, 1.7, and 2.5 kg, respectively. Cutler et al. (2013) and Durgam et al. (2014) conducted studies with active controls that revealed potentially significant weight gain (>7%) was greater for aripiprazole and risperidone than for cariprazine.

In the long-term, open-label schizophrenia and bipolar studies, 4% patients with normal hemoglobin A_{1c} baseline values developed elevated levels ($\geq$ 6.5%). In the 6-week schizophrenia trial and the 3-week bipolar mania trial of adult patients, the proportion of patients with shifts in fasting total cholesterol, LDL, HDL, and triglycerides were similar in patients treated with cariprazine and placebo. The effect on the prolactin level was minimal. There do not appear to be clinically meaningful changes in laboratory values, vital signs, or QT interval. More specifically with regard to its effect on QTc interval, at a dose three times the maximum recommended dose, cariprazine does not prolong the QTc interval to a clinically relevant extent.

Indications for Cariprazine in Child and Adolescent Psychiatry

Cariprazine is *not* FDA indicated for any psychiatric condition in children and adolescents.

Cariprazine Dose Forms Available. Capsules: 1.5, 3, 4.5, and 6 mg

Cariprazine Dosage Schedule for Schizophrenia in Adults. Cariprazine can be taken without regard to food.

Recommended dosage range is 1.5 to 6 mg/day. The starting dose of cariprazine is 1.5 mg.

The dosage can be increased to 3 mg on day 2. Depending on clinical response and tolerability, further dose adjustments can be made in 1.5-mg or 3-mg increments. Higher dosages (6 to 9 mg/day) used in the clinical trials showed early separation from placebo by the end of week 1 but carried a dosage-related risk of AEs, leading the FDA to recommend 6 mg/day as the maximum dosage in adults.

Cariprazine Dosage Schedule in Bipolar I, Manic, or Mixed Episodes in Adults. Recommended dosage range is 3 to 6 mg/day. The starting dose of cariprazine is 1.5 mg and should be increased to 3 mg on day 2. Depending on clinical response and tolerability, further dose adjustments can be made in 1.5-mg or 3-mg increments. Higher dosages (3 to 12 mg/day) used in the clinical trials evidenced significant improvement in the YMRS score by day 4 but carried a dosage-related risk of AEs, leading the FDA to recommend 6 mg/day as the maximum dosage.

Schizophrenia

U.S. Food and Drug Administration Registry Trials. The efficacy of cariprazine for the treatment of schizophrenia was established in three, 6-week, randomized, double-blind, placebo-controlled trials in patients (aged 18 to 60 years) who met (DSM-IV-TR) criteria for schizophrenia and had a PANSS score between 80 and 120 at screening and baseline. Two trials were fixed dosage; a third used two flexible dosage ranges. An active control arm (risperidone or aripiprazole) was included in the two fixed-dose trials to assess assay sensitivity. The primary efficacy measure was changed from baseline in the total score of the PANSS at the end of week 6, compared with placebo. In all three trials, cariprazine was superior to placebo.

Schizophrenia Maintenance

U.S. Food and Drug Administration Registry Trials. The efficacy of cariprazine for the maintenance treatment of adults with schizophrenia was established in a multinational, double-blind, placebo-controlled study in 200 adult patients with schizophrenia. Patients received 3, 6, or 9 mg/day of cariprazine or placebo for up to 72 weeks or until a relapse occurred. Results showed that cariprazine significantly delayed the time to relapse compared to placebo ($P = .0010$). A total of 49.5% ($N = 49/99$) of placebo-treated patients had a relapse versus 29.7% ($N = 30/101$) of the cariprazine-treated patients. The safety results were consistent with previous studies.

Bipolar I, Manic, or Mixed Episodes

Registry Trials. The efficacy of cariprazine in the acute treatment of bipolar I manic or mixed episodes was established in three, 3-week, placebo-controlled trials in patients (mean age of 39 years, range 18 to 65 years) who met DSM-IV-TR criteria for bipolar 1 disorder with manic or mixed episodes with or without psychotic features (YMRS score, ≥20). The primary efficacy measure in the three trials was a change from baseline in the total YMRS score at the end of week 3, compared with placebo. In all three trials, cariprazine was superior to placebo.

Pending Pediatric Clinical Trials

Schizophrenia

Reports of Interest. No pending pediatric clinical trials (clinical trials.gov)

Bipolar Disorder

Reports of Interest. No pending pediatric clinical trials (clinical trials.gov)

Iloperidone (Fanapt)

In May 2009, the FDA approved iloperidone for the acute treatment of schizophrenia in adults at a daily dose of 12 to 24 mg administered with or without food in bid manner initially because of its alpha-2 effects, which can cause hypotension and dizziness.

Pharmacodynamics of Iloperidone

Similar to most other atypical antipsychotics, iloperidone has high binding affinity and antagonism at serotonin 2A ($5\text{-}HT_{2A}$) and dopamine D_2/D_3 receptors; in addition, it evidences moderate affinity for dopamine D_4, serotonin $5\text{-}HT_7$, and noradrenalin alpha-1 receptors. Moderate binding affinity at $5\text{-}HT_6$, $5\text{-}HT_7$ receptors is believed to possibly enhance cognition, and $5\text{-}HT_7$ is being studied for a potential role in mood regulation and sensory processing. Iloperidone's low activity on histamine H_1 and muscarinic M_1 receptors suggests a low risk of H_1-mediated sedation and weight gain, and M_1-mediated memory/cognitive blunting, blurry vision, and urinary difficulties. Less predictable from its pharmacodynamic profile is that iloperidone has a more favorable EPS and akathisia profile than other $D_2/5\text{-}HT_{2A}$ antagonists and would be considered comparable to quetiapine in this regard. This in part may be due to the required titration to avoid orthostasis, and, if started at higher doses, the precipitation of mild EPSs could occur.

Pharmacokinetics of Iloperidone

Iloperidone is labeled for twice-a-day dosing not because of its half-life, which is 18 to 33 hours, but to minimize the potential for orthostatic hypotension during the titration phase because of its peripheral alpha-1 receptor antagonism. This early hypotensive effect seems to only last during the first few weeks of treatment, and thus the long half-life suggests that later conversion to once-a-day dosing is reasonable.

Metabolism and Elimination

Iloperidone is metabolized by the liver-specific enzyme pathways of CYP3A4 and CYP2D6. Therefore, the dosing of iloperidone should be adjusted for patients taking other medications known to inhibit CYP3A4 or CYP2D6 systems and, therefore, inhibit metabolism (e.g., increase plasma level) of iloperidone. Common scenarios among patients treated for schizophrenia would involve patients receiving adjunctive antidepressants that are CYP2D6 inhibitors such as fluoxetine, paroxetine, and venlafaxine, for which the dose of iloperidone would be reduced by 50%. CYP3A4 inhibitors such as ketoconazole or grapefruit juice would also necessitate such a reduction in iloperidone dosing. Iloperidone can be administered with or without food.

Iloperidone Dosage Schedule for Schizophrenia in Adults

The medication can be taken with or without food. The titration is as follows: day 1 = 1 mg bid; day 2 = 2 mg bid; day 3 = 4 mg bid; and day 4 = 4 mg bid. If after day 4 clinical judgment warrants an increase, titration should not exceed 2 mg twice daily (4 mg/day).

Iloperidone Dose Forms Available

Prepackaged titration packets can be utilized to carry out the first 4 days of bid dosing, which culminates in the patient achieving the lowest approved therapeutic dosage of 6 mg bid by day 4.

Tablets: 1, 2, 4, 6, 8, 10, and 12 mg. The tablets are not a long-acting formulation (Fanapt [package insert], 2017).

Tolerability and Adverse Effects of Iloperidone

In the first of the two large pivotal clinical trials conducted for FDA approval, a fairly rapid titration schedule was used to titrate iloperidone to a maximum dosage of 24 mg within 7 days, with ziprasidone used as an active control. The second trial utilized a more flexible dosing scheme, where one arm allowed dosing from 12 to 16 mg and the second arm studied dosing in the 20- to 24-mg range with risperidone used as an active control. As one might expect, the more rapid titration arms achieved modest initial greater treatment response, but at the cost of a greater side-effect burden. These trials and other large multinational trials (>570 per trial) showed that iloperidone generally had better efficacy than did placebo when using the PANSS or BPRS scores (Scott, 2009).

Of clinical importance is the observation that in the long-term flexible dose-maintenance study, the modal dose of iloperidone was 12 mg/day, suggesting that the lower end of the dose range may be therapeutic for many individuals stabilized on iloperidone. Also, in support of lower dosing is the finding that there seems to be a clinically significant dose effect with higher doses (20 to 24 mg) associated with more weight gain than did lower doses. Overall, clinical studies have also shown that iloperidone has a very favorable metabolic profile and an excellent extrapyramidal and akathisia profile in clinical trials comparable to placebo. Iloperidone is like quetiapine in that there seems to be no dose-related EPS or akathisia signal across their therapeutic dose ranges. This makes iloperidone an appealing treatment option for any patient at risk for antipsychotic-induced parkinsonism or akathisia.

In clinical studies in adults, tolerability was excellent and the rate of discontinuation from clinical trials because of adverse effects was 5.0% for iloperidone versus 5.0% for placebo. Dizziness, dry mouth, tachycardia, and orthostatic hypotension, all of which are related to early alpha-1 antagonism along with fatigue and somnolence, were the most commonly reported adverse reactions. Orthostatic hypotension and other side effects related to noradrenergic alpha-1 antagonism are more problematic with iloperidone than with most other antipsychotics. However, most of these side effects appear dose related and are transient, so they do not add to long-term burden once the initial dose-titration period is over. Although rare, priapism is related to alpha-1 antagonism and should be addressed for its potential occurrence.

Metabolic changes (hyperlipidemia, hyperglycemia) were quite favorable, and iloperidone is considered to have insignificant effects on serum lipids or glucose. Iloperidone is not likely to cause clinically significant prolactin elevation on the basis of study assessments. Although iloperidone is associated with modest weight gain, the mean change in weight from baseline across all short-term and long-term trials up to 52 weeks was 2.1 kg, which would be medically and psychologically acceptable for most patients. The extent of weight gain related to iloperidone in the pediatric population is yet to be determined.

The issue that is concerning to clinicians initially about iloperidone is its potential for QTc prolongation, which is cited in the PI in bold lettering. The PI states that in choosing among treatments, prescribers should consider the ability of Fanapt to prolong the QT interval and the use of other medications first. Iloperidone has some propensity similar to ziprasidone to prolong the QTc interval, which for some medications has been associated with a theoretic risk of arrhythmia such as torsade de pointes. The safety of iloperidone has been extensively studied in a safety study where maximal doses were used and metabolic inhibitors added. The mean QTc elevation at the maximal recommended dose of 12 mg twice a day was 9.6 ms; and when iloperidone was given as a single dose of 24 mg, the QTc elevation was 15.4 ms. When study patients were given 24 mg of iloperidone plus a full dose of a CYP2D6 inhibitor such as paroxetine 20 mg QD in combination with the CYP3A4 inhibitor ketoconazole 200 mg bid, the QTc elevation was 19 ms, which would likely be of limited clinical relevance. Thus far, the real issue of arrhythmia risk or sudden death has not been reported since iloperidone's release into the market, including overdose episodes. Similar to ziprasidone and paliperidone, the package insert for iloperidone suggests that clinicians consider the relatively greater QTc prolongation associated with these antipsychotics when considering iloperidone. In a related manner, iloperidone is contraindicated when the patient is already taking another medication with QTc elevation that meets "black box" labeling criteria such as thioridazine, pimozide, and droperidol.

It should be remembered that the recommended dose-titration schedule for iloperidone was developed for acutely ill, relapsing patients, where getting to therapeutic quickly was the priority to achieve FDA approval and that there is no known contraindication presently to the option of uptitrating at a slower rate to minimize the early onset risk of hypotension, dizziness, and tachycardia side effects. Indeed, in outpatient practice with less acute patients, this slower titration schedule seems to be common among clinicians. One should also consider the need for reinstituting the titration schedule if an individual has an interval off iloperidone of more than 3 days.

Pending Pediatric Clinical Trials (clinicaltrials.gov)

It is doubtful that the makers of iloperidone, Novartis Pharmaceuticals, will ever seek pediatric indications because the company has suspended its pediatric study "Tolerability and Pharmacokinetics of Iloperidone in Adolescent Patients." Such tolerability and PK studies are typically done before actual studies for specific conditions are initiated. Some pediatric clinicians will be enticed to consider iloperidone for its generally favorable tolerability profile, especially in the area of akathisia and other EPSs. Such a side-effect profile may be preferable in the treatment of youth with brain trauma who are often sensitive to the spectrum of EPS syndromes when antipsychotic medications are utilized. Owing to lack of pediatric studies, iloperidone should be used cautiously and not used without compelling reason in children because of the lack of clinical data and the QTc labeling precaution previously addressed.

The Use of Long-Acting Injectable Antipsychotics/Mood Stabilizers in Children and Adolescents

In adults, long-acting injectable forms of SGAs are approved for the treatment of schizophrenia, schizoaffective disorder, and BPD. However, no long-acting injectable antipsychotic/mood stabilizers (LAIs) are currently approved for use in youth despite evidence that many serious mental health disorders have their onset during childhood or adolescence (Driver et al., 2013; Kessler et al., 2007). Some experts (Chue & Emsley, 2007; Lachman, 2014; Stevens et al., 2014) have suggested that LAIs be used more frequently and earlier, particularly in nonadherent children and adolescents, because treatment adherence rates for first-episode psychosis are consistently reported to be <50%. Indeed, Hack and Chow (2001) found that, overall, children are at an even higher risk for nonadherence than are adults, with adolescents being a particularly vulnerable group. Poor insight is one of the main reasons of antipsychotic discontinuation and subsequent relapse in schizophrenia spectrum disorders (Parellada et al., 2012; Tiihonen et al., 2011) and may be more prevalent in younger youth (Parellada et al., 2011).

Although off-label, the appropriate use of long-acting injectable forms of second- and third-generation LAIs in this pediatric population is consistent with the American Academy of Child and Adolescent Psychiatry's recommendation that LAI use be considered in adolescents with schizophrenia with chronic symptoms and a history of nonadherence (McClellan et al., 2013). This recommendation is due to the strong evidence that early, comprehensive, and ongoing interventions to treat mental health disorders are important in optimizing outcomes, particularly in youth. Building evidence suggests that clinical, functional, and psychosocial decline often occurs within the first 5 years of the onset of psychosis and a longer duration of untreated illness can have a negative impact on outcome (Birchwood et al., 1998; Crumlish et al., 2009; Harris et al., 2005; Marshall et al., 2005; Perkins et al., 2005). Neurodegenerative structural changes in the brain that have been documented occur progressively during the course of schizophrenia and are thought to be associated with the duration of untreated psychosis (Emsley, Chiliza, & Asmal, 2013; Puri, 2010). Similarly, evidence suggests that the duration of medically untreated BPD is associated with poorer clinical outcomes (Medeiros et al., 2016).

LAI use may be useful in populations of youth with serious mental illness who are at risk for treatment nonadherence and relapse, but may also be useful early in treatment instead of a treatment of last resort analogous to how clozapine is underutilized in this population. Currently, there are no studies that address the issue of using LAIs for first-episode psychosis in children and adolescents. Clearly, larger controlled studies applying more rigorous study designs are needed to expand future research using LAIs in children and adolescents rather than simply extrapolating adult data to the pediatric population children, which is what we are currently forced to do.

What follows is a review of studies that are only open trials or case series/reports. However, owing to the small number of studies and their open-label nature, the findings must be interpreted cautiously. The studies cited have been restricted to those that utilized SGA LAI formulations available in 2017 in the United States.

Lytle et al. (2017) reviewed the literature from 1971 to 2015 pertaining to the use of LAIs in children and youth under the age of 18 if the studies were written in English. They identified seven reports including one open-label trial, three case reports, and three case series. No controlled trials were found. The relevant studies were published between 2007 and 2016, with only two published before 2012. Sample sizes ranged from 1 to 19 with a total of 36 individuals in all cases combined, which included those patients taking first-generation LAIs (and agents not approved in the United Sates). The age range was 11 to 17. Mean sample age was 12.1 in the open-label trial and calculated to be 14.9 in the remainder of the reports. Most patients (81%) were boys. Although the majority of reports did not comment on the race of the individuals, 19 were from Brazil, 13 were from the United States, 2 were from Spain, 1 was from Poland, and 1 was from Turkey.

Fifty percent of the primary diagnoses were BP-I, 19% were schizophrenia and 17% were bipolar spectrum disorders. The LAIs used were primarily risperidone long-acting injection (RLAI), followed by paliperidone palmitate long-acting injection (PPLAI), aripiprazole extended-release injectable, and one case with olanzapine extended release (OLAI). Most cases reported clinical improvement and the majority of individuals (82%) were reported to tolerate the medication well. The most common side effects were weight gain (mean 5.7 kg) in the RLAI open-label trial), tremor (5.6%), and oculogyric crisis (5.6%). One individual was noted to have drowsiness, difficulty focusing, and an oculogyric crisis; one individual experienced neuroleptic malignant syndrome (NMS); and one had elevated prolactin, hirsutism, and galactorrhea. Those cases that used only SGAs available in the United States are discussed in more detail here.

Boarati et al. (2013) conducted a 6-month open-label study in Brazil utilizing RLAI with 19 children and adolescents (mean age 12.1) who had a severe diagnosis of BP-I, BP-II, or BP NOS and previously used oral risperidone. Fifty-eight percent of the patients were noted to have adherence problems and 42% had failed previous oral medication trials. Five patients (26%) dropped out during the first 2 months and 14 (74%) completed the entire 6-month study. There was significant improvement in global functioning and symptom severity as measured by the Children's Global Assessment Scale 20.6 versus 42.9, $P < .0001$ and the CGI-S 5.9 versus 3.4, $P < .0001$), with improvements noted at 2 months and maintained over the remainder of the study. The most common side effects were weight gain (mean 5.7–4.1 kg) and increased appetite. Other reported side effects were high prolactin levels, mild transient tremors, and transient oculogyric crisis.

Pope and Zaara (2016) conducted a retrospective chart review on nine youth (mean age 15.4–1.0; range 14 to 17; 2 girls and 7 boys) who had been started on various LAIs during an inpatient hospitalization. All individuals were receiving an LAI for the first time that included risperidone ($N = 1$), fluphenazine ($N = 1$), paliperidone palmitate ($N = 6$), and aripiprazole ($N = 1$). Diagnoses included BP-I ($N = 1$), BP NOS ($N = 1$), schizophrenia ($N = 5$), schizoaffective disorder ($N = 1$), and mood disorder NOS ($N = 1$). Comorbid diagnoses included post-traumatic stress disorder, cannabis abuse, and ADHD. All but one patient had been on at least one other prior antipsychotic medication and had a history of nonadherence. All patients tolerated the LAIs well and showed clinical improvement with a mean decrease in CGI-S from 5.67 at admission to 2 at discharge. One patient developed EPSs that were treated with benztropine. No AEs led to discontinuation of LAI and all patients were discharged with plans to continue LAI at community mental health agencies.

Wisniewski (2012) reported on a case report from Poland of a 15-year-old male with a 2-year history of paranoid schizophrenia, frequent psychiatric hospitalizations, multiple failed trials of oral antipsychotic medications, a failed trial of RLAI, and medication nonadherence. This youth was started on OLAI 210 mg initially for 15 days and then increased to 300 mg every 2 weeks. After 2 months, he showed a reduction in positive and negative symptoms of schizophrenia as well as improved social functioning. He was reported to tolerate the medication well, with no adverse effects reported.

MANUFACTURER'S WARNING: Appropriate warning should be advised when using the olanzapine ER injection, because the usage is complicated by serious safety issues and the requirement that after receiving the injection patients must be observed for 3 hours by medical staff owing to an uncommon but serious post-injection delirium/sedation syndrome that may occur.

The PI indicates that during premarketing in ADULT clinical studies of ZYPREXA RELPREVV, AEs presented with signs and symptoms consistent with olanzapine overdose, in particular, sedation (including coma) and/or delirium, were reported in patients following an injection of ZYPREXA RELPREVV. **These events occurred in <0.1% of injections and in approximately 2% of patients who received injections for up to 46 months.** These events were correlated with an unintentional rapid increase in serum olanzapine concentrations to supratherapeutic ranges in some cases. Although a rapid and greater-than-expected increase in serum olanzapine concentration has been observed in some patients with these events, the exact mechanism by which the medication was unintentionally introduced into the blood stream is not known. Clinical signs and symptoms included dizziness, confusion, disorientation, slurred speech, altered gait, difficulty ambulating, weakness, agitation, EPSs, hypertension, convulsion, and reduced level of consciousness ranging from mild sedation to coma. Time after injection to event ranged from soon after injection to greater than 3 hours after injection. The majority of patients were hospitalized and some required supportive care, including intubation, in several cases. All patients had largely recovered by 72 hours. **The risk of an event is the same at each injection, so the risk per patient is cumulative.** It is mandatory that patients be enrolled in the ZYPREXA RELPREVV Patient Care Program to receive ZYPREXA RELPREVV treatment. Patients should be advised of the risk of post-injection delirium/sedation syndrome each time they receive an injection (see Warnings and Precautions). Patient and caregivers should be advised that after each ZYPREXA RELPREVV injection, patients must be observed at the health care facility for at least 3 hours and must be accompanied to their destination on leaving the facility. The Medication Guide should be distributed each time patients receive an injection.

Although olanzapine is an effective antipsychotic and mood stabilizer, it does have one of the greatest propensities for weight gain of all the agents in its class. Combined with the post-injection delirium/sedation syndrome SE of olanzapine ER injection, it seems likely this agent would be rarely used in patients under the age of 18.

One case series by Fu-I et al. (2009) reported on three youth, aged 11, 14, and 14, with BPD and a history of nonadherence. Each child was started on RLAI dosed at 25 mg every 2 weeks. All three children had improvement in their CGI over time with length of treatment 10, 36, and 24 weeks, respectively. The mean baseline CGI was 6.33 and mean follow-up CGI was 2.33, suggesting an overall greater than 50% improvement in clinical symptoms. The youth tolerated the medication well and no significant changes in cholesterol and prolactin levels were reported.

Another case report described a 16-year-old girl with new-onset mania with psychotic features, who was treated in an outpatient setting with RLAI 37.5 mg every 2 weeks (Patel et al., 2013). She had clinical improvement, but after the second dose of RLAI developed elevated prolactin levels, galactorrhea, and hirsutism, leading to RLAI discontinuation. Galactorrhea resolved after 1 week and hirsutism resolved after 1 month (Patel et al., 2013).

Fabrega et al. (2015) completed a small case series report from Spain on two adolescents treated with PPLAI. The first adolescent, age 14, was diagnosed with undifferentiated schizophrenia and hospitalized because of increasing negative symptoms and paranoia with concomitant total seclusion to his home for 2 years all the while refusing treatment. He was of low cognitive functioning when tested during his hospitalization. He was started on PPLAI initiated at 50 mg and later maintained at 50 mg every 28 days. He was discharged from the hospital after 17 days. One year later, he remained on medication, showed functional improvement, and had no adverse effects.

The other patient in this study was a 17-year-old boy with psychotic disorder NOS, multiple psychiatric admissions, multiple past medication trials, and treatment nonadherence. PPLAI 50 mg resulted in adverse side effects including oculogyric crisis that developed after 3 days (resolved with anticholinergic treatment), concentration difficulties, and somnolence leading to the patient declining further injections, although he was discharged from the hospital after 14 days. During a subsequent admission, he was started on zuclopenthixol decanoate 100 mg every 14 days. He subsequently reported a return in somnolence and difficulty concentrating, and was switched to the oral antipsychotic aripiprazole 15 mg/day. He again became nonadherent with subsequent paranoia and was restarted on the PPLAI in conjunction with an anticholinergic medication. No details were provided regarding the outcome of this last introduction of PPLAI.

Although these cases highlight the efficacy of LAIs, especially in cases where nonadherence issues cannot be overcome, they also evidence that fact that the clinician needs to be aware of the typical side effects associated with SGAs whether they are in oral formulations or in LAIs. Those side effects included the "usual offenders" of EPSs, increased appetite, weight gain, sedation, and endocrine side effects such as elevated prolactin and galactorrhea.

It is noteworthy that the newer SGA LAIs often have some clinical advantages over their predecessors in terms of smaller injection needle size and need for less frequent injections, for example, the case against the older RLAI (Risperdal Consta) requiring a larger needle size with an injection frequency of every 2 weeks versus the newer formulations of paliperidone palmitate (Invega Sustenna and Invega Trinza) utilizing a smaller needle size and less frequent injections of every 1 month and every 3 months, respectively. Adult trials that may allow every 6-month injection frequencies for some LAIs are under way.

The authors (Lytle et al., 2017) concluded that the literature review suggested that LAI use in youth with serious mental illness may improve clinical outcomes and adherence. Side effects of LAIs among youth are similar to those of oral preparations. However, there is a paucity of data regarding use of LAIs in youth for issues other than nonadherence to treatment. Also, the reports that currently do exist have substantial methodological limitations. Research is needed to better guide the use of LAIs in children and adolescents, especially as it pertains to possibly using LAIs early in the onset of schizophrenia or BPD or to replace oral medications that are lacking efficacy because the adult data on LAIs seems to indicate superiority in efficacy and reduced hospitalization versus oral preparations of the same agent.

The following tables summarize the second- and third-generation antipsychotic/mood stabilizer long-acting injectibles available in 2017. As stated, none of these agents are FDA approved for use in children and adolescents, so any use is off-label. This summary does not suffice as sufficient training for implementing treatment with LAIs. If treatment is initiated in the pediatric population, read the PI that describes the agent very carefully before implementation and consult with a colleague who has experience with the injectable selected. The PIs contain useful information on switching from oral antipsychotics and the management of a missed initiation or maintenance dose as well as early dosing. Coadministration of certain drugs may need to be avoided or dosage adjustments may be necessary; review drug interactions. In patients classified as CYP2D6 poor metabolizers are receiving a strong CYP3A4 inhibitor a reduction in dosing may be indicated. Once again consult the PI.

Second-Generation Antipsychotic Long-Acting Injectables

Drug	Dosage	Injection Interval	Instructions	Purpose/Side Effects	Administration Sites	Pediatric
ABILFY MAINTENA (Aripiprazole) *Requires 2-wk oral Abilify overlap*	300–400 mg	Once a month	Prefilled syringe shake for 20 s Inject, immediately store at room temperature	Schizophrenia and bipolar disorder: orthostatic hypotension tardive dyskinesia hyperglycemia	Deltoid Gluteus	Yes
ARISTADA (Aripiprazole) *Requires 3-wk overlap with oral Abilify*	441, 662, 882 mg	441–882 mg once a month. 882 mg can be given every 6 wk; 1,064 mg every 2 mo (Schizo)	Prefilled syringe tap 10× and shake 30 s Do not overtighten needle Inject in less than 10 s	Schizophrenia and bipolar disorder: orthostatic hypotension tardive dyskinesia hyperglycemia	Gluteus preferred Lower dosage can be deltoid but not preferred	No

ARIPIPRAZOLE INJECTABLE CONVERSION FROM ORAL DOSING: In conjunction with the first dose of Abilify Maintena, administer oral aripiprazole for 14 days as follows; in conjunction with the first dose of Aristada, administer current oral aripiprazole for 21 days as follows:

Abilify (PO)	Abilify Maintena (IM)	Aripiprazole lauroxil (Aristada) (IM) Dose (mg aripiprazole)	Aripiprazole lauroxil (Aristada) (IM)
10 mg/d	300 mg	441 mg (300 mg) Q monthly	Deltoid or Gluteal
15 mg/d	400 mg	662 mg (450 mg) Q monthly	Gluteal
20 mg/d	600 mg	882 mg Q 6 wk	Gluteal
15 mg/d	724 mg	1,064 mg Q 2 mo	Gluteal

Drug	Dosage	Injection Interval	Instructions	Purpose/Side Effects	Administration Sites	Pediatric
INVEGA SUSTENNA (Paliperidone) *Requires 7-d repeat after first dose. First dose is always 234, 156 mg in 7 d.*	39, 78, 117, 156, 234 mg	Once a month after initial dosing titration	Prefilled shake well	Schizophrenia and bipolar disorder: orthostatic hypotension tardive dyskinesia hyperglycemia	Deltoid Gluteus	Yes
INVEGA TRINZA (Paliperidone) Use in patients already stabilized with Sustenna at least 4 mo	273, 410, 546, 819 mg	Every 3 mo	Prefilled syringe Shake for 15 s	Schizophrenia and bipolar disorder: orthostatic hypotension tardive dyskinesia hyperglycemia	Gluteus	No

Doses for Adult Patients Adequately Treated with Invega Sustenna	
If the Last Dose of INVEGA SUSTENNA is:	**Initiate INVEGA TRINZA at the Following Dose:**
78 mg	273 mg
117 mg	410 mg
156 mg	546 mg
234 mg	819 mg

Invega 12 mg po = Invega Trinza 819 mg.
See PI for instructions on missed dosages or early dosing.
Risperidone (Risperdal) Consta is not listed as many disadvantages when compared to Paliperidone Sustenna including larger needle size and more frequent injections..

First-Generation Antipsychotics						
Drug	**Dosage**	**Injection Interval**	**Instructions**	**Purpose/Side Effects**	**Administration Sites**	**Pediatric**
Haldol Deconate	50–200 mg	Every 3–4 wk	Vials	Schizophrenia Tardive dyskinesia	Deltoid Gluteus	No
Fluphenazine Deconate	12.5–50 mg	2–3 wk	Vials	Schizophrenia	Deltoid Gluteus	No

Naltrexone Extended-Release Injectable in Opiate Addiction

Lastly in this section is a table summarizing the use of VIVITROL (naltrexone for extended-release injectable suspension) Intramuscular. Limited studies are available supporting its usage in older adolescents but given the current opiate addiction crisis that is effecting the youth of our country and the alarming mortality rate of opiates, especially when adulterated with various forms of fentanyl, it is likely its usage will continue to escalate in this population. See Chapter 11 for a detailed description of this issue.

The first-generation antipsychotic long-acting injectables are listed, but are not considered first-line injectable agents because of the following:

- Current understanding that they are more neurotoxic, especially haloperidol (Nassaralla et al., 2004)
- Inferior delivery systems resulting in less consistent dopamine/serotonin receptor blockade
- Much longer lead-in period of oral meds to achieve steady serum state before converting to injectable
- Require more frequent injections

Opioid Dependence						
Drug	**Dosage**	**Injection Interval**	**Instructions**	**Purpose/Side Effects**	**Administration Sites**	**Pediatric**
Vivitrol	380 mg	Every month	Vial preparation bring to room temperature shake well *Refrigerate*	**Must be opiate free 7–10 d** To block brain receptors for opioid dependence *Nausea, diarrhea, diaphoresis, muscle cramps, fever, goosebumps*	Gluteus	Yes 16 and over[a]

[a]It is sometimes prescribed to older adolescents on the basis of two research studies indicating its efficacy for this population (Woody et al., 2009; Marsch et al., 2005) even though it is not approved by the FDA for pediatric use.

CHAPTER 8

Antidepressant Medications

SUZIE C. NELSON AND MATTHEW J. BAKER

INTRODUCTION

With the advent of selective serotonin reuptake inhibitor (SSRI) antidepressants in the 1990s, prescribing practitioners could treat depression in children and adolescents with greater ease. Their significantly safer untoward-effects profile, in particular, the reduced risks of cardiotoxicity and lethality of overdose compared with the risks associated with tricyclic antidepressants (TCAs), changed the landscape of treating both depressive and anxiety disorders in youth. As a result, SSRIs are now the most frequently prescribed antidepressants for children and adolescents and continue to be prescribed with increasing frequency. SSRIs have also been approved for the treatment of other psychiatric disorders and are used off-label for several additional ones. Other mixed-mechanism antidepressants are also prescribed for children and adolescents for a variety of conditions, all of them with relatively safer overall characteristics than previous generations of available medications. The growing evidence base in treating childhood psychiatric conditions indicates that treatment strategies using both reasonable medication management and psychotherapy in combination is superior to either treatment modality alone. A number of large multicenter studies have contributed to these practice guidelines today.

MAJOR LANDMARK STUDIES FOR TREATMENT OF DEPRESSIVE DISORDERS

Much of what guides practice using this class of medication in children and adolescents comes from large multicenter trials examining the effects of both medication management and psychotherapy. Studies for depressive disorders include Treatment for Adolescents with Depression Study (TADS), Adolescent Depression and Psychotherapy Trial (ADAPT), and Treatment of SSRI-Resistant Depression in Adolescents (TORDIA). A summary of the characteristics of these studies is presented in Table 8.1.

Treatment for Adolescents with Depression Study

The TADS Team (2004) conducted a randomized controlled trial (RCT) in 439 patients at 13 sites (age range 12 to 17 years) with a primary diagnosis of major depressive disorder (MDD) by *Diagnostic and Statistical Manual of Mental Disorders*, Fourth

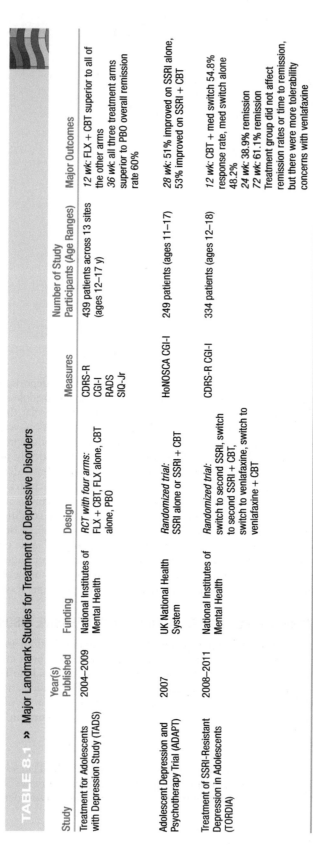

TABLE 8.1 » Major Landmark Studies for Treatment of Depressive Disorders

Study	Year(s) Published	Funding	Design	Measures	Number of Study Participants (Age Ranges)	Major Outcomes
Treatment for Adolescents with Depression Study (TADS)	2004–2009	National Institutes of Mental Health	*RCT with four arms:* FLX + CBT, FLX alone, CBT alone, PBO	CDRS-R CGI-I RADS SIQ-Jr	439 patients across 13 sites (ages 12–17 y)	*12 wk:* FLX + CBT superior to all of the other arms *36 wk:* all three treatment arms superior to PBO overall remission rate 60%
Adolescent Depression and Psychotherapy Trial (ADAPT)	2007	UK National Health System	*Randomized trial:* SSRI alone or SSRI + CBT	HoNOSCA CGI-I	249 patients (ages 11–17)	*28 wk:* 51% improved on SSRI alone, 53% improved on SSRI + CBT
Treatment of SSRI-Resistant Depression in Adolescents (TORDIA)	2008–2011	National Institutes of Mental Health	*Randomized trial:* switch to second SSRI, switch to second SSRI + CBT, switch to venlafaxine, switch to venlafaxine + CBT	CDRS-R CGI-I	334 patients (ages 12–18)	*12 wk:* CBT + med switch 54.8% response rate, med switch alone 48.2% *24 wk:* 38.9% remission *72 wk:* 61.1% remission Treatment group did not affect remission rates or time to remission, but there were more tolerability concerns with venlafaxine

CBT, cognitive-behavior therapy; CDRS-R, Children's Depression Rating Scale–Revised; CGI-I, Clinical Global Impressions–Improvement; FLX, fluoxetine; PBO, placebo; RADS, Reynolds Adolescent Depression Scale; RCT, randomized controlled trial; SIQ-Jr, Suicidal Ideation Questionnaire–Junior High School Version; SSRI, selective serotonin reuptake inhibitor.

Edition (DSM-IV) criteria (American Psychiatric Association [APA], 1994), which compared the efficacy of fluoxetine (10 to 40 mg/day) versus CBT versus fluoxetine (10 to 40 mg/day) plus CBT versus placebo (equivalent to 10 to 40 mg/day) over a 12-week period. Medication in the fluoxetine and placebo group was administered in a double-blind manner; fluoxetine was administered openly in the fluoxetine-plus-CBT group because CBT was administered unblinded.

Major outcome measures were the Children's Depression Rating Scale–Revised (CDRS-R) and the Clinical Global Impressions–Improvement (CGI-I) score. The Reynolds Adolescent Depression Scale total score and the Suicidal Ideation Questionnaire–Junior High School Version (SIQ-Jr) total score were used as secondary outcome measures. CBT was composed of a possible 15 skills-orientated 50- to 60-minute sessions on the basis of the premise that depression is "caused by or maintained by depressive thought patterns and a lack of active, positively reinforced behavioral patterns." The mean number of sessions completed was 11 in both groups with CBT. The mean fluoxetine dose in the fluoxetine-only group was 28.4 ± 8.6 mg/day and in the fluoxetine-plus-CBT group was 33.3 ± 10.8 mg/day; the mean placebo dose was 34.1 ± 9.5 mg/day.

On the basis of the improvement on the CDRS-R, combined treatment with fluoxetine and CBT was superior ($P = .001$) to treatment with placebo, but treatment with fluoxetine alone ($P = .10$) and CBT alone ($P = .40$) were not. Fluoxetine with CBT was superior to fluoxetine alone ($P = .02$) and to CBT alone ($P = .001$). Fluoxetine alone was also superior to placebo ($P = .01$). On the CGI-I Scale, rates of positive response (a rating of 1 [very much improved] or 2 [much improved]) were fluoxetine plus CBT, 71%; fluoxetine only, 60.6%; CBT only, 43.2%; and placebo 34.8%.

After patients at high risk for suicide were eliminated from the study because of exclusion criteria, 29% of the subjects had scores of >31, a level of suicidal thinking that requires prompt clinical attention on the SIQ-Jr at baseline; this decreased to 10.3% at 12 weeks and there was clinically significant improvement in suicidal thinking in all four groups. During the 12-week trial, 24 (5.5%) of the patients reported a suicide-related adverse event (AE; worsening suicidal ideation or a suicide attempt) and 7 (1.6%) of patients attempted suicide, but none was successful. Improvement in suicidality was greatest for the fluoxetine-plus-CBT group and least for the fluoxetine-only group. The authors concluded that fluoxetine is effective in the treatment of MDD and that the addition of CBT increases both clinical improvement and protection from suicidality (TADS, 2004).

The TADS participants have been followed up in a maintenance phase component from weeks 18 through 36 (Stage III) and also in a naturalistic 1-year follow-up study after the end of 36 weeks of active treatment (Stage IV) (Kennard et al., 2009; March et al., 2009). In both of these studies, the remission rates were examined. Remission is defined as a return to a symptom-free state or a near-symptom-free status. By 36 weeks, the estimated remission rates were as follows: combined treatment, 60%; fluoxetine alone, 55%; CBT alone, 64%; and overall remission rate, 60% (Kennard et al., 2009). This is a significant improvement from previous reports of the TADS group remission rates of 23% after 12 weeks (Kennard et al., 2006). In the naturalistic study, TADS treatments were stopped at 36 weeks and participants received continued treatment in the community. They were assessed by the TADS researchers at 3, 6, 9, and 12 months after completion of the initial 36-week TADS. Sixty-six percent of the original study group participated in at least one assessment and the benefits of active treatment continued during the naturalistic study period (March et al., 2009). These TADS follow-ups suggest that the majority of adolescents with depression achieve remission and that their remission can be continued with long-term treatment (Kennard et al., 2009).

Adolescent Depression and Psychotherapy Trial

The ADAPT study examined the effect of adding CBT to treatment with an SSRI (primarily fluoxetine). This study was funded by the UK National Health System and was conducted in community clinic settings. In contrast to the TADS, the authors included participants with active suicidal intent, self-harm, depressive psychosis, and/or conduct disorder. Subjects were aged 11 to 17 and had moderate to severe levels of depression.

In the ADAPT study, 510 youth were screened for participation and of those 249 were eligible for the study. All participants were offered a brief initial intervention consisting of two sessions before they were referred to the study. Some participants declined to participate in the initial intervention and were enrolled in the study. Of those who participated in the intervention, 34 of 164 improved. Youth who did not respond to the brief intervention were randomized to SSRI alone (103) or SSRI plus CBT (105). The primary SSRI used in the study was fluoxetine, which was dosed at 10 mg daily for a week and then increased to 20 mg for 5 weeks. If no response was seen by 6 weeks, the dose was increased to 40 mg; and if no response was noted by 12 weeks, then the dose was increased to 60 mg. Participants who could not tolerate fluoxetine or in whom it was ineffective were given a different SSRI. Youth were followed for 28 weeks, and response was assessed at 12 and 28 weeks. Depressive symptoms decreased, but no differences were detected between the two treatment arms. At the end of the 28-week study, 51% of those in the SSRI-alone group and 53% of those in the CBT-plus-SSRI group were much or very much improved (Goodyer et al., 2007).

Treatment of SSRI-Resistant Depression in Adolescents

The TORDIA trial was funded by the National Institute of Mental Health to provide empirical evidence to guide clinical practice when initial treatment for depression is unsuccessful. Participants aged 12 to 18 were recruited, who had not responded to an initial course of SSRI treatment. They were randomized into one of four treatments: (a) switch to a second, different SSRI (fluvoxamine, citalopram, or paroxetine); (b) switch to a different SSRI plus CBT; (c) switch to venlafaxine (150 to 225 mg); or (d) switch to venlafaxine + CBT. At the completion of 12 weeks of treatment, the groups who received CBT + medication had a response rate of 54.8%. The groups with a medication switch alone had a response rate of 48.2%. There was no difference in response rates between the study medications fluoxetine, citalopram, paroxetine, or venlafaxine (Brent et al., 2008). In a continuation study, the TORDIA study participants were continued in their treatment arm if they had responded, and nonresponders received open treatment which could consist of a switch to another antidepressant, augmentation, or addition of CBT or other psychotherapy. Of the individuals enrolled in the original study, 78.1% were followed up for another 24 weeks. They found that treatment type did not have any statistical differences and that all groups had similar remission rates. At 24 weeks, 38.9% had achieved remission. Of those who had remitted, it was more likely to occur in subjects who had a clinical response by week 12 (61.6% vs. 18.3%). Factors which predicted remission were lower rates of depression, hopelessness, anxiety, suicidal ideation, family conflict, and absence of comorbid dysthymia. The relapse rate among subjects who had initially responded by week 12 was 19.6% by week 24 (Emslie et al., 2010). The study ended at 24 weeks, and subjects were discharged to community care and naturalistically assessed at weeks 48 and 72. By week 72, 61.1% of the youth in the study had reached remission. Treatment group did not influence remission rate or time to remission. The study did find that the group assigned to SSRIs had a more rapid decline in self-reported depressive symptoms and suicidal ideation than the group assigned to venlafaxine. The venlafaxine group had a greater increase in diastolic blood pressure and pulse and had a more frequent occurrence of skin problems when compared with SSRI treatment. The authors conclude that because venlafaxine had response rates similar to that of SSRIs and more significant side effects such that a second SSRI should be selected over venlafaxine as a second-line antidepressant (Vitiello et al., 2011).

These three large studies build on earlier research on the use of fluoxetine and SSRIs in depressed youth and have advanced knowledge to guide treatment selections in depressed youth. TADS, ADAPT, and TORDIA compare the effectiveness of different treatment methods instead of comparing a treatment against placebo. Taken together, they can give physicians confidence in the continued use of medications and therapy to treat depression in adolescents.

Since the time of these larger studies, other large multicenter studies comparing medications of different classes, in addition to meta-analyses and systematic reviews, have also contributed to our understanding of how best to treat depression in youth.

Meta-analyses, Systematic Reviews, and Other Studies

Cipriani et al. (2016) assessed comparative efficacy and tolerability of antidepressants for MDD in children and adolescents with a network meta-analysis of 34 trials, including 5,260 participants and 14 different antidepressant treatments. Only fluoxetine showed statistical significance in efficacy over placebo, with a moderate effect size and was better tolerated as well. They observed relatively more discontinuations with duloxetine, imipramine, and venlafaxine because of AEs than with placebo.

Ma et al. (2014) conducted a multiple treatments meta-analysis of 21 RCTs to examine the efficacy, acceptability, and safety of CBT and medication treatments for MDD in pediatric patients. Combined fluoxetine/CBT exhibited the highest efficacy, and mirtazapine was also one of the most efficacious treatments. Fluoxetine alone was superior to CBT, other SSRIs, and placebo. Paroxetine, sertraline, escitalopram, and venlafaxine demonstrated greater acceptability than did fluoxetine and combination fluoxetine/CBT. CBT was safer than fluoxetine alone, although combination fluoxetine/CBT was less safe. Sertraline, escitalopram, venlafaxine, and paroxetine were the best tolerated, and mirtazapine and venlafaxine were the safest. The authors concluded that mirtazapine and sertraline exhibited optimally balanced safety, efficacy, and acceptability for first-line acute treatment of pediatric MDD.

Dolle et al. (2013) completed a systematic literature review, identifying more than 450 studies treating depressive disorders in children and adolescents. Although the authors felt that CBT (Cohen's d: 0.5 to 2) and interpersonal therapy (d: 0.5 to 0.6) were the recommended first choice of treatment, fluoxetine (d: 0.3 to 5.6) was also recommended, either alone or in combination with CBT.

Hetrick et al. (2012) evaluated 19 trials of newer antidepressants compared with placebo and found that overall those treated with antidepressants had lower depression severity scores and higher rates of response and remission than those treated with placebo. The effect size was deemed to be small, with a depressive symptoms reduction of 3.51 on a scale of 17 to 113. There was an increased risk of AEs and suicide-related outcome (58%, RR = 1.18) for those on antidepressants versus placebo. The authors indicated that fluoxetine might be the first-choice medication on the basis of guideline recommendations, but that the increased risk of suicide-related outcomes must be considered.

MAJOR LANDMARK STUDIES FOR TREATMENT OF ANXIETY DISORDERS AND OBSESSIVE-COMPULSIVE DISORDERS

Alongside the major studies of medications for the treatment of depression in youth, there have also been landmark studies for uses of these medications, compared to psychotherapy and alongside psychotherapy, to treat anxiety disorders and obsessive-compulsive disorder (OCD). These are summarized in Table 8.2.

TABLE 8.2 » Major Landmark Studies for Treatment of Anxiety Disorders and Obsessive-Compulsive Disease

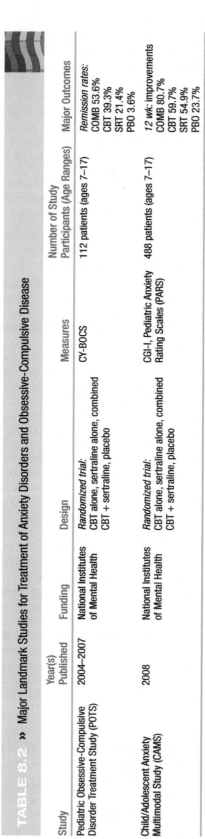

Study	Year(s) Published	Funding	Design	Measures	Number of Study Participants (Age Ranges)	Major Outcomes
Pediatric Obsessive-Compulsive Disorder Treatment Study (POTS)	2004–2007	National Institutes of Mental Health	*Randomized trial:* CBT alone, sertraline alone, combined CBT + sertraline, placebo	CY-BOCS	112 patients (ages 7–17)	*Remission rates:* COMB 53.6% CBT 39.3% SRT 21.4% PBO 3.6%
Child/Adolescent Anxiety Multimodal Study (CAMS)	2008	National Institutes of Mental Health	*Randomized trial:* CBT alone, sertraline alone, combined CBT + sertraline, placebo	CGI-I, Pediatric Anxiety Rating Scales (PARS)	488 patients (ages 7–17)	*12 wk:* improvements COMB 80.7% CBT 59.7% SRT 54.9% PBO 23.7%

CBT, cognitive-behavior therapy; CGI-I, Clinical Global Impressions–Improvement; COMB, combination of both; PBO, placebo; SRT, sertraline.

Pediatric Obsessive-Compulsive Disorder Treatment Study

The Pediatric Obsessive-Compulsive Disorder Treatment Study (POTS) was a large multisite RCT that examined the effect of CBT for OCD, sertraline, and combined treatment on improving OCD symptoms (March et al., 2004). In this study, 112 participants aged 7 to 17 were enrolled and randomly assigned to receive one of four treatment arms: (a) CBT alone, (b) medical management with sertraline, (c) combined treatment consisting of CBT and sertraline, or (d) a control condition pill placebo. In the medication groups, subjects were seen weekly and sertraline doses were started at 25 mg and adjusted upward up to 200 mg over 6 weeks. Subjects were followed up for 12 weeks. The clinical remission rate for combined treatment was 53.6%; for CBT alone, 39.3%; for sertraline alone, 21.4%; and for placebo, 3.6%. The authors conclude that children and adolescents with OCD should begin treatment with a combination of CBT and SSRI or CBT alone rather than be treated with SSRI alone initially.

In further analysis of data from the POTS, March and colleagues (2007a) examined the effects a comorbid tic disorder has on treatment outcome. In the POTS, 15% of the subjects (17 of 112) had comorbid tic disorder. In patients with a comorbid tic disorder, sertraline did not differ from placebo. Combined (sertraline + CBT) treatment remained superior and CBT alone remained superior to placebo. This study suggests that tic disorders appear to adversely affect the outcome of medication management in pediatric OCD. This suggests that youth with OCD and comorbid tics should not be treated with sertraline alone and should be offered CBT alone or in combination with sertraline as their initial treatment.

Child/Adolescent Anxiety Multimodal Study

Walkup et al. (2008) examined the use of sertraline and CBT as a treatment for children with anxiety disorders in the Child/Adolescent Anxiety Multimodal Study (CAMS). The CAMS was designed in two phases. The first phase was a 12-week trial of short-term treatment comparing CBT, sertraline, CBT + sertraline, and placebo. The second phase was a 6-month open trial of responders in the first phase. In this phase, 488 youth (mean age 10.7 ± 2.8 years) were randomized to the four treatment arms. The CBT intervention involved fourteen 60-minute sessions. The sertraline groups involved eight psychopharmacotherapy sessions and treatment with Zoloft or placebo administered on a fixed-flexible dosing schedule beginning with 25 mg/day adjusting up to 200 mg by week 8 if subjects were considered to be mildly ill or worse. Subjects receiving combination treatment received both interventions usually on the same day. Diagnosis was made using the Anxiety Disorders Interview Schedule for DSM-IV-TR, child version. Subjects who met criteria for separation, social, and/or generalized anxiety disorder (GAD) were included in the study. Improvement was assessed by treatment response on the CGI-I Scale as well as anxiety severity measures on the Pediatric Anxiety Rating Scale (PARS).

At the end of phase 1, children rated as very much or much improved on the CGI-I Scale were 80.7% for the combination therapy ($P < .001$), 59.7% for CBT ($P < .001$), and 54.9% for sertraline ($P < .001$). All three treatment arms were superior to placebo, with only 23.7% improved. Combination therapy was statistically superior to both the CBT and sertraline monotherapies. AEs included suicidal and homicidal ideation and were no more frequent in the sertraline group than in the placebo group. None of the study subjects attempted suicide. The side effects of insomnia, fatigue, restlessness, and sedation were seen more in the sertraline group than in the CBT subjects. The CAMS study has findings which have been seen in similar studies of different disorders and treatments which show that the combination of CBT and an SSRI is the most effective treatment selection for youth with internalizing (anxiety and depressive) disorders.

An analysis of remission rates seen in the CAMS trial was reported by Ginsburg et al. (2011). Remission was defined as a loss of all study-entry anxiety disorder diagnoses or by CGI-S or CGI-I measurements and varied with the loss of diagnosis having the highest remission, and the CGI-I scores have the lowest rates. They found that the combined group had the highest remission rates ranging from 46% to 68%. The sertraline group had remission rates of 34% to 46%. The CBT group had remission rates of 20% to 46%. The placebo group had remission rates of 15% to 27%. This showed that for most children in the study, some symptoms of anxiety persisted and may need additional treatment.

Piacentini et al. (2014) reported on differences between active treatment groups for response and remission rates and changes in severity of anxiety for the CAMS at weeks 24 and 36 follow-up. Acute responders maintained positive response at both time points, with combined medication and CBT treatment continuing to show superiority on some measures over monotherapy with CBT or SRT, which did not differ in efficacy. There appeared to be some convergence in efficacy between combination treatment and monotherapy during follow-up, which the authors assumed was due to greater use of concomitant treatments, such as medication and psychosocial interventions, during follow-up by the youth that had received monotherapy. The study demonstrated sustained treatment benefit from CAMS treatments.

Rynn et al. (2015) evaluated the frequency of AEs in the CAMS, comparing the frequency of AEs between children and adolescents across four treatment conditions. Subjects ages 7 to 17 years meeting DSM-IV criteria for separation anxiety disorder (SAD), GAD, or social phobia (SP) were randomized to placebo, sertraline, CBT, or both. AEs were collected by standardized inquiry and a questionnaire. No differences were found for physical and psychiatric AEs between sertraline versus placebo, although there were more total physical AEs with the sertraline-alone group than with the CBT and combination groups. All groups had higher psychiatric AEs in children ≤12 years.

Meta-analyses, Systematic Reviews, and Other Studies

Skapinakis et al. (2016) evaluated 86 RCTs in a systematic review of the clinical effectiveness, acceptability, and cost-effectiveness of pharmacologic and psychological interventions for the treatment of OCD in children, adolescents, and adults. In children and adolescents, clomipramine and all SSRIs had greater effects than did placebo, with none demonstrating relative superiority. Psychological therapies also demonstrated superiority over drug placebo. The authors also found that CBT with or without an SSRI was more likely to be cost-effective.

Skapinakis et al. (2016) systematically reviewed the clinical effectiveness and cost-effectiveness of pharmacologic and psychological interventions for the management of OCD in children, adolescents, and adults. Eighty-six RCTs were reviewed for effectiveness and 71 for acceptability. In children and adolescents, CBT and behavior therapy had greater effects than drug placebo, but did not significantly outperform psychological placebo. Fluoxetine and sertraline showed marginal statistical significance over placebo. CBT or BT combined with an SSRI was most cost-effective.

McGuire and colleagues (2015) completed a meta-analysis of CBT and serotonin reuptake inhibitors (SRIs) for child OCD, evaluating 20 RCTs. Large treatment effects were found for CBT efficacy (Hedges' $g = 1.21$), treatment response (RR = 2.72), and symptom/diagnostic remission (RR = 3.42). The number needed to treat (NNT) = 3 for treatment response and symptom/diagnostic remission for CBT. Findings across SRI trials found a moderate-to-large treatment effect for efficacy ($g = 0.50$), and a moderate effect for treatment response (RR = 1.80), and remission (RR = 2.06). NNT = 5 for treatment response and symptom/diagnostic remission with SRIs.

In a novel study to compare antidepressants of two different classes to each other and also placebo, da Costa and colleagues (2013) enrolled 30 subjects, aged 7 to 17 years, with GAD and/or SAD and/or SP in a 12-week double-blind, randomized, placebo-controlled trial of clomipramine ($N = 9$) and fluoxetine ($N = 10$). All groups showed significant improvement, and although clomipramine showed efficacy similar to that of fluoxetine, neither medication group was superior to placebo on measures of anxiety symptoms or impairment. Fluoxetine showed significant differences in some ratings of anxiety severity on the Multidimensional Anxiety Scale for Children and measures of impairment on the Children's Global Assessment Scale (CGAS) versus placebo. Overall, this study demonstrated a high placebo response rate of 77.7% and was limited by small restricted sample size, indicating larger studies of similar intervention comparison are needed.

Gorenstein et al. (2015) investigated the impact of child-focused pediatric OCD treatment on parental and family factors. Forty-three parents were evaluated after their children were randomized into group CBT or fluoxetine for 14 weeks. Findings were decreased family accommodation levels, increased cohesion, and active-recreational components of the family environment. The authors concluded that child-focused OCD treatment may positively impact family accommodation and family environment.

Gentile (2014) completed a systematic assessment of antidepressant medications in children and adolescents with non-OCD anxiety disorders. The author concluded that SP was the only condition that had been investigated by an adequate number of studies, and that venlafaxine and fluoxetine, and secondarily, fluvoxamine, are the only antidepressants that have shown convincing efficacy. The author also found that no evidence-based information definitively supports the use of antidepressants for other pediatric anxiety disorders.

SUICIDAL RISK AND ANTIDEPRESSANTS: THE BLACK BOX WARNING

Another significant event affecting the clinical use of antidepressants in the modern era has been the U.S. Food and Drug Administration (FDA) "black box" warning, which is shown on the next page. Since the FDA issued this warning for increased suicidal risk during treatment in young patients for all antidepressants in October 2004, there has been debate about the warnings and how they have affected the use of antidepressants in this population group. Several authors have examined SSRI prescription rates in many countries before and after the warnings were issued. The warnings were initially concerning paroxetine but were quickly followed by the broader warnings that continue today. Olfson and colleagues (2008) examined antidepressant prescription rates among psychiatrists, primary care physicians, and other physicians during three periods, namely, prewarning, paroxetine warning, and after the black box warnings. Youth antidepressant use during the prewarning study period increased by 36% per year ($P < .001$), which was followed by a decrease of -0.8% and -9.6% per year during the paroxetine and black box warning study periods, respectively. They noted that youth paroxetine use increased during the prewarning study period (30% per year; $P < .001$) before decreasing during the paroxetine warning study period (-44.2% per year; $P < .001$). They did not find similar changes in antidepressant use in older age groups. They found that all groups of physicians increased their use of SSRIs in youth during the prewarning period. They found that use of paroxetine decreased first by psychiatrists during the prewarning period (-23.0% per year; $P = .06$), whereas that of primary care physicians increased (+21.2% per year; $P = 1.0$). During the paroxetine warning period, use of paroxetine decreased by -49.4% per year ($P < .001$) among psychiatrists, -38.1% per year among primary care physicians, and -32.2% per year among other physicians. Kurian and colleagues (2007) found that during the 2 years before the first UK warnings in 2003, there was no change in monthly SSRI users aged 2 to 17 years with 23 new users per 10,000 persons per month. This proportion decreased by 33% in the 21 months following the UK warnings ($P < .001$). The decrease was most pronounced for antidepressants other than fluoxetine, which dropped by 54%, whereas new users of fluoxetine increased by 60%. These data suggest that warnings about the relative safety of fluoxetine in comparison with other SSRIs were heeded by practitioners. Clarke and colleagues (2012) analyzed prescription rates for antidepressants in youth at a large health maintenance organization, from 2000 through 2009. They found that the rates of antidepressant prescriptions to youth ages 10 to 17 continued to decline through 2009 as had been noted by other authors. They also found that rates of prescription refills decreased, which suggests that prescribers wanted to encourage return visits to monitor for improvement and adverse effects after the warnings were issued, which mandated close follow-up.

FDA "Black Box" Warning: Suicidality in Children and Adolescents

Note: In October 2004, the FDA directed manufacturers of antidepressant medications to add the following black box warning to their labeling: "Warning: Suicidality in Children and Adolescents—Antidepressants increased the risk of suicidal thinking and behavior (suicidality) in short-term studies in children and adolescents with major depressive disorder (MDD) and other psychiatric disorders. Anyone considering the use of (medication name) or any other antidepressant in a child or adolescent must balance this risk with the clinical needs. Patients who have started on therapy should be observed closely for clinical worsening, suicidality, or unusual changes in behavior. Families and caregivers should be advised of the need for close observation and communication with the prescriber. (Medication name) is not approved for use in pediatric patients except for patients with (Any approved pediatric claims here). (See Warnings and Precautions: Pediatric Use.)

Pooled analyses of short-term (4 to 16 weeks) placebo-controlled trials of nine antidepressants (SSRIs and others) in children and adolescents with MDD, OCD, or other psychiatric disorders (a total of 24 trials involving more than 4,400 patients) have revealed a greater risk of adverse events representing suicidal thinking or behavior (suicidality) during the first few months of treatment in those receiving antidepressants. The average risk of such events on the antidepressant was 4%, twice the placebo risk of 2%. No suicides occurred in these trials."

Furthermore, in the labeling under "Warnings," the following is indicated: "All pediatric patients being treated with antidepressants for any indication should be observed closely for clinical worsening, suicidality, and unusual changes in behavior, especially during the initial few months of a course of drug therapy, or at times of dose changes, either increases or decreases. Ideally, such observation would include at least weekly face-to-face contact with patients or their family members or caregivers during the first 4 weeks of treatment, then biweekly visits for the next 4 weeks, then at 12 weeks, and as clinically indicated beyond 12 weeks. Additional contact by telephone may be appropriate between face-to-face visits.

Adults with MDD or comorbid depression in the setting of other psychiatric illness taking antidepressants should also be observed for clinical worsening and suicidality, especially during the first few months of treatment, or at times of dose increases or decreases."

A number of international studies indicated that SSRI prescription rates declined significantly in children and adolescents while remaining either unchanged or increasing for adult populations (Dean et al., 2007; Kurdyak et al., 2007; Volkers et al., 2007). These decreases in prescription rates of SSRIs have alarmed some, who fear that depressed and anxious children would not receive treatment for their disorders.

The black box warnings have also affected research studies. The warnings were issued while the TORDIA multisite trial was recruiting subjects. Wagner et al. (2012)

describe the difficulties continuing the trial after the warnings. As a result of the paroxetine warnings, no further subjects were randomized to receive paroxetine and a citalopram arm replaced it. When additional warnings and the black box warnings were released, additional informed consents with the new warnings were required. Recruitment to the study was adversely affected following the warnings. Gibbons and colleagues (2007) analyzed dropping SSRI prescription rates in children and adolescents and compared them with youth suicide rates. U.S. and Dutch prescription rates for SSRIs were compared from 2003 to 2005, the years before and after the warnings. Suicide rates from the United States through 2004 and in the Netherlands through 2005 were compared. It was found that SSRI prescriptions for youth decreased by 22% in both the United States and the Netherlands after the warnings were issued. In the Netherlands, the youth suicide rate increased by 49% between 2003 and 2005. In the United States, the rates increased by 14% between 2003 and 2004. This was the largest year-to-year change in the suicide rate for this population ever seen since the Centers for Disease Control started collecting data.

Simon et al. (2006) provided an excellent and succinct review of the events leading up to the FDA's issuing a warning about increased suicidal risk in children and adolescents being treated with newer antidepressants. The authors identified 65,103 patients with 82,285 episodes of antidepressant treatment over a period of 12½ years ending June 30, 2003. An "episode" was defined as an outpatient antidepressant prescription filled (the index prescription) during the study period with no prior antidepressant prescription filled in the preceding 180 days and an International Classification of Diseases-Ninth Revision diagnosis of unipolar MDD, dysthymia, or depressive disorder not otherwise specified made during a treatment visit 30 days before or after the index prescription. Data were obtained from four computerized record systems, outpatient visit registration records, hospital discharge data, and mortality records (Simon et al., 2006). A total of 11,436 patients had two or more treatment episodes and 5,107 (6.2%) of the episodes occurred in patients <17 years. Females comprised 69.5% of the sample.

The authors evaluated the risks of death by suicide and serious suicide attempts (defined as leading to hospitalization), whether these risks increased during the month after starting an antidepressant, and whether the 10 newer antidepressants (bupropion, citalopram, fluoxetine, fluvoxamine, mirtazapine, nefazodone, paroxetine, sertraline, escitalopram, and venlafaxine) initially identified in the FDA warnings were associated with higher risks of serious suicidal attempts or death by suicide compared with older antidepressants.

During the 3 months before the index prescription, a total of 73 serious suicide attempts were identified. During the 6-month follow-up period after the index prescription was filled, there were 76 (93/100,000) serious suicide attempts and 31 (40/100,000) completed suicides. The probability of death by suicide was much higher in males (OR = 6.6; 95% CI = 2.9 to 14.7), but did not vary significantly with age. The probability of serious suicide attempts was not significantly different between males and females; however, it strongly correlated with younger age (Z = 3.18, P < .001) with an absolute rate of 314/100,000 (95% CI = 160 to 468) in children and adolescents and of 78/100,000 in adults (95% CI = 58 to 98).

The highest risk of serious suicide attempts was during the month before the index prescription and was primarily because of the increased risk in the 7 days preceding the index prescription; the authors attributed this to the fact that such an attempt may result in beginning treatment with antidepressants. Compared with the month before treatment, there was a decrease in serious suicide attempts during the first month after the index prescription; however, the number of attempts during the first month was greater than that in any of the following 5 months, over which a continuing gradual decline occurred. This risk of suicide death during the first month after the index prescription was not significantly higher than in the subsequent 5 months (OR = 1.2; 95% CI = 0.5 to 2.9). During the 6-month follow-up, there were a total of three suicide deaths in adolescents. The pattern of serious suicide attempts in adolescents over the 6-month period ($N = 17$) was similar to that in adults with the highest risk in the month before the index prescription, a sharp decline immediately after starting treatment and continuing to gradually decline over the next 5 months.

The authors found differences in the risks between the 10 newer antidepressants and older antidepressants (primarily tricyclics and trazodone). The risk of suicidal death over the 6-month follow-up period was 34/100,000 for the 10 newer antidepressants and 51/100,000 for the older antidepressants. The risk of serious suicidal attempts was 76/100,000 for the 10 newer antidepressants and 129/100,000 for the older antidepressants. Patients treated with the 10 newer antidepressants had the highest risk of serious suicidal behavior in the month before starting antidepressants, and the risk in the first months after the index prescription was not significantly different from that in months 2 through 5 (OR = 1.6; 95% CI = 0.9 to 3.1). Patients treated with the older antidepressants had the highest risk in the first month of treatment, which was significantly higher than in months 2 through 6 (OR = 3.6; 95% CI = 1.8 to 6.9).

The authors concluded that their data did not support the contention of increased risk of suicide deaths or serious suicidal attempts during the first month of antidepressant therapy; however, the risk of serious suicidal attempts was higher during the first week of therapy. The risk of suicide deaths appeared to be relatively constant during the first 6 months of therapy. The authors found no evidence that the newer antidepressants increased the risk of suicidal deaths or serious suicide attempts compared with the risks of older antidepressants (Simon et al., 2006).

Bridge and colleagues (2007) completed a meta-analysis of RCTs, evaluating 27 trials of pediatric MDD, OCD, and non-OCD anxiety disorders for efficacy and risk of suicidal ideation or suicide attempts with antidepressants. Pooled differences of risk significantly favored antidepressants for MDD, OCD, and non-OCD anxiety disorders. They reported the NNT (number needed to treat) to benefit was 10, 6, and 3 for treatment of MDD, OCD, and non-OCD anxiety disorders, respectively. There was also an increased risk difference of suicidal ideation and suicide attempt in all trials and indications for drug compared with placebo, with NNH (number needed to harm) = 143, without significant difference between indications, and there were no completed suicides. The authors concluded that antidepressants are efficacious for these indications, with benefits appearing much greater than risks, although varying depending on indication, age, chronicity, and study conditions.

Singh and colleagues (2013) evaluated 51 subjects who were initiated on either venlafaxine or escitalopram for MDD, finding that subjects not reporting child abuse exposure were less likely to have increased suicidality (7.6%) during the first week of antidepressant treatment when compared to subjects with low impact abuse (38.5%) and high impact abuse (58.3%). Increased suicidality was only predicted by high impact abuse after adjustment for potential confounders.

ANTIDEPRESSANT CLINICAL USE

Table 8.3 summarizes various antidepressants that are prescribed for children, adolescents, and adults. The summary includes FDA approvals per age group, formulations of medications available, starting doses, guidelines for titration, maximum doses per FDA guidelines, and other pearls for clinical practice.

SELECTIVE SEROTONIN REUPTAKE INHIBITORS

Mechanism of Action Common to the Selective Serotonin Reuptake Inhibitors

With the exception of escitalopram, which is the S-enantiomer of racemic citalopram, these SSRIs are chemically unrelated to each other or to tricyclic or tetracyclic antidepressants, or to other antidepressants currently used in clinical practice (*Physicians' Desk Reference [PDR]*, 2006). As the term SSRI suggests, at therapeutic

TABLE 8.3 » Antidepressant Preparations, Indications, and Dosage Guidelines

Medication	Available Preparations	FDA Indications	Initial Starting Dose	Typical Therapeutic Dose Range[a]	Maximum Daily Dose
Selective Serotonin Reuptake Inhibitors					
Fluoxetine	10-, 20-mg tablets (scored) 10-, 20-, 40-mg capsules 90-mg weekly capsules 20-mg/5-mL oral solution	≥8 y old: MDD ≥7 y old: OCD ≥18 y old: bulimia nervosa, panic d/o, social anxiety d/o, PMDD	*Children and adolescents:* morning dose 5 mg/d younger children for depression 10 mg/d for other indications and older children ≥18 y old: initial morning dose 20 mg/d	20 mg may be an optimal dose for treating depression 20–60 mg/d for children with OCD 20–60 mg/d for adults with OCD 60 mg/d for bulimia nervosa 20–60 mg/d for panic d/o 20 mg/d for PMDD	80 mg/d
Sertraline	25-, 50-, 100-mg tablets (scored) 20-mg/mL oral concentrate	≥6 y old: OCD; ≥18 y old: MDD, panic d/o, PTSD, PMDD, social anxiety d/o	(Either morning or evening) *Ages 6–12:* initial dose 25 mg/d *Ages 13–17:* 25–50 mg/d ≥18 y old: initial dose 50 mg/d for MDD, OCD, PMDD and 25 mg/d for panic, PTSD, social anxiety and rec'd increase to 50 mg/d after 7 d	50–200 mg/d for MDD, OCD, panic d/o, PTSD, social anxiety d/o 50–150 mg/d for PMDD	200 mg/d
Citalopram	10-, 20-, 40-mg tablets (20, 40 mg are scored) 10-mg/5-mL oral solution	≥18 y old: MDD	20 mg/d either morning or evening	20–40 mg/d	40 mg/d
Escitalopram	10-, 20-mg tablets (scored) 5-mg/5-mL oral solution	≥12 y old: MDD ≥18 y old: GAD	Morning dose 5–10 mg/d	May increase to 20 mg/d if no response to the 10-mg dose after 1 wk for adults, after 3 wk for younger adolescents	20 mg/d
Fluvoxamine	25-, 50-, 100-mg tablets (50, 100 mg are scored)	≥8 y old: OCD	*Ages 8–17:* bedtime dose 25 mg ≥18 y: initial bedtime dose 50 mg	*Ages 8–17:* 25 mg/d incremental changes up to 200 mg/d with rec to divide doses bid once above 50 mg/d ≥18 y: 50 mg/d incremental changes up to 300 mg/d with rec to divide doses bid once above 100 mg/d	*Ages 8–17:* 200 mg/d ≥18 y old: 300 mg/d

(continued)

TABLE 8.3 » Antidepressant Preparations, Indications, and Dosage Guidelines (continued)

Medication	Available Preparations	FDA Indications	Initial Starting Dose	Typical Therapeutic Dose Range[a]	Maximum Daily Dose
Paroxetine	10-, 20-, 30-, 40-mg tablets (10, 20 mg are scored) 12.5-, 25-, 37.5-mg controlled-release tablets 10-mg/5-mL oral suspension	≥18 y old: MDD, OCD, panic d/o, social anxiety d/o, PTSD, GAD	Morning dose 20 mg/d	Usual target doses for PCD, panic 40 mg/d; ranges for MDD, GAD, PTSD 20–50 mg/d	60 mg/d immediate-release tablet; 75 mg/d CR tablet; [a]differing maximums per condition
Serotonin Norepinephrine Reuptake Inhibitors					
Venlafaxine	25-, 37.5-, 50-, 75-, 100-mg IR tablets 37.5-, 75-, 150-mg XR capsules	≥18 y old: MDD for IR; MDD, GAD, social anxiety d/o, panic d/o for XR	IR dose 75 mg divided bid-tid with food XR dose 37.5–75 mg		IR max 375 mg/d XR max 225 mg/d
Duloxetine	20-, 30-, 60-mg delayed-release capsules	≥7 y old: GAD ≥18 y old: MDD, fibromyalgia, diabetic neuropathic pain, chronic musculoskeletal pain	30 mg/d	Usual target 60 mg/d	120 mg/d
Norepinephrine Dopamine Reuptake Inhibitor (NDRI)					
Bupropion	75-, 100-mg IR tablets 100-, 150-, 200-mg SR tablets 150-, 300-mg XL tablets	≥18 y old: MDD, smoking cessation, seasonal affective disorder	IR dose 100 mg bid; SR morning dose 150 mg XL morning dose 150 mg	SR target dose for depressive disorders 300 mg/d SR target for smoking cessation 150 mg/d XL target 300 mg/d	IR 450 mg/d not to exceed 150 mg per dose SR 400 mg/d not to exceed 200 mg bid XL 450 mg/d
Alpha 2-Adrenergic Antagonist					
Mirtazapine	15-, 30-, 45-mg tablets (15, 30 mg are scored) 15-, 30-, 45-mg orally disintegrating tablet	≥18 y old: MDD	15 mg at bedtime	15–45 mg/d	45 mg/d

Serotonin Agonist/Antagonists

Trazodone	50-, 100-, 150-, 300-mg tablets (scored)	≥18 y old: MDD	1.5–2 mg/kg/d divided tid, or 25 mg tid, whichever is less	25–50 mg bid-tid; aNot indicated for insomnia, but a common clinical use: start 25–50 mg QHS	6 mg/kg/d younger children; 400 mg/d outpatient; 600 mg/d inpatient; aNote: Often used for insomnia off FDA label, in which case the maximum is generally considered to be 200 mg/d
Vortioxetine	5-, 10-, 15-, 20-mg tablets	≥18 y old: MDD	10 mg/d	10–20 mg/d	20 mg/d
Tricyclic Antidepressants					
Imipramine	10-, 25-, 50-mg tablets 75-, 100-, 125-, 150-mg capsules	≥12 y old: MDD ≥6 y old: enuresis	MDD: 30–40 mg/d, or 1.5 mg/kg/d, may divide up to tid; Enuresis: 10 mg/1 h before bedtime	Depression: 25–75 mg/d or 1–3 mg/kg/d; Enuresis: 10–75 mg; dose increases may occur 10–25 mg/d weekly or 1–1.5 mg/kg/d weekly	Depression: 100 mg/d or 5 mg/kg/d; Enuresis: 50 mg/d ages 6–12; 75 mg/d ages 12+
Nortriptyline	10-, 25-, 50-, 75-mg capsules 10-mg/5-mL oral solution	≥18 y old: MDD		30–50 mg/d divided daily to four times daily, or 1–3 mg/kg/d divided tid to qid	150 mg/d; aSerum plasma level therapeutic range = 60–100 ng/mL
Amitriptyline	10-, 25-, 50-, 75-, 100-, 150-mg tablets	≥12 y old: MDD	10 mg tid + 20 mg qhs, or 1 mg/kg/d divided tid	50–100 mg/d or 1–3 mg/kg/d; Dose increases may occur 10–25 mg/d or 0.5 mg/kg/d every 2–3 d	200 mg/d or 5 mg/kg/d
Desipramine	10-, 25-, 50-, 75-, 100-, 150-mg tablets	≥18 y old: MDD	25 mg/d	25–100 mg/d	150 mg/d; aSerum plasma level therapeutic range = 100–300 ng/mL
Clomipramine	25-, 50-, 75-mg capsules	≥10 y old: OCD	25 mg/d	100–200 mg/d; During titration, divide bid and give with food	3 mg/kg/d up to 100 mg/d in first 2 wk; Maintenance 200 mg/d ages 10–17; 250 mg/d ages 18+

GAD, generalized anxiety disorder; IR, immediate-release; MDD, major depressive disorder; OCD, obsessive-compulsive disorder; PMDD, premenstrual dysphoric disorder; PTSD, posttraumatic stress disorder; SR, sustained release; XL, extended release; XR, extended release.

levels, these medications act primarily to inhibit serotonin reuptake; they also have relatively little effect on catecholaminergic (norepinephrine) reuptake mechanisms. At least five types and several subtypes of serotonin receptors with both distinct and overlapping functions have been identified in the central nervous system (Sussman, 1994a). These SSRIs have differing specificities in the serotonin receptors whose reuptake they inhibit, which explains their efficacy in treating disorders other than depression and the fact that they have somewhat different untoward effects. SSRI antidepressants also do not have clinically significant direct effects on the adrenergic, muscarinic, or histaminergic systems.

Untoward Effects Common to the Selective Serotonin Reuptake Inhibitors

The most common untoward effects of the SSRIs parallel the symptoms caused by the administration of exogenous serotonin and include headache, nausea, vomiting, diarrhea, nervousness, sleep disturbance, and sexual dysfunction (Sussman, 1994a).

Safer and Zito (2006) conducted a meta-analysis of placebo-controlled studies, which reviewed the incidence of treatment-emergent adverse events (TEAEs) of SSRIs in children, adolescents, and adults. They found that children had a two-to-three-times higher incidence of behavioral activation and vomiting than did adolescents, with adults having the lowest rates. Behavioral activation is described as restlessness, hyperkinesis, hyperactivity, and agitation. See Table 8.4 for rates of activation versus somnolence per age group (Safer & Zito, 2006). Gualtieri and Johnson (2006) conducted a retrospective chart review of 128 children and adolescents treated with SSRIs. They found that 28% developed behavioral side effects. Behavioral side effects are characterized as hyperactivity and disinhibition, which occurred in 17; anger and aggression, which occurred in 17 youth; and dysphoria and extreme emotional reactivity, which occurred in 13. They found self-injurious behavior (SIB) occurring in 12 and suicidal ideation threats or attempts occurring in 9. They analyzed the severity of the events and found that most were managed by discontinuing the medication or lowering the dose. In all, 34 of 36 youth who developed behavioral toxicity were able to continue to be treated with antidepressants after their side effects resolved with either a lower dose of the same medication or a different agent (Gualtieri & Johnson, 2006).

Zuckerman and colleagues (2007) conducted a retrospective chart review of children below 7 years of age on SSRIs. They found 39 children who were prescribed citalopram, fluvoxamine, paroxetine, fluoxetine, or sertraline. Seven patients in the sample needed to discontinue their SSRI due to AEs. One youth had gastrointestinal (GI) distress that resolved after discontinuation, and six youth developed behavioral activation which required discontinuation. In their sample, 28% of youth below 7 years of age developed AEs with behavioral activation occurring in 21% (Zuckerman et al., 2007).

SSRI-induced sexual dysfunction is of concern in adolescents, particularly due to likely underreporting of this side effect and the potential impact on treatment

TABLE 8.4 » Summary of Activation Versus Somnolence Separated by Age

	Activation		Somnolence	
	Treatment (%)	Placebo (%)	Treatment (%)	Placebo (%)
Children	10.70	3.40	3	3.40
Adolescents	2.10	1.90	11.30	5.00
Adults			16.50	7.60

Data from: Safer DJ, Zito JM. Treatment-emergent adverse events from selective serotonin reuptake inhibitors by age group: children versus adolescents. *J Child Adolesc Psychopharmacol.* 2006;16(1–2):159–169.

adherence. Sharko (2004) reviewed the literature and reported a paucity of reported cases of sexual dysfunction—only 1 male of 1,346 pediatric subjects in 31 clinical studies of SSRIs reported such an AE, erectile dysfunction. During 11 years, only eight subjects, all male, were reported to MedWatch for sexual dysfunction secondary to treatment with an SSRI: four reported loss of orgasm, three reported loss in interest, and one reported loss of physical arousal. In adults taking adequate doses of SSRIs, sexual dysfunction has been reported by 30% to 40% of patients and that this was probably a low estimate because of the difficulties many adults have in discussing sexual matters. He further speculated that the surprisingly low incidence reported was because it was even more difficult for adolescents to talk to their prescribers; in addition, scales such as the Systematic Assessment for Treatment-Emergent Events and the Side Effects Form for Children and Adolescents do not assess sexual function. In adults, it is known that relying on spontaneous self-report greatly underestimates the actual frequency of SSRI-related sexual dysfunction (Sharko, 2004). Directly asking adolescents about sex and sexual functioning is likely to be the best way to assess sexual dysfunction of our adolescent patients treated with SSRIs (Sharko, 2004); neglecting to do so is a disservice to them and may also increase rates of nonadherence with treatment.

A discontinuation syndrome has been identified for the SSRIs. Hosenbocus and Chahal (2011) reviewed the literature on discontinuation-emergent symptoms in children and adults taking SSRIs and noted that dizziness occurs in 60% of cases followed by nausea in almost 40% of adults. The most common symptoms seen in children are dizziness, lightheadedness, drowsiness, poor concentration, nausea, headache, and fatigue. These symptoms are seen when SSRIs are abruptly discontinued (Hosenbocus & Chahal, 2011). Rosenbaum et al. (1998) conducted a 4-week, prospective double-blind, placebo-substitution, discontinuation study of 242 adults receiving long-term maintenance (duration 4 to 24 months) with SSRIs for remitted depression (81 subjects on fluoxetine, 79 subjects of sertraline, and 82 subjects on paroxetine). Medication was abruptly interrupted for 5 to 8 days; 83% were randomly assigned to receive placebo and 17% to continue on their medication. Following this phase, all subjects on placebo resumed their usual maintenance dose of the SSRI they were previously taking. Two hundred twenty (91%) of the subjects completed the entire protocol. Following medication withdrawal during placebo, scores both on the Discontinuation-Emergent Signs and Symptoms (DESS) Checklist and the Symptom Questionnaire increased significantly for patients who had been on sertraline or paroxetine ($P < .001$ for both), but not for patients who were receiving fluoxetine ($P = .578$). There were many more discontinuation-emergent symptoms reported on the DESS under inquiry than reported spontaneously. Reported symptoms (ranked from most to least frequent) that occurred in at least 10% of the 185 subjects who underwent withdrawal from medication in decreasing frequency were the following: worsened mood, irritability, agitation, dizziness, confusion, headache, nervousness, crying, fatigue, emotional lability, trouble sleeping, dreaming, anger, nausea, amnesia, sweating, depersonalization, muscle aches, unsteady gait, panic, sore eyes, diarrhea, shaking, muscle tension, and chills. Overall, an SSRI discontinuation syndrome occurred in 14% of patients withdrawn from fluoxetine, 60% of patients withdrawn from sertraline, and 66% of patients withdrawn from paroxetine. There appeared to be an inverse relationship between a longer half-life and the development of discontinuation-emergent symptoms (e.g., patients abruptly discontinued from fluoxetine developed fewer discontinuation effects than did patients withdrawn from sertraline or paroxetine). In addition, patients treated with either sertraline or paroxetine were rated as having a significant increase in depressive symptoms during the withdrawal period on placebo ($P < .001$). Subjects who were taking fluoxetine did not experience this reemergence of depressive symptoms. Following restabilization on medication, there were no significant rating scale differences among the three agents (Rosenbaum et al., 1998). Discontinuation symptoms are best managed by restarting the serotonergic medication and following a more gradual taper (Hosenbocus & Chahal, 2011). In cases where SSRIs are unable to be tapered because of reemergence of symptoms, it is possible to overlap with a longer half-life SSRI such as fluoxetine. The first SSRI is tapered off slowly and then the fluoxetine can be discontinued.

Cardiac Effects

McNally and colleagues (2007) reviewed the cardiac effects of psychotropic medications in children due to their increased use in recent years, aiming to provide up-to-date clinical guidelines and risk assessment and cardiac monitoring. They discuss that the upper limit of normal QT interval when corrected for heart rate (QTc) is 450 ms in males and 460 ms in females, and that prolongation beyond 500 ms and an increase of greater than 60 ms in QTc from baseline can predict risk of developing the arrhythmia torsades de pointes. Genetic long QT syndromes, such as Jervell and Lange-Nielsen syndrome and Romano Ward syndrome, display classic symptoms of syncope, unexplained seizures, and sudden death, and are at higher risk of QT prolongation with ingestion of certain drugs. Structural heart disease, whether corrected or not, also increases prevalence of cardiac conduction abnormalities. Electrolyte abnormalities, which may result from illnesses with diarrhea or vomiting, renal tubular acidosis, or diuretic medications, may also contribute to effects from QT prolonging drugs. Higher doses of psychotropic medications may significantly affect QT changes, particularly in overdose. Other medications that affect psychotropic metabolism, including the use of other psychotropics as well as non-psychotropics, can result in QTc prolongation as well. Certain psychotropics have demonstrated more likely effects on the QTc interval, such as the atypical antipsychotics ziprasidone and clozapine, the typical antipsychotics mesoridazine, thioridazine, haloperidol, droperidol, and pimozide, TCAs, and less commonly with SSRIs and newer antidepressants aside from citalopram. The authors encourage obtaining a detailed past medical and family history in children before prescribing a psychotropic medication, specifically enquiring about a family history of sudden death, a personal or family history of unexplained syncope or seizures, a history of congenital heart disease, deafness or disorders involving electrolyte imbalance, and the use of medications that may cause electrolyte abnormalities or may impact the metabolism of other medications that may affect the QT interval. It is advised to obtain a baseline electrocardiogram (ECG) in patients with preexisting risk factors, a suspicious history, if they are taking a medication that may interact with the prescribed medication, or if the medication to be prescribed is documented to cause a prolonged QTc interval at therapeutic doses. The presence of a prolonged QTc found at baseline should prompt referral to a pediatric cardiologist. If a baseline ECG is normal but an abnormality is found after reaching steady-state concentration or after a dose change, the medication should be stopped and the child referred to a pediatric cardiologist. Parents and child patients also need to be properly informed of the risk of medication interactions, the effects of illness on electrolyte balance, and the need to contact the prescriber if other doctors plan on prescribing additional medications to the child.

Uchida and colleagues (2017) examined QTc prolongation in 49 children, aged 6 to 17 years, prescribed non-TCA medications. Medication doses of citalopram, escitalopram, fluoxetine, paroxetine, sertraline, bupropion, duloxetine, venlafaxine, and mirtazapine were standardized into "citalopram equivalent doses" based on dosing recommendations for each medication. No significant associations were found between antidepressant doses and QTc. A significant correlation was found between PR interval and daily dose in patients taking citalopram or escitalopram, although this was not present when weight-based doses were used or when corrected by age. The authors concluded that therapeutic doses of non-TCA antidepressants used in children do not seem to be associated with prolonged QTc interval or other adverse cardiovascular effects.

Use in Pregnancy and While Breastfeeding

Koren and Nordeng's (2012) review of antidepressant use in pregnancy provides a succinct risk–benefit discussion regarding treatment with both SSRIs and serotonin norepinephrine reuptake inhibitors (SNRIs) in expectant women. Considering that more than 50% of pregnancies are unplanned and that the risk of an unplanned pregnancy is likely higher in teenagers, this is a relevant concern for the treatment of this age group. These medications do cross the placenta and are excreted in breast milk. Generally, risks of cardiac malformations, primary pulmonary hypertension of the newborn, and poor neonatal adaptation syndrome are considered the most concerning; but these are also still considered to be marginal in frequency. The authors conclude in the review that if an expectant woman has a psychiatric condition that necessitates psychotropic medication treatment, then the risks of not treating the psychiatric condition outweigh the marginal risks to the developing fetus and newborn from appropriate psychotropic medication management. There is no particular difference in risk among individual SSRIs/SNRIs to the extent that sweeping recommendations for or against specific agents be made; all medications discussed in this chapter are pregnancy risk class C. Evaluating relative risks of antidepressant exposure versus neurodevelopmental risks from untreated depression in the mother would be ethically impossible to study in a prospective, randomized controlled manner. It is prudent for management to include collaboration among providers of both obstetric and mental health care for the expectant mother.

In a 2016 review of SSRI use in pregnancy, Alwan and colleagues discuss concerns about associations between medication use and miscarriage, premature delivery, other neonatal complications, cardiac defects or other birth defects, and neurodevelopmental disorders based on a small increase in absolute risk. It is difficult to separate risks associated with medication use from risks associated with the presence of the illness being treated; and risks of untreated illness must be considered. Although the increased risk is small, it is greater than the baseline complication risk, and should be considered in treatment planning. Associations with such complications are stronger with fluoxetine and paroxetine compared to other SSRIs; and SNRIs in pregnancy have been studied less than SSRIs such that fewer conclusions can be made about the risk–benefit. Authors recommended discussion of treatment options on a case-by-case basis and consideration of nonpharmacologic therapies such as psychotherapy, light therapy, and other options as part of the balance of risks, benefits, and alternatives. Those with relapsing and severe depression should continue medication if this is the best treatment option, and pharmacologic treatment should be at the lowest effective dose in such cases (Alwan et al., 2016).

Nulman and colleagues (2012) compared the neurodevelopment of children following prenatal exposure to venlafaxine, SSRIs, or untreated maternal depression. All three groups were found to have similar full-scale IQs, although the IQs of the venlafaxine and SSRI groups were significantly lower when compared to those of children of nondepressed mothers. Rates of problematic behaviors were nonsignificant, but higher in the three groups when compared to children of nondepressed mothers. Antidepressant dose and duration during pregnancy did not predict any cognitive or behavioral outcome.

Bipolar "Switching"

Jerrell and colleagues (2014) employed a retrospective cohort design to evaluate the risk of developing bipolar disorder in an ADHD cohort. Logistic regression modeling found several medications associated with a higher risk of developing bipolar disorder. They found that being treated with citalopram (aOR = 1.61), escitalopram (aOR = 1.84), fluoxetine (aOR = 2.00), paroxetine (aOR = 1.75), sertraline (aOR = 2.29), bupropion (aOR = 2.22), mirtazapine (aOR = 1.69), trazodone (aOR = 2.15), or venlafaxine (aOR = 2.37) predicted higher odds of being diagnosed with bipolar disorder. In addition, longer treatment with methylphenidate, mixed amphetamine salts, or atomoxetine (aOR = 1.01) was also associated with the risk.

Fluoxetine Hydrochloride (Prozac, Sarafem)

Fluoxetine was the first SSRI to be approved by the FDA, and there are more published reports of its use in children and adolescents than for the SSRIs that were introduced later. Fluoxetine's antidepressant effect is thought to be related to its specific and selective inhibition of serotonin reuptake by central nervous system neurons. This action appears to take place at the serotonin reuptake pump, not at a neurotransmitter receptor site, and fluoxetine appears to have no significant pharmacologic effect on norepinephrine or dopamine uptake (Bergstrom et al., 1988).

Owing to significantly less binding to muscarinic, histaminergic, and alpha-1 adrenergic receptors, there is a relative lack of anticholinergic, sedative, and cardiovascular effects of SSRIs.

The therapeutic serum levels of fluoxetine (FLX) and its major metabolite norfluoxetine (NORFLEX) in children and adolescents have been evaluated. Koelch and colleagues (2012) performed therapeutic monitoring of 71 youth aged 8 to 19 years who were being treated with fluoxetine in doses of 10 to 60 mg. They found that the serum concentrations of the active moiety (FLX + NORFLEX) ranged from 21 to 613 ng/mL. They noted that there was very high interindividual variability in the serum concentrations of FLX at each dosage level. There was no relationship between serum concentration and clinical response. The only external factor that affected serum concentration was smoking. These results are similar to therapeutic monitoring studies of fluoxetine in adults (Koelch et al., 2012).

Pharmacokinetics of Fluoxetine Hydrochloride

Peak plasma levels of fluoxetine at usual clinical doses occur after 6 to 8 hours. Food does not significantly affect the bioavailability of fluoxetine; hence, it may be administered with or without food. Fluoxetine is metabolized by the P450 2D6 system in the liver; active and inactive metabolites are excreted by the kidneys. About 95% of fluoxetine is bound to plasma proteins. The elimination half-life after chronic administration is 4 to 6 days for fluoxetine and 4 to 16 days for norfluoxetine, its active metabolite. It may take up to 4 to 5 weeks for steady-state plasma levels to be achieved, but once obtained they remain steady.

Contraindications for the Administration of Fluoxetine Hydrochloride

Known hypersensitivity to the medication is a contraindication.

Fluoxetine should not be administered to any patient who has received an monoamine oxidase inhibitor (MAOI) within the preceding 2 weeks. Because of the long half-lives of fluoxetine and its metabolites, an MAOI should not be administered sooner than 5 weeks (35 days) after discontinuing fluoxetine. The manufacturer notes that it may be advisable to wait even longer before giving an MAOI if fluoxetine has been prescribed chronically or at high doses (*PDR*, 2000).

The medication should be administered with caution if impaired liver function is present; if prescribed, a lower dose or a decrease frequency of administration should be used.

Fluoxetine is a use-in-pregnancy Category C medication and is secreted in breast milk, and hence caution is recommended for pregnant and nursing females taking fluoxetine.

Interactions of Fluoxetine Hydrochloride with Other Medications

The use of fluoxetine with other psychoactive medications has not been systematically studied. However, because it is metabolized by the P450 2D6 enzyme system, the potential exists for interactions with other medications metabolized by this system, including TCAs and other SSRIs.

When used with TCAs, their plasma levels may be significantly increased.

Agitation, restlessness, and GI symptoms have occurred when used concurrently with tryptophan.

Diazepam clearance was significantly prolonged in some patients who were administered both medications.

Elevated plasma levels and toxicity have occurred in some patients receiving carbamazepine or phenytoin when fluoxetine was added to their treatment regimes.

Untoward Effects of Fluoxetine Hydrochloride

Wernicke (1985) and Cooper (1988) have reviewed the safety and untoward effects of fluoxetine. The most frequent troublesome untoward effects are nausea, weight loss, anxiety, nervousness, insomnia, and excessive sweating.

Many of the untoward effects may be described as behavioral activation. Riddle et al. (1990/1991) reported the behavioral side effects of fluoxetine in 24 children and adolescents with various diagnoses (age range, 8 to 16 years). Mean dose was 25.8 ± 9.0 mg/day for the 12 subjects who developed fluoxetine-induced behavioral side effects, such as restlessness, hyperactivity, insomnia, an internal feeling of excitation, subtle impulsive behavioral changes, and suicidal ideation (King et al., 1991; Riddle et al., 1990/1991). Hypomania, mania, transient psychosis, and significant memory impairment have also been reported to occur in children and adolescents treated with fluoxetine (Bangs et al., 1994; Boulos et al., 1992; Hersh et al., 1991; Jafri, 1991; Jerome, 1991; Rosenberg et al., 1992; Venkataraman et al., 1992).

Simeon et al. (1990) reported that those subjects receiving fluoxetine who were depressed experienced a small but significant weight loss compared with subjects receiving placebo. Because many teenagers will be concerned about taking a medication which could cause weight gain, this could be a clinically advantageous characteristic of fluoxetine for some patients.

The effect of fluoxetine on aggression and or hostility-related events was examined in a meta-analysis (Tauscher-Wisniewski et al., 2007). Five studies were included in the analysis in which 376 children and adolescents were treated with fluoxetine compared with 255 treated with placebo. Aggression and/or hostility-related events were identified in 2.1% of youth treated with fluoxetine versus 3.1% of placebo-treated patients; this suggests that there is not an association between fluoxetine treatment and increased risk of aggression.

Reports of Interest

Fluoxetine in the Treatment of Child and Adolescent MDD

Larger multicentered landmark studies involving the use of fluoxetine and other SSRIs to treat depression were reported earlier in this chapter. Studies of fluoxetine use in youths, particularly in the early years of its use, examined smaller numbers of children and adolescents over shorter durations. Many of these youth with MDD had actually failed treatment with TCAs for numerous reasons. For example, Joshi et al. (1989) found that 10/14 children ranging in age from 9 to 15 years with major depression responded favorably within 6 weeks to fluoxetine 20 mg administered in the morning. Side effects were limited to transient nausea and hyperactivity in one patient each and did not require discontinuation of the medication.

Simeon et al. (1990) reported a 7-week, double-blind, placebo-controlled fluoxetine treatment study of 40 adolescents with major depression. Fluoxetine was gradually titrated from 20 to 60 mg/day. About two-thirds of patients in each group showed moderate to marked clinical global improvement, with significant improvement by week 3. With the exception of disturbances of sleep, all symptoms showed slightly greater improvement in subjects treated with fluoxetine than in those receiving placebo, but differences were not significant. Patients taking fluoxetine, however, experienced a small but significantly greater weight loss than those receiving placebo. Untoward effects were usually mild and transient, and none necessitated discontinuation of medication. Those most frequently reported were headache, vomiting, insomnia, and tremor.

At long-term follow up 8 to 46 months later, no significant differences were found between the fluoxetine and placebo groups, or between responders and nonresponders to the initial clinical trial. Both groups showed further overall improvement; however, there were indications that a portion of the study population was a very high risk group (Simeon et al., 1990).

Boulos et al. (1992) reported on a trial to treat 15 adolescents and young adults diagnosed with MDD who had responded unsatisfactorily to prior treatment with antidepressants, usually including tricyclics. Fluoxetine doses ranged from 5 to 40 mg daily. Of these, 64% showed at least a 50% improvement on the Hamilton Depression Rating Scale (HDRS), and 73% achieved scores of "much" or "very much improved" on the Clinical Global Impressions Scale (CGIS). Untoward effects included headache, vomiting and other GI complaints, insomnia, tremor, sweating, dry mouth, and hair loss.

Emslie et al. (1997) reported an 8-week, double-blind, randomized (stratified for age, ≤12 years or ≥13 years, and sex), placebo-controlled study of 96 children and adolescents (52 males and 44 females; age range 7 to 17 years), diagnosed by DSM-III-R (APA, 1987) criteria with nonpsychotic MDD. Following a 3-week evaluation period and a 1-week, single-blind, placebo run-in during which responders were dropped, the 96 remaining subjects were randomized to 8 weeks of treatment with placebo or fluoxetine 20 mg daily. Outcome measures included the Clinical Global Impressions–Improvement (CGI-I) subscale and the Children's Depression Rating Scale–Revised (CDRS-R). Fluoxetine was statistically better than placebo on the CGI-I; using the intent-to-treat (ITT) sample, 27 (56%) of the fluoxetine group versus 16 (33%) of the placebo group were rated much or very much improved (P = .02). After week 5, the mean CDRS-R score for the fluoxetine group became significantly lower than that for the placebo group (P = .03). Subjects initially had relatively severe and chronic symptoms of depression and, despite their overall improvement, after 8 weeks, only 15 (31%) of the fluoxetine group and 11 (23%) of the placebo group had CDRS-R scores <28, consistent with relatively complete remission of depressive symptoms. The authors concluded that fluoxetine was significantly better than placebo in acute-phase treatment of children and adolescents diagnosed with severe, persistent MDD.

Fluoxetine in the Treatment of Children and Adolescents with OCD or OCD and Tourette Disorder

Riddle et al. (1992) reported a randomized, 20-week, double-blind, placebo-controlled, fixed-dose study with crossover after 8 weeks of fluoxetine in treating 14 subjects (age range, 8.6 to 15.6 years) diagnosed with OCD by DSM-III-R criteria. Subjects received 20 mg of fluoxetine or placebo. The subjects initially receiving fluoxetine showed significant decreases on the Children's Yale–Brown Obsessive-Compulsive Scale (CY-BOCS) total score (mean decrease, 44%; P = .003), obsessions score (mean decrease, 54%; P = .009), and compulsions score (mean decrease, 33%; P = .005), and on the Clinical Global Impressions for Obsessive-Compulsive Disorder (CGI-OCD) (mean decrease, 33%, P = .0004). The subjects on placebo also showed reductions in their obsessive-compulsive symptomatology on the CY-BOCS of 27% and on the CGI-OCD of 12%, but these reductions were not significant. The most frequently reported untoward effects were insomnia, fatigue, motoric activation, and nausea. Preexisting chronic motor tics worsened in two subjects;

however, fluoxetine was continued and the tics subsided to negligible levels over the subsequent 2 years. One subject with comorbid diagnoses of MDD, separation anxiety, and oppositional disorder developed suicidal ideation, which resolved after fluoxetine was discontinued. The authors noted that 20 mg/day may be too high a dose for some children and that an initial dose of 10 mg/day of fluoxetine was the most common starting dose given to children by most child and adolescent psychiatrists. Following the crossover at 8 weeks, more of the subjects initially on fluoxetine who crossed over to placebo showed worsening. Likewise, most of the subjects who crossed over from placebo to fluoxetine showed further reductions in CY-BOCS scores. This early RCT studying treatment of OCD suggested that fluoxetine is both safe and effective in treating children and adolescents with OCD for 20 weeks (Riddle et al., 1992).

Geller and colleagues (2001) examined the effectiveness of fluoxetine in children and adolescents with OCD in a double-blind placebo-controlled study of 103 patients. Patients were initially given a 10-mg dose of fluoxetine for the first 2 weeks of treatment and then 20 mg for the next 2 weeks. Subsequent dosage titration to 40 mg or later 60 mg daily took place depending on CGI-Severity, with reductions in dose if there was difficulty tolerating the higher dose. Improvement was primarily measured with the CY-BOCS. The mean dose of fluoxetine in the treatment group was 24.6 mg. Sixteen (23%) had a final dose of 40 mg/day, and 15 (21%) had a final dose of 60 mg/day. Fluoxetine was associated with significantly greater improvement in CY-BOCS scores ($P = .26$). Patients with a 40% or greater reduction in their CY-BOCS scores were considered responders. By this criteria, 35 of 71 (49%) of the fluoxetine group and 8 of 32 (25%) of the placebo group were responders. CGI-I scales in the fluoxetine-treated group had 55% of patients rated as much or very much improved compared with 18.8% of the placebo group. Fluoxetine was well tolerated. Discontinuation due to AEs occurred in 8.5% of the fluoxetine group (headache, hyperkinesia, abnormal liver function tests, manic reaction, nervousness, or somnolence) and 6.3% of the placebo group (hyperkinesia or nervousness). The authors concluded that fluoxetine 20 to 60 mg a day was effective and well tolerated for the treatment of OCD in the pediatric population.

Fluoxetine in the Treatment of Children and Adolescents with Anxiety Disorders

Two early open-label trials paved the way for further studies of the use of fluoxetine to treat anxiety disorders in children and adolescents. Birmaher et al. (1994) followed up 21 patients (age range, 11 to 17 years) diagnosed with differing combinations of overanxious disorder, SP, and SAD, who had not responded to prior psychopharmacotherapy or psychotherapy. The mean fluoxetine dose after an average of 10 months (range, 1 to 31 months) on fluoxetine was 25.7 mg/day. Ninety-five percent of subjects showed some improvement in anxiety, with 81% rated as moderately to markedly improved on the severity and improvement subscales of the CGIS ($P = .0001$). It is important to note that in most cases, improvement did not begin until 6 to 8 weeks after initiation of fluoxetine. Although no subject fulfilled diagnostic criteria for MDD or dysthymia, the 10 patients who did have depressive symptoms also improved significantly ($P = .0001$). Untoward effects were mild and transient, and included mild headache, nausea, insomnia, and stomachache. No significant changes in pulse, blood pressure, or ECG were found, and no subject experienced agitation, manic or hypomanic symptoms, or suicidal ideation (Birmaher et al., 1994).

Fairbanks et al. (1997) treated 16 outpatients (age range, 9 to 17 years) diagnosed by DSM-III-R (APA, 1987) criteria with mixed anxiety disorders and who were unresponsive to psychotherapy. Fluoxetine was initiated at a dose of 5 mg/day and subsequently increased weekly by 5 or 10 mg/day for 6 to 9 weeks until clinical improvement occurred or to a maximum of 40 mg for subjects <12 years of age or 80 mg/day for subjects ≥12 years of age. The mean fluoxetine dose for all subjects was 35.0 ± 17.1 mg/day or 0.71 ± 0.28 mg/kg/day. The mean milligram/

kilogram/day dose was almost identical for subjects of all ages. Subjects with only one anxiety disorder responded to lower doses than did subjects with two or more anxiety disorders. Fluoxetine did not appear to aggravate the anxiety of any of the patients. The authors state that their outcome assessments found that SAD, SP, specific phobia, and panic disorder all responded favorably to fluoxetine but that GAD did not. The most common untoward effects were drowsiness, difficulty falling asleep or staying asleep, decreased appetite, nausea, abdominal pain, and a state of being easily excited or keyed up. None of the subjects was reported to have disinhibition, akathisia, suicidal or violent reactions, or hypomania.

Birmaher et al. (2003) conducted a 12-week, randomized, placebo-controlled, double-blind study to assess the efficacy and tolerability of fluoxetine in the outpatient treatment of 74 children and adolescents (age range 7 to 17 years) diagnosed by DSM-IV (APA, 1994) criteria with GAD, SP, and/or SAD; most subjects were diagnosed with more than one anxiety disorder, and 24 (32%) were also diagnosed with other non-anxiety psychiatric disorders. Fluoxetine was initiated at a dose of 10 mg/day for the first week and, if tolerated, was increased to 20 mg/day for the remaining 11 weeks of the study. No other psychiatric medications were permitted for the duration of the study.

At the end of the study, on the CGI-I Scale, 75% of the fluoxetine group versus 38.7% for the placebo group ($P = .005$) had very marked or marked improvement. Regarding AEs during the first 2 weeks, subjects on fluoxetine had significantly more AEs than those on placebo for abdominal pain, nausea, drowsiness, and headaches. For the entire duration of the study, only abdominal pain and nausea were significantly more frequent in the fluoxetine group. Subjects were more severely ill at intake (scores of >30) on the Screen for Child Anxiety-Related Emotional Disorders–Child (SCARED-C) and those with positive family histories for anxiety had a poorer clinical response to fluoxetine than did subjects without such histories. The authors concluded that fluoxetine is clinically effective and safe for the acute treatment of anxiety in this age group. They suggested that an increase in dose is indicated for patients with no or only partial clinical response after 4 to 6 weeks of treatment. In addition, they noted that mild to moderate agitation/disinhibition may be successfully treated by lowering the dose of fluoxetine in many cases (Birmaher et al., 2003).

In a 1-year follow-up of the 74 subjects in Birmaher et al.'s (2003) 12-week acute, controlled study of fluoxetine, an open-label, 1-year extension was conducted. Of the 52 analyzed completers, 42 were assigned to fluoxetine (of this group, 22 had been on fluoxetine during the acute 12-week trial and 20 had been on placebo) and 10 received no medication (of these 4 had been on fluoxetine during the 12-week acute study and 6 had been on placebo). Those subjects on fluoxetine were rated as significantly more improved than those on no medication on the SCARED–Parent Report ($P ≤ .01$), the SCARED-C ($P < .05$); the Pediatric Anxiety Rating Scale–Parent Report (PARS-P), and the PARS–Rater Report (PARS-R) ($P = .05$). The PARS–Child Report (PARS-C) was not significantly different between the fluoxetine and the placebo groups. The group showing the greatest improvement in CGI-S was the group that was on placebo during the 12-week acute trial and on fluoxetine during the 1-year open-label extension period. The results suggest that fluoxetine continues to be of benefit for the treatment of anxiety in this group of subjects for up to 15 months (Clark et al., 2005).

Fluoxetine in the Treatment of Children and Adolescents with ADHD

Gammon and Brown (1993) reported the use of fluoxetine augmentation of methylphenidate in an 8-week open trial with 32 patients (9 to 17 years old) who were diagnosed with ADHD and one or more comorbid disorders—that is, dysthymia (78%), oppositional defiant disorder (ODD; 59%), MDD (18%), anxiety disorders (18%), and conduct disorder (13%)—and who had inadequate therapeutic responses to methylphenidate alone. Addition of fluoxetine was begun with an initial dose of 2.5 or 5.0 mg/day for subjects <12 years of age and 12 years of age or older, respectively. Dose was titrated upward every 3 to 4 days in increments equal to the initial dose, to a maximum of 20 mg/day. Optimal daily dose of fluoxetine at 8 weeks ranged from 2.5 to 20 mg. The majority of subjects (19, or 59%) required 20 mg/day; six subjects (18%) received 10 to 15 mg/day; four subjects (12.5%) received 5 to 7.5 mg/day; and three subjects (9%) had optimal fluoxetine doses of 2.5 mg/day. No significant or lasting untoward effects were reported.

After 8 weeks of combined treatment, all 32 subjects showed statistically significant improvements on assessments rating attention, behavior, and affect. These improvements were also rated clinically significant in 94% (30) of the subjects. Scores on the CGAS dramatically improved ($P < .0001$). Mean scores on the Children's Depression Inventory declined from 22, which is in the clinical range for depressive symptoms, to 8, which is below that range ($P < .0001$). On the Conners Parents Rating Scale (CPRS), group means improved on all six scales; on five scales improvement was significant ($P < .001$ to $P < .0001$). There was also a marked jump in student grade point average within one marking period. Parents reported substantial improvement in hyperactivity, impulsivity, anxiety, conduct, and learning problems. Augmentation with fluoxetine also produced significant further improvement in sustaining attention and concentration and helped alleviate symptoms of anxiety, depression, irritability, and oppositionality that had not responded adequately to methylphenidate alone. More seriously affected children showed the most significant improvements (Gammon & Brown, 1993).

Fluoxetine in the Treatment of Children Diagnosed with Bulimia Nervosa

Kotler and colleagues (2003) treated 10 subjects (age range of 12 to 18 years) who were diagnosed with bulimia nervosa in an open, 8-week study with fluoxetine 60-mg/day dose. They offered subjects a 4-week supportive psychosocial treatment phase preceding the 8-week medication trial. One subject improved significantly after therapy alone and did not receive medication. Five subjects elected to start the medication phase initially. Fluoxetine was initiated at 20 mg/day and titrated to 60 mg/day by day 7 and continued for the next 7 weeks. The subjects improved having average weekly binges decrease from 4.1 to 0. Average weekly purges decreased from 6.4 to 0.9. All patients improved their CGI-I scales, with 20% rated as much improved, 50% improved, and 30% slightly improved (Kotler et al., 2003).

Fluoxetine in the Treatment of Children Diagnosed with Autism Spectrum Disorders

Given that youth with autism often have repetitive behaviors similar to those seen in OCD, it is logical to believe that SSRIs could potentially help decrease compulsive symptoms in these children. One double-blind, placebo-controlled crossover study used fluoxetine in children with autism and examined its effect on global improvement. Hollander and colleagues (2005) enrolled 45 subjects (age range 5 to 16 years) with autism spectrum disorder (ASD). They defined ASD as meeting criteria for autism, Asperger syndrome, or pervasive developmental disorder not otherwise specified (PDDNOS) by Autism Diagnostic Interview. Subjects were randomized into two acute 8-week phases separated by a 4-week washout phase. Dosage began with 2.5 mg/day of liquid fluoxetine the first week and was then titrated up for the next 2 weeks up to a maximum dose of 0.8 mg/kg/day by the end of week 4. This dose was maintained for the remainder of the 8-week phases. Clinical response was assessed by CY-BOCS and CGI-AD (Clinical Global Improvement Scale Adapted to Global Autism) assessments. The dosage range of fluoxetine used was 2.4 to 20 mg. Their analysis showed that low-dose fluoxetine was superior to placebo in the treatment of repetitive behaviors by CY-BOCS compulsion scale. The effect size was in the moderate-to-large range (0.76). The improvement in CGI autism scores was only slightly superior to that of placebo in the fluoxetine group. They did not detect any increase in suicide subscale measures, and anxiety/nervousness on fluoxetine was less than on placebo. The authors attribute the lack of side-effect differences between placebo and fluoxetine groups to their low doses and slow titration schedule. This contrasts with other studies which have found that SSRI treatment in ASD children frequently has increased side effects of behavioral activation (hyperactivity and agitation), aggression, and suicidal ideation (West et al., 2009).

Fluoxetine in the Treatment of Children Diagnosed with Selective (Elective) Mutism

Black and Uhde (1994) treated 15 subjects (age range 6 to 11 years) who were diagnosed with elective mutism with fluoxetine in a double-blind, 12-week study. Fluoxetine was given at a dose of 0.2 mg/kg/day for the first week, increased to 0.4 mg/kg for the second week, and further increased to 0.6 mg/kg for the final 10 weeks of the study. The mean maximum dose of fluoxetine was 0.60 to 0.62 mg/kg/day or 21.4 mg/day (range, 12 to 27 mg/day). Both groups showed significant improvement from baseline over time in elective mutism, anxiety, and social anxiety as rated by parents, teachers, and clinicians. The fluoxetine group improved significantly more than the placebo group on parents', but not on teachers' or clinicians' ratings of mutism and clinical global improvement. This was consistent with earlier findings that children with elective mutism show improvements in the home setting before that in school and in clinic settings. The authors noted that, although statistically significant, the improvements were modest and that the subjects continued to show serious impairments in their functioning. Untoward effects were minimal (Black & Uhde, 1994).

Dummit et al. (1996) reported a 9-week, open-label study of fluoxetine in the treatment of 21 children (age range, 5 to 14 years) who met DSM-IV (APA, 1994) criteria for selective mutism and comorbid avoidant disorder or SP. Efficacy was assessed by ratings of the CGAS and the Liebowitz Social Anxiety Scale. Subjects rated themselves on the social behavior scale, and parents rated their children on the same scale. Initially, fluoxetine was begun at a dose of 1.25 mg/day and gradually increased. The mean optimal daily dose of fluoxetine was 28.1 mg/day or 1.1 mg/kg/day, and the dose ranged from 20 to 60 mg/day. Overall scores on all indicators indicated significant improvement on all rating scales ($P < .001$ for clinicians' and subjects' self-ratings and $P < .005$ for parental ratings). After 9 weeks, 16 of 21 (76%) subjects were rated as "improved" by their psychiatrist. Treatment outcome was inversely related to age, with 14 of 15 children <10 years improving to a clinically meaningful degree and only 2 of the 6 children ≥10 years old doing so. Four children developed excitement and behavioral disinhibition, which resulted in three of them discontinuing the medication and in dose reduction in the fourth child. Most untoward effects were transient, and none was reported during the final week of treatment. The authors recommended a relatively low initial dose of 5 to 10 mg/day because of the possibility of behavioral activation and also noted that complete remission of the elective mutism often required more than 9 weeks of treatment, even in the marked treatment responders.

Sertraline Hydrochloride (Zoloft)

Sertraline hydrochloride is an SSRI that is chemically unrelated to other antidepressants currently in use. Clinical effect is presumed to be related to its inhibition of neuronal serotonin uptake. It has only very weak effects on norepinephrine and dopamine reuptake. *In vitro*, sertraline has no significant affinity for alpha-1, alpha-2, or beta-adrenergic, cholinergic, gamma aminobutyric acid (GABA), dopaminergic, histaminergic, 5-HT_{1A}, 5-HT_{1B}, or 5-HT_2 serotonergic, or benzodiazepine receptors. Chronic administration of sertraline is thought to downregulate norepinephrine receptors.

Pharmacokinetics of Sertraline Hydrochloride

Peak plasma levels of sertraline hydrochloride are reached between 4.5 and 8.4 hours after ingestion. Food increases the availability of sertraline slightly and peak blood levels are higher and are reached more quickly. Dosage, however, does not require adjusting, and sertraline may be taken with or without food. During the first pass, sertraline undergoes extensive N-demethylation in the liver to form N-desmethylsertraline, which has a half-life of 62 to 104 hours but is significantly less pharmacologically active than sertraline. Both sertraline and N-desmethylsertraline subsequently undergo oxidative deamination followed by reduction, hydroxylation, and glucuronide conjugation. The average termination half-life of plasma sertraline is about 26 hours. Steady-state plasma levels at a given dose occur within about 7 days. The medication and metabolites are excreted in about equal amounts in the feces and urine, although all unmetabolized sertraline (about 13%) is found in the urine.

Data provided by the manufacturer suggest that patients in the pediatric age range, 6 through 17 years old, metabolize sertraline with slightly greater efficacy than do adults. Nevertheless, because of their lower body weights, lower doses than that prescribed for adults may be advisable (*PDR*, 2000).

Alderman et al. (1998) explored single 50-mg-dose and steady-state (200 mg/day) pharmacokinetics of sertraline in 61 patients (age range, 6 to 17 years). The authors found that all pharmacokinetic parameters for serum sertraline and des-methylsertraline levels were similar for their patients and those reported for adults when corrected for weight. They concluded that the titration regimen recommended for adults was suitable and safe.

In their study of 92 children and adolescents prescribed sertraline for the treatment of OCD, March et al. (1998) reported that trough plasma levels of sertraline and its active metabolite desmethylsertraline, normalized for body weight, did not correlate significantly with age, sex, or clinical response.

Axelson et al. (2002) reported that the pharmacokinetics of sertraline varied significantly in adolescents (mean age 15.1; range 13.1 to 17.9 years) according to dose. The mean steady-state half-life at 50 mg/day was 15.3 ± 3.5 hours compared with 20.4 ± 3.4 hours at a dose of 100 to 150 mg/day. Because of this, they recommended that sertraline should be administered twice daily if adolescents were receiving <200 mg daily. The authors also measured platelet serotonin reuptake inhibition. They found that after 2 weeks' treatment with 50 mg/day of sertraline, platelet serotonin uptake was <70% in six of nine subjects and concluded that most adolescents need sertraline doses higher than 50 mg daily to achieve an adequate therapeutic response.

Alderman et al. (2006) reported the tolerability and efficacy of long-term sertraline use up to 200 mg/day in children and adolescents (age range 6 to 18 years). Over the 24-week study period, no significant age or gender effects or age-by-gender interactions were observed in sertraline values. Mean sertraline plasma concentrations normalized for dose and body weight did not differ significantly by age or gender. This study suggests that long-term treatment with sertraline in children and adolescents results in dose-normalized plasma concentration similar to that seen in adults.

Contraindications for the Administration of Sertraline Hydrochloride

Known hypersensitivity to sertraline hydrochloride is a contraindication.

Because of a possibility for serious, life-threatening reactions when administered simultaneously with an MAOI, the use of sertraline in combination with an MAOI is contraindicated. At least 14 days should elapse after stopping an MAOI before administering sertraline. On the basis of the half-life of sertraline, at least 14 days should elapse following its discontinuation before administering an MAOI.

Untoward Effects of Sertraline Hydrochloride

The most common side effects of sertraline in premarketing controlled studies included nausea, insomnia, diarrhea, ejaculatory delay, and somnolence. March et al. (1998) reported in a multicenter, 12-week, placebo-controlled trial of 187 children and adolescents (age range, 6 to 17 years) that four untoward effects occurred significantly more frequently in the subjects receiving sertraline: insomnia (37% vs. 13%; $P < .001$); nausea (17% vs. 7%, $P = .05$); agitation (13% vs. 2%, $P = .005$); and tremor (7% vs. 0%, $P = .01$). Additional untoward effects that occurred in at least 2% of the patients of the March et al. study and at least at twice the rate reported in patients on placebo were hyperkinesia, twitching, fever, malaise, purpura, weight loss, impaired concentration, manic reaction, emotional lability, abnormal thinking, and epistaxis (*PDR*, 2000). There is one case report of serotonin syndrome occurring in a 9-year-old boy following administration of a single 50-mg dose of sertraline (Phan et al., 2008).

Effects of Sertraline on the Heart

Wilens et al. (1999) prospectively assessed cardiovascular functions (vital signs and ECG parameters) of the 187 children and adolescents diagnosed with OCD and treated with sertraline ($N = 92$) or placebo ($N = 95$), as discussed later in the report by March et al. (1998). Baseline data were contrasted with data from weeks 1, 4, and 12 of the study. There were no clinically significant differences in supine or standing heart rates or systolic or diastolic blood pressures between the two groups. There were no significant differences in PR, QRS, or QTc, and no significant new developments of sinus arrhythmias, nodal abnormalities, or intraventricular conduction abnormalities with the exception of two subjects on sertraline who developed a QTc interval of >440 ms ($P = .05$); no subject developed a QTc interval of >460 ms. The authors concluded that monotherapy with sertraline in doses of up to 200 mg/day in healthy children and adolescents was not associated with any symptomatic or asymptomatic clinically significant cardiovascular untoward effects, but cautioned that the sample size precluded conclusions regarding small differences or rare events.

Reports of Interest

Sertraline in the Treatment of Children and Adolescents with OCD

Skarphedinsson et al. (2015) conducted an RTC examining the effectiveness of add-on sertraline (SRT) versus continued CBT in children and adolescents who have not responded to an initial course of CBT for OCD. Fifty-four subjects (ages 7 to 17 years), who had been classified as nonresponders after 14 weekly sessions of CBT, were randomized to SRT or CBT for 16 weeks. Twenty-one of 28 participants completed CBT, whereas 15 of 22 participants completed SRT. No significant between-group differences were found for SRT versus continued CBT.

March et al. (1998) reported a multicenter randomized double-blind, placebo-controlled 12-week, parallel-group trial of sertraline versus placebo in 187 patients diagnosed with OCD by DSM-III-R criteria. There were 107 children aged 6 to 12 years, of whom 53 received active medication and 54 were given placebo, and 80 adolescents aged 13 to 17 years, of whom 39 received active medication and 41 were given placebo. The four main dependent-outcome measures for efficacy were the CY-BOCS, the National Institute of Mental Health Global Obsessive-Compulsive Scale (NIMH GOCS), and the NIMH Clinical Global Impressions–Severity of Illness (CGI-S) and CGI-I rating scales. Subjects had at least moderate impairment and absence of significant depression. Sertraline was initiated at 25 mg/day for children and 50 mg/day for adolescents and titrated upward by 50 mg weekly for 4 weeks, until a maximum of 200 mg/day or the maximum tolerated dose was achieved. Patients then continued to receive this dosage for weeks 5 through 12 of the study. Mean dose of sertraline at endpoint was 167 mg/day for the 92 subjects on sertraline.

Patients receiving sertraline improved significantly more than did patients on placebo on the CY-BOCS ($P = .005$), the NIMH GOCS ($P = .02$), and the CGI-I Scale ($P = .002$). Untoward effects reported were described earlier; the authors note they may have increased because the protocol required the dose to be titrated upward so rapidly. There was no evidence that sertraline caused clinically significant changes in vital signs, laboratory values, or ECG.

March et al. (1998) concluded that sertraline appears to be a safe and effective short-term treatment for OCD in this age group. There was no significant difference in the untoward effects of sertraline in children compared with those in adolescents. The authors recommended an initial sertraline dose of 50 mg/day, titrated over a period of 6 to 8 weeks to reach maximum doses in partial or nonresponders. For an adequate clinical trial, sertraline should be taken for at least 10 to 12 weeks.

Sertraline in the Treatment of Children and Adolescents with OCD or Depression

Alderman et al. (1998) treated 29 children and 32 adolescents diagnosed by DSM-III-R (APA, 1987) criteria with OCD ($N = 16$), MDD ($N = 44$), or both ($N = 1$) for 5 weeks with sertraline titrated to 200 mg/day. Efficacy was assessed by ratings of the CY-BOCS, the NIMH GOCS, and the CGI-S and CGI-I scales.

At the end of the 5 weeks on sertraline, scores on the CY-BOCS for the 17 patients diagnosed with OCD decreased significantly from baseline (24.9 vs. 12.9; $P < .001$), scores on the NIMH GOCS declined significantly from baseline (10.2 vs. 6.7; $P < .001$), and scores on the CGI-S declined from 4.8 to 2.8 ($P < .001$). Ratings on the CGI-S for the 41 patients with depression who completed the 5-week period on sertraline declined significantly from 4.8 to 2.8 ($P < .001$). Overall, 51 subjects reported at least one untoward effect, but most were mild or moderate: headache (21%), nausea (21%), insomnia (21%), somnolence (15%), dyspepsia (12%), and anorexia (12%). Medication was discontinued in three of the children with depression because of the development of moderate hyperactivity in one, nervousness attributed to family stress in another, and severe self-mutilation in the third. The authors concluded that their results suggest that sertraline, administered as recommended for adults, is safe and effective in the treatment of subjects 6 to 17 years of age diagnosed with OCD or MDD.

Sertraline in the Treatment of Children and Adolescents with Major Depression

McConville and colleagues (1996) found in an open-label sertraline trial of 13 inpatients (3 males and 10 females; age range, 12 to 18 years) with MDD that at a dose range was 25 to 200 mg/day, mean ratings on the three scales (Ham-D, Montgomery-Asberg Depression Scale [M-ADS], and CGI-D) measuring depressive symptoms decreased significantly from premedication baseline to 12 weeks ($P < .001$ in all cases), with 11 of the 13 patients experiencing a decrease of more than 50% in their Ham-D scores. Because of a sharp drop in depressive symptoms during the first week on sertraline, which was attributed to placebo or non-medication effects (e.g., hospitalization), authors also analyzed changes from the end of treatment week 1 to the end of treatment week 12. All were still significant (Ham-D, $P = .027$; M-ADS, $P = .022$; and CGI-D, $P = .029$). The most frequent untoward effects at 12 weeks were insomnia (69%), drowsiness (61%), weight change (46%), nightmares (39%), loss of appetite (31%), and headache (31%). In this early small inpatient study, authors concluded that sertraline was a promising medication for the treatment of adolescent MDD (McConville et al., 1996).

Ambrosini et al. (1999) reported the combined data of six university-affiliated outpatient clinics that treated 53 adolescents (age range, 12.2 to 19.8 years), diagnosed with MDD with sertraline in a 10-week, open-label, acute-phase study. Thirty-seven subjects (70%) had a single episode and 16 (30%) had recurrent MDD; the mean duration of the index depressive episode was 78 ± 79 weeks, and most subjects had moderate ($N = 29$ [55%]) or severe ($N = 22$ [42%]) symptoms by DSM-III-R criteria (APA, 1987). Severity of illness and efficacy were rated on the Schedule for Affective Disorders and Schizophrenia (SADS), HDRS, the CGAS, Beck Depression Inventory (BDI), and the CGI-S and CGI-I scales. The mean sertraline dose at week 6 was 93.3 ± 20 mg/day and at week 10 was 127.2 ± 45 mg/day.

By week 2, there was significant improvement over baseline ($P = .0001$) in scores on the HDRS, the 17-item depression rating scale (part of the Mini-SADS), the BDI, and the CGI-S. Response rates improved with time throughout the study. The response rate on the 17-item scale, the most sensitive indicator of depressive symptoms, increased from 55% of subjects at 6 weeks to 76% by 10 weeks. On the HDRS, 26 (55.3%) subjects had a reduction in their scores by at least 50% by week 10. Response did not correlate with the age of the subject or baseline severity of depressive symptoms. Twenty-two of the 26 responders completed the additional 12-week period on sertraline, during which they maintained their improvement or improved further. Untoward effects occurred in about 10% of the patients and were usually mild to moderate in severity, including headache (36%), insomnia (26%), nausea (17%), dizziness (15%), flulike symptoms (13%), diarrhea (13%), fatigue (11%), agitation (11%), and somnolence (11%). No patient developed manic symptoms. The only patient to discontinue sertraline did so because of akathisia.

The authors concluded that their data suggested that sertraline in doses of up to 200 mg/day was efficacious and safe in treating chronically depressed adolescent outpatients with moderate to severe MDD. They emphasized that, in the acute phase of treatment, it is important to administer sertraline for at least 10 weeks and that improvement can continue even after 10 weeks (Ambrosini et al., 1999).

Wagner et al. (2003) reported on the results of two multicenter randomized, double-blind placebo-controlled trials that were conducted at 53 sites that examined the use of sertraline for MDD. The study enrolled 367 children and adolescents aged 6 to 17 years. Subjects met the diagnostic criteria for MDD as defined by DSM-IV and as determined by K-SADS-PL at the first and third visits of a 2-week screening period. The mean dose of patients who completed 10 weeks of double-blind treatment was 131 mg/day of sertraline and 144 mg/day of placebo equivalent.

Treatment outcomes were assessed with the CDRS-R and CGI-S. The sertraline-treated group experienced statistically significant greater improvement than placebo patients on the CDRS-R total score. They had a mean change at week 10 of −30.24 versus −25.83, respectively, $P = .001$. Sixty-nine percent of sertraline-treated patients compared with 59% of placebo patients were considered responders ($P = .05$).

Sertraline was generally well tolerated by the study subjects. The four AEs that occurred in at least 5% of the sertraline-treated subjects with an incidence of at least twice that of placebo were diarrhea, vomiting, anorexia, and agitation. Serious adverse events (SAEs) were seen in seven sertraline-treated patients and in six placebo patients. Suicide attempts were seen in two sertraline subjects and in two placebo subjects. Suicidal ideation was seen in three sertraline subjects. Aggressive reaction was seen in one sertraline subject. Medical hospitalization occurred in one sertraline subject and in four placebo subjects.

The authors concluded that their pooled analysis demonstrates that sertraline is an effective and well-tolerated short-term treatment for children and adolescents with MDD. They note that their study showed a medication–placebo difference similar to that found by Emslie and colleagues (2002) with fluoxetine.

Rynn and colleagues (2006) followed up the subjects in this study in a long-term (24 week) open-label observational extension study. Two hundred twenty-one of 299 patients in the original study chose to continue. All patients were initially dosed with 50 mg of sertraline regardless of their final study-medication dose taken. Doses were flexibly titrated in the range of 50 to 200 mg/day. Subjects who had received placebo in the initial study received their first dose of sertraline in the extension study. By the conclusion of the study, the mean daily dose was 109.9 mg/day. They found that patients continued to improve. The mean overall CDRS-R score at endpoint was 29.4 (SD ± 12.62), which is indicative of mild depressive symptomatology. By the end of the study, 86% of patients were considered CDRS-R responders and 58% had CDRS-R scores indicative of remission of their depressive symptoms. They had 18 subjects discontinue their medicine related to sertraline, 9 from AEs, 1 from a laboratory abnormality (elevated liver function test), and 8 from lack of efficacy.

Sertraline Hydrochloride in the Treatment of Children Diagnosed with Anxiety

Rynn et al. (2001) examined the treatment of children with GAD with sertraline in a randomized placebo-controlled trial. They enrolled 22 children and adolescents aged 5 to 17 who met DSM-IV criteria for GAD according to the Anxiety Disorders Interview Schedule for Children–Revised and who also had a Hamilton Anxiety Rating Scale score over 16. Sertraline was dosed 25 mg the first week and increased to 50 mg in the second. Subjects were followed up with nine weekly medication management visits for the 9-week treatment phase. They were not allowed to participate in CBT, but were allowed to continue other psychotherapies in which they had been participating. At the end of the evaluation period, subjects receiving sertraline showed improvement in Hamilton Anxiety Scale (Ham-A) total score, and CGI-S and CGI-I scales showed significant improvement with sertraline treatment when compared with that in the placebo group. Ninety percent of the patients who received sertraline were rated as improved (10 of 11) compared with only 10% of the placebo group (1 of 11). Two patients in the sertraline group were rated as markedly improved, representing a likely remission rate of 18%. This study was limited by small sample size and relatively low sertraline dose (50 mg) in older adolescents, but points to the usefulness of sertraline for youth with GAD.

Sertraline Hydrochloride in the Treatment of Children Diagnosed with Selective Mutism

Carlson et al. (1999) treated five outpatients (one male and four females; age range, 5 to 11 years) diagnosed with selective mutism by DSM-IV (APA, 1994) criteria in a 16-week, double-blind, placebo-controlled trial of sertraline within a replicated multiple-baseline/across-participants research design. There were four randomly ordered treatment phases: no medication for 2 weeks, placebo for 2 to 6 weeks, 50 mg/day of sertraline for 2 weeks, and 100 mg/day of sertraline for 6 to 10 weeks (subjects who were assigned to longer placebo periods had a respectively shorter time on 100 mg/day of sertraline). Selective mutism had been present from 2 to 7 years in the subjects. Subjects had no comorbid psychiatric conditions, no prior pharmacologic treatment of their selective mutism, or ongoing psychotherapy, although all five had previously had behavioral therapy and three had had individual psychotherapy. Efficacy was determined by ratings on goal attainment scaling to quantify the progress toward a target behavior, for example, speaking; both parents and teachers rated children on this scale. CGI-S ratings adapted for mutism, anxiety, and shyness were completed by parent, teacher, and psychiatrist. Improvement in speaking occurred within a few days of beginning sertraline in four of the five subjects as rated by parents. Two of the five subjects were speaking in school and no longer met criteria for selective mutism after <10 weeks of receiving sertraline. Parents of a third subject taking 50 mg/day of sertraline reported that their daughter was speaking in school and in other settings at follow-up 20 weeks after the study. Untoward effects were minimal and did not require dose reduction. The results suggest that sertraline may be useful in treating selective mutism in this age group.

Sertraline Hydrochloride in the Treatment of Children Diagnosed with Post-traumatic Stress Disorder

Given its effectiveness in adults, researchers have sought to show that sertraline is also helpful as a psychopharmacologic intervention in children and adolescents. The effectiveness of sertraline in the treatment of post-traumatic stress disorder (PTSD) was examined in a double-blind placebo-controlled trial by Robb et al. (2010), which yielded negative results. In this multicenter trial, youth who met criteria for PTSD after a 2-week assessment period were enrolled in the 10-week trial and given either flexible doses of sertraline (50 to 200 mg/day) or a placebo. One hundred thirty-one patients were randomized to receive sertraline or placebo. The study found that there was no difference on the UCLS PTSD-I (University of California Los Angeles Post-Traumatic Stress Disorder Index) scores between the sertraline and the placebo group. Both groups had improvement in the assessment measures, but the placebo group had more improvement than did the sertraline group. An interim analysis of the study data was performed, and the study was stopped for futility after 81.8% of the initially planned subject group was enrolled.

Another study by Cohen et al. (2007) found little benefit to adding sertraline to an already established effective treatment for PTSD in children: trauma-focused cognitive behavior therapy (TF-CBT). In this study, 25 females aged 10 to 17 were randomly assigned to receive TF-CBT + placebo or TF-CBT + sertraline for 12 weeks. Both groups had significant improvement in their PTSD and clinical outcome measures. No differences were found in most measures except that the CGI ratings suggested a slight improvement in the sertraline TF-CBT group. The authors conclude that sertraline could have caused some improvement in comorbid depression symptoms.

Stoddard et al. (2011) examined the effect of sertraline to prevent PTSD in burned children. In this study, 26 children aged 6 to 20 years who were admitted to a pediatric burn center were screened and randomized to receive either sertraline dosed between 25 and 150 mg or placebo in a double-blind placebo-controlled design. The subjects who received sertraline had no difference in child-reported symptoms from their peers who received placebo. The sertraline group did show a greater decrease in parent-reported symptoms over the course of the study. This suggests that sertraline may prevent the emergence of PTSD symptoms in children.

Citalopram Hydrobromide (Celexa)

The SSRI citalopram hydrobromide is a racemic bicyclic phthalane derivative that is chemically unrelated to other SSRIs or to tricyclic, tetracyclic, and other antidepressants.

Citalopram has minimal effects on the neuronal reuptake of norepinephrine and dopamine. It has no or very low affinity for 5-HT_{1A}, 5-HT_{2A}, dopamine D_1, and D_2, alpha-1, alpha-2, or beta-adrenergic, histamine H_1, GABA, muscarinic, cholinergic, and benzodiazepine receptors.

Pharmacokinetics of Citalopram Hydrobromide

Food does not affect the bioavailability of citalopram hydrobromide. Peak serum levels occur about 4 hours after ingestion. With once-daily dosing, steady-state plasma levels occur in approximately 1 week and are about 2.5 times the concentration observed after a single dose.

Metabolism occurs primarily by N-demethylation in the liver, with CYP3A4 and CYP2C19 being the primary enzymes involved. The parent compound is at least eight times more active than its metabolites, suggesting that they do not play a significant role clinically. Mean terminal half-life is about 35 hours.

Contraindications for Administration of Citalopram Hydrobromide

Known hypersensitivity to citalopram hydrobromide is a contraindication.

Because of a possibility of serious, life-threatening reactions when administered simultaneously with an MAOI, it is recommended that the medication not be used in combination with an MAOI. At least 2 weeks should elapse after stopping citalopram before administering an MAOI and, conversely, after stopping an MAOI before administering citalopram.

Untoward Effects of Citalopram Hydrobromide

Dry mouth, increased sweating, nausea, diarrhea, somnolence or insomnia, ejaculatory disturbance (in 6%, usually ejaculatory delay) have been reported in individuals taking citalopram.

In 2011, the FDA issued safety warnings concerning the use of citalopram. At higher doses, citalopram can cause abnormal changes to the electrical activity of the heart. These changes, known as prolongation of the QT interval, can lead to fatal changes in the heart's rhythm. The risk increases with higher dosing of citalopram and the maximum dose was lowered to 40 mg from 60 mg. They also recommend monitoring of ECG and electrolytes in cases where citalopram is an essential to treatment at higher doses. Baseline potassium and magnesium measurement and periodic monitoring are recommended as hypokalemia and/or hypomagnesemia can increase risk of QTc prolongation (Silva, 2012).

Klein-Schwartz et al. (2012) performed an 11-year retrospective analysis of national poison center data for children younger than age 6 who had ingested SS-RIs. Following citalopram ingestion, pediatric patients were noted to have a higher occurrence of seizures and cardiac toxicity, specifically conduction disturbances and other ECG changes, compared to ingestions of other SSRIs. Children generally develop minimal toxicity with SSRI ingestions, and the overall hazard of all SSRIs compared to other antidepressants is lower. The hazard index for citalopram was 2.8-fold higher than that for other SSRIs, which mirrors trends of hazard indices for overdose in adults. This relative difference was not enough to result in recommendations to triage outpatient pediatric citalopram ingestions differently from other SSRIs. In addition, this review did not identify dose thresholds for predicting either seizures or cardiac toxicity.

Advantages of Citalopram Hydrobromide

There was no clinically significant difference between placebo and citalopram on cardiac parameters, including electroconductivity from baseline ECG. The only significant difference was a mean decrease in cardiac rate of 1.7 beats per minute.

Reports of Interest

Citalopram Hydrobromide in the Treatment of Children and Adolescents Diagnosed with MDD

Wagner et al. (2004b) conducted a randomized double-blind placebo-controlled trial of citalopram in the treatment of children and adolescents with major depression. Citalopram was initiated at 20 mg/day with the potential to increase to 40 mg after week 4 if clinically necessary. The overall mean citalopram dose was 24 mg/day. Outcome was assessed with change in baseline of CDRS at week 8 or termination from the study. Secondary measures included the CGI-I. A total of 178 patients were enrolled in the study. Citalopram treatment showed statistically significant improvement on CDRS when compared with placebo as early as week 1. Improvements continued at every observation point to the end of the study. The difference in response rate at week 8 between placebo (24%) and citalopram (36%) was statistically significant. Side effects were mild with nausea, rhinitis, and abdominal pain occurring in only ≥10% of citalopram-treated patients. There were no reports of mania in this study. Two placebo-group patients were discontinued form the study because of aggravated depression, and two patients on citalopram had agitation, requiring discontinuation from the study. ECG results, laboratory values, and weight did not have any clinically significant change.

Shirazi and Alaghband-Rad (2005) conducted an open-label trial of citalopram in children and adolescents with depression in Iran. In their trial, 30 children aged 8 to 17 were enrolled. Subjects diagnosed with MDD were given citalopram 10 to 40 mg for 6 weeks. Outcomes were measured using the HDRS and CGAS. They found improvement in HDRS and CGAS in the moderate (50% to 70% improvement) to large (>70% improvement) range in 91.7% of the children in the study. They also noted that most subjects showed improvement in symptoms 102 weeks after onset of medication. They did have five subjects (16.7%), three boys and two girls, with a mean age of 12.6, develop mania, which required them to discontinue the medication. These subjects were all taking 20 mg of citalopram from the beginning of the study and developed mania by the second week. The authors caution against using citalopram because of this high switch rate to mania.

Citalopram Hydrobromide in the Treatment of Children and Adolescents Diagnosed with OCD

Thomsen (1997) treated 23 subjects (age range 9 to 18 years) diagnosed with OCD by DSM-III-R (APA, 1987) criteria with citalopram in a 10-week, open-label study. An initial dose of 10 mg of citalopram was given approximately 2 weeks after referral and gradually titrated to a target dose of 40 mg/day. The mean dose of citalopram at the end of the 10 weeks was 37.0 ± 0.8 mg/day, with a dose range of 10 to 40 mg/day. Efficacy was assessed by ratings on the Y-BOCS or its version for children (CY-BOCS) <15 years old, the Children's Assessment Schedule, and the CGAS. Posttreatment (10-week) ratings on the Y-BOCS or CY-BOCS improved significantly over baseline (mean scores declined from 30.1 to 20.9; $P = .001$). Improvement in social functioning was reflected by scores on the CGAS, which improved significantly from baseline to posttreatment ratings (mean scores increased from 59.1 to 71.0; $P = .001$). Overall, however, only six patients improved sufficiently so as to no longer meet the diagnostic criteria for OCD, and they continued to have symptoms of subclinical OCD. Mild untoward effects were reported by 13 subjects; dry mouth, headache, and tremor were transient, resolving within a few weeks. Restlessness occurred in four patients, increased anxiety in two patients, and erectile dysfunction in one patient. The findings suggested that citalopram may be effective and well tolerated in children and adolescents diagnosed with OCD at doses of up to 40 mg/day.

Alaghband-Rad and Hakimshooshtary (2009) reported on their results of a randomized controlled clinical trial of citalopram versus fluoxetine in children and adolescents with OCD. Twenty-nine subjects aged 7 to 18 with OCD were enrolled in the study and randomized to receive either citalopram 20 mg or fluoxetine 20 mg. They chose to compare citalopram to fluoxetine as the effectiveness of fluoxetine to treat pediatric OCD had been demonstrated in prior studies (Geller et al., 2001; Riddle et al., 1992). The study lasted 6 weeks and outcome was measured with the CY-BOCS and the CGI. At the conclusion of the study, each group demonstrated significant improvement in their CY-BOCS scores from baseline ($P < .01$), but they did not find any improvement in CGI. They also did not show any differences in safety or efficacy between citalopram and fluoxetine. They did have one subject receiving citalopram drop out after having a hypomanic episode; another subject who received fluoxetine also had a hypomanic episode.

Citalopram Hydrobromide in the Treatment of Children and Adolescents Diagnosed with Autism Spectrum Disorder

King and colleagues (2009) investigated the efficacy of citalopram in a placebo-controlled trial of children with ASD. One hundred forty-nine youth 5 to 17 years old were randomized to receive citalopram ($N = 73$) or placebo ($N = 76$). Subjects were included if they met criteria for an ASD which included autism, Asperger disorder, or PDDNOS. Citalopram was administered in the liquid version and was started at 2.5 mg/day and increased by 2.5 mg/week initially and then 5 mg/week increments to a maximum of 20 mg/day. Subjects were followed up for 12 weeks and improvement was measured by CGI and CY-BOCS modified for pervasive developmental disorders (PDDs). The authors hypothesized that youth with high levels of repetitive behaviors would respond to citalopram in a model similar to OCD response. At the conclusion of the study, no significant difference was found in response between the citalopram and placebo groups. The citalopram group did have more side AEs. Increased energy level, impulsiveness, decreased concentration, hyperactivity, stereotypy, diarrhea, insomnia, and dry skin were seen more often in the citalopram group. They also had two subjects on citalopram have seizures. One subject had a preexisting seizure disorder and was able to remain in the study with an increased dose of anticonvulsants. The other subject developed a prolonged seizure and continued to have frequent seizures after citalopram was discontinued and was withdrawn from the study. This trial does not support the use of citalopram for the treatment of repetitive behavior in children with ASDs and also questions the safety of these medications in this diagnostic group.

Escitalopram Oxalate (Lexapro)

Escitalopram oxalate is the pure S-enantiomer, the active isomer, of racemic citalopram, an SSRI.

Pharmacokinetics of Escitalopram Oxalate

Escitalopram oxalate may be taken with or without food. Maximum plasma levels occur about 5 hours after ingestion of the medication. Escitalopram oxalate has a half-life of about 27 to 32 hours. Steady-state plasma levels occur in approximately 1 week at a given dose. Escitalopram oxalate is metabolized primarily through demethylation by the hepatic enzymes CYP3A4 and CYP2C19. About 18% is excreted in the urine.

Contraindications for the Administration of Escitalopram Oxalate

Hypersensitivity to escitalopram oxalate, any of its inactive ingredients, or citalopram is a contraindication to its administration. Because escitalopram is the active isomer of racemic citalopram, the two medications should not be administered together.

Escitalopram oxalate should not be coadministered with an MAOI or within 14 days of treatment with an MAOI being discontinued. At least 14 days should elapse after stopping escitalopram oxalate therapy before administering an MAOI.

Untoward Effects of Escitalopram Oxalate

Untoward effects include GI disorders, especially nausea (15%), insomnia (9%), somnolence (6%), increased sweating (5%), fatigue (5%), and decreased appetite (3%). Sexual untoward effects in males include ejaculation disorder (12%, most of which was accounted for by delayed ejaculation), decreased libido (6%) and impotence (3%); in females, they include decreased libido (3%) and anorgasmia (3%). Of note, untoward effects were approximately twice as frequent in patients treated with 20 mg of escitalopram daily compared with patients treated with 10 mg daily.

No significant ECG changes were reported. There is a report of prolonged QTc interval change in a 14-year-old girl with escitalopram overdose (Scharko & Schumacher, 2008). The youth ingested 200 mg of escitalopram and her QTc the day after ingestion was 450 ms. Two days after ingestion, it was 469 ms and normalized later that day to 420 ms.

Reports of Interest

Escitalopram Oxalate in the Treatment of Children and Adolescents Diagnosed with MDD

Findling et al. (2013) evaluated the efficacy, safety, and tolerability of escitalopram 10 to 20 mg/day in adolescents (ages 12 to 17) with MDD in a 16- to 24-week multisite extension study following an 8-week randomized, double-blind, flexible-dose, placebo-controlled trial. Patients maintained the same randomized group and dosage during the extension; primary efficacy was evaluated with the CDRS-R, whereas secondary efficacy utilized the CGI-I. Safety was evaluated with AE reports and the Columbia-Suicide Severity Rating Scale (C-SSRS). Total score improvement on CDRS-R was significantly greater for escitalopram than for placebo, and both response and remission rates were significantly higher for escitalopram than for placebo. Headache, insomnia, vomiting, influenza-like symptoms, diarrhea, and urinary tract infection were more frequent in the treatment group than with placebo, although these were mild to moderate and most were not felt to be related to the study drug. Suicidal behavior and/or ideation was 10.9% for placebo and 14.5% for escitalopram.

Wagner and colleagues (2006) conducted a double-blind randomized placebo-controlled trial of escitalopram in the treatment of pediatric depression. Study participants were screened and enrolled if their CDRS-R score was at least 40 at the initial screening and baseline visits; this scale also served as the primary outcome measure. The study enrolled 268 patients; 104 children aged 6 to 11 years and 160 adolescents aged 12 to 17 years were randomized to receive either escitalopram or placebo. Escitalopram dose was 10 mg for the first 4 weeks and then flexibly dosed to 10 to 20 mg/day depending on clinical response and tolerability of the study medication. Eighty-two percent of the subjects completed the 8-week study. Escitalopram did not significantly improve CDRS-R scores when compared with placebo at endpoint for the total group. When the data were analyzed for adolescents only (12 to 17 years), escitalopram significantly improved CDRS-R scores in this group alone. The lack of efficacy in younger patients is attributed to the high placebo response rate (52.3%). Headache and abdominal pain were the only AEs in >10% of the escitalopram group. Potential suicide-related events were observed in one patient on escitalopram and two on placebo. One subject on placebo had a manic reaction and no patients on escitalopram were observed to have mania. There were no completed suicides in the study. This was the first double-blind study of escitalopram that suggested some efficacy in adolescents but not children.

Emslie and colleagues (2009) completed a randomized, double-blind, placebo-controlled multisite trial of escitalopram in the treatment of adolescent depression. Three hundred sixteen adolescents aged 12 to 17 were randomized to receive placebo (158) or escitalopram (158). The escitalopram dose was initiated at 10 mg/day for the first 3 weeks and then increased to 20 mg/day at the end of week 3 or 4. Response was assessed using the CDRS-R. At the conclusion, 83% of the study subjects completed the 8 weeks of double-blind treatment. Improvement seen in the escitalopram group was significant when compared with the placebo group. The CDRS-R score for the escitalopram group was -22.1 versus -18.8 for placebo, $P = .22$. AEs seen in the escitalopram group, which occurred in at least 10% of the patients, were headache, menstrual cramps, insomnia, and nausea. Only influenza-like symptoms occurred in at least 5% of the escitalopram group and at least twice the incidence of placebo (7.1% vs. 3.2%). Discontinuation rates caused by AEs were 2.6% for escitalopram and 0.6% for placebo. There were 12 AEs that were considered to be suggestive of self-harm; 6 occurred in each group (3.8% of placebo and 3.9% of escitalopram patients). In the Emslie and colleagues study, escitalopram was effective and well tolerated in the treatment of depressed adolescents. This positive study, along with others, led the FDA to approve escitalopram for the treatment of depression in adolescents in March 2009.

Escitalopram Oxalate in the Treatment of Children and Adolescents Diagnosed with PDDs

Owley et al. (2005a) assessed the effectiveness of escitalopram in the treatment of 28 subjects (25 males and 3 females; age range 6 to 17 years) who were diagnosed with PDDs (autistic disorder, 20 [71%]; Asperger disorder, 5 [18%]; and PDDNOS, 3 [11%]) in a 10-week, open-label forced-titration study. Inclusion criteria included a score of >12 on the Irritability Subscale of the Aberrant Behavior Checklist–Community Version (ABC-CV). The primary outcome measures were the CGI-S Scale and the ABC-CV. A subject with a reduction of >50% on the ABC-CV irritability subscale was defined as a "responder."

Escitalopram was initiated at a dose of 2.5 mg daily with forced weekly increases to 5, 10, 15, and 20 mg as of the fifth week. If predetermined problems with sleep or significant increases in irritability or hyperactivity on the subscales of the ABC-CV occurred, the dose was reduced to that of the preceding week and maintained there for the duration of the study. At endpoint, the mean daily dose of escitalopram was 11.1 ± 6.5 mg with a range of 0 mg/day (a subject who developed disinhibition and aggression on the lowest permitted dose of 2.5 mg was dropped from the study) to 20 mg/day. The authors noted that some patients might be able to tolerate only doses as low as 1 mg/day without developing AEs. Of the 18 subjects for whom AEs were reported, who required reduction in dose to that of the preceding week, irritability was primarily responsible in 7, hyperactivity in 6, and both irritability and hyperactivity in 5. No subjects reported suicidal ideation, and there was no evidence of increased SIB or sleep difficulties. The responder rate was 17/28 (61%). On the ABC-CV Rating Scale, scores at week 10 were significantly improved on the Irritability, Lethargy, Stereotypy, and Hyperactivity subscales at $P < .001$ and on the Inappropriate Speech subscale at $P = .035$; the ABC-CV total score was also significant at $P < .001$. CGI-S mean score at baseline was 5.2 ± 1.0 and at endpoint was 4.6 ± 1.2 ($P < .001$). The authors concluded that escitalopram was useful in treating some common symptoms present in PDD and that controlled studies should be undertaken for such subjects.

Fluvoxamine Maleate (Luvox)

Fluvoxamine maleate is an SSRI that belongs to a new chemical series, the 2-aminoethyloxime ethers of aralkylketones. It is chemically unrelated to other SSRIs and clomipramine. In *in vitro* studies, the fluvoxamine exhibited no significant affinity for histaminergic, alpha- or beta-adrenergic, muscarinic, or dopamine receptors.

Pharmacokinetics of Fluvoxamine Maleate

Food does not significantly affect the bioavailability of fluvoxamine. In volunteers, peak plasma concentrations at steady state occurred between 3 and 8 hours after ingestion of the medication and revealed nonlinear pharmacokinetics for single doses of 100, 200, and 300 mg, with higher doses resulting in disproportionately higher plasma levels (e.g., plasma levels of 88, 283, and 546 ng/mL, respectively). The mean plasma half-life at steady state for young adults taking 100 mg/day was 15.6 hours.

Labellarte et al. (2004) reported on the multiple-dose pharmacokinetics of fluvoxamine maleate in 16 children (9 males and 7 females) and 18 adolescents (9 males and 9 females) being treated for OCD. They measured serum levels >12 hours after 12 or more consecutive doses of 25, 50, 100, and 150 mg of fluvoxamine. Maximum daily dose was 200 mg/day for children and 300 mg/day for adolescents, given in two doses 12 hours apart. Compared with adolescents, children had higher mean peak plasma concentrations, higher mean area under the plasma concentration–time curve, and lower apparent oral clearance; at a dose of 50 mg twice daily, adjusted mean serum level for children was 182.45 versus 67.50 ng/mL for adolescents ($P \le .05$). Compared with male children, female children had higher mean peak plasma concentration, higher mean area under the plasma concentration–time curve and reported more AEs. Adolescents had pharmacokinetics similar to those reported for adults on 150-mg, twice-daily doses. These data suggest that children, especially female children, have a higher exposure to fluvoxamine at a given dose than do adolescents and adults.

Smokers metabolize fluvoxamine maleate about 25% faster than do nonsmokers.

Contraindications for Fluvoxamine Maleate Administration

Known hypersensitivity to fluvoxamine maleate is a contraindication.

Coadministration of terfenadine, astemizole, or cisapride with fluvoxamine maleate is contraindicated. This is because fluvoxamine maleate is likely to be a potent inhibitor of P450 3A4 isoenzyme, which would cause increased levels of the previously mentioned medications and result in the lengthening of the QT interval, which has been associated with torsade de pointes–type ventricular tachycardia and fatalities.

Because of a possibility for serious, life-threatening reactions when administered simultaneously with an MAOI, the use of fluvoxamine maleate in combination with an MAOI is contraindicated. At least 14 days should elapse after stopping an

MAOI before administering fluvoxamine maleate. On the basis of the half-life of fluvoxamine maleate, at least 14 days should elapse following its discontinuation before administering an MAOI.

Interactions of Fluvoxamine Maleate with Other Medications

Benzodiazepines should be coadministered with great caution. Plasma levels and half-life of alprazolam were approximately doubled when it was given together with fluvoxamine, resulting in decreased psychomotor performance and memory; if coadministered, the dose of alprazolam should be reduced by at least 50% and gradually titrated to the lowest effective dose. Coadministration of diazepam is not recommended, as fluvoxamine maleate reduces its clearance and that of its major metabolite N-desmethyldiazepam, and clinically significant increases would be expected.

Many other potential interactions, particularly with medications that inhibit or are metabolized by cytochrome P450 isoenzymes, have been reported (package insert).

Untoward Effects of Fluvoxamine Maleate

The most frequently reported untoward effects were somnolence, insomnia, dry mouth, nervousness, tremor, nausea, dyspepsia, anorexia, vomiting, abnormal ejaculation, asthenia, and sweating. As decreased appetite and weight loss can occur with fluvoxamine, these parameters should be monitored.

Reports of Interest

Fluvoxamine Maleate in the Treatment of OCD

Riddle and colleagues (2001) studied the safety and efficacy of fluvoxamine in treating OCD in 120 subjects aged 8 to 17 in a double-blind, placebo-controlled, multicenter trial, over 10 weeks. Subjects with comorbidities were excluded from the study. The primary outcome measure was change from the baseline CY-BOCS total score. Dose range was 50 to 200 mg/day, with children aged 8 to 12 receiving a mean daily dose of 157 ± 55 mg by week 10 and adolescents 13 to 17 years old receiving a mean dose of 170 ± 46 mg by week 10. Mean CY-BOCS scores in the fluvoxamine group were statistically lower than in the placebo group at weeks 1, 2, 3, 4, 6, and 10 in the study. Defining response as a 25% reduction in the CY-BOCS scores, 42% of the fluvoxamine group were responders while 26% of the placebo group were responders. Further analysis showed that there was a higher proportion of responders in the younger age group, which may have been due to the dose limitation of 200 mg/day in the adolescents. AEs occurring in at least 10% of study participants (placebo-adjusted rate) were insomnia and asthenia; other AEs included dyspepsia, hyperkinesia, somnolence, and agitation. Vital sign abnormalities in the study included weight gain and decreases in both diastolic and systolic blood pressure, but these were observed in both study groups. None of the AEs or physical examination findings were considered serious. The authors concluded that fluvoxamine was well tolerated and efficacious in treating OCD in children and adolescents and commented on the similarity of mean CY-BOCS score reductions in this study and the March et al. (1998) study of sertraline to treat OCD (Riddle et al., 2001).

Fluvoxamine Maleate in the Treatment of Adolescents Diagnosed with MDD or OCD

Apter et al. (1994) reported treating 20 adolescent inpatients 13 to 18 years of age who were diagnosed with MDD ($N = 6$) or OCD ($N = 14$) with fluvoxamine in an 8-week, open-label protocol. Inclusion criteria for the six patients with depression included lack of response to a TCA, additional symptoms of suicidality, impulsivity or affective instability, or a comorbid major psychiatric diagnosis. Comorbidities in the MDD group included borderline personality and conduct disorders and bulimia. Comorbidities in the OCD group included Tourette syndrome (TS), schizophrenia, and anorexia nervosa. Fluvoxamine was increased by 50 mg weekly until either a therapeutic result was obtained or untoward effects prevented further increase. Doses ranged from 100 to 300 mg/day (mean, 200 mg/day). Sixteen patients completed the study, and four dropped out because of untoward effects; for the latter four patients, the last ratings while on medication were used in analyzing the data.

All six patients with MDD improved significantly on the BDI ($P < .0002$), but only two of the four patients with comorbid MDD and borderline personality disorder showed clinically significant decreases in impulsivity and suicidality.

As a group, the 14 patients with OCD improved significantly on the Yale–Brown Obsessive-Compulsive Scale (Y-BOCS) ($P < .0001$). Of note, statistically significant improvement over baseline ratings on the Y-BOCS did not occur until week 6, and there was further improvement at week 8.

All subjects developed at least some mild untoward effects compared with baseline ratings on the Dosage Record Treatment-Emergent Symptom Scale. Fluvoxamine initially caused some activating untoward effects, such as insomnia, hyperactivity, agitation, excitement, anxiety, and hypomania. These were mild and transient in most cases; however, one patient with a family history of bipolar disorder who developed hypomania was dropped during the fifth week. Nausea, tremor, and dermatitis occurred in about 75% of subjects; in one case, the medication had to be discontinued because of itchy maculopapular dermatitis. No changes in heart rate, blood pressure, ECG, or routine laboratory tests were reported. No patient showed a significant increase in ratings on the Suicide Potential or Overt Aggression Scales (Apter et al., 1994).

Fluvoxamine Maleate in the Treatment of Children and Adolescents Diagnosed with Anxiety Disorders

Walkup et al. (2001) reported findings of a multisite, double-blind, placebo-controlled trial of fluvoxamine in the treatment of 128 subjects (age range, 6 to 17 years) who were diagnosed with SP, SAD, or GAD and treated for 8 weeks with fluvoxamine or placebo. Fluvoxamine was titrated on an individual basis to a maximum of 300 mg/day. Efficacy was determined by ratings on the PARS and the CGI-I Scale. Fluvoxamine-treated subjects had significantly improved ratings on the PARS compared with subjects on placebo ($P < .001$). Their PARS scores decreased by 9.7 ± 6.9 points, whereas the placebo group had a decrease of 3.1 ± 4.8 points. On the CGI-I, 76% of subjects on fluvoxamine were rated as responders versus only 29% on placebo ($P < .001$). These data suggest that fluvoxamine may be an effective treatment for children and adolescents diagnosed with these three anxiety disorders.

Paroxetine Hydrochloride (Paxil), Paroxetine Mesylate (Pexeva)

Paroxetine hydrochloride, an SSRI, is the hydrochloride salt of a phenylpiperazine compound. Its chemical structure is unrelated to that of other SSRIs and antidepressants currently in use. Studies suggest that its antidepressant action and clinical efficacy in obsessive-compulsive, panic, and social anxiety disorders are related to its being a highly potent selective inhibitor of neuronal serotonin reuptake. In addition, paroxetine has only a very weak effect on the neuronal reuptake of norepinephrine and dopamine. Paroxetine has little affinity for muscarinic alpha-1-, alpha-2-, beta-adrenergic; dopamine (D_2); 5-HT_1, 5-HT_2; and histamine (H_1) receptors.

Pharmacokinetics of Paroxetine Hydrochloride

Food slightly increases bioavailability of paroxetine; it increases maximum plasma levels and decreases the time to reach peak plasma concentration from about 6.5 to 5 hours. Paroxetine may be administered with or without food without dosage adjustment. Paroxetine is extensively metabolized in the liver, in part by the P450 2D6 enzyme system. Its principal metabolites have only one-fiftieth the potency of the parent compound in inhibiting serotonin reuptake. About two-thirds of the medication is excreted in the urine and one-third in the feces. Serum half-life $(T_{1/2})$ is approximately 21 hours. Steady-state plasma levels usually occur within 10 days.

Findling et al. (1999) studied paroxetine pharmacokinetics in 30 children and adolescents (age range, 6 to 17 years; mean age, 11.2 ± 2.9 years), 15 of each sex, who were being treated for a diagnosis of MDD. The mean half-life of paroxetine in this age group was 11.1 ± 5.2 hours, considerably shorter than that in adults; however, steady-state plasma levels were still achieved with once-daily dosing.

There has been great interest in the role of all SSRIs in contributing to suicidal thoughts and behaviors in children and adolescents. Paroxetine was the first SSRI to have suicide concerns identified. The FDA issued a statement about the possibility of paroxetine increasing risk of suicidal thinking in children below 18 years of age in June 2003. The FDA recommended that paroxetine not be used to treat depression in children and adolescents, and similar warnings were issued by the United Kingdom's Chairman of the Committee on Safety of Medicines (Duff, 2003; FDA, 2003). A full discussion of the issue was discussed earlier in this chapter. An analysis of all subjects treated with paroxetine and placebo in double-blind trials was completed by Apter et al. (2006). One thousand one hundred ninety-one children and adolescents who received paroxetine or placebo in double-blind studies were blindly reviewed; incidents of AEs were reviewed and cases of suicidal or nonsuicidal behavior were examined. Incidence rates were calculated for suicide-related events and for rating scale items assessing suicidality. The authors found that suicide-related events occurred more often in paroxetine (22 of 642, 3.4%) than in placebo groups (5 of 549, 0.9%). Except for one child, all suicide-related events occurred in adolescents over 12. The authors conclude that adolescents treated with paroxetine showed an increased risk of suicide-related events.

Contraindications for the Administration of Paroxetine Hydrochloride

Known hypersensitivity to paroxetine hydrochloride is a contraindication.

Because of a possibility of serious, life-threatening reactions when administered simultaneously with an MAOI, the use of paroxetine in combination with an MAOI is contraindicated. At least 14 days should elapse after stopping an MAOI before administering paroxetine. On the basis of the half-life of paroxetine, at least 14 days should elapse following its discontinuation before administering an MAOI.

Untoward Effects of Paroxetine Hydrochloride

In clinical trials, between 16% and 20% of patients discontinued taking paroxetine for the following reasons: asthenia, sweating, nausea, decreased appetite, somnolence, dry mouth, dizziness, insomnia, tremor, nervousness, ejaculatory and other male sexual disturbances, and female sexual disorders.

Findling et al. (1999) reported that 2 (6.7%) of their 30 subjects (mean age, 11.2 ± 2.9 years) diagnosed with MDD and treated with paroxetine developed hypomania, requiring discontinuation of the medication. In both cases, the hypomanic symptoms remitted without complications following discontinuation.

Reports of Interest

Paroxetine in the Treatment of Children and Adolescents with MDD

Le Noury et al. (2016) analyzed the safety and relapse rates of paroxetine or imipramine versus placebo in a 6-month extended treatment phase following an 8-week double-blind RCT of adolescents with unipolar major depression. Thirty-one percent of patients on paroxetine and imipramine were responders after the initial trial compared with 39% on placebo. Forty-one percent of initial responders to paroxetine relapsed compared to 26% of patients taking imipramine and 21% of patients on placebo. Paroxetine had 211 AEs compared with 147 AEs with imipramine and 100 on placebo. The continuation phase was not felt to offer support for longer term efficacy of either paroxetine or imipramine.

Le Noury et al. (2015) reanalyzed a 2001 study by Keller and colleagues that compared the efficacy and safety of paroxetine and imipramine with placebo for treating adolescents with unipolar major depression. They found that contrary to the original study findings, efficacy of paroxetine and imipramine was not statistically significant or clinically significantly different from placebo for any primary or secondary outcome. Increases in clinically significant harms, such as suicidal ideation and behavior in the paroxetine group and cardiovascular problems in the imipramine group, were also identified by Le Noury and colleagues on their analysis of the data.

Berard et al. (2006) conducted a 12-week, prospective, international (10 different countries), multicenter (33 centers), randomized, double-blind, placebo-controlled, flexible-dose, parallel-group study of the safety and efficacy of paroxetine in the treatment of outpatient adolescents, age range 12 to 19 years, diagnosed with unipolar major depression by DSM-IV criteria. In these, 286 met study criteria and were randomly assigned at a 2:1 ratio to paroxetine ($N = 187$) or to placebo ($N = 99$). This was the first major depressive episode for approximately 83% of the subjects. Paroxetine was initiated at a dose of 20 mg daily, with a final dose range of 20 to 40 mg/day. During the study, 55 (30.2%) of the paroxetine group (including 11.8% because of AEs and 4.9% for lack of efficacy) and 24 (25.8%) of the placebo group (including 7.1% because of AEs and 6.5% for lack of efficacy) withdrew from the study.

Subjects meeting "responder" criteria on the Montgomery-Åsberg Depression Rating Scale included 60.5% of the paroxetine group and 58.2% of the placebo group, which did not differ significantly ($P = .70$) or clinically. On the K-SADS-L, the paroxetine group had a decrease of 9.3 points and the placebo group of 8.9 points, which did not differ significantly ($P = .62$) or clinically. Regarding secondary measures of efficacy, the two groups did not differ significantly on the CGI-S, the Mood and Feelings Questionnaires, or the BDI; however, the CGI-I Scale showed a significant difference between the groups. A rating of 1 (very much improved) or 2 (much improved) was present at endpoint for 69.2% of the paroxetine group versus 57.3% of the placebo group ($P = .045$). Further analysis by age subgroup indicated that this significance was contributed mainly by subjects 16 years or older.

AEs were also not statistically different between the paroxetine and placebo groups, being reported in 69% of the paroxetine group and 59.1% of the placebo group. The most frequent AEs reported in the paroxetine group were nausea, headache, dizziness, somnolence, decreased appetite, infection, and asthenia; only decreased appetite was statistically more frequent compared with the placebo group. AEs related to suicidality occurred in 4.4% of the paroxetine group and 2.1% of the placebo group, which was not statistically different ($P = .502$). Suicidal attempts were reported in three (1.7%) of the paroxetine group and two (2.1%) of the placebo group with no statistical difference between the groups ($P = 1.000$).

The authors concluded that there were no significant statistical or clinical differences between paroxetine and placebo in treating this group of adolescents diagnosed with MDD on the primary outcome variables; however, the CGI-I rate was significantly greater for the paroxetine group. They also suggested that adolescents >16 years may respond more favorably to paroxetine than do younger adolescents. The authors commented that paroxetine in the doses used (20 to 40 mg/day) was generally well tolerated in this age group (Berard et al., 2006).

Emslie et al. (2006) treated 206 subjects 7 to 17 years old with MDD with paroxetine or placebo for 8 weeks. In a randomized multicenter double-blind placebo-controlled trial, patients eligible for the study were randomized to receive paroxetine (10 to 50 mg) or placebo. A total of 73.4% of subjects completed the 8-week study. It was noted that a higher percentage of patients withdrew from the paroxetine group (30.7%) than did the placebo group (22.5%). This pattern was not evident in the 7- to 11-year-old subgroup, but was evident in the adolescent subgroup. The doses used in the paroxetine group were 20.4 mg/day throughout the study (18.9 mg/day for children and 21.8 mg/day for adolescents). Outcomes were measured by CDRS-R rating changes from baseline to 8 weeks as well as improvement in CGI-I scores and change from baseline of illness of the CGI-S scores. The study did not find any differences in depression rating scales between the paroxetine and placebo group. CDRS-R total score adjusted mean changes from baseline for patients receiving paroxetine and placebo were −22.58 (SE 1.47) and −23.38 (SE 1.60). It was noted that AEs of suicidal behavior and/or ideation while taking paroxetine was 1.92% versus placebo 0.98%. The authors conclude that paroxetine was not shown to be more efficacious than placebo for treating pediatric MDD.

Paroxetine in the Treatment of Children and Adolescents Diagnosed with Dysthymia

In a small open-label study, Nobile and colleagues (2000) treated seven subjects diagnosed by DSM-III-R (APA, 1987) criteria with dysthymia, primary type, without comorbidity for MDD, for 3 months. Efficacy was assessed by ratings on the HDRS, the CGI-S Scale, and the CGI-I Scale. Dosage range was 10 to 40 mg daily. Clinical improvement of responders was noted within the first month of treatment and the improvement continued over the course of treatment. The mean dose of paroxetine after 3 months was 20.12 mg/day. Five (71%) of the seven completers (two subjects withdrew during the first month, one female participant was noncompliant and another female participant stopped because of nausea and stomachaches) were "responders." The five responders were maintained on medication and reassessed 6 months after beginning paroxetine; all five showed further improvement on the Ham-D (mean 6-month score was 1.2 ± 2.17), and all five were rated with "no disease" on the CGI-S and "very much improved" on the CGI-I. The most common untoward effects were nausea and stomachache (28.6%). Sedation, insomnia, behavioral activation, and inappropriate behavior were reported by one patient each. The authors noted that their data suggest that paroxetine is effective in the treatment of dysthymia in this age group and merits further study (Nobile et al., 2000).

Paroxetine in the Treatment of Children and Adolescents Diagnosed with OCD

Rosenberg et al. (1999) conducted a 12-week, open-label trial of paroxetine in treating 20 outpatients (9 males and 11 females; ages 8 to 17 years) diagnosed with OCD by DSM-IV criteria (APA, 1994) and having a CY-BOCS rating of >16. The criterion for a positive response was a reduction of OCD symptom severity by >30% on the CY-BOCS.

The initial dose of paroxetine was 10 mg/day and could be titrated upward by a maximum increase of 10 mg every 2 weeks to a daily maximum of 60 mg or until good clinical response or until untoward effects prevented further increase. At the end of the study, subjects showed significant ($P = .001$) improvement on the CY-BOCS, the CGAS, and the CGI. Patients also showed a significant decrease in anxiety ($P = .008$). Of clinical interest, one of the two subjects with tic-related OCD failed to improve and the other, diagnosed with Tourette disorder, had a worsening of OCD symptoms and a doubling of tic severity consonant with the earlier studies suggesting that tic-related OCD may be less responsive to specific SRIs. Overall, paroxetine was considered safe and effective in treating these particular subjects.

Gilbert et al. (2000) used volumetric magnetic resonance imaging (MRI) to measure and compare thalamic volumes in 21 psychotropic-naïve subjects (7 males and 14 females; age range, 8.08 to 17.33 years) diagnosed by DSM-IV (APA, 1994) criteria with OCD whom they were treating with paroxetine with 21 matched healthy controls. After baseline assessment, including MRI, 13 of the 21 subjects were treated with paroxetine 10 mg/day that was titrated to a maximum of 60 mg/day depending on clinical response; mean dose of paroxetine after 12 weeks was 51.00 ± 8.76 mg/day (range, 40 to 60 mg/day). Subjects did not receive CBT or psychotherapy other than supportive or family therapy. On the basis of CY-BOCS ratings, 7 of the 10 subjects were considered responders, having a 30% or greater improvement in their scores. At baseline, thalamic volumes of treatment-naïve patients with OCD were significantly greater than those of controls ($P = .01$). Thalamic volume in the 10 patients with OCD decreased significantly (19% mean reduction in volume) after 12 weeks' treatment with paroxetine ($P = .01$) and was no longer significantly different from that of the controls ($P = .76$). Reduction in thalamic volume correlated with significantly lower scores on the CY-BOCS, but the dose of paroxetine did not correlate with final thalamic volume. Repeat MRIs were also obtained in eight medication-free controls about 12 weeks after baseline; they showed less variation (a mean of $\pm5.6\%$ of baseline) in volume, suggesting that the greater change in the paroxetine group was a real phenomenon. The authors' preliminary findings suggest that treatment-naïve children diagnosed with OCD have serotonergic abnormalities that result in increased thalamic volumes. During the 12-week period of treatment with paroxetine, significant reduction in thalamic volume and clinical improvement in OCD symptomatology occurred.

Geller et al. (2004) conducted a prospective, multicenter, 10-week, randomized, double-blind, placebo-controlled, flexible-dose, parallel-group trial to evaluate the efficacy and safety of paroxetine hydrochloride in treating 203 children aged 7 to 11 and adolescents aged 12 to 17 who were diagnosed with OCD by DSM-IV criteria. The primary measure of efficacy was the change from baseline to the week 10 last-observation-carried-forward endpoint in total score on the CY-BOCS.

About one-third (33.7%) of the paroxetine group and 23.8% of the placebo group did not complete the study. AEs (10.2%; $N = 10$) were the most common reason for this in the paroxetine group, and lack of efficacy (13.3%; $N = 14$) was the most common reason in the placebo group. The average length of treatment for the paroxetine group was 60 days and for the placebo group 64 days. The final mean dose of paroxetine for children was 25.4 mg/day and for adolescents was 36.5 mg/day.

The paroxetine group improved significantly more than the placebo group on the CY-BOCS total score (-8.75 vs. -5.34 points, $P = .002$). Patients with higher initial CY-BOCS scores had greater changes from baseline than did patients with lower initial scores ($P = .002$) and children had greater changes from baseline than adolescents ($P < .001$). In addition, the three secondary measures utilizing the CY-BOCS for paroxetine were all statistically superior to those for placebo and the other three were numerically but not significantly superior.

The most frequently reported AEs in the paroxetine group were headache (24.5%), abdominal pain (17.3%), nausea (16.3%), upper respiratory infection (12.2%), somnolence (12.2%), motor hyperactivity (12.2%), and trauma (physical and accidental injuries) (10.2%); of these, only hyperactivity and trauma occurred at least twice as frequently as in the placebo group. Overall, 10.2% (eight children and two adolescents) of the paroxetine group and 2.9% of the placebo group discontinued treatment because of an AE. During treatment discontinuation, that is, the period of medication taper or follow-up during the first 2 weeks off the medication, patients who were taking paroxetine experienced nausea (2.5%) and vomiting (3.8%) compared with 1.1% and 0%, respectively, of patients who were on placebo.

The authors concluded that paroxetine had a modest overall effect in reducing symptoms on the CY-BOCS and was significantly more efficacious than was placebo. Its tolerability and safety profile were similar to those observed with other SSRIs in children and adolescents being treated for OCD.

Paroxetine in the Treatment of Children and Adolescents Diagnosed with Social Anxiety Disorder

Wagner et al. (2004a) conducted a 38-center, randomized, double-blind, placebo-controlled 16-week study of paroxetine in a total of 322 children (age 8 to 11) and adolescents (age 12 to 17) who met DSM-IV (APA, 1994) criteria for social anxiety disorder. Paroxetine was begun at a dose of 10 mg and could be increased at weekly intervals to a maximum of 50 mg/day; after week 2, dose could be reduced to the prior dose in the event of an AE. At the end of the study, subjects whose daily dose was 20 mg or more were tapered off by reducing the dose by 10 mg weekly. The primary outcome measure (efficacy endpoint) was a rating of 1 (very much improved) or 2 (much improved) on the CGI-I Scale.

At week 16, the mean dose of paroxetine for all subjects was 32.6 mg/day; for children it was 26.5 mg/day, and for adolescents it was 35.0 mg/day. Of the subjects in the paroxetine group, 77.6% (125/161) met criteria for responders versus 38.3% (59/154) of subjects in the placebo group ($P < .001$). The benefit of paroxetine was apparent within 4 weeks. Paroxetine also showed statistically more clinical benefit than did placebo ($P < .001$) on five secondary outcome measures, which included specific scales for social anxiety.

Most AEs were of mild to moderate intensity. AEs that possibly occurred as a result of treatment in >5% of subjects on paroxetine and at a rate at least twice that of placebo were as follows: insomnia, 14.1% versus 5.8% ($P = .02$); decreased appetite, 8.0% versus 3.2% ($P = .11$); and vomiting, 6.7% versus 1.9% ($P = .07$). Rates of nervousness, hyperkinesia, asthenia, and hostility also met the preceding criteria in children but not in adolescents; rates of somnolence and insomnia met these criteria in adolescents but not in children (P values were not given). The authors concluded that paroxetine was effective in treating children and adolescents diagnosed with social anxiety disorder (Wagner et al., 2004a).

SELECTIVE SEROTONIN AND NOREPINEPHRINE REUPTAKE INHIBITORS

Venlafaxine Hydrochloride (Effexor)

Venlafaxine hydrochloride is chemically unrelated to other available antidepressants. Its antidepressant effects are thought to be due to its potent inhibition of the reuptake of neuronal serotonin and norepinephrine and weak inhibition of dopamine uptake (a serotonergic noradrenergic reuptake inhibitor). Venlafaxine does not have significant affinity for muscarinic, histaminergic, or alpha-1 adrenergic receptors.

Pharmacokinetics of Venlafaxine Hydrochloride

Food has no significant effect on the bioavailability of venlafaxine. The medication is extensively metabolized by the liver to O-desmethylvenlafaxine, the major metabolite, which is clinically active. Mean terminal elimination half-life is approximately 11 hours. Steady-state serum concentrations are achieved within approximately 3 days of multidose administration. The primary route of excretion of venlafaxine and its metabolites is through the kidneys.

Contraindications for Venlafaxine Hydrochloride Administration

Known hypersensitivity to the medication is a contraindication.

Because of a possibility of serious, life-threatening reactions when administered simultaneously with an MAOI, it is recommended that the medication not be used in combination with an MAOI. At least 2 weeks should elapse after stopping an MAOI before administering venlafaxine. On the basis of the half-life of venlafaxine, at least 7 days should elapse following its discontinuation before administering an MAOI.

Significant hepatic or renal disease may markedly decrease elimination of the medication and increase serum levels. If the clinician elects to use venlafaxine, adjustment of dosage may be necessary.

Use with caution in patients with depression having a history of hypomania or mania, as activation of either could occur.

Untoward Effects of Venlafaxine Hydrochloride

Among the most commonly reported untoward effects are anxiety, nervousness, somnolence or insomnia, nausea, anorexia, initial dose-dependent weight loss, constipation, increased sweating, dry mouth, dizziness, abnormal ejaculation/ orgasm, and impotence. A sustained increase in supine diastolic blood pressure, which appeared to be dose related has been reported in some patients treated with venlafaxine. Many other untoward effects have been reported.

Electrocardiogram Changes

Administration of regular venlafaxine resulted in no treatment-emergent conduction abnormalities compared with those of placebo, but the mean heart rate was increased by 4 beats per minute compared with that over baseline. On Effexor XR (brand name extended-release preparation), however, the QTc interval increased by 4.7 ms over baseline, compared with a decrease of 1.9 ms for placebo. Heart rate increased by 4 beats per minute over baseline on Effexor XR compared with an increase of 1 beat per minute over baseline for placebo.

Reports of Interest

Venlafaxine Hydrochloride in the Treatment of Major Depressive Disorder

Emslie and colleagues (2007) reported on the use of venlafaxine in two placebo-controlled trials. In this report, the results of two similar trials comparing venlafaxine to placebo were combined. Three hundred sixty-seven subjects were enrolled: 183 were assigned to receive placebo, and 184 were assigned to receive venlafaxine ER. Venlafaxine ER was dosed at 37.5 mg for the first week. Titration to max doses of 112.5 mg daily, 150 mg daily, or 225 mg daily were based on weight. The mean daily dose of venlafaxine ER was 97.1 mg/day. Among children (7 to 11 years), the mean dose was 80.4 mg/day, and among adolescents (12 to 17 years), the mean dose was 109.2 mg/ day. Outcomes were measured using the CDRS-R score. The pooled data did not show any statistically significant differences between venlafaxine ER and placebo on the CDRS-R. Analysis of the pooled data showed that adolescents 12 to 17 had greater improvement on the CDRS-R with venlafaxine ER than with placebo (-24.4 vs. -19.9; $P = .22$). Children did not show any clinically significant improvement in CDRS-R scores. AEs commonly seen were anorexia and abdominal pain. There were more hostility and suicide-related events in the venlafaxine ER–treated subjects than in the placebo-treated subjects. There were no completed suicides. The authors conclude that venlafaxine ER may be an effective treatment in depressed adolescents, but not in children with depression.

Venlafaxine Hydrochloride in the Treatment of Anxiety in Children and Adolescents

March and colleagues (2007b) reported on a double-blind placebo-controlled trial of venlafaxine ER to treat pediatric social anxiety disorder. In this study, 293 subjects aged 8 to 17 who met criteria for social anxiety disorder were randomized to receive either venlafaxine ER or placebo over 16 weeks. Venlafaxine was titrated from 37.5 mg to a maximum of 225 mg/day depending on weight and clinical response over the length of the study. The primary measures of response were the social anxiety scale, child or adolescent version (SAS-CA) and the CGI-I scores. The authors found that when compared with placebo, ITT random regression analysis indicated a statistically significant advantage for venlafaxine ER ($P = .001$) on the SAS-CA. On the CGI-I, 56% of the venlafaxine ER–treated subjects responded, which was superior to placebo at 37%. Three patients on venlafaxine ER and none on placebo developed treatment-emergent suicidality, and there were no completed suicides. The authors conclude that venlafaxine ER is an effective and fairly well-tolerated treatment for generalized social anxiety disorder in children and adolescents.

Venlafaxine Hydrochloride in the Treatment of ADHD in Children and Adolescents

Ghanizadeh and colleagues (2013) completed a systematic review of non-controlled and controlled trials of venlafaxine in children and adolescents with ADHD. Three uncontrolled trials and two double-blind controlled clinical trials were evaluated.

The authors found that venlafaxine appeared effective for treating ADHD and that rates of some adverse effects were less than those documented for methylphenidate. One of the controlled trials found no difference in efficacy between venlafaxine and methylphenidate, whereas the other trial reported lower efficacy for venlafaxine. The most common adverse effects were headache, insomnia, and nausea. Larger and more robust clinical trials were recommended to further evaluate venlafaxine's efficacy, safety, and tolerability in treating ADHD.

Olvera et al. (1996) conducted a 5-week, open-label trial of venlafaxine in the treatment of 16 subjects (15 males and 1 female; age range, 8 to 16 years) diagnosed with ADHD without comorbid depression by DSM-IV (APA, 1994) criteria to assess efficacy, dose range, and untoward effects. Efficacy was determined by ratings on the CPRS and the Conners, Continuous Performance Test (CPT). The mean dose of venlafaxine for the 10 completers was 60 mg/day or 1.4 mg/kg/day given in two or three divided doses. Overall, 7 (44%) of the 16 subjects improved on the CPRS. At the end of 5 weeks, mean ratings on the CPRS impulsivity factor improved significantly ($P = .008$), and mean ratings on the CPRS hyperactivity index improved significantly ($P = .003$); there were no significant changes in mean ratings on the CPRS conduct factor. Cognitive symptoms of ADHD as reflected in omission or commission errors or reaction time on the CPT showed no significant improvement. The most common untoward effects were drowsiness (8/16, 50%), nausea (6/16, 37.5%), irritability (5/15, 33%), and behavioral activation (worsening of hyperactivity in 5/15, 33%). The authors concluded that low doses of venlafaxine appeared to be effective in reducing behavioral but not cognitive symptoms of ADHD, but that behavioral activation may be of concern (Olvera et al., 1996).

Findling et al. (2007b) conducted a 2-week open-label trial of venlafaxine in the treatment of ADHD in 38 males aged 5 to 17 years. The authors wanted to examine changes in symptom severity, tolerability, and pharmacodynamics of venlafaxine in youths with ADHD. The study was conducted with three dosing strata per age group: 0.5, 1.0, and 2.0 mg/kg/day maintained for the 2 weeks of the study. At the end of the study, parent ADHD rating scale-IV (ARS-IV) scores were improved over baseline in total inattentive and hyperactive-impulsive subscores ($P < .001$). Teacher ARS-IV ratings for total symptoms were improved over baseline ($P = .03$). Inattentive symptoms were improved ($P = .02$), but hyperactivity-impulsivity symptoms did not reach statistical significance ($P = .06$). When response was defined by a CGI-S score of 1 or 2, only 5% of study subjects were classified as responders; 2 of 17 adolescents and none of the 21 children had responded. No difference in response was found among the dosing levels. No subjects discontinued because of AEs. No suicidal behaviors were observed or reported in the study. Considering that venlafaxine requires at least 4 weeks to see an antidepressant response in adults, the length of this trial was likely inadequate to see treatment effects. The authors conclude that this open trial shows that venlafaxine may offer some benefit and appears relatively safe for the short-term treatment of ADHD.

Duloxetine Hydrochloride (Cymbalta)

Duloxetine hydrochloride is a potent inhibitor of serotonin and norepinephrine reuptake and a weak inhibitor of dopamine reuptake. It has little to no significant activity at H1-histaminergic, alpha-adrenergic, or muscarinic receptors.

Pharmacokinetics of Duloxetine Hydrochloride

Duloxetine may be taken with or without food and does not affect the maximum plasma concentration, but delays it and decreases the amount absorbed by about 10%. Because the capsules contain enteric-coated pellets that prevent the medication from degrading in the stomach, there is a median delay of about 2 hours until absorption begins. Evening doses are absorbed up to 3 hours more slowly and cleared up to 33% more rapidly than are morning doses. Maximum plasma levels occur about 6 hours after ingestion of the medication.

Duloxetine hydrochloride has a half-life of about 12 hours (range 8 to 17 hours). Steady-state plasma levels occur after about 3 days at a given dose. Duloxetine is extensively metabolized primarily by the hepatic P450 enzymes CYP2D6 and CYP1A2. About 70% is eliminated in the urine and 20% through the feces.

Lobo et al. (2014) compared pediatric and adult pharmacokinetics for duloxetine, finding that children and adolescents with MDD had similar pharmacokinetics, although estimates of clearance and volume of distribution were higher in the pediatric population than in adults, and average steady-state duloxetine concentrations were approximately 30% lower in pediatric patients than in adults. Dose, body surface area, and race produced statistically significant but not clinically meaningful effects.

Contraindications for the Administration of Duloxetine Hydrochloride

Hypersensitivity to duloxetine hydrochloride or its components is a contraindication to its administration. Concomitant use with MAOIs is contraindicated. It should not be prescribed to patients with uncontrolled narrow-angle glaucoma. Duloxetine should not be coadministered with thioridazine.

Duloxetine should not be coadministered with an MAOI or within 14 days of treatment with an MAOI being discontinued. At least 5 days should elapse after stopping duloxetine therapy before administering an MAOI.

Interactions of Duloxetine Hydrochloride with Other Medications

CYP1A2 inhibitors are expected to increase duloxetine plasma levels; for example, fluvoxamine increases maximum plasma levels by 2½ times and the serum concentration by up to 6 times. Quinolone antibiotics should also be avoided for the same reason.

Potent CYP2D6 inhibitors also are expected to increase duloxetine plasma levels, for example, 20 mg of paroxetine daily reportedly increased plasma levels caused by 40 mg daily of duloxetine by 60%; fluoxetine and quinidine would also be expected to increase plasma levels of duloxetine.

Duloxetine, itself, is a moderate inhibitor of CYP2D6. Coadministration of duloxetine with other medications that are extensively metabolized by CYP2D6, which have a narrow therapeutic index such as the TCAs nortriptyline, amitriptyline, imipramine, and desipramine; phenothiazines, and type 1C antiarrhythmics should be avoided if possible because of potentially dangerous increases in their serum levels. If coadministered, TCA serum levels should be monitored closely. Coadministration with thioridazine is contraindicated because of the risk of ventricular arrhythmias and sudden death that has been associated with elevated thioridazine levels.

Untoward Effects of Duloxetine Hydrochloride

The most common untoward effects reported in adult placebo-controlled clinical trials were nausea (20% vs. 7%), dry mouth (15% vs. 6%), constipation (11% vs. 4%), fatigue (8% vs. 4%), decreased appetite (8% vs. 2%), somnolence (7% vs. 3%), and increased sweating (6% vs. 2%). Duloxetine was associated with a mean blood pressure increase of 2 mm Hg systolic and 0.5 mm Hg diastolic compared with levels with that of placebo.

Reports of Interest

Duloxetine in the Treatment of Major Depression

Two large studies evaluating safety and efficacy of duloxetine for treating MDDs in youth, comparing both to placebo and to fluoxetine, were conducted over a 36-week period. Atkinson et al. (2014) utilized a flexible-dose method in children (ages 7 to 11) and adolescents (ages 12 to 17) with MDD. Three hundred and thirty-seven subjects were randomized to receive duloxetine 60 to 120 mg/day, fluoxetine 20 to 40 mg/day, or placebo. Emslie et al. (2014) studied duloxetine fixed dose in children (ages 7 to 11) and adolescents (ages 12 to 17) with MDD. Four hundred and sixty-three patients received either duloxetine 60/day mg, duloxetine 30 mg/day, fluoxetine 20 mg/day, or placebo. Both studies used the CDRS-R as the primary outcome measure. In the fixed-dose design, the C-SSRS, and TEAEs were also formally assessed. Neither active drug separated significantly ($P < .05$) from placebo at 10 weeks on CDRS-R in both studies; thus, trial results were inconclusive. There were no significant differences on SAEs between duloxetine or fluoxetine groups compared with the placebo groups. There were also no clinically significant ECG abnormalities or completed suicides or deaths in these studies. Another finding of both studies was that much larger proportions of subjects in all study arms (duloxetine, fluoxetine, and placebo) showed improvement in suicidal ideation (ranging from 69% to 100% of subjects in their respective groups) compared to the number of subjects reporting worsening of suicidal ideation (ranging from 5.2% to 9.4% of subjects in the groups).

Subsequently, a 2015 pooled analysis of these duloxetine studies examined safety and tolerability further. Significantly more patients discontinued due to AEs due to duloxetine treatment (8.2%) than due to placebo (3.1%). The proportion of patients who reported at least one TEAE did not differ among the groups (63%, 62%, 62%, respectively), nor did the proportion of TEAE reporting when comparing children aged 7 to 11 to adolescents aged 12 to 17. The most commonly reported side effects were nausea and other GI events, headache, and dizziness. Patients on duloxetine had a mean pulse increase of 3 beats per minute, and mean blood pressure increase of <2.0 mm Hg. Although there was a 2% to 3% decrease in weight percentile during the acute treatment phase, most patients tended toward baseline weight percentile during the extended treatment phase (Emslie et al., 2015).

Prakash and colleagues (2012) conducted an open-label study on the use of duloxetine in pediatric patients with major depression. The study was conducted as a 32-week, single-arm, flexible-dose, open-label study. Patients were started with duloxetine at 20 mg/day or 30 mg/day, based on weight. The dose was then flexibly escalated from 20 to 30 to 60 to 90 to 120 mg daily over the 8-week dose-titration phase. During the 12-week extended safety trial, dose could again be titrated within the range of 20 to 120 mg depending on the investigator's discretion. Seventy-two patients were enrolled in the study and, of those, 58 (80.6%) completed the 10-week dose-titration phase, 48 (66.7%) completed the 18 weeks of acute treatment, and 42 (58.3%) completed an additional 12 weeks of extended treatment. The study enrolled 31 children 7 to 12 years and 24 adolescents 13 to 17 years. The majority of patients (55/72; 76%) required dose escalation to higher doses of duloxetine (60, 90, or 120 mg/day).

Four patients (5.6%) discontinued because of TEAE. Three had nausea/vomiting, rash, or reemergence of ADHD. A fourth patient on duloxetine 120 mg/day discontinued after 5 months of treatment because of irritability. The most common TEAEs were seen in the acute treatment period. Nausea was reported in 25% of the total study population. Females experienced nausea 40%, vomiting 17.1%, and dizziness 14.3%, more frequently than did males. Headaches were seen in 13.9% of the study subjects. SAEs were seen in five patients (6.9%) six times, which required hospitalization during the study and occurred during the acute treatment period. Two patients had SIBs, one felt to be nonsuicidal and one felt to be suicidal. One patient abruptly stopped duloxetine (90 mg) and had worsening of depression. One patient had worsening of ODD while on 30 mg/day. Another patient experienced viral gastroenteritis on 60 mg/day. Overall, one nonfatal suicidal attempt occurred and two patients (2.8%) experienced worsening of suicidal ideation. The study included 19 patients with suicidal ideation at baseline and 17 (90%) reported improvement in suicidal ideation. Half of the patients experienced clinically significant elevation in blood pressure which, in most cases (58%), was transient.

The study did show improvement in depression measures by the end of the acute and extension treatment phases, as measured by CGI-S and CDRS-R scores. A total of 43/72 (59.7%) of subjects achieved remission at the end point of the 18-week acute treatment phase. The authors suggest that this study shows duloxetine is generally well tolerated in pediatric patients at doses from 30 to 120 mg daily. They did observe transient elevations in blood pressure in many patients, which may be clinically significant. The pharmacokinetic results suggest that adjustment of total daily dose (TDD) based on body weight may not be necessary for pediatric patients and TDDs lower than that used in adults may not be indicated.

Duloxetine in the Treatment of GAD

Strawn et al. (2015) evaluated the safety, efficacy, and tolerability of duloxetine in children and adolescents (ages 7 to 17) with GAD. Two hundred seventy-two patients were treated with flexible-dose duloxetine (30 to 120 mg/day) or placebo for 10 weeks, followed by open-label dosing for 18 weeks. Measures used were the PARS, CGI-S Scale, CGAS, and C-SSRS. Laboratory, ECGs, and vital signs were also monitored. Duloxetine demonstrated statistically significant reduction in anxiety symptoms compared to placebo on the PARS. Although there were statistically greater pulse rates, weight differences, AEs due to GI symptoms, oropharyngeal pain, dizziness, cough, and palpitations in the duloxetine group, there was no significant difference in systolic or diastolic blood pressure or in discontinuation between the active medication and placebo groups.

Desvenlafaxine (Pristiq)

Two recent trials of desvenlafaxine versus placebo for treatment of MDD have not demonstrated statistical significance from placebo, although one was considered to be a failed trial because it also did not replicate previously established efficacy for fluoxetine. Atkinson and colleagues (2018) compared placebo to low-exposure desvenlafaxine or high-exposure desvenlafaxine in 109 children aged 7 to 11 and 254 adolescents aged 12 to 17. Subjects met DSM-IV-TR criteria for MDD and had baseline CDRS-R total scores >40. Primary efficacy endpoint was CDRS-R score at 8 weeks, and CGI-I and CGI-S scales were also examined. Safety was also evaluated to determine which children had adverse effects and C-SSRS scores were followed. There was no statistically significant difference in comparing placebo to either treatment group, and incidence of adverse effects was similar among the groups. Although a safe and generally tolerated medication, efficacy was not demonstrated in this study. In a similarly designed study but with an additional comparison treatment arm of fluoxetine, Weihs and colleagues (2018) found that neither desvenlafaxine nor the reference medication fluoxetine separated from placebo such that conclusions could not be made regarding efficacy.

Findling et al. (2014) completed an 8-week, multicenter, open-label, fixed-dose study of desvenlafaxine to evaluate its safety and tolerability in the treatment of 20 children and 20 adolescents with MDD. Children (ages 7 to 11) were administered 1 to 100 mg/day and adolescents (ages 12 to 17) were administered 25 to 200 mg/day, and followed in a 6-month flexible-dose extension study. Four children and three adolescents withdrew because of AEs; most commonly reported were upper abdominal pain (15%), headache (15%) in children, and somnolence (30%), nausea (20%), upper abdominal pain (15%), headache (15%) in adolescents. Oppositional behavior in one child was the single SAE reported, and there were two adolescents who reported suicidal ideation at time of screening and one who reported suicidal ideation after screening. No statistically significant changes in blood pressure were reported but there were slight increases in pulse rates among children and adolescents.

NOREPINEPHRINE AND DOPAMINE REUPTAKE INHIBITORS

Bupropion Hydrochloride (Wellbutrin, Zyban)

Bupropion hydrochloride is an antidepressant of the aminoketone class. It is not related chemically to the tricyclics, tetracyclics, or other known antidepressants.

Pharmacokinetics of Bupropion Hydrochloride

Peak plasma concentrations are usually reached in about 2 hours. The metabolism of bupropion is extensive and complex. Following peak serum levels, there is a biphasic decline; average half-life of the second (postdistributional) phase is 14 hours (range, 8 to 24 hours). Several metabolites are pharmacologically active and have long half-lives. Six hours after a single-dose, plasma bupropion levels are about 30% of peak concentration.

On the basis of a study of 19 subjects (11 males and 8 females; age range 11 to 17, mean age 15.2 ± 1.8 years) who were treated with bupropion sustained release (SR) for diagnoses of ADHD ($N = 16$) and depressive disorders ($N = 16$) which were comorbid in 13 subjects, Daviss et al. (2005) reported that youths metabolize bupropion SR to active metabolites faster than do adults and that bupropion SR should be given to subjects in this age group in divided doses.

Contraindications for Bupropion Hydrochloride Administration

Known hypersensitivity to bupropion hydrochloride and seizure disorders are contraindications.

A current or prior diagnosis of bulimia or anorexia nervosa is also a contra-indication because a higher incidence of seizures is reported when bupropion is administered to such patients.

Bupropion should not be administered concurrently with an MAOI. At least a 14-day period off MAOIs should precede initiation of treatment with bupropion hydrochloride.

Concurrent administration with any medication that reduces the seizure threshold is a relative contraindication.

Interactions of Bupropion Hydrochloride with Other Medications

Relatively few data are available on interactions of bupropion hydrochloride with other medications. Increased adverse experiences were reported when the medication was administered concomitantly with L-dopa. MAOIs may increase the acute toxicity of bupropion.

Although bupropion is not metabolized by the CYP2D6 enzyme, the medication and its metabolite, morpholinol, inhibit this enzyme *in vitro*. Therefore, extreme caution should be exercised when coadministering any medication metabolized by that enzyme, and initial dosage should be as low as possible.

Untoward Effects of Bupropion Hydrochloride

Of particular clinical concern is the finding that seizures have been associated with about 4 (0.4%) per 1,000 patients treated with bupropion at doses of 450 mg/day or less. This is about four times the incidence of seizures reported with other approved antidepressants, and the incidence of seizures increases with higher daily doses. Conversely, Clay et al. (1988) note that the positive effects of bupropion on memory performance may be unique among antidepressants and that other antidepressants either have no effect or a negative effect on memory performance.

During the first few days of treatment, agitation, motor restlessness, and insomnia frequently occur; starting at a lower dose and making increments gradually helps to minimize these effects.

The most common untoward effects were reported to be agitation, dry mouth, insomnia, headache, nausea, vomiting, constipation, and tremor.

Ferguson and Simeon (1984) reported no adverse (or positive) effects on cognition on a cognitive battery in 17 children with attention-deficit disorder (ADD) or conduct disorders who were treated in an open trial with bupropion.

Reports of Interest

Bupropion Hydrochloride in the Treatment of Children with Comorbid ADHD and Depression

Daviss and colleagues (2001) investigated the effectiveness and tolerability of bupropion SR in 24 adolescents (aged 11 to 16 years) with comorbid ADHD and either MDD, dysthymic disorder, or both. Subjects began with a 2-week, single-blind placebo lead-in and subsequently received up to 10 weeks of active treatment with bupropion SR with a flexible-dose titration schedule. No subjects discontinued medication because of side effects. Fifty-eight percent of subjects ($N = 14$) were rated as responders in both depression and ADHD, with 29% of responders ($N = 7$) in depression only and 4% ($N = 1$) in ADHD only. Compared with the initial ratings on placebo, parent ($P < .0005$) and children ($P = .016$) depression ratings improved significantly. Parent ADHD ratings were significantly improved as well ($P < .0005$), but not teacher ratings ($P = .8$). Functional impairment improved significantly as well ($P < .0005$). The authors concluded effectiveness for bupropion SR in adolescents with comorbid ADHD and depression, but noted the need for randomized, placebo-controlled studies.

Bupropion Hydrochloride in the Treatment of Children Diagnosed with ADHD

A systematic review of clinical trials of bupropion for ADHD demonstrated its efficacy, three of which found efficacy comparable to methylphenidate, because there was a lack of statistically significant treatment effects between the two medications ($P > .05$). It also reported on the large double-blind, placebo-controlled multicenter study that found smaller effect sizes for bupropion than on methylphenidate (see discussion of Conners et al. [1996] later). The systematic review concluded that there is some evidence that bupropion can be considered as a nonstimulant alternative for management of ADHD among youth, and some evidence also supports its use for those who have ADHD comorbid with conduct, substance use, or depressive disorders. Conclusions are considered with caution because of the relatively limited database (Ng, 2017).

Jafarinia et al. (2012) compared the safety and efficacy of treatment with bupropion or methylphenidate in a 6-week randomized double-blind study of 44 children, aged 6 to 17, which met DSM-IV-TR criteria for ADHD. Bupropion was dosed at 100 to 150 mg/day, whereas methylphenidate was dosed at 20 to 30 mg/day. Symptoms were measured with the Teacher and Parent Attention-Deficit/Hyperactivity Disorder Rating Scale-IV at baseline, week 3, and week 6 of treatment. No significant difference in symptoms was found between the two groups at each time point. Parent scales revealed that 75% of the bupropion group and 90% of the methylphenidate group achieved response by week 3 ($P = .212$), and 90% of each treatment group achieved response by week 6 (Fisher's exact test $P = 1.0$). Teacher scales showed that 30% of the bupropion group and 50% of the methylphenidate group showed response by week 3 ($P = .197$), and responses by week 6 were 40% and 60%, respectively ($P = .206$). Although the methylphenidate group showed a higher frequency of headache, other side effects were not significantly different between the groups; the most common side effects among both groups were decreased appetite and insomnia. There were no SAEs in either treatment group. The authors concluded that bupropion and methylphenidate have comparable safety and efficacy for children with ADHD.

Stuhec et al. (2015) reviewed 28 clinical trials to evaluate the comparative efficacy and tolerability of different ADHD medications. Efficacy, determined by standard mean difference (SMD) compared to placebo, was small for bupropion (SMD = -0.32), modest for atomoxetine (SMD = -0.68), and methylphenidate (SMD = -0.75), and high for lisdexamfetamine (SMD = -1.28). Treatment discontinuation was

statistically lower than placebo for methylphenidate while not statistically different for bupropion, atomoxetine, or lisdexamfetamine. Their analysis indicated that
overall all-cause treatment discontinuation was related to lack of efficacy rather than
because of adverse effects, and bupropion had the lowest acceptability for continuation. The authors commented that tolerability and other comorbidity factors may
play a role in choosing a nonstimulant to treat ADHD; and as particular focus of
the meta-analysis was bupropion, they concluded in part that more double-blind
randomized trials evaluating bupropion are needed.

Clay et al. (1988) reported that bupropion hydrochloride was safe and efficacious
in treating prepubertal children diagnosed with ADHD. Thirty prepubertal children
diagnosed with ADHD were enrolled in a double-blind, placebo-controlled study and
individually titrated to optimal doses of bupropion (Clay et al., 1988). Optimal doses
ranged from 100 to 250 mg/day. Subjects receiving bupropion showed statistically
significant improvement on the CGI-I and CGI-S Rating Scales, on the Self-Rating
Scale, and on digit symbol and delayed recall on the Selective Reminding Test. No
significant improvement was reported on the Conners Parent Questionnaire and
the Conners Teacher Questionnaire. The only serious side effect noted was an allergic rash in two children. The authors' clinical impression was that children with
additional prominent symptoms of conduct disorder responded particularly well to
bupropion. They also noted that some children who had previously not responded
satisfactorily to stimulants had a good response to bupropion.

Casat et al. (1989) administered bupropion to 20 children and placebo to 10
children in a parallel-groups design, double-blind comparison study. All subjects
were diagnosed with ADHD. Decreases in symptom severity and overall clinical
improvement were noted in physician ratings, and there was a significant decrease
in hyperactivity in the classroom settings on the Conners Teacher Questionnaire.

Barrickman et al. (1995) conducted a 16-week, double-blind crossover-design
study comparing bupropion with methylphenidate (MPH) in the treatment of 15
outpatients (12 males and 3 females; age range, 7 to 16 years) who were diagnosed
with ADHD by DSM-III-R (APA, 1987) criteria. Following an initial 2-week washout
period, subjects were randomly assigned to bupropion or MPH for a 6-week treatment period. This was followed by another 2-week washout; subjects then received
the alternative medication for the next 6 weeks. Efficacy was determined by ratings
on the Iowa-Conners Abbreviated Parent and Teacher Questionnaires (ICQ-P and
ICQ-T), the CGI-I Scale, the CGI-S Scale, and side effects scale. The final mean dose
of bupropion was 140 ± 146 mg/day (range, 50 to 200 mg/day) or 3.3 ± 1.2 mg/kg/
day (range, 1.4 to 5.7 mg/kg/day). The final mean dose of MPH was 31 ± 11 mg/
day (range, 20 to 60 mg/day) or 0.7 ± 0.2 mg/kg/day (range, 0.4 to 1.3 mg/kg/day).
Treatment with both bupropion and MPH resulted in significantly lower scores on
the ICQ-P ratings and the ICQ-T ratings when compared with baseline ($P < .001$).
There was no significant difference between the two medications, and the order in
which they were given was not significant. Ratings on some of the individual factors
on the ICQ improved significantly more on methylphenidate (e.g., attention on the
ICQ-P, suggesting that MPH was slightly more effective than bupropion. Untoward
effects were minimal, were usually transient, and occurred primarily during the first
2 weeks of treatment: drowsiness, fatigue, nausea, anorexia, dizziness, "spaciness,"
anxiety, headache, and tremor. Bupropion appears to be a useful treatment option
for treating ADHD, but may be slightly less effective than MPH overall and have
somewhat more, although usually mild, untoward effects.

Conners et al. (1996) conducted a multisite, 6-week, parallel-group randomized,
double-blind comparison of bupropion hydrochloride ($N = 72$) and placebo ($N = 37$)
in 109 children diagnosed with ADDH by DSM-III criteria (APA, 1980a); none of
the subjects had comorbid MDD. Age range was 6 to 12 years; two-thirds were
in the third grade or below. Daily maximum doses of 150, 200, and 250 mg were
permitted for subjects weighing 20 to 30 kg, 31 to 40 kg, and >40 kg, respectively.

Teachers noted significant improvement in hyperactivity and conduct problems after the third day on medication. Parents rated restless-impulsive behavior and conduct problems as significantly improved only at the end of the 4-week treatment period. CGI ratings by clinicians at the four settings were not significant when their data were pooled. At the end of the study, when all subjects had completed a week on placebo, teachers' ratings showed no difference between the placebo and medication groups. The authors also reported modest improvement in cognitive functions of attention and memory retrieval. Although the bupropion group improved below the subject selection cutoff of 15 points on the hyperactivity index, the degree of improvement was less than that typically found with the treatment of the standard stimulants. Overall, untoward effects were infrequent. There were no clinically important differences in vital signs, ECG, or laboratory values between the two groups. Six patients on bupropion developed abnormal electroencephalograms (EEGs), including three who developed spike-and-wave discharges. No patient had evidence of clinical seizure activity during treatment. Bupropion hydrochloride appears to be a possible second-line treatment for children diagnosed with ADHD, although the magnitude of clinical improvement appears to be less than what is typical for standard stimulants, and there is some concern about AEs on the EEG and increased seizure potential (Conners et al., 1996).

Although confirmation of these findings is needed, bupropion may be an alternative treatment for ADHD that does not respond to standard therapies.

Bupropion Treatment of Adolescents Diagnosed with ADHD and Comorbid Substance Abuse and Conduct Disorder

Riggs et al. (1998) treated in a 5-week, open-label study using bupropion 13 nondepressed adolescent males (age range, 14 to 17 years) diagnosed with ADHD by DSM-IV (APA, 1994) criteria, who were residing in a long-term, unlocked facility for treatment of their comorbid substance abuse and conduct disorders. Efficacy was determined by ratings on the Conners' Teacher Rating Scale-39 (CTRS-39), the CGI-S, and the CGI-I scales. Bupropion was started at a dose of 100 mg twice daily and increased to 100 mg given three times daily after 7 days for the final 4 weeks of the study. Final dose of all subjects was 300 mg/day (dose range, 3.9 to 5.6 mg/kg/day). Subject mean score on the CTRS-39 declined significantly by 13% ($P \leq .01$); the mean CGI-S score improved by 39% ($P < .002$); and the mean CGI-I score was rated "much" or "very much improved" for seven subjects and "minimally improved" for the remaining six. Untoward effects were reported by seven (54%) of the adolescents; most were mild and transient. One subject, however, developed hypomanic symptoms during the fifth week of the study. The symptoms resolved within 1 week after discontinuing bupropion. These initial data suggest that bupropion may be a useful treatment for such adolescents.

Bupropion in the Treatment of Comorbid ADHD and Chronic Motor Tic Disorder or Tourette Disorder

Spencer et al. (1993b) reported that bupropion exacerbated tics in four children with ADHD and comorbid TS. All four patients had been initially treated with stimulants, when two patients with preexisting symptoms of ADHD and TS experienced worsening of their tics and the other two developed tics and TS. Bupropion was subsequently prescribed as a possibly effective alternative treatment for children diagnosed with ADHD who did not respond satisfactorily to stimulants or could not tolerate their untoward effects. All four children experienced an exacerbation of tics over a period ranging from almost immediately to 2 months. The tics rapidly improved to pretreatment levels when bupropion was discontinued. The authors suggest that bupropion may not be a useful alternative to stimulants in treating patients with comorbid ADHD and TS.

Bupropion SR has been shown to be efficacious in treating nicotine dependency in adolescents, whether this co-occurred with ADHD or not. For a full discussion of its efficacy in this population, see Chapter 11.

OTHER ANTIDEPRESSANTS

Mirtazapine (Remeron)

Mirtazapine has a tetracyclic chemical structure unrelated to other antidepressants in use. Preclinical studies showed that it acts as an antagonist at central presynaptic alpha-2-adrenergic inhibitory autoreceptors and heteroreceptors, resulting in an increase in central noradrenergic and serotonergic activity. Mirtazapine is a potent antagonist of 5-HT_2 and 5-HT_3 receptors, but has no significant affinity for 5-HT_{1A} and 5-HT_{1B} receptors. It is also a potent antagonist of histamine (H_1) receptors, which may cause its prominent sedative effects. Mirtazapine is a moderate peripheral alpha-1-adrenergic antagonist, which may cause the orthostatic hypotension that sometimes occurs. The medication also has moderate antagonistic properties at muscarinic receptors, which may explain the relatively low incidence of anticholinergic effects associated with its use.

Pharmacokinetics of Mirtazapine

Food has a clinically insignificant effect on the rate and bioavailability of mirtazapine. It is rapidly absorbed, with peak plasma concentrations occurring about 2 hours after ingestion. It is extensively metabolized in the liver by demethylation and hydroxylation followed by glucuronide conjugation. Serum half-life ranges between 20 and 40 hours and is significantly longer in females (mean, 37 hours) than in males (mean, 26 hours). Steady-state plasma levels occur within 5 days at a given dose. Elimination is about 75% via urine, with most of the remainder being excreted in the feces.

Contraindications for the Administration of Mirtazapine

Known hypersensitivity to the medication is a contraindication.

Because mirtazapine was associated with the development of severe neutropenia in about 0.1% of patients in premarketing clinical trials, whenever a patient develops sore throat, fever, stomatitis, or other signs of infection and has a low white blood cell count, mirtazapine should be discontinued and the patient closely monitored.

Because of a possibility of serious, life-threatening reactions when administered simultaneously with an MAOI, it is recommended that the medication not be used in combination with an MAOI. At least 2 weeks should elapse after stopping an MAOI before administering mirtazapine. Likewise, depending on the half-life of mirtazapine, at least 2 weeks should elapse following its discontinuation before administering an MAOI.

Untoward Effects of Mirtazapine

Somnolence occurred in more than one-half of patients administered mirtazapine and resulted in discontinuation of treatment in 10.4% of 453 subjects in a controlled 6-week trial (package insert). Other untoward effects included increased appetite, weight gain, dizziness, dry mouth, and constipation. Many other untoward effects have been reported.

Report of Interest

Mirtazapine in the Treatment of Social Phobia

Mrakotsky and colleagues (2008) conducted an open-label pilot trial of the effectiveness of mirtazapine in children and adolescents with SP. The authors enrolled 18 children aged 8 to 17 who met DSM-IV-TR criteria for social anxiety disorder.

They initiated mirtazapine at 15 mg/day and increased to 30 mg after 1 week. The target maximum dose was 0.58 mg/kg/day or the lesser of 45 mg/day. Eight patients were on their target maximum dose of 0.8 mg/kg/day. Primary outcomes were symptom improvement depending on clinician rating and self-report as well as tolerability. Fifty-six percent of youth (10/18) responded to treatment and 17% (3/18) achieved full remission. They did find that SP symptoms increased during the first 2 weeks of treatment along with symptoms of anxiety and depression. The side effects seen were increased sleepiness in the morning and irritability, which were felt to be mild. By the final visit, 2 of 18 patients had moderate to severe AEs of headaches and sleepiness. No suicidal ideation or suicide attempts were reported. Four patients discontinued because of AEs. The authors conclude that this study provides some evidence for the use of mirtazapine as a treatment for pediatric SP and encourage further studies.

Trazodone Hydrochloride (Desyrel)

Trazodone hydrochloride is chemically unrelated to tricyclic, tetracyclic, and other currently approved antidepressant agents. Although it is a serotonin reuptake inhibitor, it is unlike the SSRIs in that its metabolites have significant effects on other neurotransmitter systems and their receptors (Cioli et al., 1984). It is approved for the treatment of adults diagnosed with major depressive episode, both with and without prominent symptoms of anxiety. Although trazodone's antidepressant activity is not fully understood, it inhibits serotonin reuptake in the brain in animals and potentiates behavioral changes induced by 5-hydroxytryptophan. It also blocks H_1-histaminergic and alpha1-adrenergic receptors. Trazodone is more commonly used "off-label" as a low-dose sedative hypnotic for youth with depression and anxiety (Owens et al., 2010).

Pharmacokinetics of Trazodone Hydrochloride

It is recommended that trazodone be ingested soon after eating. When taken in this manner, up to 20% more of the medication may be absorbed than when taken on an empty stomach, and maximum serum concentration is achieved more slowly (in about 2 hours rather than 1 hour) and with a lesser peak. This appears to diminish the likelihood of developing dizziness and/or lightheadedness.

Trazodone is eliminated through the liver (about 20% biliary) and the kidneys (about 75%). Elimination is biphasic: the initial half-life is between 3 and 6 hours, which is followed by a second phase with a half-life of between 5 and 9 hours.

Contraindications for Trazodone Hydrochloride Administration

Known hypersensitivity to the medication is a contraindication.

Interactions of Trazodone Hydrochloride with Other Medications

Increased phenytoin levels have been reported when administered concomitantly with trazodone.

Trazodone should not be administered with MAOIs because the effects of their interaction are unknown.

Untoward Effects of Trazodone Hydrochloride

The most common side effects include drowsiness, dizziness or lightheadedness, dry mouth, and nausea or vomiting.

Priapism, which has necessitated surgical intervention and resulted in some cases of permanent impairment of sexual functioning, has been reported (incidence, about 1:15,000). Male patients with a prolonged or inappropriate erection should be told to discontinue trazodone immediately and contact their physician or, if it persists, to go to an emergency room.

Trazodone in the Treatment of Children and Adolescents with Significant Aggression

Zubieta and Alessi (1992) reported an open study of 22 inpatients (18 males and 4 females; age range, 5 to 12 years) with severe, treatment-refractory behavioral disturbances. They were diagnosed with disruptive behavioral and mood disorders often with comorbidity. Six of the children continued to receive neuroleptics for psychotic symptoms during the trial of trazodone. An initial dose of 50 mg of trazodone at bedtime was begun on an average of 23 ± 20 days after admission. It was titrated over a period of about 1 week to the maximum dose tolerated and given three times daily. The 13 children designated as responders received a mean dose of 185 ± 117 mg/day (4.8 ± 1.7 mg/kg/day) of trazodone for a mean of 27 ± 13 days. The seven nonresponders received a mean dose of 158 ± 70 mg/day (4.7 ± 2.0 mg/kg/day) for a mean of 24 ± 11 days. The most frequent AE was orthostatic hypotension (50%), but this effect diminished over a few days and did not require clinical intervention; 27% of children reported drowsiness; 9%, nervousness; and 9%, anger. Dizziness, increased fatigue, and nocturnal enuresis each occurred in one child (4.5%).

Target symptoms that improved most frequently were impulsivity, hyperactivity, "involvement in dangerous activities," cruelty to people, frequency of physical fights, arguing with adults, and losing one's temper. Improvement of symptoms usually occurred within a few days of the initial administration of trazodone, as contrasted with the several weeks of continuous administration typically required for its antidepressant effects to occur. In a telephone follow-up 3 to 14 months later (mean, 8.8 ± 4.2 months), 9 of the 13 responders were successfully contacted. Eight of the children continued to receive a mean trazodone dose of 241 ± 128 mg/day (range, 100 to 800 mg/day). Trazodone was the only medication being taken at follow-up, the neuroleptics that three children were taking at discharge having been withdrawn within 2 months of discharge. Overall, parents rated their children's improvement at 70 ± 20 (range, 50 to 90) on a subjective overall rating of efficacy scale ranging from 0 to 100 (Zubieta & Alessi, 1992). Trazodone appears to be a potentially useful medication in treating acute and chronic behavioral disorders that have not responded to other treatments and merits further investigation.

Ghaziuddin and Alessi (1992) noted the relationship of the expression of aggression and decreased levels of serotonin in the central nervous system and the successful use of trazodone to control aggressive behavior in adults with organic mental disorders. They administered trazodone to three boys who were 7, 8, and 9 years old with primary diagnoses of severe disruptive behavioral disorders; two of the boys were hospitalized. Trazodone was initiated at doses of 25 mg once or twice daily and increased gradually. Improvement of symptoms was noted within 7 to 10 days at a mean dose of 3.5 mg/kg/day of trazodone (about 75 mg/day). In all three cases, marked deterioration of behavior occurred upon discontinuing the medication and aggressiveness decreased to former treatment levels once medication was resumed. One boy had no reported untoward effects; one experienced mild sedation during the first week, but this remitted with no change in dosage. The third experienced spontaneous erections on 100 mg/day; because of concerns about reported priapism, dosage was reduced to 75 mg daily and behavioral control deteriorated. When 1,000 mg daily of L-tryptophan (which has been subsequently withdrawn from the commercial market) was added, behavior markedly improved again. No ECG changes were noted in any of the boys. The authors note that further studies will be needed to determine the efficacy and safety of trazodone in treating aggressive children.

Trazodone for the Treatment of Insomnia in Youth with Major Depression

Shamseddeen and colleagues (2012) examined the use of trazodone as an adjunctive sleep aid in the TORDIA study described earlier. In the TORDIA trial, participants were randomly assigned to one of four treatments after an unsuccessful initial SSRI treatment. All participants in the study received sleep hygiene education. The study allowed for the addition of a sleep agent in a nonblinded manner because it was felt that residual sleep disturbance was a common symptom in adolescents who failed to have their depression remit in acute-phase treatment (Vitiello et al., 2011). Of the 334 youth enrolled in the study, 58 (17%) received at least one adjunctive sleep medication depending on the pharmacotherapist's clinical judgment. One sleep medication was used in 48 of the subjects, 8 received two medications, and 2 were prescribed three different medications. The most frequently prescribed sleep medication was trazodone, which was prescribed for 33, and antihistamines were prescribed to 20. GABA-acting nonbenzodiazepines were prescribed to 11; two agents were used—zolpidem ($N = 10$) or eszopiclone ($N = 1$).

Youth who received trazodone were six times less likely to respond than those who received no sleep medication. Subjects who received trazodone were three times more likely to experience self-harm. None of the subjects (0 of 13) cotreated with trazodone, and either paroxetine or fluoxetine, had an improvement in their depression. Subjects treated with hypnotics other than trazodone had similar rates of depression response and self-harm events as did subjects who received no sleep medication. The authors suggest that, based on their findings, the use of trazodone for the management of sleep difficulties in adolescent depression should be reevaluated. They recommend that future research on the management of sleep disturbance in adolescent depression be conducted.

Vilazodone (Viibryd)

Gaw and colleagues (2018) completed a retrospective analysis of single-substance exposures with vilazodone in children under age 6 from 2011 to 2016 using data from the National Poison Data System. Seven hundred and fifty-three vilazodone ingestions in children <6 years old were reported, with 49% experiencing one or more clinical effects. The median dose associated with major effects was 50 mg versus 40 mg for moderate effects. With higher dose exposures, there was an increased proportion admitted to a health care facility as well as experiencing serious outcomes. Younger age at exposure had higher risk of hospital admission and serious outcomes, including coma, seizures, ataxia, and hallucinations or delusions. The authors concluded that off-label use of vilazodone in children under 6 years should be discouraged until further research can establish adequate safety.

Russell and colleagues (2017) completed a retrospective observational case series analysis of both single and polysubstance SSRI exposures in children under 6 years of age that were reported to the National Poison Data System. A total of 11,384 SSRI exposures in children <6 years old were reported from January 2012 to June 2016. Of all exposures, 5.9% involved vilazodone, but represented the highest proportion of health care facility admissions compared with other SSRIs. Children exposed to vilazodone also have higher odds of experiencing a major or moderate outcome in single (25.2%) and polysubstance exposures (35.6%) compared to other SSRIs, including seizure and coma, which were more common with vilazodone exposures.

Vortioxetine Hydrobromide (Brintellix)

Vortioxetine hydrobromide is a serotonin antagonist–agonist, with antagonism at the 5-HT_3, 5-HT_{1D}, and 5-HT_7 receptors, partial agonism at the 5-HT_{1B} receptor, and is also a 5-HT_{1A} agonist. It also inhibits 5-HT reuptake. It binds with high affinity to the 5-HT transporter, but not with high affinity to the norepinephrine or dopamine transporters.

Pharmacokinetics of Vortioxetine Hydrobromide

Pharmacologic properties are thought to be from the parent compound. Studies in adults indicate that the mean terminal half-life is about 66 hours. Steady-state plasma concentrations are typically reached within about 2 weeks. Administration with or without food does not appear to affect pharmacokinetics.

Contraindications for Vortioxetine Administration

Known hypersensitivity to vortioxetine or components of the brand name medication are contraindications.

Vortioxetine should not be administered concurrently with an MAOI. At least a 14-day period off MAOIs should precede initiation of treatment with vortioxetine.

Interactions of Vortioxetine with Other Medications

It is recommended to reduce the vortioxetine dose by half when it is coadministered with a strong CYP2D6 inhibitor. Likewise, it is also recommended to increase the dose when coadministered with a 2D6 inducer for more than 14 days, but the maximum dose in such cases should not exceed three times the original dose. If coadministration with the 2D6 inducer ceases, the dose or vortioxetine should be returned to the original dose within 14 days.

Untoward Effects of Vortioxetine

The most common untoward effect was nausea, followed in frequency by diarrhea, dry mouth, dizziness, constipation, vomiting, flatulence, abnormal dreams, and pruritis.

Report of Interest

Vortioxetine Safety and Tolerability

Findling and colleagues (2017) utilized a 14-day open-label prospective study of 48 child and adolescent patients to evaluate the pharmacokinetics and tolerability of single and multiple doses of vortioxetine, ranging from 5 to 20 mg, in children and adolescents with a depressive or anxiety disorder. Pharmacokinetics were found to be proportional to dose in both age groups, although maximum plasma concentration was 30% to 40% lower in adolescents than in children. Most AEs were mild and consistent with observations in adult patients. The authors concluded that efficacy and safety trials could be performed with these doses in pediatric populations. Findling and colleagues (2018) completed a 6-month open-label extension study of vortioxetine in this population using the same dosing to evaluate the long-term safety and tolerability of this medication in the pediatric population. Forty-one patients continued in this open-label extension with 95% ($N = 39$) continuing their previous dose. Fifty-one percent ($N = 21$) withdrew during this study because of administration ($N = 8$), AEs ($N = 4$), and lack of efficacy ($N = 3$). Eighty-five percent had one or more AEs, 86% of which were of mild to moderate severity. Headache (27%), nausea (20%), dysmenorrhea in 19% of females, and vomiting (15%) were the most common reported. Twelve percent ($N = 5$) reported a severe AE, including suicidal ideation ($N = 5$), nonsuicidal SIB ($N = 2$), and nonfatal suicide attempt ($N = 1$). Severe AEs were not considered related to study medication. The authors concluded that the dosing strategy of 5 to 20 mg/day of vortioxetine appears safe, well tolerated, and suitable for future clinical studies in the pediatric population.

TRICYCLIC ANTIDEPRESSANTS

Indications for TCAs in Child and Adolescent Psychiatry

FDA-approved indications for the use of TCAs in children and adolescents, such as for depression, OCD, and enuresis are summarized in Table 8.3. In some cases, these earlier FDA approvals are based on more limited data than are available for medications in greater use currently. For example, a review of the literature on the use of TCAs in children and adolescents with major depression found them to be clinically effective in several open studies, but no double-blind placebo-controlled study has reported that tricyclics were superior to placebo (Ambrosini et al., 1993).

In general, the use of TCAs in children and adolescents has diminished greatly with the availability of newer antidepressants and other treatments. Given the significant risk of death when taken in overdose, concerns about cardiotoxicity with general use, and availability of other treatment options which are better tolerated, TCAs are rarely considered as first-line treatments for childhood mental health disorders.

TCAs in the Treatment of Children Diagnosed with Enuresis

A Cochrane database systematic review of 64 trials (4,071 children) involving the use of TCAs to treat enuresis found the TCAs imipramine, desipramine, and amitriptyline to be more effective than placebo for treatment of enuresis, although treatment effects were not sustained after medication was discontinued. Imipramine was the TCA most commonly used to treat enuresis in these trials. Treatment gains were measured by fewer wet nights per week and also the ability to have at least 14 consecutive dry nights. There was not enough evidence to determine effectiveness among the different tricyclics and there was also not enough evidence to determine effectiveness of given doses of tricyclics. Imipramine combined with oxybutynin outperformed imipramine alone. Imipramine combined with desmopressin did not differ from imipramine alone, but was more effective than desmopressin alone. The combination of desmopressin and oxybutynin outperformed the tricyclics, as did bed alarms. Imipramine was more effective than simple behavioral interventions and diet restriction but less effective than complex behavioral interventions such as a three-step program. Bed alarms showed a better rate of maintaining treatment gains following discontinuation of the intervention (Caldwell et al., 2016).

TCAs in the Treatment of Children and Adolescents Diagnosed with ADHD

A Cochrane database systematic review evaluating the efficacy of TCAs for ADHD included findings from six RCTs with a total of 216 participants, five of which were comparisons of desipramine to placebo and one of nortriptyline to placebo. Two of the desipramine trials included comparisons with clonidine and clomipramine or methylphenidate. Two included subjects who had comorbid tics. They found that desipramine and nortriptyline appeared to improve the core symptoms of ADHD, but the evidence supporting their use was low (Otasowie et al., 2014).

Although the treatment of ADHD is not an approved indication, TCAs were previously among the second-line medications most frequently prescribed in treating patients diagnosed with ADHD who have not responded to stimulant medication; they were used as the drug of first choice by some clinicians when comorbid diagnoses such as depression or anxiety disorder are present (Green, 1995). The use of TCAs has significantly decreased since the reports of sudden death with their use and the introduction of the SSRI antidepressants. Of the TCAs, imipramine hydrochloride (IMI) and desipramine hydrochloride (DMI) are the best studied and were the most frequently used, although nortriptyline hydrochloride, amitriptyline hydrochloride, and the antiobsessional drug, clomipramine hydrochloride, have also been found to be effective. Overall, DMI appears to have a lower risk of untoward effects than IMI, amitriptyline, and clomipramine (Biederman et al., 1989a); however, cardiotoxicity is a major concern (see later discussions). There are few studies on long-term safety and efficacy of the TCAs in treating ADHD (Green, 1995).

The mechanism of action of TCAs in ADHD is different from that in depression. Optimal doses are usually considerably lower, and the onset of clinical response is rapid (Donnelly et al., 1986; Linnoila et al., 1979), although one study required 3 to 4 weeks for subjects treated with DMI to show significant clinical improvement compared with subjects receiving placebo (Biederman et al., 1989b). When used to treat ADHD, tricyclics improve mood and decrease hyperactivity, but usually are sedating and do not appear to improve concentration (Wender, 1988). TCAs have also been reported to cause small but significant declines in motor performance, which are usually of limited clinical significance (Gualtieri et al., 1991).

The preponderance of published studies strongly suggests that TCAs are effective in the treatment of ADHD. In fact, in the early 1970s, some authors considered IMI to be the drug of choice in treating ADHD (Huessy & Wright, 1970; Waizer et al., 1974). Most double-blind studies comparing TCAs with a stimulant, a placebo, or both have found that both drugs are superior to placebo; however, the stimulant drug is usually equal or superior to the tricyclic on most of the clinically significant measures of improvement and, overall, the literature suggests that stimulants are superior (Campbell et al., 1985; Klein et al., 1980; Pliszka, 1987; Rapoport & Mikkelsen, 1978b).

Parallel to the situation with stimulants, there is evidence that patients diagnosed with ADHD may not respond to one TCA but may have a markedly positive response to another. For example, Wilens et al. (1993b) found that 31 (70%) of 44 subjects who had had unsatisfactory responses to desipramine subsequently had positive responses to nortriptyline.

One difference noted in several studies relates to the longer serum half-lives of the TCAs compared with those of methylphenidate and dextroamphetamine; the therapeutic effects last longer with the tricyclics, and behavior after school and in the evenings of subjects receiving tricyclics is typically rated better by parents and others than behavior of subjects on the stimulants, because clinical efficacy is not lost by late afternoon or early evening (Green, 1995; Yepes et al., 1977).

Pharmacokinetics of TCAs

About 7% of the general population has a genetic variation that results in decreased activity of the drug-metabolizing enzyme cytochrome P450 2D6 (*PDR*, 1995). Such individuals metabolize TCAs more slowly than usual and may develop toxic serum levels at therapeutic doses of <5 mg/kg. Individuals taking the same oral dose of desipramine have been reported to have up to a 36-fold variation in plasma levels (*PDR*, 1995).

There may be large interindividual variations in steady-state plasma levels of tricyclics and their metabolites, although intraindividual levels are usually reproducible and correlate linearly with dose. Preskorn et al. (1989a) reported that steady-state IMI plus DMI levels varied 22-fold (from 25 to 553 ng/mL) among 68 hospitalized children, aged 6 to 14 years, who were prescribed a fixed daily dose of 75 mg of IMI to treat major depression ($N = 48$) or enuresis ($N = 20$); likewise, Biederman et al. (1989b) found that DMI serum levels varied up to 16.5-fold when fixed doses of DMI were administered.

Potter et al. (1982) found that about 5% of 47 subjects, including 32 enuretic males aged 7 to 13 years, were deficient DMI hydroxylators and that such subjects had two to four times the steady-state concentrations of either IMI or DMI per unit dose as the general population. Preskorn et al. (1989b) warned that persons who metabolize tricyclics slowly may develop central nervous system toxicity, which may be confused with worsening of depression, or severe cardiotoxicity when taking conventional doses of tricyclics and that deaths have occurred. Because of these variables, it is necessary to obtain plasma levels to avoid treatment failures for subtherapeutic levels or possible toxic effects from excessive levels.

Dugas et al. (1980) have recommended administering TCAs to children in two or three divided doses daily if more than 1 mg/kg/day is given to avoid or minimize untoward effects related to peak serum levels. Long-acting preparations (e.g., imipramine pamoate capsules) are designed for once-daily dosing; their use is not recommended in children and younger adolescents because of their high unit potency and the greater sensitivity of this age group to cardiotoxic effects.

Table 8.5 summarizes the development of symptoms of central nervous system toxicity. Preskorn et al. (1989b) have urged that therapeutic drug monitoring of TCAs be considered a routine standard of care for patients receiving these drugs.

TABLE 8.5 » Evolution of Central Nervous System Tricyclic Antidepressant Toxicity

Affective Symptoms	Motor Symptoms	Psychotic Symptoms	Organic Symptoms
Mood	Tremor	Thought disorder	Disorientation
↓Concentration	Ataxia	Hallucinations	↓Memory
Lethargy	Seizures[a]	Delusions	Agitation
Social withdrawal			Confusion

[a]Seizures typically occur late but can occur earlier in the evolution.

From Preskorn SH, Jerkovich GS, Beber JH, et al. Therapeutic drug monitoring of tricyclic antidepressants: a standard of care issue. *Psychopharmacol Bull.* 1989;25:281–284.

TCA Discontinuation/Withdrawal Syndrome

Some children experience a flulike withdrawal syndrome, with GI symptoms including nausea, abdominal discomfort and pain, vomiting, headache, and fatigue. These symptoms result from cholinergic rebound and may be considered a cholinergic overdrive phenomenon. Ryan (1990) noted that because of their rapid metabolism of tricyclics, some prepubertal children and younger adolescents may show daily withdrawal effects if they receive their entire daily tricyclic medication in one dose; hence, it may be necessary to divide the medication into two or three doses.

When maintenance medication is discontinued, tapering the medication down over 10 days to 2 weeks rather than abruptly withdrawing the medication will usually avoid the development of a clinically significant withdrawal syndrome. The clinician is cautioned that in patients with poor compliance, who in essence may undergo periodic self-induced acute withdrawals, the resulting withdrawal syndrome may be confused with untoward effects of the medication, inadequate treatment, or worsening of the underlying condition.

As an example, gradual taper of nortriptyline in one study yielded only 6 of 30 youths experiencing withdrawal symptoms; in all cases symptoms were mild, and in five subjects they were limited to the GI system (stomachache, nausea, and/or emesis).

Contraindications for TCA Administration

Known hypersensitivity to TCAs is an absolute contraindication.

TCAs are contraindicated in children and adolescents with cardiac conduction abnormalities.

TCAs should not be administered concomitantly with an MAOI. At least 14 days must pass after discontinuing an MAOI before administering a TCA.

Tricyclics may lower the seizure threshold and should be used with caution in individuals with seizure disorder.

TCAs may activate psychotic processes in patients with schizophrenia.

Interactions of TCAs with Other Drugs

Hyperpyretic crises or severe convulsive seizures may occur in patients receiving MAOIs and TCAs simultaneously.

Anticholinergic effects of TCAs may be additive with those of antipsychotics and result in central nervous system anticholinergic toxicity.

The central nervous system depressive effects of TCAs may be additive with those of alcohol, benzodiazepines, barbiturates, and antipsychotics.

TCAs may diminish or reverse the efficacy of antihypertensive agents.

Cigarette smoking may decrease the efficacy of TCAs.

Untoward Effects of TCAs

TCAs and Cardiotoxicity

Reports of Sudden Death

Sudden deaths have been reported in children taking TCAs. Although many of these deaths have not been proved to be cardiac related, cardiac arrhythmias, particularly tachyarrhythmias and torsade de pointes, are suspected.

Certain circumstances may increase the risk of the occurrence of torsade de pointes and/or sudden death in association with the use of drugs that prolong the QTc interval, including (a) bradycardia; (b) hypokalemia or hypomagnesemia; (c) concomitant use of other drugs that prolong the QTc interval; and (d) presence of congenital prolongation of the QT interval (*PDR*, 2005, p. 2611).

Reports of sudden death spanning from the 1970s to the early 1990s revealed that for the cases, TCAs were prescribed for a variety of indications including ADHD and enuresis. Reported cases included administration of desipramine and imipramine often with plasma levels in the therapeutic or subtherapeutic ranges, although in the case of a 6-year old girl, her dose had been raised to 14.7 mg/kg/day. Some cases involved recent increase in the dose, whereas others did not; and in some cases the events leading to death included physical exertion (Saraf et al., 1974; "Sudden Death," 1990). Several publications, reports, editorials, and commentaries rapidly followed the reports of these deaths. It became clear how little was known about the cardiac effects of tricyclics in prepubertal and even older subjects. The response was to be even more cautious when administering tricyclics not only to children but also to adolescents (Geller, 1991). In particular, it was recommended that a rhythm strip be obtained at baseline, during titration of medication, and at maintenance levels emphasizing measurement of the QTc to aid in identifying potentially vulnerable children (Riddle et al., 1991). Elliott and Popper (1990/1991) recommended obtaining ECGs at baseline, at a dose of about 3 mg/kg/day, and at a final dose of not >5 mg/kg/day. They also suggested using the following parameters as guidelines for cardiovascular monitoring in children and adolescents receiving TCAs:

PR interval: <210 ms
QRS interval: widening to no more than 30% over baseline
QTc interval: <450 ms
Heart rate: maximum of 130 beats per minute
Systolic blood pressure: maximum of 130 mm Hg
Diastolic blood pressure: maximum of 85 mm Hg

Although a more conservative viewpoint would be to obtain an ECG after each dose increase, Elliott and Popper (1990/1991) have pointed out that simply increasing the frequency of ECG monitoring does not necessarily reduce the risk of sudden death.

Cardiovascular toxicity of TCAs is of concern in all age groups, but especially in children and younger adolescents. Of particular concern is the slowing of cardiac conduction as reflected on the ECG by increases in PR and QRS intervals, cardiac arrhythmias, tachycardia, and heart block.

Although there was an initial speculation that children are more sensitive to cardiotoxic effects of TCAs than are adolescents and adults because of the relative efficiency with which they convert TCAs to potentially cardiotoxic 2-OH metabolites (Baldessarini, 1990), subsequent studies did not support this. Wilens et al. (1992) studied steady-state serum concentrations of DMI and 2-OH-DMI (OHDMI) in 40 child, 36 adolescent, and 27 adult psychiatric patients. Serum levels of DMI per weight-corrected (milligram/kilogram) dose rose from 50 ng/mL in children (age range, 6 to 12 years), to 56 ng/mL in adolescents (age range, 13 to 18 years), and to 91 ng/mL in adults (age range, 19 to 67 years). Contrary to expectations, OHDMI levels also increased with age from 17 ng/mL in children to 20 ng/mL in adolescents, and to 26 ng/mL in adults. The results did not support the hypothesis that children would develop relatively higher levels of OHDMI than adolescents and adults because of more efficient hepatic oxidative metabolism of DMI. Children either were more efficient in clearing both DMI and OHDMI than were adults or absorbed DMI relatively inefficiently. In fact, the data supported the clinical impression that children and adolescents usually require higher milligram/kilogram doses of DMI than do adults to reach similar serum DMI and OHDMI concentrations (Wilens et al., 1992).

These findings were consistent in a subsequent study by Wilens and colleagues (1993a). Children and adolescents showed no significant associations between serum drug and metabolite levels and heart rate or conduction (PR and QRS) intervals, although there was a weak relationship between sinus tachycardia and higher total DMI plus OHDMI levels. About 10% of the subjects had combined DMI plus OHDMI serum levels of 250 ng/mL or greater, which may increase risk of cardiovascular toxicity. They recommended monitoring serum levels and obtaining a baseline ECG and ECGs with increases in daily dose of >3 mg/kg (Wilens et al., 1993a).

Because routine ECGs may not record infrequent cardiac arrhythmias, Biederman et al. (1993) examined 24-hour ECG recordings and echocardiographic findings in 35 children and 36 adolescents receiving long-term (1.5 ± 1.2 years) DMI therapy for psychiatric disorders. Compared with untreated healthy children, subjects' ECGs had significantly higher rates of single or paired premature atrial contractions and runs of supraventricular tachycardia and a decreased rate of sinus pauses and junctional rhythm. DMI levels correlated significantly only with paired premature atrial contractions. All echocardiographic findings but one were normal; the abnormal one was thought to be caused by a pericardial effusion of viral origin and not drug related. Overall, the data supported earlier impressions that treatment with DMI is associated with minor and benign cardiac effects (Biederman et al., 1993).

In a subsequent study designed to further evaluate the cardiac effects of DMI on autonomic input to the heart, Walsh et al. (1999) obtained 24-hour ECGs from 42 subjects; 12 subjects were 7 to 18 years of age, and 30 subjects were between 19 and 66 years old. The authors assessed cardiac autonomic input using spectral analysis of the RR interval variability to determine heart rate variability. Pretreatment (off-medication) ECGs were done before administration of DMI in 41 cases. The ECG on DMI was done at optimal clinical dose, but 5 mg/kg/day could not be exceeded. The authors reported that DMI treatment was associated with a significant increase in heart rate and significant decreases in RR interval variability at all frequencies. DMI had no selective effect on the ratio of high-frequency bands, which are thought to reflect parasympathetic input, to low-frequency bands, which are thought to reflect sympathetic input. Hence, DMI had no impact on cardiac sympathetic/vagal (parasympathetic) balance. Although the RR interval variability was greater in the younger age group both with DMI and off medication, the magnitude of the effect of DMI on RR interval variability was similar in children, adolescents, and adults. The authors noted that the decrease in cardiac vagal modulation with DMI theoretically should increase the risk of arrhythmia because parasympathetic input to the heart generally protects against the development of arrhythmias. However, they did not resolve the issue as to whether DMI treatment would significantly increase the risk of developing a life-threatening arrhythmia.

The preceding studies appear to conclude that TCAs in the usual clinical dose range (<5 mg/kg/day) and at the usual serum drug and metabolite levels (250 to 300 ng/mL or less of DMI plus OHDMI) are usually associated with minor and clinically benign effects on cardiac function in all age ranges. They further suggest that children and adolescents are not at significantly greater risk for developing such effects compared with adults. Although the number of sudden deaths is small, the causal mechanism(s) are unknown and no specific cardiac finding has any known predictive value; clinically, it is considered prudent to monitor both ECG changes and serum drug and metabolite levels and to keep them within recommended parameters whenever TCAs are prescribed.

Amitai and Frischer (2006) used the large database of the American Association of Poison Control Centers (AAPCC) Toxic Exposure Surveillance System (TESS) for the 20-year period, 1983 to 2002, to determine the relative risk of death that was associated with the ingestion of desipramine compared with other TCAs (amitriptyline [AMI], imipramine, nortriptyline, and doxepin) in younger children (<6 years old) and older children and adolescents (6 to 17 for years 1983 to 1992 and 6 to 19 for years 1993 to 2002). (The case fatality rate [CFR] was defined as the ratio of the number of deaths divided by the number of exposures, an exposure being a report to the AAPCC-TESS concerning an individual ingestion of a drug or toxin.) The authors reported that there was a total of 24 deaths in the younger group and 144 deaths in the older group during these 20 years; most ingestions in the younger group were thought to be accidental, whereas those in the older group were usually intentional or "suicide." The authors noted that poisoning fatalities are vastly underreported to poison control centers and that the actual number of fatalities is much higher. The CFR for desipramine was significantly higher than that of the other four drugs in both groups ($P \leq .001$). Specifically, the CFR for desipramine exceeds that for amitriptyline by 7- to 8-fold, for doxepin by 4-fold; for imipramine by 6- to 12-fold; and for nortriptyline by 7- to 10-fold. The authors concluded that the reports on sudden death in children treated with desipramine coupled with its increased lethality compared with other TCAs when ingested accidently or in a suicide attempt indicate that restrictions should be placed on the use of desipramine in children and adolescents (Amitai & Frischer, 2006).

Other Untoward Effects of TCAs

Untoward effects to the central nervous system may include drowsiness, EEG changes, seizures, incoordination, anxiety, insomnia and nightmares, confusion secondary to anticholinergic toxicity, delusions, and worsening of psychosis.

TCAs may cause blood dyscrasias; if a patient develops fever and sore throat during treatment with tricyclics, a complete blood count should be taken.

Anticholinergic untoward effects may include dry mouth, blurred vision, and constipation.

Changes in libido, both increases and decreases, have been reported; gynecomastia and impotence have also been reported.

Preskorn et al. (1988) reported that cognitive toxicity was associated with supratherapeutic plasma levels of tricyclics.

TCAs, including clomipramine, may cause acute psychotic episodes if inadvertently administered to some individuals with schizophrenia who have been incorrectly diagnosed.

Clinical Monitoring and the Use of TCAs

Baseline studies that should be completed before initiating treatment with a TCA include sitting and supine blood pressure, complete blood count with differential, electrolytes, thyroid function tests, blood urea nitrogen, serum creatinine, urinalysis with osmolality, liver function tests, and an ECG.

Several investigators have noted that in clinical practice an absolute upper-dose maximum for TCAs is not very useful because of the marked intersubject variability in pharmacokinetics (e.g., metabolism and elimination) and the fact that, although children as a group tend to metabolize and/or eliminate TCAs more rapidly than do older adolescents and adults, some children, perhaps genetically slow hydroxylators, may reach very high serum levels on doses well below the recommended maximum (Biederman et al., 1989b). Hence, careful clinical monitoring, including serum levels, is essential.

Imipramine Hydrochloride (Tofranil), Imipramine Pamoate (Tofranil-PM)

Because imipramine hydrochloride has been the most widely used clinically and has been more thoroughly studied in children and adolescents than the other tricyclics, it will serve as the prototype.

Untoward Effects of Imipramine

Imipramine (IMI) has many untoward effects, some of which are potentially life-threatening. Cardiovascular effects, including arrhythmias, tachycardia, blood pressure changes, impaired conduction and heart block, and a decreased seizure threshold, are particularly worrisome.

IMI in the Treatment of Enuresis

Although the pharmacologic treatment of enuresis has been shown to be effective (Poussaint & Ditman, 1965; Rapoport et al., 1980b), it should not be employed until possible organic etiologies have been ruled out by appropriate physical examination and tests. It should be emphasized that behavioral therapies (e.g., conditioning with an alarm and pad apparatus) are the treatments of choice for functional enuresis. There is a tendency for some children to become tolerant of IMI's antienuretic effects, and many children relapse after medication withdrawal. Desmopressin acetate (a synthetic analog of the natural hormone, arginine vasopressin) nasal spray or tablets may be effective in some cases of enuresis that do not respond satisfactorily to other treatments.

IMI's antienuretic effect occurs rapidly and appears to be unrelated to its antidepressant effects; it may directly inhibit bladder musculature and increase outlet resistance (American Medical Association, 1986). It also appears that the IMI plus DMI plasma level required for the effective treatment of enuresis is lower than that required for treating MDD. DeGatta et al. (1984) treated 90 enuretic patients, aged 5 to 14 years, with IMI and reported that the minimum efficient serum concentration of IMI plus DMI in most cases was 80 ng/mL. However, about 20% of the subjects did not respond satisfactorily to IMI even with adequate serum levels.

Fritz et al. (1994) reviewed prior studies of plasma levels of IMI and DMI, its metabolite, in enuretic children treated with IMI and reported on levels in 18 additional patients. The therapeutic efficacy of IMI was moderately but significantly related to increasing levels of milligram/kilogram dosage. Intersubject plasma combined IMI and DMI levels varied at least sevenfold at every dosage. The combined IMI and DMI levels at 2.5 mg/kg averaged 136.0 ng/mL (range, 35 to 170 ng/mL) for complete responders, 116 ng/mL (range, 37 to 236 ng/mL) for partial responders, and 96.0 ng/mL (range, 60 to 157 ng/mL) for nonresponders. The authors noted that despite the lack of a clear therapeutic window, serum-level monitoring is useful in identifying subjects with low serum levels and suboptimal responses. In such cases, the dose of IMI may be raised before concluding that the medication is ineffective. Knowledge of the serum level is essential, however, to avoid the danger of further dose increases resulting in toxic serum levels in nonresponsive subjects who have relatively high serum levels.

A trial of IMI may occasionally be indicated when safer and more efficacious methods have failed and the symptom is psychologically a handicap or distressing to the patient, or perhaps when rapid control is essential to permit a child to go to summer camp or to travel.

The most frequent untoward effects reported in the treatment of enuretic children with IMI are nervousness, sleep disorders, tiredness, and mild GI disturbances (*PDR*, 1995). DeGatta et al. (1984) reported that 40% of their 90 enuretic subjects had at least one side effect; 42% had loss of appetite, 16% had light sleep, 11% had abdominal pains, 8% had dry mouth, and 8% had headaches.

In clinical practice, initial ECGs often have not been done for the treatment of enuresis because the final total daily dosage of IMI usually remains below 2.5 mg/kg and the risk of cardiotoxicity is low. In the light of the several sudden deaths reported in children receiving TCAs, even in usual doses, the author recommends a baseline ECG to screen for cardiac abnormalities that may increase the risk of conduction disorders secondary to tricyclic administration. It is suggested that bedwetters who void soon after falling asleep benefit if IMI is given earlier and in divided doses (e.g., 25 mg in midafternoon and 25 mg before bedtime) (*PDR*, 1995). A maximum dose of 2.5 mg/kg should not be exceeded because of the possibility of developing

ECG abnormalities. Doses of more than 75 mg/day do not increase efficacy and do increase untoward effects (*PDR*, 1995).

IMI in the Treatment of Childhood (Prepubertal) MDD

IMI and nortriptyline were the only tricyclics approved by the FDA for investigational use in the treatment of MDD in children 12 years of age and younger. FDA guidelines for ECG changes during treatment with either drug were as follows:

1. The PR interval should not exceed 0.21 second.
2. Resting heart rate should be <130 beats per minute.
3. The QRS interval should not exceed 0.02 second more than the baseline interval.

The blood pressure of children receiving IMI, which can both elevate the blood pressure and produce orthostatic hypotension, should not be permitted to exceed 145/95 mm Hg (Geller & Carr, 1988). IMI levels above 5 mg/kg are not usually permitted in investigational protocols (Hayes et al., 1975).

In a double-blind placebo-controlled study investigating the use of IMI in 38 prepubescent children diagnosed with MDD, there was no significant difference between response to IMI (56%; 9 of 16 subjects) and response to placebo (68%; 15 of 22 subjects). Further examination of total maintenance plasma levels (IMI plus DMI) in 30 prepubescent children resulted in a positive correlation between plasma level and clinical response. The authors reported that a maintenance total plasma level of 150 ng/mL was the most important differentiating point between responders and nonresponders. Eighty-five percent (17) of 20 subjects whose values were above 150 ng/mL had positive responses, but only 30% (3) of 10 children with lower values responded positively. The authors also found nothing, including dosage, that predicted plasma levels (Puig-Antich et al., 1987). This is consonant with the finding that combined IMI and DMI steady-state plasma levels varied sixfold (from 56 to 324 ng/mL) in 11 boys receiving 75 mg/day of IMI (Weller et al., 1982).

These authors also reported that the following untoward effects were found in more than 30% of the children treated with IMI: excitement, irritability, nightmares, insomnia, headache, muscle pain, increased appetite, abdominal cramps, constipation, vomiting, hiccups, dry mouth, bad taste in the mouth, sweating, flushed face, drowsiness, dizziness, tiredness, and restlessness. Similar untoward effects were present in the placebo group, although at lower frequencies. The untoward effects were severe enough in 17 of the 30 children to prevent upward titration to 5 mg/kg/day; cardiac side effects were responsible in 10 of these cases. Nine children had increases in the PR interval to the maximum, and one child's resting heart rate reached 130 beats per minute. No child on placebo showed ECG changes from baseline, whereas nearly every child receiving IMI had at least minor changes (Puig-Antich et al., 1987).

Preskorn et al. (1987) reported a double-blind, randomly assigned, placebo-controlled study of 22 hospitalized, prepubertal children with depression aged 6 to 12 years; IMI was found to be statistically better than placebo ($P < .05$) by 3 weeks, when IMI plus DMI plasma levels were monitored to adjust dosage of IMI to reach a therapeutic range of 125 to 250 ng/mL. Total plasma levels below 125 ng/mL yielded a response rate only somewhat better than placebo, and levels above 250 ng/mL were associated with a lower response rate and an increased incidence of toxic untoward effects. The latter included prolongation of intracardiac conduction, increased blood pressure and heart rate, and mental confusion. The authors conducted a prior study in which clinicians were unaware of plasma levels and further increased dosages, resulting in some children developing total IMI plus DMI plasma levels >450 ng/mL, the antidepressant response was poor, and several children developed toxic confusion that was incorrectly interpreted as a worsening of the depressive condition. This underscored the importance of monitoring plasma drug levels because a reduction in dosage, not an increase, would be indicated.

On the basis of their own data and those of Puig-Antich et al. (1987), Preskorn et al. (1989a) concluded that plasma IMI plus DMI levels ranging from 125 to 250 ng/mL were both efficacious and safe in treating MDD in children. These authors suggested using an initial oral dose of 75 mg IMI daily and then determining the combined plasma concentration of IMI plus DMI 7 to 10 days later, when steady-state levels would be expected. On the basis of their experience, 78% of children initially had plasma levels outside of the therapeutic range; 66% were below 125 ng/mL and 12% were above 250 ng/mL. Because intraindividual plasma levels were reproducible and linearly correlated with dose, the authors used the following formula to adjust the dosage:

New dose = (initial dose/initial level) × desired level

The desired level was 185 ng/mL, the midpoint of the optimal range. Using this strategy, 84% of their patients achieved levels within the therapeutic range. The remaining 16% had subtherapeutic levels, possibly requiring additional adjustments (Preskorn et al., 1989a).

IMI in the Treatment of Comorbid Prepubertal MDD and Conduct Disorder

Puig-Antich (1982) reported that 16 of 43 prepubertal males accepted for treatment of MDD had a codiagnosis of conduct disorder. These subjects did not differ on significant demographic and clinical variables from subjects diagnosed with MDD only. Approximately one-third of each group had auditory hallucinations consistent with Research Diagnostic Criteria (RDC) for psychotic subtype major depression. A history of major depression was found to precede the onset of conduct disorder in 14 (87%) of the 16 cases. Thirteen of the 16 patients who completed the study had a full antidepressant response between 5 and 18 weeks after beginning medication. Although this was a double-blind study, only one patient had a full response during the 5-week double-blind period; the others received either IMI openly or were switched to DMI and titrated upward. Dosage of 5 mg/kg/day was the desired dosage, but doses above and below this were administered; exact dosage was not reported for these patients. Of particular interest, however, was the fact that 11 of the 13 boys who definitely recovered from the major depression also experienced total remission of their conduct disorders. In a majority of cases, conduct disorders reappeared following recurrence of another major depressive episode. In six of these patients, who were treated with the same drug and dosage associated with remission, conduct disorders persisted in two (33%) following remission of the depressive symptoms. Puig-Antich (1982) emphasized the potential importance of treating these comorbid disorders and avoiding the recurrence of the depression during childhood and adolescence in significantly improving the prognosis of this subgroup of conduct disorders, which appear to develop following the onset of major depression.

IMI in the Treatment of Adolescent MDD

Thirty-four adolescents with MDD treated with IMI in an open study with monitoring of plasma IMI levels showed some differences from prepubescent children (Ryan et al., 1986). IMI was titrated to a dose of 5 mg/kg/day; the adolescents had an overall positive response rate of 44% (15) of 34, but there was no relationship between positive response and higher plasma IMI levels. Another difference between the adolescents and prepubertal children with MDD was that, as a group, nonpsychotic subjects did not respond more favorably than the psychotic subtype. The authors hypothesized that adolescents with MDD were less responsive to IMI because of an antagonistic effect of sex hormones, levels of which increase during adolescence (Ryan et al., 1986).

Strober et al. (1990) treated 35 adolescents (mean age, 15.4 years; age range, 3 to 18 years) openly with IMI; they had been hospitalized and diagnosed by RDC criteria with MDD with at least probable certainty. Ten of the adolescents also met criteria for delusional subtype. After failing to improve after 1 week's hospitalization, subjects were treated for 6 weeks with IMI. Six (17.7%) of the 34 subjects who completed the study were unable to achieve the target dose of 5 mg/kg/day because of untoward effects. Average daily dose was 222 ± 49 mg/day, and steady-state IMI plus DMI levels varied 11-fold (mean, 237 ± 168 ng/mL; range, 79 to 888 ng/mL). Eight (33%) of the 24 nondelusional subjects and 1 (10%) of the 10 delusional subjects were considered responders, suggesting greater refractoriness in patients with psychotic features. None of the responders had a plasma IMI plus DMI level below 180 ng/mL, but the difference between responders and nonresponders was not significant. Overall, only 10 (29.4%) patients were rated very much improved or much improved on the CGI-I Scale.

IMI in the Treatment of ADHD

A considerable body of literature attests to the clinical efficacy of IMI in the treatment of ADHD, although most studies find stimulants superior (for review, see Campbell et al., 1985; Rapoport et al., 1974, 1978c). Wender (1988) noted that when used to treat ADHD, tricyclics improve mood and decrease hyperactivity but usually are sedating and do not appear to improve concentration.

The mechanism of action of IMI in ADHD is different from that in depression; it is rapidly effective, and lower doses are often required. Mean dosages reported in the literature have ranged from 20 to 173.7 mg/day. The development of tolerance by some children to the therapeutic effects of IMI within about 6 weeks presents difficulties.

In a double-blind, placebo-controlled, crossover-design study of 30 hyperactive children, Werry et al. (1980) found IMI to be statistically more effective than methylphenidate in its overall therapeutic effect. Untoward effects of IMI, however, were greater and more troublesome than those of methylphenidate. Methylphenidate was given in doses of 0.40 mg/kg; IMI was given in doses of 1 and 2 mg/kg/day. The authors found few significant differences between the two IMI doses, but thought that the lower dose resulted in a slightly better clinical response and milder side effects (Werry et al., 1980).

A 1-year follow-up study of 76 hyperactive boys treated with IMI or methylphenidate found that significantly more subjects on IMI discontinued the medication because of lack of benefit or untoward effects, but that subjects in both treatment groups who continued on either drug improved equally (Quinn & Rapoport, 1975). The large dropout rate is a considerable clinical disadvantage in using IMI. It appears that tolerance to IMI may develop, resulting in deterioration after an initial improvement (Gross, 1973; Klein et al., 1980; Quinn and Rapoport, 1975; Waizer et al., 1974).

IMI in the Treatment of Separation Anxiety Disorder (School Phobia/School Refusal)

Over the course of three decades several studies, including some double-blind, placebo-controlled studies, examined the efficacy of IMI to treat SAD and school phobia. In the examination of 35 children with school phobia, doses ranging from 100 to 200 mg/day did not result in regular return to school after 3 weeks in the study protocol, but did result in significant separation from placebo with more regular return to school in 6 weeks (Gittelman-Klein & Klein, 1971). Next, IMI doses of 75 to 200 mg/day were effective for school phobia in a group of children ages 6 to 14, with responses seen at doses of 125 mg/day and maximum response in 6 to 8 weeks. Some children with severe separation anxiety without school phobia responded with doses as low as 25 to 50 mg/day (Klein et al., 1980). In a group of 21 children ages 6 to 14 who were identified as treatment refractory to 1 month of vigorous behavioral therapy, treatment with IMI was not significantly different than with placebo, with 50% improvement in both groups in this study. However, the IMI group had no untoward effects such as irritability, dry mouth, and dizziness (Klein et al., 1992).

Finally, Bernstein and group (2000) conducted a double-blind, placebo-controlled study of 63 adolescents (mean age, 13.9 ± 3.6 years; 38 females, 25 males) with school refusal and comorbid anxiety and MDD, over 8 weeks randomized to either IMI or placebo; in addition, all subjects received concurrent, manual-based, monitored CBT. Efficacy was assessed by clinicians using the Anxiety Rating for Children–Revised (ARC-R) and CDRS-R. At completion of the study, mean IMI dose was 182.3 ± 50.3 mg and the mean IMI plus DMI blood level was 151.2 ± 90.2 µg/L; nine subjects had levels <150 µg/L, including three with no detectable drug or metabolite; the mean IMI plus DMI level was 58.0 ± 51.4 µg/L. Subjects receiving IMI with concomitant CBT improved significantly more than did subjects on placebo and CBT in weekly hours of school attendance and in decreased depression as rated on the CDRS-R. There were no significant differences between the groups on the ARC-R and two self-report measures; thus, despite improvement, subjects still had significant symptoms. Similar to such studies examining SSRIs in combination with CBT, this work suggests that a multimodal approach (i.e., CBT plus pharmacotherapy) results in a superior response. Only a little more than half of the subjects receiving IMI plus CBT were attending school 75% of the time (Bernstein et al., 2000).

Nortriptyline Hydrochloride (Pamelor)

Untoward effects of nortriptyline and other TCAs were discussed earlier in the introduction to the TCAs. Untoward effects of nortriptyline are also discussed later in the summaries of its use in children and adolescents.

Nortriptyline Dosage Schedule for Children and Adolescents

Pharmacokinetic studies of TCAs in adults have shown that their elimination half-lives are sufficiently long to permit the frequent practice of giving a single bedtime dose once titration is completed (Rudorfer & Potter, 1987). Geller et al. (1987b), however, noted that 41 children, aged 5 to 12 years, had a significantly shorter mean nortriptyline plasma half-life (20.8 ± 7.2 hours; range, 11.2 to 42.5 hours) than did 32 adolescents aged 13 to 16 years (31.1 ± 19.8 hours; range, 14.2 to 76.6 hours). Geller et al. (1985) also found that correlations between the milligram/kilogram dose of nortriptyline and steady-state plasma levels were not significant in 33 children and adolescents aged 5 to 16 years. The clinical significance of these data, including the interindividual variation of half-life by as much as six- or sevenfold, prompted Geller et al. (1987b) to advise that nortriptyline should be administered twice daily for all patients up to 16 years of age and that plasma-level monitoring is essential to ensure achieving therapeutic plasma nortriptyline levels.

Geller et al. (1985) have used a single test dose of nortriptyline to predict steady-state plasma levels and to determine the initial dose of nortriptyline and presented tables suggesting daily doses to reach therapeutic nortriptyline plasma levels (Table 8.6).

To use this method, the clinician must have access to a laboratory that can reliably assay nortriptyline levels of <20 ng/mL. To use this table clinically, Geller et al. (1985) and Geller and Carr (1988) suggested the following:

1. At 9:00 AM, administer a single dose of 25 mg to patients aged 5 to 9 years or 50 mg to patients aged 10 to 16 years.
2. Twenty-four hours later (9:00 AM the next day), draw blood to determine the plasma nortriptyline level.
3. Use the table to determine the suggested medication dose for the patient's nortriptyline level and age.
4. Seven days later, determine plasma nortriptyline level 9 to 11 hours after a dose. If the level is not in the therapeutic range (60 to 100 ng/mL), adjust the dosage using the following equation (Geller & Carr, 1988):

Day 7 plasma levels/current dose = 80 ng/mL/adjusted dose

TABLE 8.6 » Suggested Nortriptyline Hydrochloride Dose Schedules for Children and Adolescents	
24-h Plasma Level (ng/mL)	Suggested Total Daily Dose (mg)
Predicted doses from 24-h plasma levels after a single dose of 25 mg administered to 5- to 9-y-olds.[a]	
6–10	50–75
11–14	35–40
15–20	25–30
21–25	20
Predicted doses from 24-h nortriptyline plasma levels after a single dose of 50 mg administered to 10- to 16-y-olds.[a]	
10–14	75–100
15–19	50–75
20–24	40–50
25–29	35
30–34	30
35–40	25
>40	20

[a]Total daily dose should be divided and given twice daily because of relatively short half-life.

Adapted from Geller B, Cooper TB, Chestnut EC, et al. Child and adolescent nortriptyline single dose kinetics predict steady state plasma levels and suggested dose: preliminary data. *J Clin Psychopharmacol.* 1985;5:154–158.

Reports of Interest

Nortriptyline in the Treatment of MDD in Children and Adolescents

Geller et al. (1985, 1986, 1987a, 1987b, 1989, 1990, 1992) have studied pharmacokinetic parameters of nortriptyline and its use in treating children and adolescents diagnosed with MDD. There are no double-blind, placebo-controlled studies establishing nortriptyline's superiority over that of placebo in treating MDD in children or adolescents.

In an open study of 22 children aged 6 to 12 treated in an outpatient setting for MDD, Geller et al. (1986) found that therapeutic efficacy correlated with nortriptyline plasma levels. Responders had significantly higher mean milligram/kilogram daily doses (1.02 ± 0.21 mg/kg; range, 0.64 to 1.57 mg/kg) than nonresponders (0.82 ± 0.51 mg/kg; range, 0.40 to 2.01 mg/kg). The mean nortriptyline steady-state plasma level was also higher in responders (60.31 ± 20.90 ng/mL; range, 18.8 to 111.5 ng/mL) than in nonresponders (30.86 ± 17.64 ng/mL; range, 12 to 54.3 ng/mL). All subjects with steady-state nortriptyline plasma levels of at least 60 ng/mL responded. At the end of the 8-week protocol, seven of the eight nonresponders recovered when the dose was increased to achieve steady-state nortriptyline plasma levels of 60 to 100 ng/mL. Overall, 21 of the 22 subjects had good clinical response with minimal and transient side effects, and all ECGs remained within recommended parameters for prepubertal children (Geller et al., 1986).

Geller et al. (1989, 1992) enrolled 72 prepubescent children, aged 6 to 12 years, who were diagnosed with MDD, nondelusional type, by RDC (Spitzer et al., 1978) and DSM-III (APA, 1980a) criteria in a double-blind, placebo-controlled study of the efficacy of nortriptyline. The children were chronically depressed: 96% had been ill for at least 2 years, and 50% had MDD for 5 or more years before entering the study. Both the nortriptyline and the placebo groups had a low rate of positive response (30.8% on nortriptyline and 16.7% on placebo), and there was no significant difference between them. There was no significant correlation between mean nortriptyline plasma level and response. Because of the poor response rate and the unlikelihood of finding a statistical difference between the placebo and active groups if the protocol were completed, Geller et al. (1989, 1992) stopped their study at this point.

Geller et al. (1990) enrolled 52 postpubertal adolescents, aged 12 to 17 years and diagnosed with MDD by RDC (Spitzer et al., 1978) and DSM-III (APA, 1980a) criteria in a random-assignment, double-blind, placebo-controlled study of nortriptyline. Subjects had scores on the CDRS and the Kiddie Global Assessment Scale, placing them in the severe range of pathology. Mean nortriptyline plasma level was 91.1 ± 18.3 ng/mL. The results of the study showed such a low rate of response to nortriptyline that the study was terminated early. Only 1 (8.3%) of 12 subjects receiving nortriptyline responded, whereas 4 (21.1%) of the 19 subjects on placebo responded. (The one responder to nortriptyline went on to have a bipolar course.)

Nortriptyline in the Treatment of Children and Adolescents Diagnosed with ADHD

Saul (1985) treated 60 patients diagnosed with ADD (age range, 9 to 20 years) with nortriptyline. They were initially prescribed stimulant medication but responded poorly and were switched to nortriptyline. Fifty-four (90%) of the 60 subjects had positive responses. Satisfactory clinical response usually occurred at 50 mg daily; 75 mg/day was the maximum dose given. Within 5 to 6 weeks, typically there was a marked change in attitude followed by an increase in attention span and a decrease in impulsivity. The most clinically significant untoward effects at the initial dose were dizziness and sleepiness; their inconvenience was minimized by administering the medication around bedtime.

Prince et al. (2000) conducted a two-phase, 9-week, controlled study of 35 subjects (28 males and 7 females; mean age, 9.8 ± 2.6 years) diagnosed with ADHD by DSM-IV (APA, 1994) criteria. During the first 6-week, open-label phase, subjects were administered nortriptyline in divided doses (before school and after dinner) that were individually titrated up to a maximum of 2 mg/kg/day over the first 2 weeks. Mean nortriptyline dose at the end of week 4 was 79 ± 36 mg/day or 1.9 mg/kg/day, with a mean serum nortriptyline concentration of 81 ± 66 ng/mL (range, 10 to 316 ng/mL). At the end of 6 weeks, the mean nortriptyline dose was 77 ± 35 mg/day or 1.8 mg/kg/day. Thirty-two subjects completed the first phase; two subjects had dropped out because of untoward effects and one because of nonresponse. By the end of week 6, there was an overall mean reduction in the ADHD symptom checklist of 53% ($P < .001$); 29 subjects (84%) had reductions of >30% of their baseline ratings. Opposition defiant symptoms also significantly decreased by 48% ($P < .001$) during the 6-week open phase, with 25 subjects (71%) having a >30% reduction compared with baseline ratings. There was no significant correlation between dose or serum level of nortriptyline and improvement in ADHD or opposition symptoms.

Twenty-five of the 29 responders elected to participate in the 3-week double-blind discontinuation phase; of the 23 subjects who completed this phase, 12 had been randomized to nortriptyline and 11 to placebo. The subjects who continued to receive nortriptyline had significantly lower scores on the DSM-IV ADHD checklist compared with subjects receiving placebo ($P < .04$). Overall, subjects randomized to nortriptyline maintained their clinical improvements in ADHD and ODD symptoms, whereas those randomized to placebo had a significant re-exacerbation of these symptoms and their week-9 ratings were not significantly different from baseline. During the study, heart rate increased by 18% ($P < .05$), but there were no clinically significant changes in blood pressure, in PR, QRS, QTc, or any new ECG abnormality. The data suggest that nortriptyline is efficacious in treating both ADHD and oppositional symptoms in ADHD and ADHD with comorbidity (Prince et al., 2000).

Nortriptyline in Comorbid ADHD and Chronic Motor Tic Disorder or TS

In a retrospective study of 12 children and adolescents (age range, 5 to 16 years; mean, 10.9 ± 1.0 years) diagnosed with ADHD and comorbid chronic motor tic disorder ($N = 2$) or TS ($N = 10$), Spencer et al. (1993c) reported that 8 (67%) subjects were rated as being markedly or very much improved ($P = .01$) in their movement disorders, and 11 (92%) were rated much or very much improved ($P = .0001$) in their ADHD symptoms. The average dose of nortriptyline was 105 ± 11.7 mg/day or 2.8 ± 0.3 mg/kg/day. Mean serum nortriptyline level was 122.7 ± 12.1 ng/mg for the 10 patients for whom such values had been determined. There were few untoward effects. The only cardiac symptom was a mild tachycardia in one patient; no clinically significant changes occurred in EEGs.

Amitriptyline Hydrochloride (Elavil, Endep)

Amitriptyline hydrochloride is a tertiary amine TCA. Although the TCAs block reuptake of both norepinephrine and serotonin, evidence suggests that the tertiary amine tricyclics block the reuptake of serotonin more than the reuptake of norepinephrine, whereas the secondary amine tricyclics may block norepinephrine uptake more than serotonin uptake.

Pharmacokinetics of Amitriptyline Hydrochloride

Untoward effects of amitriptyline were discussed earlier in "Untoward Effects of TCAs" as well as in the summaries of its use in children and adolescents later.

Reports of Interest

Historical early studies on the use of amitriptyline in youth have yielded nonsignificant results or difficulty with tolerability. In a 1977 study comparing amitriptyline, methylphenidate, and placebo, although amitriptyline was comparable to methylphenidate in reducing hyperactivity and aggression in both the home and school environments, the doses of amitriptyline sufficiently high to control symptoms could not be tolerated. Sedation remained a problem throughout the 2-week period on amitriptyline. Studies examining efficacy of amitriptyline in prepubertal children with MDD (Kashani et al., 1984), adolescents with MDD (Kramer & Feiguine, 1981), and adolescents with treatment-resistant MDD (Birmaher et al., 1998) did not yield significant results compared to placebo.

Desipramine Hydrochloride (Norpramin, Pertofrane)

Desipramine is a secondary amine TCA. Although the TCAs block reuptake of both norepinephrine and serotonin, evidence suggests that the secondary amine tricyclics block the reuptake of norepinephrine more than the reuptake of serotonin, whereas tertiary amine tricyclics may block serotonin uptake more than norepinephrine uptake.

Pharmacokinetics and Adverse Effects of Desipramine Hydrochloride

Pharmacokinetics and adverse effects of DMI, including sudden death, were discussed earlier under "Pharmacokinetics of TCAs" and "Untoward Effects of TCAs" and later under the "Reports of Interest" for DMI that follow.

Reports of Interest

Desipramine Hydrochloride in the Treatment of Adolescent MDD

Two studies demonstrated similar findings when examining efficacy of desipramine compared to placebo to treat MDD in adolescents. Neither study demonstrated significant differences between DMI and placebo on primary outcome measures; thus, efficacy was not demonstrated. However, significant adverse effects necessitating discontinuation of DMI occurred in both studies, including allergic-type pruritic maculopapular rash, GI complaints, laryngospasm, and orthostatic hypotension (Boulos et al., 1991; Kutcher et al., 1994).

Desipramine Hydrochloride in the Treatment of Enuresis

Rapoport et al. (1980b) found that 75 mg of DMI at bedtime had a short-term antienuretic effect that was not statistically different from that of IMI.

Desipramine Hydrochloride in the Treatment of ADHD

Garfinkel et al. (1983) studied 12 males (mean age, 7.3 years; range, 5.9 to 11.6 years) who were diagnosed with ADD and required day hospital or inpatient treatment for the severity of their symptoms of impulsiveness, inattention, and aggression. The subjects received placebo, methylphenidate, DMI, and clomipramine in a double-blind, crossover experiment. The mean dose of DMI was 85 mg/day and did not exceed 100 mg/day or 3.5 mg/kg/day for any subject. Methylphenidate was significantly better than the other three in improving overall classroom functioning as rated on the Conners Scale by teachers ($P < .005$) and program child care workers ($P < .001$).

Two open and long-term studies demonstrated significant improvement in severe ADD in adolescents and also in children with ADD. The adolescent group consisted of 12 youths who had responded poorly to or did not tolerate stimulants. After 4 weeks and at a mean daily dose of 1.57 mg/kg (range, 0.58 to 2.63 mg/kg), 11 of the 12 patients improved, and 5 were rated "much" or "very much" improved on the CGI Scale. At 52 weeks, optimal daily doses ranged from 0.93 to 5.95 mg/kg. Nine patients sustained their improvement for more than 6 months, and 8 of these were rated "much" or "very much" improved. Plasma levels for a given dose varied as much as 10-fold. Untoward effects were most troublesome during the first month; drowsiness (50%); postural dizziness (25%); weight loss and/or decreased appetite (25%); headache (16%); insomnia (8%); and racing thoughts (8%). The untoward effects lessened in all cases following reduction in dosage (Gastfriend et al., 1984). Subsequently, 18 children diagnosed with ADD were treated with DMI for 4 to 52 weeks. Doses at 4 weeks ranged from 0.7 to 4 mg/kg/day (mean, 2.0 ± 0.9 mg/kg/day); on later follow-up, doses were significantly higher, ranging from 1.3 to 6.3 mg/kg/day. Improvement at follow-up time (mean time at follow-up, 22.9 ± 15.9 weeks) was also significantly greater than at 4 weeks. Although there was sufficient time for tolerance to medication to have developed, it was not observed (Biederman et al., 1986).

Biederman et al. (1989a, 1989b) reviewed earlier work in this area and studied the efficacy of DMI in treating 42 children and 20 adolescents diagnosed with ADD with hyperactivity ($N = 60$) or without hyperactivity ($N = 2$). Sixty-nine percent of their subjects had responded poorly to earlier treatment with stimulants. The subjects were randomly assigned to a 6-week, double-blind, parallel-group, placebo-controlled protocol. Desipramine was titrated upward to an average daily dose of 4.6 ± 0.2 mg/kg, a relatively high dose. Patients treated with DMI had statistically significant improvement in symptoms rated on the Conners Abbreviated Parent and Teacher Questionnaires, compared with subjects receiving placebo ($P = .0001$). The patterns of improvement were similar in adolescents and children. There was no significant relationship between serum DMI levels and clinical response, making the designation of an optimal level inappropriate. Some subjects who improved had serum levels below 100 ng/mL. About one-fourth of the patients had high levels, between 300 and 900 ng/mL; of this group, 80% (12 of 15) improved (Biederman et al., 1989b).

Untoward effects were usually mild and were more frequent in subjects receiving DMI than in the placebo group ($P < .05$); overall, there was no discernible relationship between serum level and untoward effects. Symptoms included dry mouth (32%), decreased appetite (29%), headache (29%), abdominal discomfort

(26%), tiredness (25%), dizziness (23%), and insomnia (23%). Although no subjects developed any clinically apparent cardiovascular signs or symptoms, cardiovascular and ECG untoward effects, such as increased diastolic blood pressure, tachycardia, and conduction abnormalities, were statistically more frequent in subjects receiving DMI. There was a suggestion that ECG changes occurred more frequently at higher serum DMI levels. Of special interest is the fact that in contrast to reports of rapid improvement of subjects with ADD in response to IMI, subjects in this study required 3 to 4 weeks to show significant clinical improvement with DMI as compared with placebo (Biederman et al., 1989b).

Biederman et al. (1989b) suggested that a steady-state serum DMI level between 100 ng/mL and a maximum of 300 ng/mL is probably efficacious and safe for most children and adolescents, but that some patients will require daily doses >3.5 mg/kg/day to reach these serum levels. They estimated that optimal doses range between 2.5 and 5 mg/kg/day. The authors (Biederman et al., 1989b) recommended the following parameters as being more clinically relevant in the titration of DMI than accepting an arbitrary maximum limit in dose (e.g., 5 mg/kg):

1. The DMI serum level should be kept under 300 ng/mL.
2. The PR interval on the ECG should be <200 ms.
3. The QRS interval on the ECG should be <120 ms.

Desipramine shows some promise as an alternative medication for children and adolescents diagnosed with ADHD who have unsatisfactory responses to other indicated medication options for ADHD. Gualtieri et al. (1991) reported that DMI improved long-term memory performance, analogous to that reported with stimulants, when used in treating children diagnosed with ADHD. Its use requires strict clinical monitoring, including ECG and serum levels, because of its pharmacokinetics and cardiotoxicity.

Coadministration of Desipramine Hydrochloride and Methylphenidate in the Treatment of ADHD with Symptoms of MDD or Comorbid MDD

Rapport et al. (1993) studied the separate and combined effects of methylphenidate and DMI on cognitive functions in 16 hospitalized children (aged 7 years, 9 months to 12 years, 10 months) diagnosed with ADHD and MDD, ADHD with symptoms of MDD, or MDD with symptoms of ADHD. Following a 2-week baseline period, subjects received placebo, DMI, three dose levels of methylphenidate (10, 15, and 20 mg), and combined methylphenidate and DMI at each of the methylphenidate levels. Desipramine was begun at 50 mg/day and increased by 25 mg every 2 days, unless untoward effects prevented the increase and until plasma levels between 125 and 225 mg/mL were reached, because earlier studies had suggested this to be the range of maximum therapeutic efficacy in prepubertal children. Methylphenidate alone improved vigilance, both drugs had positive effects on short-term memory and visual problem solving, and the combination of both drugs affected learning of higher order relationships. The effects of these drug conditions on mood and behavior were not reported.

In a separate report concerning the same subjects, Pataki et al. (1993) detailed the untoward effects of methylphenidate and DMI alone and in combination in a subset of 13 patients. The mean final dose of DMI during combined administration with methylphenidate was 148 mg/day (range, 75 to 300 mg/day) or 4.4 mg/kg/day (range, 2.5 to 6.6 mg/kg/day). The mean plasma DMI level during combined administration with methylphenidate was 170 ng/mL (range, <50 to 228 ng/mL for the 11 subjects for whom it was available). Because methylphenidate is reported to inhibit hepatic enzymes that metabolize tricyclics, DMI plasma levels alone and when coadministered with methylphenidate were compared. The mean final plasma level of DMI when administered alone was 159 ng/mL, compared with a level of 170 ng/mL when administered in combination with methylphenidate, and the difference in plasma levels was not significant. On individual bases, however, the most extreme variations were found in a subject who received 75 mg of DMI daily (2.9 mg/kg/day) in combination with methylphenidate and had a plasma level of 158 ng/mL and another subject who received 300 mg of DMI daily (6.6 mg/kg/day) that resulted in a plasma level of 146 ng/day.

Untoward effects were more frequent in the combined DMI and methylphenidate treatment than in any of the other conditions: nausea (17% vs. 8% in the 40 mg/day methylphenidate group), dry mouth (42% vs. 8% in the 40 mg/day methylphenidate and the DMI-alone groups), and tremor (8% vs. none in any other group). The combination of DMI and methylphenidate resulted in an increase in ventricular heart rate that was significantly greater than that in the other conditions; however, this increase was not in a range that would place the children at clinical risk according to the pediatric cardiologist. Three children had sinus tachycardia on ECG: all three occurred during the combined drug treatment but were not thought to be of clinical significance by the pediatric cardiologist.

The authors concluded that, clinically, the untoward effects of combined DMI and methylphenidate treatment were not significantly greater than those for DMI alone; untoward effects were similar to those during administration of DMI alone, and there was no evidence that the addition of methylphenidate increased DMI levels significantly (Pataki et al., 1993). This study was conducted on a very small number of patients, and much larger samples are needed before definitive conclusions may be reached.

Desipramine Hydrochloride in Comorbid ADHD and Chronic Motor Tic Disorder or TS

Although stimulants are the treatment of choice in ADHD, they may exacerbate tics. Hence, problems arise when children have preexisting tic disorders or when they develop tics while being treated with stimulants. Indeed, some authorities recommend not giving stimulants to children with a family history of tics or Tourette disorder.

Riddle et al. (1988) noted that Tourette disorder and ADHD coexist in approximately 50% of children who are referred for evaluation of Tourette disorder and that between 20% and 50% of such patients develop worsening of their tics if treated with stimulants. The authors treated seven children with DMI, aged 7 to 11 years, all of whom had diagnoses of ADHD and various tic disorders. Desipramine was begun at 25 mg daily and increased by 25 mg every 2 to 3 days to a maximum of 100 mg, or a lower level when clinical improvement was satisfactory or untoward effects prevented further increase. Four children improved "remarkably," and one child "moderately" when rated on the CGI-I Scale. Two children were considered nonresponders. Six children showed no change in the status or severity of their tics. One child's intermittent eye-blinking became persistent after 3 weeks of DMI; this had also occurred in this patient during a previous trial of methylphenidate (Riddle et al., 1988).

In a retrospective study of 33 children and adolescents (age range, 5 to 17 years; mean, 12.0 ± 0.6 years) diagnosed with chronic motor tic disorder or TS, 30 of whom had comorbid ADHD, Spencer et al. (1993a) reported that 27 (82%) of the 33 had significant improvement ($P = .0001$) in their movement disorders and 24 (80%) of the 30 with ADHD had significant improvements ($P = .0001$) in their ADHD symptoms when treated with DMI. The average dose of DMI was 127 ± 9.8 mg/day or 3.5 ± 0.3 mg/kg/day. Mean serum DMI level was 132 ± 16 ng/mg for the 22 patients for whom such values had been determined. Untoward effects, rash (one) and abdominal pain (one), caused two patients to withdraw prematurely from the study, precluding their inclusion in the analysis of data. The study was discontinued in four patients because of untoward effects: nausea and vomiting (one), irritability and agitation (two), and worsening of a tic (one). Eight subjects (24%) had asymptomatic cardiac abnormalities including new onset of incomplete right bundle branch block (four), junctional rhythms (two), benign ectopic atrial contractions on Holter monitor (one), and an increase in the QTc interval (one).

Clomipramine Hydrochloride (Anafranil)

Clomipramine is an antiobsessional drug that belongs to the class of TCAs. Clomipramine itself has potent inhibitory effects on the neuronal reuptake of serotonin as compared with neuronal reuptake of norepinephrine; however, its primary metabolite, desmethylclomipramine, effectively inhibits norepinephrine uptake.

Flament et al. (1987) studied the actions of clomipramine on peripheral measures of serotonergic and noradrenergic function in children and adolescents diagnosed with OCD. They compared 29 such children and adolescents (mean age, 13.9 ± 2.5 years; range, 8 to 18 years) with controls and found that a high pretreatment level of platelet serotonin was a strong predictor of a favorable clinical response and that clomipramine treatment produced a very marked decrease in platelet serotonin concentration in all patients ($P < .0001$). Clomipramine treatment also produced a trend toward reduction in platelet monoamine oxidase activity ($P = .11$) and increased peripheral noradrenergic function. The plasma level of norepinephrine in standing subjects increased significantly ($P < .008$). These data suggest that clomipramine's inhibition of serotonin uptake may be essential to its antiobsessional effect (Flament et al., 1987).

Pharmacokinetics of Clomipramine Hydrochloride

Clomipramine has a long half-life. The mean half-life of a single 150-mg dose is 32 hours, and the mean half-life of its major metabolite, desmethylclomipramine, is 69 hours. Steady-state serum levels usually occur within 1 to 2 weeks at a given daily dosage. Children and adolescents <15 years of age had significantly lower plasma concentrations for a given dose compared with adults (package insert). Dugas et al. (1980) reported that peak plasma clomipramine levels were achieved 3 to 4 hours after ingestion in the three children they studied and reported an apparent plasma terminal half-life of 11.9 to 17.3 hours. The bioavailability of clomipramine is not significantly affected by ingestion with food, and administering it during initial titration in divided doses with meals helps to reduce GI side effects. Clomipramine is metabolized largely into its major bioactive metabolite, desmethylclomipramine; both compounds are ultimately metabolized into their glucuronide conjugates by the liver. The metabolites are excreted through the bile duct and the kidneys.

Contraindications for the Administration of Clomipramine Hydrochloride

Known hypersensitivity to clomipramine hydrochloride is a contraindication.

Untoward Effects of Clomipramine Hydrochloride

The most significant risk of clomipramine appears to be the development of seizures. Risk for seizures is cumulative; and, for doses up to 300 mg/day, increased from 0.64% at 90 days to 1.45% at 1 year. Other untoward effects that occur in children and adolescents include somnolence, tremor, dizziness, headache, sleep disorders, increased sweating, dry mouth, GI effects (constipation and dyspepsia), anorexia, fatigue, cardiovascular effects (postural hypotension, palpitations, tachycardia, and syncope), abnormalities of vision, urinary retention, dysmenorrhea in females, and ejaculation failure in males (package insert). Because of reports of blood dyscrasias, a complete blood cell count should be determined in patients who develop fever and sore throat during the course of treatment.

Dugas et al. (1980) reported in their study of 8 children and 28 adolescents who were administered clomipramine for enuresis or depressive symptomatology that the incidence of untoward effects was clearly related to the clomipramine plasma concentration. Untoward effects occurred in about 15% to 20% of patients with plasma clomipramine levels below 60 ng/mL and were present in more than 90% of cases with serum levels above 90 ng/mL. Hypotension occurred only in cases with serum levels above 80 ng/mL. No discernible relationship was found between untoward effects and plasma levels of desmethylclomipramine.

There are few published studies on the use of clomipramine in children and adolescents diagnosed with OCD. Those of Flament et al. (1985, 1987) and of Leonard et al. (1989) include some children below the age of 10 years and are summarized here.

Clomipramine was found to be significantly superior to placebo in a placebo-controlled, double-blind, crossover study of 19 subjects whose ages ranged from 10 to 18 years (mean, 14.5 ± 2.3 years) who were diagnosed with severe primary OCD (Flament et al., 1985). The dose range was 100 to 200 mg/day (mean, 141 ± 30 mg/day). The experimental data suggested that clomipramine has a direct antiobsessional action that is independent of any antidepressant effect. In fact, 10 of the subjects had been previously treated with other tricyclics without significant benefit. Flament et al. (1987) increased the number of their subjects to 29 (mean age, 13.9 ± 2.5 years; range, 8 to 18 years) and reported the continued efficacy of clomipramine; the mean daily dose of clomipramine was 134 ± 33 mg/day.

Leonard et al. (1989) compared the efficacy of clomipramine and DMI in the treatment of severe primary OCD in 49 child and adolescent subjects (31 males and 18 females) (mean age, 13.86 ± 2.87 years; range, 7 to 19 years) in a 10-week crossover-design study. Administration of clomipramine was begun at 25 mg/day for children weighing 25 kg or less and at 50 mg/day for subjects weighing more than 25 kg. Dosage was increased weekly by an amount equal to each subject's initial dose. Maximum dosage did not exceed 250 mg/day or 5 mg/kg/day. The mean dose of clomipramine at week 5 was 150 ± 53 mg/day, with a range of 50 to 250 mg/day. Clomipramine was markedly superior to desipramine DMI in decreasing obsessive-compulsive symptoms on several rating scales. In addition, 64% of patients who improved significantly when initially on clomipramine experienced relapse following the crossover to DMI; this was a relapse rate similar to that for placebo in the preceding Flament et al. (1985) study. The most common side effects reported were dry mouth, tremor, tiredness, dizziness, difficulty sleeping, sweating, constipation, poor appetite, and weakness.

Leonard et al. (1991) reported that, of the 48 children completing the preceding 1989 study, 28 (58%) were still receiving maintenance clomipramine 4 to 32 months later. Twenty-six of these patients agreed to participate in an 8-month double-blind study in which DMI was substituted for clomipramine. At the time of entry to the protocol, subjects' daily doses of clomipramine ranged from 50 to 250 mg (mean dose, 134.7 ± 58.2 mg/day or 2.4 ± 0.6 mg/kg/day). Subjects continued to receive clomipramine at their maintenance level for 3 months, at which time DMI was substituted for clomipramine for the next 2 months. For the final 3-month period, all subjects received clomipramine. Twenty subjects completed the study. Eight of nine patients (89%) randomly assigned to DMI relapsed during the 2-month period, whereas only 2 (18%) of 11 patients remaining on clomipramine relapsed. The authors noted that the eight patients who relapsed on DMI experienced symptom improvement to previous levels within 1 month of clomipramine being reinstituted. This is clinically important because it suggests that a significant percentage of children and adolescents need long-term drug treatment to prevent recurrence of obsessive-compulsive symptoms; however, if relapse occurs when an attempt to discontinue clomipramine is made, comparable clinical control can usually be regained upon reinstating clomipramine.

DeVeaugh-Geiss et al. (1992) reported a multicenter trial in which 60 children and adolescents, aged 10 to 17 years, diagnosed with OCD were administered clomipramine in a 10-week, double-blind, fully randomized, parallel-groups, placebo-controlled study. Thirty-one patients were assigned to the clomipramine group and 29 to the placebo group; except for an excess of males in the clomipramine group, they were comparable. Placebo was administered to all patients under single-blind conditions for the first 2 weeks. During the active drug stage, the initial daily dose was 25 mg of active drug or placebo; over the next 2 weeks, this dose was titrated to either 75 or 100 mg daily depending on weight. Subsequent increases to a maximum of 3 mg/kg/day or 200 mg were permitted at the discretion of the investigator. Twenty-seven subjects in each group completed the study. Untoward effects were typical of the TCAs. The patients receiving clomipramine improved significantly compared with those in the placebo group. On the Y-BOCS, the clomipramine group had a mean reduction in score of 37% and the placebo group a reduction of 8% ($P < .05$), and on the NIMH Global Scale, the groups had reductions of 34% and 6%, respectively ($P < .05$).

Evidence suggests that clomipramine is effective for children and adolescents with severe OCD; however, the FDA has not approved for advertising it as effective and safe in treating children <10 years of age.

Clomipramine Hydrochloride in the Treatment of ADHD

Garfinkel et al. (1983) compared the clinical efficacy of methylphenidate, DMI, and clomipramine in a double-blind, placebo-controlled, crossover study of 12 males (mean age, 7.3 years; range, 5.9 to 11.6 years) diagnosed with ADD who required day hospital or inpatient treatment for severe impulsiveness, attention deficit, and aggression. The mean dose of clomipramine was 85 mg/day and did not exceed 100 mg or 3.5 mg/kg/day for any subject. Methylphenidate was significantly better than the other three in improving overall classroom functioning as rated on the Conners Scale by teachers ($P < .005$) and program child care workers ($P < .001$). Clomipramine, however, was significantly better than DMI in reducing scores reflecting aggressivity, impulsivity, and depressive/affective symptoms. On the basis of these data, clomipramine would merit further study in treating children and adolescents with ADHD who do not respond satisfactorily to stimulant medication.

Clomipramine Hydrochloride in the Treatment of Autistic Disorder

Gordon et al. (1993) conducted a double-blind comparison of clomipramine, DMI, and placebo in 30 subjects (20 males and 10 females; age range, 6 to 23 years; mean, 10.4 ± 4.11 years) diagnosed with autistic disorder to assess the efficacy of clomipramine in treating obsessive-compulsive and stereotyped motor behaviors. During the initial 2-week, single-blind, placebo washout period, two patients were dropped, one because of positive response and the other because of a refusal to take pills. Fourteen subjects were randomly assigned to a 10-week, double-blind, crossover comparison of clomipramine and placebo, and the other 14 subjects were randomly assigned to a similar comparison of clomipramine and DMI. Two patients were dropped from each group—a 23-year-old man on placebo because of violent outbursts, a 7-year-old girl on clomipramine secondary to a grand mal seizure, and two others for extraneous reasons. The 12 patients in the clomipramine/placebo comparison group showed significantly reduced autistic behaviors ($P = .0001$), anger/uncooperativeness ($P = .0001$), hyperactivity ($P = .001$), but not speech deviance ($P = .27$) in week-5 ratings on the 14-item Autism Relevant subscale of the CPRS while receiving clomipramine. These subjects also had a significant improvement in obsessive-compulsive symptoms ($P = .001$) and overall improvement on the Efficacy Index of the CGI Scale ($P = .0001$) during the period on the active drug. The 12 patients in the clomipramine/DMI comparison group improved significantly more during the period on clomipramine than during the period on DMI on week-5 ratings on the Autism Relevant subscale of the CPRS ($P = .0003$) and anger/uncooperativeness ($P = .008$). The two drugs were not significantly different on the hyperactivity factor, but both were better than placebo; clomipramine showed a trend toward improvement on the speech factor compared with DMI ($P = .08$). Obsessive-compulsive symptoms improved significantly more with clomipramine

($P = .001$), and clomipramine was superior to DMI on the Efficacy Index of the CGI Scale ($P = .005$). The authors noted that SIBs such as hitting, kicking, biting, and pinching, which were present in four patients who had not responded to intensive behavioral and drug interventions in two cases, improved significantly in all four subjects when they were receiving clomipramine. Untoward effects of clomipramine were usually minor, and they were not significantly different from those of placebo or DMI. However, dosage of clomipramine was reduced in one patient because of prolongation of QTc interval to 450 ms and in another because of severe tachycardia (Gordon et al., 1993).

Five patients who continued to be maintained on clomipramine underwent a double-blind placebo substitution for 8 weeks between months 5 and 12 of maintenance therapy. Four (80%) of the five worsened during the period on placebo, but regained former clinical improvement when clomipramine was reinstated (Gordon et al., 1993).

Clomipramine Hydrochloride in the Treatment of Enuresis

Dugas et al. (1980) administered clomipramine to 10 enuretic children. A therapeutic effect was observed at plasma clomipramine concentrations of 20 to 60 ng/mL, whereas lower and higher levels were associated with lack of therapeutic efficacy or untoward effects. In a later report, the sample was increased to 31 enuretic children (Morselli et al., 1983). Of the 21 who had good therapeutic outcomes, 16 (76%) had plasma steady-state clomipramine concentrations >15 ng/mL, whereas only 3 of the 10 nonresponders had such high plasma levels. The plasma-level differences between the responders and the nonresponders were significant ($P < .05$).

Clomipramine Hydrochloride in the Treatment of Depressive Symptoms

Dugas et al. (1980) treated 1 boy, 8.5 years old, and 25 adolescents, 13 to 19 years old, who had significant depressive symptomatology with clomipramine. Clomipramine doses ranged from 0.24 to 2.93 mg/kg/day. Sixteen patients received other psychoactive medication simultaneously. Twelve of the 26 patients responded positively. Final diagnoses of these patients were school phobia (3), anorexia nervosa (6), manic-depressive psychosis (1), depression (5), and depressive reactions in behavior disorders or borderline personalities (11). Two patients had no therapeutic response, 1 had a minimal response, 11 had moderate improvement, 3 had "good" results, and 9 had excellent results. The patients diagnosed with anorexia responded least favorably; only two had a good response, whereas four of the five diagnosed with depression had excellent responses. Similar plasma levels of clomipramine were present in both responders and nonresponders; however, nonresponders had proportionally higher levels of desmethylclomipramine.

Clomipramine Hydrochloride in the Treatment of School Phobia (Separation Anxiety)

Berney et al. (1981) treated 52 children diagnosed with school refusal, which consisted of a neurotic disorder with a marked reluctance to attend school for at least 4 weeks' duration and was frequently associated with depressive features. The study was double blind and placebo controlled and lasted for 12 weeks. Forty-six patients, aged 9 to 14 years, completed the study; 19 were on placebo and 27 were on clomipramine. The total daily dosage of clomipramine was titrated slowly to 40 mg/day for 9- and 10-year-olds; 50 mg/day for 11- and 12-year-olds; and 75 mg/day for 13- and 14-year-olds. There was no evidence that clomipramine was superior to placebo in reducing separation anxiety and neurotic behavior or being specific for depression. The authors, however, noted that they used proportionally lower doses of clomipramine than the doses used in studies reporting its efficacy in treating school phobia/separation anxiety.

9

CHAPTER

Antiepileptic Mood Stabilizers and Lithium Carbonate

JULIA C. JACKSON AND NATOSHA S. OSANSANYA

LITHIUM CARBONATE (LITHOTABS, ESKALITH, LITHANE, LITHOBID) AND LITHIUM CITRATE (CIBALITH-S)

Currently, lithium carbonate is approved by the U.S. Food and Drug Administration (FDA) for the treatment of manic episodes of bipolar disorders and for maintenance therapy of bipolar patients. Lithium carbonate is FDA approved for persons 12 years of age and older; however, pediatric approval was based solely on literature supporting its use in adults with bipolar disorder. Over the past three decades, lithium carbonate has been investigated in the treatment of many child and adolescent disorders, but especially in the treatment of children with severe aggression directed toward self or others, children with bipolar or similar disorders, and behaviorally disturbed children whose parents are known lithium responders. One major impetus for this research was that typical antipsychotic agents, which were historically used often to control severe behavioral disorders and sometimes mania, not only could cause cognitive dulling when used in sufficient dosage to control symptoms but also carried significant risk of causing tardive dyskinesia when used on a long-term basis (Platt et al., 1984).

Pharmacokinetics of Lithium Carbonate

The lithium ion is readily absorbed from the gastrointestinal tract and is most commonly administered in the form of lithium carbonate (Li_2CO_3), a highly soluble salt. Peak plasma concentrations occur within 2 to 4 hours, and complete absorption takes place within approximately 8 hours (Baldessarini, 1990). Approximately 95% of a single dose of lithium is excreted by the kidneys, with up to two-thirds of an acute dose being excreted within 6 to 12 hours. The serum half-life is approximately 20 to 24 hours. Depletion of the sodium ion causes a clinically significant degree of lithium retention by the kidneys. Steady-state serum lithium levels typically occur within 5 to 8 days of repeated identical daily doses of lithium carbonate. Although lithium pharmacokinetics differs considerably among individuals, they are fairly stable over time for a given person (Baldessarini & Stephens, 1970).

Vitiello et al. (1988) and Malone et al. (1995) studied the pharmacokinetics of lithium carbonate in children. Both discovered a trend toward a shorter elimination half-life and a significantly higher total renal clearance of lithium. Findling et al. (2010) discovered similar results in 39 youth with bipolar-I disorder, although they determined that fat-free mass explained most of the variability in volume of distribution and clearance parameters. The conclusion that lithium clearance correlates well with fat-free mass is important given that obesity is often seen in children taking psychotropic medication.

Contraindications for Lithium Carbonate Administration

Administration of lithium carbonate is relatively contraindicated in individuals with significant renal or cardiovascular disease, severe debilitation, severe dehydration, or sodium depletion because these conditions are associated with a very high risk of lithium toxicity. Patients with such disorders should be thoroughly assessed, usually in consultation with the person providing medical care, before beginning lithium therapy.

Except under urgent circumstances, adolescents who are likely to become pregnant should not be administered lithium; this is particularly true of those in early pregnancy. Although recent data support that cardiac teratogenicity, including Ebstein anomaly, is likely to be small with *in utero* lithium exposure, fetal echocardiography is recommended between 16 and 20 weeks gestation in all cases of first-trimester lithium exposure (*PDR*.net, 2017). Nursing should not be undertaken during treatment with lithium because lithium is excreted in human milk.

Significant thyroid disease is a relative contraindication to lithium carbonate therapy; however, with careful monitoring of thyroid function and the use of supplemental thyroid preparations when necessary, it may be used when other drugs are not effective and the potential benefits outweigh the risks.

Interactions of Lithium Carbonate with Other Drugs

There are several reports that increased neuroleptic toxicity with an encephalopathic syndrome, or neuroleptic malignant syndrome may occur when lithium and neuroleptics are used concomitantly, but this has usually been seen with high doses. The simultaneous use of lithium and neuroleptic agents, however, may be indicated in some cases of mania or schizoaffective psychoses, and many patients have received both a neuroleptic and lithium with no untoward effects.

Elevations in lithium serum concentration and increased risk of neurotoxic lithium effects may occur when carbamazepine and lithium are used simultaneously because carbamazepine decreases lithium renal clearance. Use of calcium channel blockers in conjunction with lithium treatment has resulted in neurotoxicity, including ataxia, tremors, and gastrointestinal symptoms.

Many other drugs may increase or decrease serum lithium levels by influencing its absorption or excretion by the kidneys. For example, cyclooxygenase-2 inhibitors, nonsteroidal anti-inflammatory drugs, metronidazole, enalapril, and losartan increase plasma lithium levels. By contrast, sodium bicarbonate, alkalinizing agents, and xanthine preparations lower serum lithium concentrations. Frequent serum drug monitoring should be employed when these types of medications are used together.

Lithium Toxicity

One major difficulty associated with the administration of lithium carbonate is its low therapeutic index; lithium toxicity is closely related to serum lithium levels and may occur at doses of lithium carbonate close to those necessary to achieve therapeutic serum lithium levels. Adverse effects or side effects are those unwanted symptoms that occur at therapeutic serum lithium levels, whereas toxic effects occur when serum lithium levels exceed therapeutic levels. However, this is not absolute, because patients who are unusually sensitive to lithium may develop toxic signs at serum levels below 1.0 mEq/L (*Physicians' Desk Reference* [PDR], 2000).

Lithium toxicity may be heralded by diarrhea, vomiting, mild ataxia, coarse tremor, muscular weakness and fasciculations (twitches), drowsiness, sedation, slurred speech, and impaired coordination. Patients and/or their caretakers must be made familiar with the symptoms of early lithium toxicity and instructed to discontinue lithium immediately and contact their physician if such signs occur. Increasingly severe and life-threatening toxic effects, including cardiac arrhythmias and severe central nervous system difficulties such as impaired consciousness, confusion, stupor, seizures, coma, and death, may occur with further elevations in serum lithium levels.

No specific treatment for lithium toxicity is available. If signs of early lithium toxicity appear, the drug should be withheld, lithium levels determined, and the medication resumed at a lower dosage only after 24 to 48 hours. Severe lithium toxicity is life threatening and requires hospital admission, treatments to reduce the concentration of the lithium ion, and supportive measures.

Lithium's low therapeutic index and its pharmacokinetics make it necessary to administer lithium carbonate tablets or immediate-release capsules in divided doses, usually three or four times daily, to maintain therapeutic serum levels without toxicity. Even controlled-release tablets must be administered every 12 hours. It is essential that a laboratory capable of determining serum lithium levels rapidly and accurately be readily available to the clinician. For accuracy and serial comparisons, determinations of serum lithium levels should be made when lithium concentrations are relatively stable and at the same time each day. Typically, blood is drawn 12 hours after the last dose of lithium and immediately before the morning dose (trough level).

Although some patients who are unusually sensitive to lithium may exhibit toxic effects at serum levels below 1 mEq/L, for most patients mild to moderate toxic effects occur at serum levels between 1.5 and 2 mEq/L and moderate-to-severe reactions occur at levels of 2 mEq/L and above.

Lithium decreases sodium reuptake by the renal tubules; hence, adequate sodium intake must be maintained. This is especially important if there is significant sodium loss during illness (e.g., sweating, vomiting, or diarrhea) or because of changes in diet or elimination of electrolytes. The importance of adequate ingestion of ordinary table salt and fluids should be emphasized. Caution during hot weather or vigorous exertion is also advised, because additional salt loss and concomitant dehydration secondary to pronounced diaphoresis may cause serum lithium levels of patients on maintenance lithium to increase and move into the toxic range. This may also be true of sweating caused by elevated body temperature secondary to infection or heat without exercise (e.g., sauna), but some evidence suggests that heavy sweating caused by exercise may result in lowered rather than in elevated serum lithium levels. Jefferson et al. (1982) studied four healthy athletes who were stabilized on lithium for 1 week before running a 20-km race. At the end of the race, the subjects were dehydrated, but their serum lithium levels had decreased by 20%. The authors found that the sweat-to-serum ratio for the lithium ion was approximately four times greater than that for the sodium ion. These authors concluded that strenuous exercise with extensive perspiration was more likely to decrease rather than increase serum lithium levels, and patients were more likely to require either no change or an increase, rather than a decrease, in dosage of lithium to maintain therapeutic levels. The authors do caution, however, that any conditions that significantly alter fluid and electrolyte balance, including strenuous exercise with heavy sweating, should be carefully monitored with serum lithium levels.

Untoward Effects of Lithium Carbonate

Lithium carbonate is frequently reported to have adverse effects early in the course of treatment, although most diminish or disappear during the first weeks of treatment. Studies show that side effects are more likely to occur in pediatric versus adult patients (Campbell et al., 1984a, 1991).

Early adverse effects include fine tremor (unresponsive to antiparkinsonism drugs), polydipsia, and polyuria that may occur during initial treatment and persist or be variably present throughout treatment. Nausea and malaise or general discomfort may initially occur, but usually subside with ongoing treatment. Weight gain, headache, and other gastrointestinal complaints such as diarrhea may also occur. Taking lithium with meals or after meals or increasing the dosage more gradually may be helpful in controlling gastrointestinal symptoms.

Later adverse effects are often related to serum level, including levels in the therapeutic range; these include continued hand tremor that may worsen, polydipsia, polyuria, weight gain and edema, thyroid and renal abnormalities, dermatologic abnormalities (including acne), fatigue, leukocytosis, and other symptoms. As serum levels increase, toxicity increases and other, more severe untoward effects, discussed earlier under toxicity, appear.

The most common adverse effects of lithium carbonate in 61 children, aged 7 to 17 years and diagnosed with bipolar-I disorder were nausea (66.7%), headache (65%), vomiting (55%), dizziness (36.7%), diarrhea (30%), upper abdominal pain/tremor (26.7%), and somnolence (18.3%) (Findling et al., 2011). This study involved an 8-week open-label trial of lithium with starting doses of either 300 mg twice daily or 300 mg thrice daily. Similarly, in a later trial of lithium in youth, the most common adverse effects were vomiting (45%), nausea (43%), and headache (36%) (Findling et al., 2015).

Abnormalities in renal functioning (diminution of renal concentrating ability) and morphologic structure (glomerular and interstitial fibrosis and nephron atrophy) have been reported in adults on long-term lithium maintenance. Vetro et al. (1985) reported that after 1 year of lithium treatment, one child developed polyuria with daytime enuresis and impaired renal concentration. Other parameters of renal function did not change, and polyuria ceased within a few days of lithium being discontinued. Five other children on long-term lithium therapy showed transient albuminuria that remitted spontaneously, and discontinuation of treatment was not necessary (Vetro et al., 1985). At least four cases of nephrotic syndrome related to pediatric lithium treatment have been reported (Peterson et al., 2008; Sakarcan et al., 2002). In the cases, discontinuation of lithium resulted in resolution of symptoms. Given that reemergence of proteinuria has been reported during lithium rechallenge, this should be avoided (Peterson et al., 2008). Peterson et al. (2008) argue that because the use of lithium in the pediatric population is likely to increase, periodically monitoring for urine protein, particularly during the first year of treatment, is reasonable.

Lithium may also interfere with thyroid function. Vetro et al. (1985) reported that two children developed goiter with normal function after 1.5 to 2 years of lithium therapy. Findling et al. (2011) revealed that 4 out of 61 pediatric patients experienced a treatment-emergent thyroid-related adverse event during an 8-week open-label trial of lithium—hypothyroidism ($N = 1$) and elevated thyroid-stimulating hormone (TSH) levels ($N = 3$). Furthermore, three patients experienced significant changes in levels of antithyroglobulin AB and thyroid peroxidase ($N = 1$) and increased thyrotropin levels ($N = 2$) (Findling et al., 2011). A retrospective study showed that lithium treatment in 61 adolescent patients was associated with increased TSH levels, although only one patient's TSH level rose above the level considered to be clinically significant (>10 mU/L) (Amitai et al., 2014). In a cross-sectional study, 30 adolescent patients with mean lithium levels of 0.74 mmol/L for 1 year or more had higher thyroid volumes and TSH levels compared to adolescents taking other mood-stabilizing medication (Sethy & Sinha, 2016). T_3 and T_4 levels were normal in both groups, leading investigators to conclude that long-term lithium treatment may result in subclinical hypothyroidism, and that laboratory and ultrasonography monitoring should be considered when prescribing lithium to adolescent patients (Sethy & Sinha, 2016).

Neuroleptic malignant syndrome has been reported in a few patients who were administered neuroleptic drugs and lithium simultaneously.

Dostal (1972) reported specific adverse effects of lithium in 14 developmentally delayed adolescent males that interfered with patient management despite significant therapeutic gains. Polydipsia, polyuria, and nocturnal enuresis were so severe as to alienate staff who cared for the youngsters. These symptoms remitted within 2 weeks of discontinuing lithium (Dostal, 1972).

Premedication Work-up and Periodic Monitoring for Lithium Treatment

Routine Laboratory Tests

Complete Blood Cell Count with Differential

Lithium frequently causes a clinically insignificant and reversible elevation of white blood cells (WBCs), with counts commonly between 10,000 and 15,000 cells/mm^3. The lithium-induced leukocytosis characteristically shows neutrophilia (increased polymorphonuclear leukocytes) and lymphocytopenia (Reisberg & Gershon, 1979). Thus, leukocytosis can usually be differentiated from the one caused by infection because the increase in neutrophils is in more mature forms, whereas in infection younger forms predominate. Lithium may also increase platelet counts. Lithium-induced leukocytosis has in fact shown to be medically advantageous in some patient scenarios. For example, Mattai et al. (2009) discovered that six pediatric patients experienced a 66% increase in absolute neutrophil count after lithium was added to their clozapine regimen, which bolstered support for the use of lithium to manage clozapine-induced neutropenia.

Serum Electrolytes

Serum electrolyte levels should be determined, in particular to verify that sodium ion levels are normal, because hyponatremia decreases lithium excretion by the renal tubules.

Pregnancy Test

Lithium crosses the placenta, and data from birth registries suggest teratogenicity with abnormalities, including cardiac malformations, especially Ebstein anomaly. Lithium is relatively contraindicated during pregnancy, especially during the first trimester. Infants born to mothers taking lithium appear to be at increased risk for hypotonia, lethargy, cyanosis, and electrocardiogram (ECG) changes (United States Pharmacopeial Dispensing Information [USPDI], 1990). All females who could be pregnant should be tested before initiation of lithium therapy and warned that, because of lithium's teratogenic potential for the fetus, they should take care not to become pregnant while taking the medication.

Renal Function Tests

Baseline assessment of renal functioning is essential because the kidney is the primary route of elimination of lithium. For healthy children and adolescents, a baseline serum creatinine, blood urea nitrogen level, and urinalysis are usually adequate and should be monitored every 3 to 6 months during lithium therapy (Kowatch & DelBello, 2003). If kidney disease is suspected or abnormalities are found, a more thorough evaluation, including tests such as urinalysis (including specific gravity), 24-hour urine volume, and 24-hour urine for creatinine clearance and protein, should be performed and the patient should be referred to a nephrologist if necessary.

Thyroid Function Tests

Lithium causes thyroid abnormalities primarily by decreasing the release of thyroid hormones. This causes such findings as euthyroid goiter; hypothyroidism; decreased triiodothyronine (T_3), thyroxine (T_4), and protein-bound iodine levels; and elevated ^{131}I and TSH levels between 5% and 15% of patients receiving long-term lithium therapy (Jefferson et al., 1987). Recommended baseline studies include T_4 and TSH levels. Hypothyroidism resulting from lithium treatment is thought to be related to preexisting Hashimoto thyroiditis, suggesting that determining antithyroid antibodies as part of the work-up may also be useful (Rosse et al., 1989). Thyroid function tests should be monitored every 3 to 6 months throughout lithium treatment (Kowatch & DelBello, 2003). If there is a suggestion of thyroid abnormality during symptom-based or laboratory screening, consultation with an endocrinologist should be considered.

Cardiovascular Function Tests

Various cardiac conduction and repolarization abnormalities (e.g., bradycardia) and reversible ECG abnormalities have been reported in a large percentage of adults receiving lithium. ECG changes commonly include benign, reversible T-wave changes (flattening, isoelectricity, and inversion of T waves), which are dose dependent, and an increase in the PQ interval (Jefferson et al., 1987). It has been hypothesized that lithium's cardiotoxic effects result from its displacing and substituting for intracellular potassium. Gathering a thorough cardiac history including the presence or absence of palpitations, slow or rapid heart rate, dizziness, preexisting heart disease, or a family history of significant cardiac pathology such as prolonged QT syndrome or sudden cardiac death, is important when determining whether an otherwise safe medication could be harmful to particular patient (Singh et al., 2016). A baseline ECG should be obtained routinely in patients >40 years of age or those who have any history or clinical suggestions of cardiovascular disease. Although not considered mandatory in young, healthy patients, a baseline ECG is justifiable and useful to have for comparison, should cardiovascular abnormalities develop at some later time. If patients have or develop cardiac abnormalities, frequent ECG monitoring should be done in consultation with a cardiologist.

Calcium Metabolism Tests

Lithium may increase renal calcium reabsorption, resulting in hypocalciuria (Jefferson et al., 1987). Lithium may also cause hyperparathyroidism with hypercalcemia and hypophosphatemia, with resulting decreased bone formation or density in children. If abnormal results occur, parathyroid hormone (parathormone) levels may be determined. Lithium may also replace calcium in bone formation, especially in immature bones (USPDI, 1990). A baseline calcium level should be determined in children and adolescents, but a baseline parathormone level is not usually recommended.

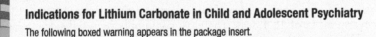

Indications for Lithium Carbonate in Child and Adolescent Psychiatry

The following boxed warning appears in the package insert.

NOTE: WARNING—Lithium toxicity is closely related to serum lithium levels and can occur at doses close to therapeutic levels. Facilities for prompt and accurate serum lithium determinations should be available before initiating therapy.

Lithium carbonate is FDA approved for the treatment of manic episodes of bipolar illness and maintenance therapy of manic-depressive patients, with a history of mania, who are at least 12 years of age. Significant normalization of manic symptomatology may require up to 3 weeks of lithium carbonate therapy; hence, concomitant use of antipsychotic medication may be initially required for more rapid control of manic symptoms. See subsequent text regarding titration of dose and recommended serum lithium levels.

(continued)

Indications for Lithium Carbonate in Child and Adolescent Psychiatry (*continued*)

Lithium Dosage Schedule

- *Children up to 11 years of age:* Not recommended (see subsequent text for studies done in this patient population).
- *Adolescents at least 12 years of age and adults:* Dosage must be individually regulated according to clinical response and serum lithium levels. As noted earlier, the pharmacokinetics of lithium carbonate makes it necessary to administer the total daily dose in smaller doses administered three or four times daily if immediate-release tablets or syrup is used, or twice daily if controlled-release capsules are used, to minimize risk of reaching toxic serum levels of lithium. (More detailed information on administering, titrating, and monitoring lithium in children and adolescents is found in the subsequent text.)

Lithium Carbonate Dose Forms Available

- *Eskalith CR/Lithium Carbonate/Lithium/Lithobid Oral Tablet ER:* 300, 450 mg
- *Eskalith/Lithium/Lithium Carbonate Oral Capsule:* 150, 300, 600 mg
- *Lithium/Lithium Carbonate Oral Tablet:* 300 mg
- *Syrup (lithium citrate):* 8 mEq/5 mL (8 mEq of lithium is equivalent to 300 mg of lithium carbonate)

Titration of Lithium Dosage (Ages 12 and Up)

Typically, doses of approximately 1,800 mg/day will achieve the serum lithium levels necessary to control symptoms during acute mania (between 1 and 1.5 mEq/L). During long-term maintenance, serum lithium levels usually range between 0.6 and 1.2 mEq/L; this usually requires a divided daily dose between 900 and 1,200 mg (GlaxoSmithKline, 2003). Berg et al. (1974), however, reported that a 14-year-old girl and her father, who were both diagnosed with bipolar manic-depressive disorder, required daily doses of lithium as high as 2,400 mg to achieve therapeutic levels.

Schou (1969) noted that early untoward effects, such as nausea, diarrhea, muscle weakness, thirst, urinary frequency, hand tremor, and a dazed feeling, may be caused by a too rapid rise in serum lithium levels. Lithium is a gastric irritant. A low initial dose of lithium taken after meals, which slows absorption, and gradual increases in dose will often avert the development of these symptoms. When they develop, they usually subside spontaneously within a few days.

Serum lithium levels should be monitored twice weekly during the acute manic phase and until both serum level and clinical condition have stabilized. In the maintenance phase of therapy during remission, serum lithium levels should be monitored every 3 to 6 months (Kowatch & DelBello, 2003). Lithium levels should be drawn 12 hours after the last dose and before the subsequent dose.

Patel et al. (2006) treated 27 adolescents (12 to 18 years old) with an initial lithium carbonate dose of 30 mg/kg/day (twice-daily dosing; maximum starting dose of 600 mg PO twice daily), during a 6-week open-label trial of lithium for the treatment of bipolar depression. Seventy percent of subjects achieved a therapeutic level of 1.0 to 1.2 mEq/L over a mean of 18.4 days. The most commonly reported side effects were headache (74%), nausea/vomiting (67%), polyuria (33%), stomachache (30%), polydipsia (26%), and abdominal cramps (19%). Almost all of the side effects were judged to be mild to moderate in severity, and the authors concluded that lithium carbonate was relatively well tolerated in this trial (Patel et al., 2006).

Use of Lithium Carbonate in Children Below 12 Years of Age

The therapeutic dosages of lithium carbonate used in treating children above 5 years of age with various disorders do not differ significantly from those used in treating older adolescents and adults, and the principles of administration are essentially the same (Campbell et al., 1984a).

Weller et al. (1986) published a guide for determining the initial total daily lithium dose for prepubertal children 6 to 12 years of age. The guide and summary of how it is used are presented in Table 9.1. Lower initial doses should be used for children diagnosed with mental retardation or organicity (central nervous system damage) (E. B. Weller, personal communication, 1990).

The purpose of this guide is to reach therapeutic serum lithium levels (0.6 to 1.2 mEq/L) as rapidly as possible using currently available tablet strengths without undue risk of reaching toxic serum levels. The authors administered lithium to 10 subjects diagnosed with manic-depressive illness and 5 subjects diagnosed with conduct disorder (CD), following these guidelines. About 13 of the 15 subjects had serum lithium levels in the therapeutic range after only 5 days of treatment. Side effects were reported to be minimal, primarily mild nausea, abdominal pain, polydipsia, polyuria, and increase in preexisting enuresis. Most were transient, and none required discontinuation of lithium. As discussed earlier, some adverse effects of lithium appear to be related to excessively rapid increases in serum lithium level. It remains to be determined whether the use of the proposed lithium dosage guide will cause significantly more adverse effects or will increase their severity more than would a more gradual titration of lithium. In cases where very rapid control of symptoms is critical, however, it may be proved to be especially useful.

Findling et al. (2011) likewise studied lithium dosing in children and adolescents suffering from bipolar-I disorder. In this 8-week trial, outpatients aged 7 to 17 years were started on lithium 300 mg twice daily (if <30 kg) or 300 mg twice or thrice daily (for children >30 kg). Doses were then increased by 300 mg/week unless one of the following stop criteria occurred: a therapeutic response was obtained (Clinical Global Impressions–Improvement [CGI]-I Scale score ≤2 and a 50% decrease in Young Mania Rating Scale [YMRS] score from baseline), youth experienced significant adverse effects, doses exceeded 40 mg/kg/day, or the serum lithium level was expected to be >1.4 mEq/L. As mentioned previously, the most commonly observed side effects during this trial were nausea (66.7%), headache (65%), vomiting (55%), dizziness (36.7%), diarrhea (30%), upper abdominal pain/tremor (26.7%), and somnolence (18.3%). The authors concluded that lithium was well tolerated and exhibited similar side-effect profiles in all dosing arms of the study, which led them to conclude that lithium dosed at 300 mg thrice daily (with an additional 300-mg increase during the first week), followed by 300-mg weekly increases until one or more stop criteria are met will be used in upcoming randomized placebo-controlled trials (Findling et al., 2011).

Reports of Interest

Lithium has been widely looked at over the years for the treatment of pediatric bipolar disorder (PBD). Older studies consisted primarily of case reports, chart reviews, and

TABLE 9.1 » Lithium Carbonate Dosage Guide for Prepubertal School-Aged Children			
Weight (kg)	8 AM Dose (mg)	12 Noon Dose (mg)	6 PM Dose (mg)	Total Daily Dose (mg)
<25	150	150	300	600
25–40	300	300	300	900
40–50	300	300	600	1,200
50–60	600	300	600	1,500

Dose specified in schedule should be maintained at least 5 days with serum lithium levels drawn every other day 12 hours after ingestion of the last lithium dose until two consecutive levels appear in the therapeutic range (0.6 to 1.2 mEq/L). Dose may then be adjusted depending on serum level, side effects, or clinical response. Do not exceed 1.4 mEq/L serum level. Lower initial dose should be used for children diagnosed with mental retardation or organicity.

From Weller EB, Weller RA, Fristed MA. Lithium dosage guide for prepubertal children: a preliminary report. *J Am Acad Child Psychiatry*. 1986;25:92–95.

only a few small double-blind placebo-controlled trials, although studies completed over the past decade, including larger open and double-blinded controlled trials, have offered increased clarity regarding the efficacy and tolerability of lithium in the treatment of PBD.

Lithium Carbonate in the Treatment of Youth Bipolar Disorder

Geller et al. (1998) conducted a 6-week, double-blind, placebo-controlled, parallel-groups study comparing lithium and placebo in the treatment of 25 outpatients (16 males and 9 females; mean age, 16.3 ± 1.2 years) diagnosed by *Diagnostic and Statistical Manual of Mental Disorders, Third Edition–Revised* (DSM-III-R) (American Psychiatric Association [APA], 1987) criteria with a bipolar disorder or major depressive disorder with one or more predictors of future bipolar disorder and substance dependency disorder. After 3 weeks, the percentage of positive weekly random urine tests was significantly lower in the lithium group than in the placebo group (P = .042). When symptoms of mania and mood symptoms' persistence were studied specifically, however, lithium did not separate from placebo. The ratings of untoward effects on the acute lithium side effects scale showed that lithium was well tolerated. Only polyuria and polydipsia occurred significantly more frequently in the lithium group than in the placebo group. The authors concluded that lithium may be effective for the treatment of adolescents with bipolar disorder and a comorbid substance use disorder (SUD), although acknowledged that further research was needed with larger sample sizes and longer treatment durations.

In this trial, the mean age of onset of substance abuse disorders was approximately 6 years after the mean age of onset of subjects' mood disorders. Subjects did not have to agree to stop their substance abuse to participate in the study. About 13 subjects were assigned to the lithium group; of these, 10 completed the study. About 12 were assigned to the placebo group and 11 completed the study.

Efficacy was determined by ratings on the Children's Global Assessment Scale (CGAS) and random weekly urine drug assays. "Responders" were required to have a score of ≥65. Lithium was initiated with a 600-mg dose and was titrated to yield a serum lithium level between 0.9 and 1.3 mEq/L. The total dose was divided and given at 7:00 AM and 7:00 PM daily. The subjects on lithium improved significantly more than those on placebo depending on predefined response criteria. Six (60%) of the ten completers on lithium were "responders," compared with 1 (9.1%) of the 11 completers on placebo (P = .024). The mean daily lithium dose for the 10 completers was 1,733 ± 428 mg; the responders' daily dose was significantly higher (1,975 ± 240 mg) than that of the nonresponders (1,368 ± 399 mg; P = .02), but there was no significant difference in their serum lithium levels (responders, 0.88 ± 0.27 mEq/L vs. nonresponders, 0.85 ± 0.3 mEq/L).

Kafantaris et al. (2003) conducted a 4-week, open trial of lithium carbonate in treating acute mania in 100 adolescents (mean age, 15.23 years; age range, 12 to 18 years; 50 males, 50 females) who were diagnosed with bipolar-I disorder, met DSM-IV criteria for a current manic or mixed episode, and had a score of ≥16 on the YMRS. Attention-deficit/hyperactivity disorder (ADHD) was a codiagnosis in 31% of patients. At the end of week 4, all the ratings showed significant improvement (P < .001). Sixty-three patients met responder criteria by the end of week 2. Remission of manic symptoms (YMRS score < 6) occurred in 26 patients by week 4 and only 4 of the 23 patients with suicidal ideation at baseline had such symptoms by week 4. The authors reported that the presence of baseline psychotic features (with antipsychotic treatment), prominent depressive symptoms, comorbid diagnoses including ADHD, early onset of mood disorders, and severity of mania at initial presentation and hospitalization did not significantly impact a response to lithium at week 4. Adverse effects present at week 4 ratings in >10% of patients included weight gain (1 to 12 lb), 55.3%; polydipsia, 33.3%; polyuria, 25.5%; headache, 23.5%; tremor, 19.6%; gastrointestinal pain, 17.6%; nausea, 15.7%; vomiting,

13.7%; anorexia, 13.7%; and diarrhea, 13.7%. The study authors concluded that lithium appeared efficacious in the treatment of adolescent mania when used with or without concomitant antipsychotic medication (Kafantaris et al., 2003).

In this trial, immediate-release lithium was rapidly titrated to therapeutic serum levels between 0.6 and 1.2 mEq/L using Cooper's technique (Cooper et al., 1973). Subjects ($N = 46$) with severe aggression and/or psychosis were treated concomitantly with antipsychotics. Mean lithium serum level at the end of week 1 was 0.90 ± 0.25 mEq/L; at endpoint (week 4), the mean serum level was 0.93 ± 0.21 mEq/L and the mean dose was 1,355 ± 389 mg/day.

Subjects were rated weekly on the YMRS, Hamilton Depression Rating Scale (17-item), Brief Psychiatric Rating Scale (BPRS), CGI-I Scale, and the CGAS. Responders were defined as having both a decrease of >33% from baseline YMRS score and a ≤2 rating (much or very much improved) on the CGI-I.

Findling et al. (2006a) conducted a prospective, 8-week, open-label outpatient lithium plus divalproex combination therapy trial for 38 patients aged 5 to 17 years with bipolar type I or II. The enrolled patients had a mean age of 10.5 years, were previously stabilized with lithium plus divalproex, and subsequently relapsed during treatment with either medication as monotherapy. During the randomized maintenance monotherapy trial, half of the patients received divalproex (target serum concentrations of 0.6 to 1.2 mmol/L), and the other half received lithium (target serum concentrations of 0.6 to 1.2 mmol/L). If subjects evidenced mood relapse by the unblinded physician monitor during the monotherapy phase, they were enrolled in the restabilization study and treated with both lithium and divalproex at doses previously required to achieve stabilization. At the end of the 8-week restabilization study, a significant decline in YMRS, Children's Depression Rating Scale–Revised (CDRS-R), CGAS, and the Clinical Global Impressions-Severity (CGI-S) scores were discovered in almost all of the enrolled patients. The authors thus concluded that most youth who initially stabilize with a combination of lithium and divalproex, and subsequently destabilize with monotherapy treatment alone, can be effectively restabilized with prior effective doses of lithium and divalproex.

In this trial, outcome measures included the CDRS-R and the YMRS. The CGI-S was used to assess bipolar symptom severity, and the CGAS was used to determine overall functioning at both home and school. Of the 38 patients enrolled in the restabilization phase, 35 completed all 8 weeks (92.1%), whereas 2 withdrew consent and 1 was lost to follow-up. No patients ended the study because of medication intolerance.

Limitations of the study include its open-label design, short trial duration, and subjects with comorbid diagnoses such as ADHD were allowed to receive concomitant pharmacotherapy, which may have facilitated symptom reduction during the trial, independent of the study medications (Findling et al., 2006a).

Pavuluri et al. (2006) studied 38 youth, ages 4 to 17 years, with a history of preschool-onset bipolar disorder during a 12-month open-label trial. All subjects received lithium as monotherapy. The authors concluded that a large percentage of youth with a history of preschool-onset bipolar disorder were either nonresponders or only partial responders to lithium when used as monotherapy. Subsequent augmentation of lithium with risperidone in these cases was judged to be effective and well tolerated during the trial (Pavuluri et al., 2006). In this trial, response was defined as a ≥50% decrease from baseline YMRS score. Patients who did not adequately respond to lithium monotherapy after 8 weeks, and those with symptom relapse after an initial positive response, were provided risperidone augmentation for up to 11 months. Of the 38 subjects treated with lithium monotherapy, 17 responded positively and 21 required risperidone augmentation. The response rate for youth treated with both lithium and risperidone was 85.7%. Predictors of inadequate response to lithium monotherapy included the presence of comorbid ADHD, high symptom severity at baseline, history of sexual or physical abuse, and preschool age (Pavuluri et al., 2006).

Only one study looked at lithium treatment for youth with bipolar depression (Patel et al., 2006). In this 6-week open-label study, 27 adolescents with an episode of depression associated with bipolar-I disorder were treated with lithium 30 mg/kg (twice-daily dosing), which was adjusted to achieve therapeutic serum lithium levels between 1.0 and 1.2 mEq/L. Study results revealed a large effect size of 1.7, a lower response rate of 48%, and a remission rate of 30%. Side effects were deemed to be of mild to moderate severity, and lithium was judged to be relatively well tolerated in this study. Study authors concluded that depending on this positive open-label study, lithium may be effective for the treatment of depression in adolescents with bipolar disorder. Future controlled studies are needed to replicate these findings, however. In this trial, efficacy measures included the CDRS-R and the CGI Scale for Bipolar Disorder (CGI-BP), response rates were defined as ≥50% reduction in CDRS-R score, and remission rates were defined as a CDRS-R score ≤28 and a CGI-BP Improvement score of 1 or 2 (Patel et al., 2006).

Mitsunaga et al. (2011) sought to study morphometric characteristics of the subgenual cingulate cortex (SGC), which has been implicated in the pathophysiology of mood disorders. Twenty bipolar disorder youth with a mean age of 14.6 years, and 20 age- and gender-matched controls without bipolar disorder underwent high-resolution magnetic resonance imaging. Although no differences were discovered in SGC volumes between subjects with bipolar disorder and healthy controls, further analysis revealed that subjects with bipolar disorder with prior mood stabilizer exposure, compared with subjects without prior mood stabilizer exposure and to healthy controls, had significantly increased SGC volumes. This finding led the authors to conclude that mood stabilizer exposure may be correlated with increases in SGC size. The authors describe many limitations to the aforementioned study, however, including a small sample size, concomitant use of atypical antipsychotic medication by study subjects, which may or may not have neurotrophic properties of its own, and the presence of comorbid ADHD in study subjects, a diagnosis which currently has unknown effects on SGC size (Mitsunaga et al., 2011).

Geller et al. (2012) studied 279 antimanic medication-naive subjects, aged 6 to 15 years, with *DSM-IV* bipolar-I disorder (manic or mixed phase) in a randomized controlled trial assessing response to lithium, risperidone, or divalproex sodium. Study results revealed statistically significant higher response rates for risperidone (68.5%) versus both lithium (35.6%) and divalproex sodium (24.0%). Lithium versus divalproex sodium response rates did not differ significantly. The authors concluded that risperidone is more efficacious than lithium or divalproex sodium for the initial treatment of childhood mania (Geller et al., 2012). In this trial, blinded independent evaluators conducted all assessments. Medications were increased weekly only if there was inadequate response and if the medication remained well tolerated. Maximum doses of lithium carbonate, divalproex sodium, and risperidone were 1.1 to 1.3 mEq/L, 111 to 125 µg/mL, and 4 to 6 mg, respectively, and primary outcome measures were the Clinical Global Impressions for Bipolar Illness Improvement–Mania and the Modified Side Effects Form for Children and Adolescents (Geller et al., 2012).

Goldstein et al. (2013) prospectively examined predictors of first-time SUDs in 167 youth aged 12 to 17 with bipolar disorder. Multiple variables were examined in relation to the first onset of a SUD, and participants were periodically interviewed for a period of 4.25 ± 2.11 years. The authors determined that first-onset SUD occurs after a mean of 2.7 ± 2 years from intake, and that lifetime alcohol experimentation at intake was most predicative of a first-onset SUD. The authors also concluded that lithium exposure in the preceding 12 weeks correlated with a lower likelihood of developing a SUD, although they caution that the study was observational and naturalistic, substance use was based exclusively on self-report, and there were no comparison samples of youth without bipolar disorder (Goldstein et al., 2013).

Findling et al. (2015) studied 81 youth (ages 7 to 17 years) with PBD I in an 8-week multicenter, randomized, double-blind, placebo-controlled trial comparing lithium to placebo. The authors concluded that lithium was superior to placebo in reducing manic symptoms, was generally well tolerated, and was not associated with weight gain. In this trial, the primary efficacy measure was the YMRS, although overall CGI-I scores also favored lithium. Lithium was started at either 600 or 900 mg/day depending on weight. The mean daily dose for patients aged 7 to 11 years was 1,292 ± 420 mg, and for patients aged 12 to 17 years the mean daily dose was 1,716 ± 606 mg. Side effects were mild to moderate, with the most common including vomiting (45%), nausea (43%), and headache (36%). Although promising, the authors concluded that because of the trial's short duration conclusions about lithium's long-term efficacy in patients with PBD cannot be made (Findling et al., 2015).

Lithium Carbonate in the Maintenance Treatment of Youth Diagnosed with Bipolar Disorder

Kafantaris et al. (2004), using a 2-week blinded discontinuation study design, randomized 40 prior lithium responders to either lithium or placebo. Before the randomized discontinuation phase, lithium responders received 4 weeks of open-label lithium treatment, which yielded average serum lithium levels of 0.99 ± 0.21 mEq/L. During the discontinuation phase, 19 adolescents were maintained on lithium monotherapy and 21 received placebo after a 3-day lithium taper. Study authors reported no statistic difference in mood exacerbation rates between lithium monotherapy (52.6%) and placebo (61.9%) and concluded that lithium may be ineffective for maintenance treatment of adolescent bipolar disorder (Kafantaris et al., 2004). Study limitations including small sample sizes and a relatively short open-label treatment lead-in phase prevent firm conclusions from being drawn, and additional studies are needed.

Findling et al. (2005) compared lithium carbonate and valproic acid in the maintenance treatment of youth diagnosed with bipolar disorder and found no clinically significant differences between the two drugs for this indication. This study is summarized in the section on valproic acid (Findling et al., 2005).

Lithium Carbonate in the Treatment of Youth with Severe Mood Dysregulation

Severe mood dysregulation (SMD) is defined as a syndrome encompassing severe nonepisodic irritability and hyperarousal in youth (Liebenluft et al., 2003). In 2009, Dickstein et al. studied lithium for the treatment of youth aged 7 to 17 years with SMD in a randomized double-blind placebo-controlled trial. Subjects who met SMD criteria were gradually weaned off all of their outpatient psychiatric medication, in an inpatient setting, for a total of four drug half-lives. This was followed by a 2-week single-blind placebo run-in phase, after which only those who continued to meet SMD criteria ($N = 25$) were randomized to either lithium or placebo for the 6-week double-blind randomized controlled trial. The primary clinical outcome measure was a CGI-I score of <4 by the end of the trial. Results revealed not only a relatively small rate of improvement in the lithium group but also no significance between group differences in outcome measures. This led the authors to conclude that lithium may not be effective for youth with chronic irritability and hyperarousal. However, given the small sample size, these findings should be considered preliminary (Dickstein et al., 2009).

Lithium Carbonate in the Treatment of Disorders with Severe Aggression, Especially When Accompanied by Explosive Affect, Including Self-Injurious Behavior

In a double-blind, placebo-controlled study of 61 treatment-resistant hospitalized children (age range, 5.2 to 12.9 years) diagnosed with undersocialized aggressive CD, both haloperidol and lithium were found to be superior to placebo in ameliorating behavioral symptoms (Campbell et al., 1984b). Optimal doses of lithium carbonate ranged from 500 to 2,000 mg/day (mean, 1,166 mg/day); corresponding serum levels ranged from 0.32 to 1.51 mEq/L (mean, 0.99 mEq/L). The authors noted that lithium caused fewer and milder untoward effects than did haloperidol and that these effects did not appear to interfere significantly with the children's daily routines. There was also a suggestion that lithium was particularly effective in diminishing the explosive affect and that other improvements followed (Campbell et al., 1984b).

Campbell et al. (1995) reported a double-blind, placebo-controlled study that was designed to replicate their 1984 study. Fifty treatment-resistant inpatients (46 males and 4 females; mean age, 9.4 ± 1.8 years; age range, 5.1 to 12.0 years) diagnosed with CD, under socialized aggressive type by *DSM-III* (APA, 1980a) criteria and having chronic severe explosive aggressiveness were treated with lithium carbonate only or placebo. Following a 2-week, placebo baseline period during which baseline assessments were conducted and placebo responders were eliminated, the 50 remaining subjects were randomly assigned to placebo ($N = 25$) or lithium ($N = 25$) for a 6-week period; this was followed by 2 weeks of posttreatment placebo. On the Global Clinical Judgments (Consensus) Scale (GCJCS), 68% (17/25) of subjects on lithium were rated as moderately or markedly improved while only 40% (10/25) of subjects on placebo were so rated ($P = .003$). Further refining this measure, 40% (10/25) of the subjects of lithium were "markedly" improved versus only 4% (1/25) of the subjects on placebo. The CGI-I scores after 6 weeks were also significantly better for the lithium group ($P = .044$); although it was not significant whether the lithium group improved more on the CGI-S. The authors concluded that these data supported the conclusions of their earlier study and that lithium carbonate can be efficacious in treating children with CD and explosive aggressiveness who have not responded to psychosocial treatments or medication with methylphenidate or standard neuroleptics.

In this trial, efficacy was assessed by ratings on the GCJCS, Children's Psychiatric Rating Scale (CPRS), CGI, CGI-S, and CGI-I Scales, Conners Teacher Questionnaire, and the Parent–Teacher Questionnaire. Lithium carbonate was begun at 600 mg/day and titrated individually over a 2-week period with a maximum permitted dose of 2,100 mg/day or serum lithium of 1.8 mEq/L or equivalent saliva lithium level. The mean optimal dose of lithium was 1,248 mg/day (range, 600 to 1,800 mg/day); the mean serum lithium level was 1.12 mEq/L (range, 0.53 to 1.79 mEq/L); and the mean saliva lithium level was 2.5 mEq/L (range, 1.45 to 4.44 mEq/L) (Campbell et al., 1995).

Vetro et al. (1985) treated 17 children, aged 3 to 12 years, with lithium, who were hospitalized for hyperaggressivity, active destruction of property, severely disturbed social adjustment, and unresponsiveness to discipline. Ten of the children had not responded to prior pharmacotherapy, including haloperidol and concomitant individual and family therapy. Lithium carbonate was titrated slowly over 2 to 3 weeks to achieve serum levels in the therapeutic range (0.6 to 1.2 mEq/L). Mean serum lithium level was 0.68 ± 0.30 mEq/L. The authors reported that 13 of the children improved enough that their abilities to adapt to their environment could be described as good, and their aggressivity had been reduced to tolerable levels. Three of the four cases that did not improve had poor compliance in taking the medication at home. The authors also noted that these children usually required continuous treatment with lithium for longer than 6 months.

DeLong and Aldershof (1987) reported that rage, aggressive outbursts, and, interestingly, encopresis responded favorably to lithium pharmacotherapy in children with behavioral disorders associated with a variety of neurologic and medical diseases, including mental retardation.

Lithium Carbonate in the Treatment of Children and Adolescents Diagnosed with Conduct Disorder

Rifkin et al. (1997) studied 33 inpatients aged 12 to 17 years diagnosed with CD for 2 weeks and concluded that lithium did not appear helpful for this indication. In this study, lithium or placebo was administered in a double-blind manner. Lithium was adjusted to a blood level of 0.6 to 1.0 mmol/L and the authors concluded that there was no correlation between the lithium blood level and the score on the Overt Aggression Scale (OAS). The short duration of the trial was acknowledged as a limitation (Rifkin et al., 1997).

By contrast, Malone et al. (2000) conducted a 6-week, double-blind, placebo-controlled, parallel-groups study comparing lithium carbonate and placebo in the treatment of 40 inpatients (33 males and 7 females; mean age, 12.5 years; age range, 9.5 to 17.1 years) who were diagnosed with CD by *DSM-III-R* (APA, 1987) criteria and hospitalized for chronic, severe aggressive behavior. Eighty-six inpatients entered the study; however, 46 were eliminated during the initial 2-week single-blind placebo baseline; 40 of this group did not meet the protocol's aggression criteria. All 40 remaining subjects entered the 4-week treatment phase and completed the protocol; 20 subjects were assigned randomly to each group.

Efficacy was determined by ratings on the GCJCS, the CGI, and the OAS. On the GCJCS, 16 (80%) of the lithium group versus six (30%) of the placebo group were rated as "marked" or "moderately" improved on the criterion for responders ($P = .004$). Significantly more of the lithium group were also rated as responders on the CGI (17 [30%] vs. 4 [20%] of the placebo group; $P = .004$). On the OAS, the lithium group continued to show improvement over the 4-week period, whereas the placebo group showed an initial decline at week 1 but then remained rather stable. The lithium group's mean decrease from baseline was significantly greater than that of the placebo group, with a significant interaction between treatment group and time ($P = .04$). Although untoward effects were frequent, they were usually mild and similar for both placebo and lithium groups. Only three adverse effects occurred significantly more on lithium: nausea in 12 of 20, vomiting in 11 of 20, and urinary frequency 11 of 20 ($P \leq .05$ in all cases). The authors noted that the aggressive behavior of 40 (47.1%) of their initial 85 subjects improved significantly during the first 2 weeks secondary to hospitalization and treatment with placebo alone. For the 40 subjects who remained aggressive and entered the medication phase of the protocol, lithium was a safe and effective treatment. The authors noted that determining the long-term efficacy and safety of lithium in such subjects will require further research.

In this study, lithium was initiated with a 600-mg dose; serum lithium levels were determined 24 hours later, and an initial target dose was calculated for each subject using a nomogram. Subsequent lithium doses were increased by 300 mg daily and given in three equal doses to reach the target dose. At the end of the study, optimal mean lithium dose was $1,425 \pm 321$ mg/day (range, 900 to 2,100 mg/day) with a mean steady-state therapeutic lithium level of 1.07 ± 0.19 mmol/L (range, 0.78 to 1.55 mmol/L) (Malone et al., 2000).

Lithium Carbonate in the Treatment of Children and Adolescents Diagnosed with Autism

Siegel et al. (2014) completed a retrospective chart review of 30 child and adolescent patients diagnosed with autism spectrum disorder per *DSM-IV-TR* criteria who were prescribed lithium for mood symptoms such as elevated mood, mania, hypersexuality, or decreased need for sleep. Forty-three percent of patients were rated as improved on the CGI-I Scale, which rose to 71% when two or more pretreatment mood symptoms were present. The authors concluded that the presence of mania or euphoric/elevated mood was most correlated with an improved rating. In this study, mean lithium blood levels and length of treatment were 0.70 mEq/L and 29.7 days, respectively. Almost half of the patients experienced side effects, however, to include vomiting (13%), tremor (10%), fatigue (10%), irritability (7%), and enuresis (7%). The authors concluded that although lithium may be of interest in patients with autism with mood symptoms, a relatively high rate of medication side effects warrants caution. Other limitations of the study include its retrospective and uncontrolled design (Siegel et al., 2014).

ANTIEPILEPTIC MOOD STABILIZERS

Currently, there is robust clinical interest in the off-label use of antiepileptic drugs to treat psychiatric disorders in children and adolescents; however, their safety and efficacy in treating these disorders remains to be fully elucidated. In addition to ongoing research clarifying the question of efficacy and tolerability of antiepileptic medication in youth, research designed to delineate which specific disorders, symptoms, and patients or subgroups of patients are most likely to respond well to antiepileptic medication would be of clear value (e.g., patients with various abnormal electroencephalogram (EEG) findings and patients who are mentally disabled or have other evidence of abnormal central nervous system functioning compared with affectually or behaviorally disordered patients without signs of central nervous system dysfunction).

Valproic Acid (Depakene); Divalproex Sodium (Valproic Acid and Valproate Sodium [Depakote; Depacon])

Note: The FDA has directed the manufacturers of valproic acid and its derivatives (e.g., divalproex sodium and valproate sodium) to label their products with the following black box warning. *Hepatotoxicity*: Hepatic failure resulting in fatalities has occurred in patients receiving valproic acid. Experience has indicated that children below the age of 2 years are at a considerable increased risk of developing fatal hepatotoxicity, especially those with congenital metabolic disorders, those with severe seizure disorders accompanied by mental retardation, and those with organic brain disease. When valproic acid products are used in these patient groups, they should be used with extreme caution and as a sole agent. The benefits of therapy should be weighed against the risks. Above this age group, experience in epilepsy has indicated that the incidence of fatal hepatotoxicity decreases considerably in progressively older patient groups. These incidents usually have occurred during the first 6 months of treatment. Serious or fatal hepatotoxicity may be preceded by nonspecific symptoms such as malaise, weakness, lethargy, facial edema, anorexia, and vomiting. In patients with epilepsy, a loss of seizure control may also occur. Patients should be monitored closely for appearance of these symptoms. Liver function tests should be performed prior to therapy and at frequent intervals thereafter, especially during the first 6 months. *Teratogenicity*: Valproate (VPA) can produce teratogenic effects such as neural tube defects (e.g., spina bifida), craniofacial defects, and limb malformations. Accordingly, the use of VPA products in women of childbearing potential requires that the benefits of its use be weighed against the risk of injury to the fetus. *Pancreatitis*: Cases of life-threatening pancreatitis have been reported in both children and adults receiving VPA. Some of the cases have been described as hemorrhagic with a rapid progression from initial symptoms to death. Cases have been reported shortly after initial use as well as after several years of use. Patients and guardians should be warned that abdominal pain, nausea, vomiting, and/or anorexia can be symptoms of pancreatitis that require prompt medical evaluation. If pancreatitis is diagnosed, VPA should ordinarily be discontinued. Alternative treatment for the underlying medical condition should be initiated as clinically indicated.

In addition to the black box warnings described, in 2008 the FDA issued an alert advising providers to monitor patients who are taking or starting antiepileptic medication for any changes in behavior that could indicate the emergence of depression or worsening suicidal thoughts or behavior (*PDR*.net, 2008).

Valproic acid and divalproex sodium (a stable coordination compound of valproic acid and valproate sodium) both dissociate to the VPA ion in the gastrointestinal tract and have antiepileptic properties. These drugs are indicated for the treatment of simple and complex absence seizures and adjunctively in patients with multiple seizure types, which include absence seizures. Divalproex sodium has also been approved by the FDA for advertising as safe and effective for adults in the treatment of acute mania associated with bipolar disorder and for migraine prophylaxis in adults aged 65 years or younger (*PDR*.net, 2017).

Pharmacokinetics of Valproic Acid

Following oral administration, valproic acid and divalproex sodium dissociate to the VPAion, which is the active agent, in the gastrointestinal tract. Administration of valproic acid with food may slow the absorption rate, but does not interfere with clinical efficacy. Food does not significantly affect the total amount of VPA absorbed and may be helpful in reducing gastrointestinal irritation in some patients.

Peak plasma concentration usually occurs within 1 to 4 hours for immediate-release valproic acid, within 3 to 5 hours for delayed-release divalproex, and within 4 to 17 hours for extended-release (ER) divalproex tablets (*PDR*.net, 2017). Valproic acid is metabolized almost entirely by the liver; the metabolites are excreted primarily in the urine. Plasma VPA half-life is between 6 and 16 hours; the more rapid metabolism rates occur most frequently in patients receiving valproic acid and other antiepileptics that induce enzymes that increase the metabolism rate of valproate.

In a retroactive chart review of 16 males (age range, 5 to 14 years; mean age, 9.3 years) hospitalized for mood stabilization, Good et al. (2001) found that a relatively conservative total loading dose of 15 mg/kg/day of divalproex sodium given in two equal doses resulted in therapeutic trough plasma VPA levels on day 5 of therapy in 13 (81.3%) cases. The initial dose was calculated for one subgroup using actual weight and for a second subgroup using adjusted ideal body weight (IBW). For the latter group, Adjusted IBW = IBW + 40% (current weight − IBW). All subjects were also taking atypical antipsychotics, and some were taking stimulants as well during this period. The authors noted several findings of clinical interest: Of the eight patients experiencing untoward effects (mostly sedation and nausea), six (75%) had VPA plasma levels of >90 μg/mL. Patients who were ≥15% over IBW and who were dosed according to actual body weight were significantly more likely to have supratherapeutic (>120 μg/mL) VPA plasma levels than normal-weight subjects or overweight subjects whose doses were determined by adjusted IBW. On the basis of this study, it would seem prudent to calculate and use adjusted IBW for significantly overweight children and adolescents if it is decided to administer a loading dose of VPA to rapidly achieve therapeutic plasma levels.

Contraindications for Valproic Acid Administration

Valproic acid can cause severe hepatotoxicity, including fatal hepatic failure. Children below 2 years of age, and patients with mitochondrial disease or carnitine deficiency are at increased risk. It should not be administered to anyone with hepatic disease, significant liver dysfunction, or known hypersensitivity to the drug.

Because valproic acid has been reported to cause teratogenic effects in the fetus, it should be administered with caution to women who are likely to become pregnant, and they should be warned to notify their physician immediately if they become pregnant.

Interactions with Other Drugs

VPA may potentiate the action of central nervous system depressants such as alcohol and benzodiazepines.

Coadministration with clonazepam may induce absence seizures in patients with a history of absence-type seizures.

Coadministration with risperidone (4 mg/day) did not affect the predose or average plasma concentrations and exposure area under the curve (AUC) of VPA (a total of 1,000 mg administered in three divided doses), but there was a 20% increase in VPA peak plasma concentration after concomitant administration of risperidone.

Ambrosini and Sheikh (1998) have reported two cases in which coadministration of valproic acid and guanfacine resulted in significantly increased levels of valproic acid. It was suggested that this was secondary to drug–drug competition at the level of hepatic glucuronidation.

Other drug interactions have been reported.

Untoward Effects of Valproic Acid

The most serious side effects of valproic acid are hepatic failure and pancreatitis, which can be fatal. Hepatic failure occurs most frequently within the first 6 months of treatment. Children below 2 years of age are at increased risk. The risk of hepatotoxicity decreases considerably as patients become progressively older. Hence, liver function must be monitored carefully and frequently, especially during the first 6 months of treatment. Cases of pancreatitis while taking valproic acid have been reported after initial use as well as after several years of use. Patients should be educated to monitor for symptoms of abdominal pain, nausea, vomiting, and/or anorexia while taking valproic acid.

Hyperammonemic encephalopathy has also been reported with valproic acid treatment. Ammonia level should be checked in all patients experiencing episodes of confusion while taking valproic acid.

Valproic acid has a known ability to cause neutropenia, thrombocytopenia, and macrocytic anemia, hence patients taking valproic acid should have a complete blood count checked periodically throughout treatment.

Nausea, vomiting, and indigestion may occur early in treatment with valproic acid and usually are transient. Mood stabilizers including valproic acid have been associated with relevant weight gain, which should be monitored and addressed. Sedation may occur, and untoward psychiatric effects such as emotional upset, depression, psychosis, aggression, hyperactivity, and behavioral deterioration have been reported.

Amitai et al. (2015) completed a retrospective naturalistic study on the effects of long-term valproic acid treatment in 104 adolescent inpatients, and discovered that platelet counts decreased and mean TSH and triglyceride levels increased. Despite this there were no serious adverse effects, leading investigators to conclude that long-term valproic acid treatment is safe for inpatient adolescent psychiatry populations. Many of the adolescents in this study were taking more than one psychotropic medication, which was a limitation in this study. Mean valproic acid blood levels were 65.81 ± 22.18 μg/mL and the mean duration of treatment was 98.7 ± 135.94 days. The study authors recommended that baseline thyroid function labs along with metabolic and hematologic parameters should be completed before and throughout treatment.

Avari (2016) reported a case of an adolescent male hospitalized for paranoia and disorganized thinking and speech. His symptoms responded to a trial of quetiapine, although residual irritability persisted prompting his provider to add valproic acid (initial dose of 250 mg, titrated up to 1,000 mg daily over 2 weeks, resulting in a blood level of 88 μg/mL). His irritability and aggression acutely worsened following the addition of valproic acid, and ammonia levels, chemistries and liver function test were normal. When VPA was discontinued, his irritability and aggression subsided (Avari, 2016).

VPA and Polycystic Ovaries

Isojarvi et al. (1993) published an article noting that there was an association between VPA use in treating epileptic women and polycystic ovaries and hyperandrogenism (elevated serum testosterone concentrations). The finding was more pronounced in women who had begun treatment with valproate before 20 years of age than in women who began VPA treatment at 20 years of age or older. Sussman and Ginsberg (1998) published a critical review of VPA and polycystic ovary syndrome (PCOS), concluding that the available evidence suggests that early and long-term treatment with valproic acid is a causal or precipitating factor in the development of PCOS in epileptic women, particularly if they are overweight; relative risk factors for nonepileptic adolescents are at present unknown. Johnston (1999) basically concurs. Piontek and Wisner (2000) have suggested clinical guidelines for the appropriate clinical management of women with reproductive capacity who are treated with VPA. Although risk of PCOS does not preclude the use of valproic acid/divalproex sodium in adolescent females, risks and benefits must be discussed, informed consent obtained, and careful monitoring maintained. Further research is needed to clarify this issue.

Indications for Valproic Acid/Divalproex Sodium in Child and Adolescent Psychiatry

NOTE: Before prescribing see black box warning information on page 312.

Valproic acid, valproate sodium, and divalproex sodium are approved for use alone or in combination (see exception to this in patients <2 years of age in boxed warning at the beginning of chapter) with other drugs in treating patients with simple and complex absence seizures or as an adjunctive agent in patients with multiple-type seizures, which include absence seizures. Valproic acid is additionally approved for the treatment of acute mania and migraine prophylaxis in adults. It has not been evaluated for safety and efficacy in either treating pediatric mania or in the prophylactic treatment of pediatric migraine headache and is not approved by the FDA for such advertising.

Dosage Schedule

- *Children <2 years of age:* Contraindicated for any indication.

Treatment of Epilepsy

- *Children ≥2 years of age, adolescents, and adults:*
  An initial daily dose of 15 mg/kg is recommended. Weekly increases of 5 to 10 mg/kg/day until seizures are controlled or untoward effects prevent further increases are recommended. The maximum recommended daily dose is 60 mg/kg. Amounts >250 mg/day should be administered in divided doses.

Treatment of Acute Mania (Divalproex Sodium Only)

- *Children and adolescents:* Not indicated.
- *Adults:*
  An initial divided daily dose of 750 mg is recommended, followed by rapid titration to achieve satisfactory clinical response or reach total (trough) plasma VPA levels of 50 to 125 µg/mL, which are usually associated with clinical efficacy. The maximum recommended dosage is 60 mg/kg/day. Titration can usually be completed within 14 days.
  Plasma levels of total VPA between 50 and 100 µg/mL are usually considered to be the therapeutic range for epilepsy (and for off-label psychiatric uses); however, in the treatment of acute mania, levels up to 125 µg/mL are recommended.

Prophylactic Treatment of Migraine Headache (Divalproex Sodium Only)

- *Children and adolescents:* Not indicated.
- *Adults aged 65 years and younger:* An initial 250-mg dose of divalproex sodium administered twice daily is recommended. Some patients have benefited from doses as high as 1,000 mg/day; however, higher doses showed no evidence of increased benefit in clinical trials.

Dosage Forms Available (Valproic Acid, Depakene)

- *Capsules:* 250 mg
- *Syrup:* 250 mg/5 mL dispensed in 16-oz bottles

Dosage Forms Available (Divalproex Sodium, Depakote)

- *Sprinkle capsules:* 125 mg
- *Delayed-release tablets (Depakote):* 125, 250, and 500 mg
- *Extended-release tablets (Depakote-ER):* 250 and 500 mg. This formulation permits once-a-day dosing

Dosage Forms Available (Valproate Sodium)

- *Injectable (Depacon):* 100 mg/mL dispensed in 5-mL single-dose vials

Reports of Interest

Divalproex has been shown to be effective in open studies of youth with bipolar disorder. Papatheodorou et al. (1995) reported an open-label, 7-week study in which the efficacy and safety of divalproex sodium was assessed in the treatment of 15 subjects (2 males and 13 females; mean age, 17.3 years, with 10 subjects being 15 to 18 years old and 5 being 19 or 20 years old) who were diagnosed by *DSM-III-R* (APA, 1987) criteria with bipolar disorder, in an acute manic phase. The 13 completers' ratings on the Modified Mania Rating Scale (MMRS), BPRS, Global Assessment Scale (GAS), and CGI were all very significantly lower ($P < .0001$ for all four scales) than at baseline. An analysis of variance (ANOVA) found a significant reduction in the MMRS within 1 week on valproex ($P < .016$), which continued throughout the treatment period. Overall, untoward effects were benign and their frequency was reported to decrease over the duration of the study, with a very low number being reported at the end of the study. Liver function tests remained normal, except for one patient with transiently elevated enzyme levels that reverted to normal without change in dosage. Study authors concluded that divalproex sodium is safe and efficacious in the acute (short-term) treatment of mania in adolescents, although this study was limited by its open-label design and small sample size. In this trial, efficacy was evaluated using ratings on the MMRS, the BPRS, the GAS, the CGI Scale, and the Valproic Acid Side Effects Scale. Following a 2-day entry phase during which baseline evaluations were performed, subjects began 7 weeks of treatment with divalproex sodium. Medication was administered in three divided doses and individually titrated. Thirteen patients completed the 7-week study; one patient was discontinued for lack of clinical response and one patient withdrew because of "subjectively intolerable sedation and dizziness." All 13 completers required some additional medication for symptom control (e.g., agitation) during the study. Mean dose at the end of 7 weeks was 1,423.08 mg/day (range, 750 to 2,000 mg/day) and the mean serum valproic acid level (12 to 14 hours after the evening dose and before the morning dose) was 642.85 ± 183.08 μmol/L (range, 360 to 923 μmol/L) (Papatheodorou et al., 1995).

Kowatch et al. (2000) studied 42 outpatients with bipolar disorder who were randomized to receive divalproate, lithium, or carbamazepine for 6 weeks in a nonblind manner. The divalproate response rate was calculated at 53% compared with a response rate of 38% for both lithium and carbamazepine. This small study demonstrated that divalproate may be beneficial in the treatment of youth with bipolar disorder. (The mean study subject age was 11.4 years. Response was defined as having a reduction of ≥50% on YMRS scores from baseline; Kowatch et al., 2000.)

Wagner et al. (2002) studied divalproex sodium in an open-label study for the treatment of 40 bipolar patients aged 7 to 19 years. The duration of this open-label study varied from 2 to 8 weeks, depending on treatment response. The mean serum VPA level at the final visit was 83.4 μg/mL. Sixty-one percent of subjects showed a ≥50% improvement in Mania Rating Scale scores, leading the authors to conclude that divalproex sodium may be effective in the treatment of youth with bipolar disorder. The most common side effects noted were headache, nausea, vomiting, diarrhea, and somnolence. All side effects were judged to be in the mild-to-moderate-severity range, and laboratory data results were unremarkable. Notably, 43% of study subjects required adjunctive medication to control symptoms such as agitation, irritability, insomnia, and restlessness (Wagner et al., 2002).

Pavuluri et al. (2005) studied divalproex sodium in pediatric mixed mania during a prospective 6-month open trial involving 34 subjects with a mean age of 12.3 years. The primary outcome measures were the YMRS and the CDRS-R. Response rate, defined as both ≥50% change from baseline YMRS score and ≤40 score on the CDRS-R at the end of the study, was reported as 73.5%. Similar to findings in

Wagner et al. (2002), approximately 65% of subjects completing Pavuluri's study required acute adjunctive medications (Pavuluri et al., 2005).

Redden et al. (2009) conducted a 6-month open-label study assessing the safety of divalproex sodium ER in 9- to 17-year-old subjects with a diagnosis of bipolar-I disorder. One hundred and nine subjects completed the study. The most common adverse effects were weight gain (16%), nausea (9%), and increased appetite (8%). Asymptomatic elevations in mean plasma ammonia levels were observed. The mean YMRS score decreased 12.4 points from baseline to final visit, equating to a 56% response rate. The authors concluded that divalproex sodium ER was generally well tolerated in youth with acute mania, with a side-effect profile similar to that of adults (Redden et al., 2009).

In contrast to the apparent positive findings reported in many open-label studies of divalproex sodium for the treatment of PBD, the few controlled studies done are less encouraging. In a large double-blind, randomized pilot study, DelBello et al. (2006) discovered that quetiapine was superior to divalproex sodium for the acute treatment of adolescent mania. In this study, 50 adolescents with bipolar-I disorder, manic, or mixed episode were randomized to quetiapine (400 to 600 mg daily) or divalproex sodium (serum levels of 80 to 120 μg/mL) for 28 days. The primary outcome measure was the change in YMRS score across the study period. The authors concluded that quetiapine is at least as effective as divalproex sodium in this study population and may result in a quicker reduction of manic symptoms than does divalproex sodium. The rates of adverse effects did not differ significantly between the two study medications (DelBello et al., 2006).

Findling et al. (2007a) conducted a double-blind, placebo-controlled trial of divalproex monotherapy for the treatment of symptomatic youth judged to be at high risk of developing bipolar disorder. Subjects were between the ages of 5 and 17 years, met *DSM-IV* criteria for bipolar disorder not otherwise specified (NOS) or cyclothymia, and had at least one natural parent with bipolar illness. Fifty-six subjects were randomly assigned to either divalproex sodium or placebo. The mean serum divalproex sodium concentration at the end of the study was 78.8 μg/mL. At the end of the study, there was no significant difference in outcome measures between divalproex sodium and placebo. Both groups, however, did exhibit significant decreases in depression and mania as well as improvement in psychosocial functioning. The authors concluded that the relatively high response rates seen in both groups during this study were similar to response rates reported in prior open-label trials of divalproex sodium. These findings led them to question whether positive response rates seen during open-label trials were due to divalproex sodium *per se* versus placebo (Findling et al., 2007a).

Wagner et al. (2009) studied divalproex ER for the treatment of youth with bipolar disorder in a large double-blind, randomized, placebo-controlled trial. In this study, 150 patients aged 10 to 17 years were randomized to placebo or divalproex ER titrated to a serum concentration of 80 to 125 μg/mL. The primary outcome measure was change in YMRS score. The response rate for divalproex ER, defined as ≥50% reduction in YMRS scores, was 24%, which was lower than the response rates reported during previous trials of divalproex in PBD. No statistically significant difference between the divalproex-ER-treated patients and the placebo-treated patients was found during this trial. The incidence of adverse effects between the two study arms was similar. The authors concluded that this study does not provide support for the use of divalproex ER in the treatment of youth with bipolar-I disorder, although they caution that future studies are needed to replicate or refute their findings (Wagner et al., 2009).

Pavuluri et al. (2010a) conducted a 6-week, double-blind randomized trial of risperidone versus divalproex in 66 patients with PBD. Subjects were randomized to either risperidone (0.5 to 2 mg daily) or divalproex (60 to 120 μg/mL). Outcome measures included the YMRS and the CDRS-R. The study authors reported that the risperidone group showed more rapid improvement than did the divalproex group ($P < .05$), with response rates based on YMRS of 78.1% for risperidone and 45.5% for divalproex, which was a significant difference. The dropout rate for the risperidone group was 24%, compared with 48% in the divalproex group. Increased irritability was the most common reason for dropout in the latter group.

Geller et al. (2012) reported similar findings during an 8-week randomized controlled trial of risperidone, lithium, or divalproex sodium for the initial treatment of bipolar-I disorder, manic or mixed phase, in children and adolescents. In this trial, the Treatment of Early Age Mania recruited 279 antimanic medication-naive subjects with a mean age of 10.1 years. Subjects received a titrated schedule of lithium, divalproex sodium, or risperidone to mean doses of 1.09 mEq/L, 113.6 µg/mL, and 2.57 mg, respectively. Primary outcome measures were the Clinical Global Impressions for Bipolar Illness Improvement–Mania and the Modified Side Effects Form for Children and Adolescents. Higher response rates occurred with risperidone versus lithium (68% vs. 35.6%, $P < .001$) as well as with risperidone versus divalproex sodium (68% vs. 24%, $P < .001$). Response rates between lithium and divalproex sodium did not differ significantly. The authors concluded that risperidone was more effective than lithium or divalproex sodium, but was associated with potentially severe metabolic side effects (Geller et al., 2012).

Kowatch et al. (2015) completed a 6-week double-blind, placebo-controlled trial comparing valproic acid and risperidone in 46 children aged 3 to 7 years who were diagnosed with bipolar-I disorder. Primary outcome measures include a ≥50% decrease in YMRS score from baseline, or a CGI-I score of 1 or 2. Investigators determined that risperidone demonstrated clear efficacy over placebo ($P = .008$), whereas valproic acid did not ($P = .50$). In this trial, subjects were tapered off of current medication upon study entry and were randomized to monotherapy treatment with risperidone, placebo, or valproic acid. The mean valproic acid level was 81 µg/mL and investigators cautioned that this may have limited the response to this medication; whereas risperidone's mean daily dose was 0.5 mg daily. The valproic acid–treated group experienced statistically but not clinically significant decreases in unconjugated bilirubin and albumin, total red blood cells, hemoglobin, and hematocrit, whereas the risperidone group experienced statistically but not clinically significant increases in unconjugated bilirubin, gamma-glutamyltransferase, cholesterol, and prolactin levels. Study authors also discovered a potential relationship between valproic acid and increased mood lability in this patient population (28% of VPA-treated subjects) (Kowatch et al., 2015).

Valproic Acid Versus Lithium in the Maintenance Treatment of Children and Adolescents Diagnosed with Bipolar Disorder

Findling et al. (2005) conducted a double-blind study to determine whether divalproex sodium (DVPX) or lithium was superior as the only drug in maintenance treatment of 139 subjects (age range 5 to 17 years; mean age 10.8 ± 3.5 years; 93 [66.9%] males, 46 [33.1%] females) who were diagnosed with bipolar I (131, 94.2%) or bipolar II (8, 5.8%) disorder and stabilized on a combination of lithium carbonate and valproex sodium during acute treatment. Sixty subjects who met remission criteria (CDRS score < 40, YMRS score < 12.5, and a CGAS score > 51) for a minimum of 4 weeks were than randomized to monotherapy with either lithium ($N = 30$) or divalproex ($N = 30$) for up to 76 weeks; subjects were dropped from the study if they violated protocol or required additional clinical intervention. Subjects were tapered off the nonmaintenance/discontinued drug over a period of 8 weeks to minimize discontinuation rebound relapse. The authors concluded there was no clinically significant difference between lithium and valproex monotherapy in maintaining the youth who were stabilized on combination lithium/valproex therapy for bipolar disorder. In this trial, subjects maintained on lithium were maintained at lithium serum concentrations between 0.6 and 1.2 mmol/L and those on VPA were maintained with plasma concentrations between 50 and 100 μg/mL. Primary measures of effectiveness were time to premature discontinuation due to emerging mood symptoms of relapse, *or* premature discontinuation for any reason.

Median survival time to mood relapse for subjects on lithium was 114 ± 57.4 days for lithium and 112 ± 56 days for subjects on valproex and was not statistically different ($P = .55$); overall, 38 (63.3%) subjects relapsed. There was also no significant difference between the lithium and valproex groups in the 12 (20%) who dropped out for any reason ($P = .72$). At the study's conclusion, the mean lithium serum level was 0.84 ± 0.3 mmol/L and the mean VPA plasma level was 75.3 ± 29.4 μg/mL (Findling et al., 2005). Only six subjects (10%), three in each treatment group completed the 76-week protocol, a vivid indication of the chronic and debilitating course of PBD.

Regarding adverse effects, comparing lithium with valproex, emesis (30% vs. 3%), enuresis (30% vs. 6.7%), and increased thirst (16.5% vs. 0%) were significantly more frequent in the lithium group; other frequent adverse effects, which were not significantly different between lithium and valproex were headache (13.3% vs. 23.3%), tremor (20.0% vs. 16.7%), stomach pain (10.0% vs. 23.3%), nausea (16.7% vs. 6.7%), diarrhea (13.3% vs. 6.7%), and decreased appetite (10% vs. 10%) (Findling et al., 2005).

Valproic Acid in the Treatment of Aggression in Children and Adolescents

Few studies have looked at valproic acid's efficacy in treating aggression specifically. Blader et al. (2009) studied the efficacy of divalproex in the treatment of children with ADHD and aggression refractory to stimulant monotherapy. Children aged 6 to 13 years were eligible to participate if they had a diagnosis of ADHD and either oppositional defiant disorder (ODD) or CD. Children with coexisting mood, anxiety, and psychotic disorders, or pervasive developmental disorders (PDDs), Tourette syndrome, and mental retardation were excluded from the study. The Retrospective Modified OAS was used to measure severity of aggression. Parents completed this scale at baseline and weekly during the study. The Conners' Global Index–Parent Version measured severity of ADHD symptoms. During the study's lead-in phase, 74 participants received open stimulant treatment for 5 weeks. Those whose aggression persisted despite optimal control of ADHD symptoms during the lead-in phase were randomly assigned to receive double-blind, flexibly dosed divalproex or placebo along with their stimulant for 8 weeks. Given that 31 participants' aggression remitted during the lead-in phase, 10 withdrew from the study, and 3 exhibited low adherence, a total of 30 children were able to be randomized to take either divalproex or placebo. All participants received weekly behavioral therapy throughout. Target serum divalproex levels were between 80 and 110 mg/L. The mean serum valproic acid level during the study was 68.11 mg/L. By the end of the study, the authors concluded that a significantly higher percentage of children receiving divalproex during the trial (57%) met aggression remission criteria compared with those assigned to placebo (15%). This study is limited by its small sample size, and additional studies are clearly needed to more accurately estimate valproic acid's efficacy in the treatment of aggression in children with ADHD and comorbid ODD or CD (Blader et al., 2009).

Barzman et al. (2006) studied the efficacy of quetiapine versus divalproex for the treatment of impulsivity and reactive aggression in adolescents with comorbid bipolar disorder and a disruptive behavior disorder (ODD or CD). Thirty-three adolescents were randomized in a double-blind manner to 28 days of quetiapine 400 to 600 mg daily or divalproex (serum level 80 to 120 μg/mL). The primary measure of efficacy was the change in the Positive and Negative Syndrome Scale (PANSS) Excited Component (EC). The authors reported that there was no significant difference in the PANSS EC scores between the two treatment groups and thus stated that both medications appear to have similar efficacy in the treatment of impulsivity and reactive aggression in children with bipolar disorder comorbid with ODD or CD (Barzman et al., 2006). The absence of a placebo arm in this study is a notable limitation. Further studies are needed to replicate these findings.

Divalproex Sodium in the Treatment of Adolescents with Disruptive Behavioral Disorders

In an open-label, 5-week study, Donovan et al. (1997) treated 10 outpatient adolescents (8 males and 2 females; age range, 15 to 17 years) with divalproex sodium who were diagnosed by *DSM-III-R* (APA, 1987) criteria with disruptive behavioral disorders (7, CD; 2, ODD; and 1, ADHD). Most had comorbid drug abuse or dependency (5, marijuana abuse; 3, marijuana dependency; and 1, alcohol abuse). All 10 subjects had severe unpredictable mood swings and a low threshold/high amplitude for dyscontrol once irritable, with frequent and severe temper tantrums ("explosive mood disorder"), which preceded drug abuse by at least 1 year. Efficacy was determined depending on multiple informants' (subjects, parents, and teachers) reports of temper outbursts and mood lability and the Global Assessment of Functioning (GAF; Axis V of the *DSM-III-R* diagnoses) Scale.

Divalproex sodium was initiated at a dose of 250 mg/day and titrated to 1,000 mg/day over a period of 2 to 4 weeks. The mean plasma VPA level after receiving 1,000 mg/day of divalproex for 1 week was 75 μg/mL (range 45 to 113 μg/mL). At the end of the fifth week, all 10 subjects showed significant improvement on all three measures; 9 subjects had no temper outbursts during the fifth week, and 6 subjects had no significant mood lability. Their mean number of temper outbursts decreased from 6.5 ± 4.5 at baseline to 0.1 ± 0.3 after 5 weeks. The mean mood lability score (0 = least to 4 = greater frequency, duration, and autonomy of mood swings) decreased from 3.8 ± 0.4 at baseline to 0.5 ± 0.7 after 5 weeks. The mean GAF score improved from 37.8 ± 7.0 at baseline to 65.7 ± 10.2 after 5 weeks. Divalproex was well tolerated, with only two patients reporting mild sedation and transient nausea. There were no serious untoward effects, and liver function tests showed no significant changes. Improvements were maintained while on medication during follow-up; however, five subjects independently discontinued medication for at least 5 days and rapidly relapsed; improvement recurred within a few days of resuming medication. A sixth patient took medication sporadically during follow-up and maintained gains for approximately 6 weeks, when partial relapse occurred. These data suggest that divalproex sodium may be safe and efficacious in such adolescents, although further studies should be undertaken (Donovan et al., 1997).

Donovan et al. (2000) conducted a 12-week, randomly assigned, double-blind, placebo-controlled, crossover study of divalproex sodium in the treatment of 20 outpatients (16 males and 4 females; mean age, 13.8 ± 2.4 years; age range, 10 to 18 years), all of whom were diagnosed with CD or ODD by *DSM-IV* (APA, 1994) criteria and chronic explosive temper (more than four episodes monthly of rage, property destruction, or fighting with minimal provocation) and mood lability (multiple daily unpredictable shifts in mood from normal to irritable and withdrawn to boisterous behavior). Four subjects were diagnosed with comorbid ADHD and six with marijuana abuse. Efficacy was assessed by ratings on the Modified OAS and on six items from the anger-hostility subscale of the Symptom Checklist-90 (SCL-90); it was decided *a priori* that "responders" had to have a $\geq 70\%$ reduction from baseline scores on both rating scales. The first 6 weeks of the study consisted of a parallel-groups design, with 10 subjects randomly assigned to VPA or placebo. Divalproex was gradually titrated to 10 mg/lb/day over the first 2 weeks; if the plasma level of VPA was <90 μg/mL at that time, a single increase of 250 mg/day was added. (To preserve the blind, a similar number of increases were made in the placebo group.) Doses ranged from 750 to 1,500 mg/day, and the mean plasma VPA level was 82.2 ± 19.1 μg/mL. At the end of this 6-week phase, 8 (80%) of the 10 patients receiving divalproex were rated as responders versus no responders in the 10 subjects on placebo ($P < .001$). Seventeen subjects completed phase I (during the first 2 weeks, one subject on divalproex dropped out as he was incarcerated for parole violation and two subjects on placebo dropped out for lack of clinical improvement). Fifteen subjects (eight responders to divalproex and seven nonresponders to placebo) entered the crossover phase of the study (weeks 7 to 12), and all completed it. Six (86%) of the seven placebo nonresponders during phase I responded to divalproex during phase II. Six of the eight responders to divalproex during phase I began relapsing between 1 and 2 weeks into phase II, and at the end of week 12, their average Modified OAS score had worsened to only 33% over baseline and their average anger-hostility scores on the subscale of the SCL-90 declined to 27% over baseline. Of the 15 subjects completing the entire study, 12 met "responder" criteria only during the medication phase, suggesting that divalproex is significantly better than placebo ($P = .003$) in this population.

Steiner et al. (2003) studied 71 youth with CD in a 7-week randomized controlled trial comparing treatment response to low dose (up to 250 mg/day) or high dose (between 500 and 1,500 mg/day or a plasma level between 50 and 120 µg/mL) of divalproex sodium. Sixty-six percent of subjects previously committed violent offenses including manslaughter, robbery, rape, or assault with a deadly weapon. At study exit, a blinded clinician rated subjects according to the CGI-S, and estimated symptom improvement compared to the CGI-S at study entry. Investigators found that subjects receiving a high dose of divalproex sodium were more likely to be rated as markedly improved, and also self-reported improved impulse control ($P < .05$) and restraint ($P < .06$). Study authors concluded that although this study provides preliminary support for short-term efficacy of divalproex sodium in the treatment of CD, larger and longer term studies are needed to fully understand the role divalproex sodium may play in a comprehensive treatment plan for CD.

Valproic Acid in the Treatment of Children and Adolescents Diagnosed with Mental Retardation and Mood Disorders

Kastner et al. (1990) reported treating three patients with valproic acid, a 16-year-old male with moderate mental retardation and two girls with profound mental retardation (ages 8 and 13 years). All three patients had symptoms of a comorbid mood disorder, including self-injurious behaviors such as face gouging and head banging, irritability, aggressiveness, hyperactivity, sleep disturbance, and paroxysms of crying. All had unsatisfactory responses to trials of several other medications. All three patients showed excellent response to valproic acid and at follow-up had maintained their gains for 7 to 10 months. Maintenance doses were 2,700 mg/day (plasma level, 109 µg/mL) for the 16-year-old, 3,000 mg/day (plasma level, 75 µg/mL) for the 13-year-old, and 1,500 mg/day (plasma level, 111 µg/mL) for the 8-year-old. The authors noted that the plasma levels were high or just above the typical therapeutic upper range and that no hepatic abnormalities developed in their patients.

In a 2-year prospective study, Kastner et al. (1993) administered valproic acid to 21 patients diagnosed with mental retardation who also had behavioral symptoms of irritability, sleep disturbance, aggressive or self-injurious behavior, and behavioral cycling that were interpreted as symptomatic of an affective disorder. Eighteen patients completed the study. (Two were lost to follow-up, and one developed acute hyperammonemia and was dropped from the study.) Twelve of the patients completing the study were 18 years old or younger; the degree of mental retardation ranged from moderate to profound. Valproic acid was titrated upward until symptoms remitted or untoward effects prevented further increase, to plasma levels between 50 and 125 µg/mL. Patients' ratings on the CGI-S Scale after 2 years on medication were significantly improved ($P < .001$) from ratings at baseline. Patients with a diagnosis of epilepsy or a suspicion of seizures correlated with a positive response ($P < .005$). Of note, 9 of the 10 patients who were receiving neuroleptic drugs at the beginning of the study were no longer being prescribed these drugs at the study's completion.

Hellings et al. (2005) conducted a double-blind, placebo-controlled study to evaluate the efficacy of VPA in treating aggressive symptoms in 30 subjects (20 male and 10 female; age range 6 to 20 years) who were diagnosed with a PDD by *DSM-IV* criteria (27 were diagnosed with autistic disorder, 1 with PDDNOS, and 2 with Asperger disorder). Comorbid diagnoses, with the exception of Tourette disorder were permitted. No other psychotropic medications or antiseizure medications were permitted. Subjects exhibited significant aggression toward themselves or others, or to property, a minimum of three times weekly. Twenty-six subjects had intelligence quotients (IQs) in the mentally retarded range. Subjects were randomly assigned to liquid placebo ($N = 14$) or liquid VPA ($N = 16$) for a period of 8 weeks, following a 1-week lead-in on placebo. In the VPA group, the liquid placebo was gradually replaced by liquid VPA beginning with a 250 mg/5 mL dose. VPA liquid (250 mg/5 mL) was added every 3 days to reach a target dose of 20 mg/kg/day. A psychiatrist not involved in ratings adjusted the VPA to achieve trough plasma levels of 70 to 100 µg/mL after measurement at the end of 2 and 4 weeks. Mean VPA trough plasma levels were 75.5 µg/mL at week 4 and 77.8 µ/mL at week 8.

There were no statistically significant differences between the two groups on the primary outcome measure, the Aberrant Behavior Checklist–Community (ABC-C) Scale ($P = .65$), or the secondary outcome measures, the CGI-Isubscale ($P = .16$), and the OAS ($P = .96$). The CGI-S subscale also showed no statistic difference between the groups ($P = .96$).

Adverse effects were usually mild. One subject on VPA developed a rash and dropped out of the study. Increased appetite was the only adverse effect that was significantly greater in the VPA group ($P = .03$). Gastrointestinal complaints, sedation, headache, chills, and fever did not differ. Two subjects on VPA had elevations of ammonia above the normal range of 21 to 50 µmol/L, and the parent of one of these subjects reported cognitive slowing and slurred speech at times (ammonia was 98 µmol/L at the end of the study).

The authors noted that there was high intrasubject variability with large differences in the frequency and severity of aggression in different weeks, and high intersubject variability with large standard deviations for each of the outcome measures, which weakened study power. Following completion of the study, 10 subjects on VPA elected to continue on the drug and 6 on placebo elected to an open trial of VPA. Ten of these 16 subjects continued to demonstrate a positive and sustained response. The authors concluded that although this study did not demonstrate efficacy of VPA, there might be a subgroup of aggressive children and adolescents with PDD who respond favorably to VPA and that a larger, multisite study is indicated.

Hollander et al. (2006) studied divalproex sodium for the treatment of repetitive behaviors in autism in an 8-week double-blind placebo-controlled trial involving 13 patients with autism spectrum disorder (ASD). The average age of subjects was 9.5 years (12 subjects were child/adolescent patients and 1 subject was 40 years old). Nine subjects were randomized into the treatment group and four into the placebo group. The primary outcome measure was the Children's Yale-Brown Obsessive Compulsive Scale (C-YBOCS), Compulsion subscale. The mean serum divalproex level at the end of the study was 58.23 ± 21.63 µg/mL. Authors reported a significant improvement in repetitive behavior scores for subjects taking divalproex (average improvement of 0.889 points), and a worsening of behavior scores with patients taking placebo (average worsening of 2.5 points). A large effect size of $d = 1.53$ was reported for divalproex sodium. Ultimately, none of the patients in the placebo group maintained or improved their C-YBOCS scores, whereas 77% of the divalproex group did. There were no statistically significant differences in adverse effects between the two study groups. The authors concluded that this study provides preliminary support for the successful use of divalproex sodium in the treatment of repetitive behaviors in patients with ASD (Hollander et al., 2005).

However, the small sample size and short study duration are important limitations to consider with this study.

Hollander et al. (2010) also conducted a 12-week randomized double-blind, placebo-controlled trial studying the efficacy of divalproex sodium for the treatment of irritability in 27 youth with ASDs. Primary outcome measures included the (CGI-I) Scale focusing on irritability and the irritability subscale of the ABC. Sixteen subjects were randomized to active treatment and 11 subjects to placebo. The study authors reported that 62.5% of the subjects randomized to active treatment showed a reduction in irritability according to CGI-I scores versus only 9.09% in the placebo arm. Analysis of ABC–irritability subscale scores revealed that subjects receiving divalproex sodium benefited from a drop of >0.53 points/week compared with subjects who were randomized to placebo. It was noted that treatment responders had higher mean VPA levels (89.77 µg/mL) than nonresponders (64.33 µg/mL). Response noted per the CGI-I Scale was found to be dose dependent in this study. For example, subjects with VPA levels between 87 and 110 µg/mL showed a 100% response rate, whereas subjects with levels <87 µg/mL had a reduced response rate of 60%. Subjects with VPA levels >110 µg/mL experienced the lowest response rate (33%). Divalproex sodium was well tolerated overall, with side effects ranging from mild to moderate, and no serious adverse events were reported. The study authors concluded that this study suggests that VPA may be beneficial for the treatment of irritability associated with ASD, although larger studies are needed to support or refute the findings (Hollander et al., 2010).

Carbamazepine (Tegretol; Carbatrol; Equetro)

Note: The FDA has directed that black box warnings be added to the labeling of carbamazepine products indicating that the risk of developing *aplastic anemia and agranulocytosis* is five to eight times greater than in the general population, although the incidence is very low. Most cases of leukopenia do not progress to the more serious aplastic anemia or agranulocytosis. However, complete pretreatment hematologic testing should be obtained as a baseline. If low or decreased WBC or platelet count occurs during treatment, close monitoring should be implemented and discontinuing carbamazepine should be seriously considered if there is any evidence of bone marrow depression. Carbamazepine also carries the risk for *serious dermatological reactions* including toxic epidermal necrolysis (TEN) and Stevens—Johnson syndrome (SJS). These reactions are estimated to occur in 1 to 6 per 10,000 new users in countries with predominantly Caucasian populations. The risk for TEN and SJS is estimated to be approximately 10 times higher in some Asian countries. Studies in patients with Chinese ancestry revealed a strong association between the human leukocyte antigen (HLA)-B*1502 allele and the risk of developing serious dermatologic reactions while taking carbamazepine. It is recommended that patients with at-risk ancestry be screened for the presence of HLA-B*1502 before initiating carbamazepine treatment. Patients who are positive for this allele should not be treated with carbamazepine unless the benefit carefully outweighs the risk.

In addition to the black box warnings described, in 2008 the FDA issued an alert advising providers to monitor patients who are taking or starting antiepileptic medication for any changes in behavior that could indicate the emergence of depression or worsening suicidal thoughts or behavior (*PDR*.net, 2017).

Carbamazepine is an anticonvulsant indicated for the treatment of psychomotor and grand mal seizures. It is also a specific analgesic for trigeminal neuralgia.

Pharmacokinetics of Carbamazepine

Peak serum levels occur 4 to 5 hours after ingestion of standard carbamazepine tablets. Initial serum half-life values range from 25 to 65 hours; however, carbamazepine is an autoinducer of its own metabolism. Autoinduction stabilizes over 3 to 5 weeks at a fixed dose, with half-life decreasing to 12 to 17 hours. In children, there is a poor correlation between dose and serum level of carbamazepine.

Contraindications for Carbamazepine Administration

Known hypersensitivity to carbamazepine or tricyclic antidepressants, a history of previous bone marrow depression, and the ingestion of a monoamine oxidase inhibitor within the previous 14 days are contraindications. Coadministration with nefazodone or lurasidone is also contraindicated.

Interactions of Carbamazepine with Other Drugs

Carbamazepine is both a CYP3A4 substrate and an inducer. As such, it will reduce plasma levels of other CYP3A4 substrates (clozapine, benzodiazepines, hormonal contraceptives, warfarin, etc.). Other CYP3A4 inhibitors will raise carbamazepine levels (cimetidine, azoles, macrolides, etc.). When coadministered with risperidone (6 mg/day) over a 3-week period, plasma concentrations of risperidone and 9-hydroxyrisperidone were decreased by approximately 50%. Plasma levels of carbamazepine did not appear to be affected. Carbamazepine also reduces serum levels of haloperidol and aripiprazole.

When coadministered with olanzapine, carbamazepine in doses of 200 mg twice daily caused an approximately 50% increase in the clearance of olanzapine. This was thought to be secondary to carbamazepine's being a potent inducer of CYP1A2 activity. Higher daily doses of carbamazepine may cause an even greater increase in olanzapine clearance.

Carbamazepine serum levels are markedly reduced by the simultaneous use of phenobarbital, phenytoin, or primidone.

Increased lithium serum concentrations and increased risk of neurotoxic lithium effects may occur when carbamazepine and lithium are used simultaneously because carbamazepine decreases lithium renal clearance.

The FDA has advised that carbamazepine may lose up to one-third of its potency if stored under humid conditions such as in a bathroom. Supplies should be kept tightly closed and in a dry location.

Untoward Effects of Carbamazepine

The most frequently reported untoward effects are dizziness, drowsiness, unsteadiness, nausea, and vomiting. These are more likely to occur if treatment is not begun with the low doses recommended. As noted earlier, aplastic anemia and agranulocytosis, although rare, have been reported. Hence, a complete baseline hematologic evaluation must be done and complete blood cell count with differential and platelets must be repeated and monitored closely throughout the treatment. Liver dysfunction, cardiovascular complications, and hyponatremia have been reported.

Carbamazepine is classified as pregnancy category D and should not be prescribed to those who are pregnant or nursing. Carbamazepine use in pregnancy has been associated with neural tube defects, craniofacial abnormalities, growth retardation, and cardiac defects. The North American Antiepileptic Drug Pregnancy Registry noted that major congenital malformations occurred in 3% out of approximately 1,000 women exposed to carbamazepine in the first trimester, translating to a relative risk of 2.7 (CI: 1,7) compared to those not taking carbamazepine (*PDR.net*, 2017).

Pleak et al. (1988) reported that adverse behavioral and neurologic reactions developed in 6 of their 20 male subjects, aged 10 to 16, who were diagnosed with various disorders, but primarily with ADHD and CD, and who were participating in an ongoing protocol evaluating the efficacy of carbamazepine in treating severe aggressive outbursts in child and adolescent inpatients. The untoward effects included a severe manic episode in a 16-year-old, hypomania in a 10-year-old, and increased irritability, impulsivity, and aggressiveness and/or worsening of behavior in two subjects aged 14 and 15. Two 11-year-old boys developed EEG abnormalities, with sharp waves and spikes. One of these boys improved behaviorally, but had his first two absence seizures in several years. The authors caution that patients must be monitored carefully for the development of adverse neuropsychiatric effects.

Amstutz et al. (2013) replicated associations between HLA-B*1502 and HLA-A*3101 and carbamazepine-induced hypersensitivity reactions, including SJS and drug-induced hypersensitivity syndrome, in diverse pediatric populations in North America. Forty-two youth with carbamazepine hypersensitivity reactions and 91 youth tolerant to carbamazepine were studied. Researchers concluded that HLA-A*3101 was not significantly associated with SJS, but was significantly associated with other carbamazepine-induced hypersensitivity reactions. By contrast, in this study HLA-B*1502 was strongly associated with SJS and not with other carbamazepine-induced hypersensitivity reactions. Importantly, not all children with the identified genetic variants developed hypersensitivity reactions. The authors suggested that the safest approach is to test for both variants, regardless of ancestry, when considering carbamazepine use in youth, although they cautioned that additional studies are needed (Amstutz et al., 2013).

Carbamazepine and the Induction of Mania

Three additional cases of carbamazepine-induced mania have been reported in children (Myers & Carrera, 1989; Reiss & O'Donnell, 1984). Myers and Carrera speculated that when adverse behavioral effects such as irritability, insomnia, agitation, talkativeness, and prepubescent hypersexuality occur with carbamazepine administration, they may be symptoms of an unrecognized hypomania or mania.

Indications for Carbamazepine

Carbamazepine is approved for use in patients at least 6 years of age for the treatment of various seizure types. Patients diagnosed with partial seizures with complex symptomatology (psychomotor or temporal lobe) tend to benefit the most from carbamazepine, but patients with generalized tonic-clonic (grand mal) seizures or a mixed seizure pattern may also improve. Absence (petit mal) seizures are not controlled by carbamazepine. Patients with trigeminal and glossopharyngeal neuralgias have shown reduction in pain when treated with carbamazepine. Carbamazepine is approved for treatment of acute mania and mixed episodes associated with bipolar-I disorder for adults only (*PDR*.net, 2017).

Carbamazepine Dosage Schedule

The following are doses recommended for treatment of epilepsy. It is recommended that carbamazepine be taken with meals.

- *Children under 6 years of age:* 10 to 20 mg/kg/day bid or tid. Increase the dose weekly to achieve optimal clinical response, tid or qid. The maximum daily dose is 35 mg/kg/24 hours.
- *Children 6 through 12 years of age:* Begin with a dose of 100 mg twice daily (or 50 mg four times daily if suspension is used). The dose may be increased weekly by increments of 100 mg (bid regimen for carbamazepine XR, and a tid or qid regimen for other formulations) to obtain optimal response. The daily dose should not usually exceed 1,000 mg. Usual maintenance daily dose is 400 to 800 mg.
- *Patients > 12 years old:* Begin with a dose of 200 mg twice daily (or 100 mg four times daily if suspension is used). The dose may be increased weekly by increments of 200 mg as clinically indicated to obtain optimal response. Carbamazepine XR tablets may be dosed bid, whereas all other preparations should be dosed tid or qid. The daily dose should not usually exceed 1,000 mg for children ages 12 to 15, or 1,200 mg daily for children older than 15 years. Usual maintenance daily dose is 800 to 1,200 mg. Usual therapeutic carbamazepine plasma levels are 4 to 12 μg/mL.

Carbamazepine Dose Forms Available

- *Tablets:* 200 mg
- *Chewable tablets:* 100 mg
- *Suspension:* 100 mg/5 mL
- *Extended-release tablets (Tegretol-XR):* 100, 200, and 400 mg
- *Extended-release capsules (Carbatrol; Equetro):* 100, 200, and 300 mg

▌ *Reports of Interest*

Carbamazepine Use for Nonspecific Pediatric Behavioral Symptoms

Remschmidt (1976) reviewed data from 28 clinical trials (seven double-blind and 21 open studies) with a total of >800 nonepileptic child and adolescent subjects who were treated with carbamazepine. Positive clinical results were found for target symptoms of hyperactivity or hypoactivity, impaired concentration, aggressive behavioral disturbances, and dysphoric mood disorders. In addition to these behavioral effects, Remschmidt suggested that these patients experienced positive mood changes, increased initiative, and decreased anxiety.

Puente (1976) reported an open study in which carbamazepine was administered to 72 children with various behavioral disorders who did not have evidence of neurologic disease. Fifty-six children completed the study. The usual optimal dose was 300 mg/day (range, 100 to 600 mg/day). Carbamazepine was given for an average of 12 weeks (range, 9 to 23 weeks). Twenty symptoms were rated on a severity scale at the beginning and end of the treatment. Individual symptoms were present in as many as 55 and in as few as 2 of the 56 children. Over the course of treatment, a decrease in symptom expression of 70% or more occurred in 17 of 20 symptoms in at least 60% of the subjects. Interestingly, all 6 children (100%) with night terrors responded positively, as did 16 (94%) of the 17 children with other sleep disturbances. Anxiety, present in 47 children, improved in 34 (72%). Enuresis improved in 8 of 9 children (89%), and aggressiveness, present in 46 children, improved in 32 (70%). The most frequent untoward effects were transient drowsiness (20%), nausea and vomiting (4%), and urticaria (4%).

Carbamazepine in the Treatment of Juvenile-Onset Bipolar-I Disorder

Woolston (1999) reported three cases diagnosed with bipolar-I disorder whom he treated successfully with carbamazepine. One case, a 16-year-old female, experienced several cycles of mania followed by depression managed with various neuroleptics and lithium for approximately 4 years. The patient was noncompliant with lithium at least three times, resulting in manic episodes within a month that were followed by severe depression. Following the last of these episodes, she was started on carbamazepine, 150 mg/day, which was increased to 300 mg/day 3 weeks later and continued at that dosage. Her serum carbamazepine level was 7 µg/mL. The patient became euthymic within 3 weeks and remained so on 300 mg/day of carbamazepine over the next 4 years, with the exception of three brief hypomanic episodes that responded to the addition of a short course of haloperidol 1 mg/day. No untoward effects were reported and blood counts and liver function remained within normal limits.

A 14-year-old male with mania treated with lithium for approximately 2 years discontinued lithium because it made him tired and dysphoric. He subsequently developed another manic episode. Carbamazepine was initiated at a dose of 100 mg/day and was increased to 200 mg/day 5 days later. His mania improved significantly within 15 days and he did not experience the unpleasant symptoms he associated with lithium. His carbamazepine serum level was 8 µg/mL. He remained euthymic on carbamazepine 200 mg/day for the next 3 years with serum levels ranging from 6 to 9 µg/mL. No untoward effects were reported and blood counts and liver chemistries remained normal throughout his treatment.

The third case was a 12.5-year-old girl, also diagnosed with spastic cerebral palsy and mild mental retardation. She was treated briefly with risperidone for persistent euphoric mood, decreased need for sleep, and intermittent hallucinations. After 3 weeks, she had increased manic symptoms with flight of ideas, pressured speech, motor restlessness, and nearly continuous visual hallucinations with poor reality testing. Risperidone was discontinued and carbamazepine 100 mg/day was started. After 1 week, she showed improvement in sleep and reality testing and experienced no untoward effects. Carbamazepine was increased to 200 mg/day. Six days later, hallucinations remitted, she was euthymic, had no evidence of a thought disorder, and her normal sleep pattern returned. Her serum carbamazepine level was 8 µg/mL. The patient was continued on maintenance carbamazepine, 200 mg/day. Over the next 2 years, she developed two brief periods of hypomania, both of which responded rapidly to an additional 50 mg of carbamazepine. She remained euthymic on her final maintenance daily dose of 300 mg of carbamazepine.

Craven and Margaret (2000) reported a case of a 16-year-old boy with cerebral palsy and comorbid bipolar disorder who had a favorable response to carbamazepine treatment. At the age of 9 years, this patient began to experience mood instability. His mood varied between depression and inappropriate elation, and he spoke of seeing monsters. During depressive episodes, he would refuse to eat and would become uncommunicative. Extensive medical work-ups were negative. He was initially diagnosed with a depressive disorder. A trial of imipramine proved ineffective and so was discontinued. A trial of Prozac was then started, which resulted in restlessness, insomnia, and an objectively elated mood. His diagnosis was later changed to bipolar disorder and carbamazepine 200 mg twice daily was started. Within 1 month of starting carbamazepine, his mood returned to baseline, and at the time of the case report, he was reported to have remained stable for a period of 18 months (Craven & Margaret, 2000).

Davanzo (2003) conducted a retrospective review of clinical changes during the hospitalization of 44 preadolescent bipolar youth, who were treated with lithium, carbamazepine, or divalproex sodium. Four trained clinicians, who were blinded to the treatment group, reviewed daily progress notes and discharge summaries and rated them according to the CGI-I Scale. Length of hospitalization, severity of illness at admission, and comorbidity did not differ between treatment groups. Each group approached serum therapeutic levels for their respective medication at day 7 of hospitalization. The author reported that the mean CGI-I scores were systematically higher, or worse, for carbamazepine compared with those of lithium and divalproex. This difference was statistically significant by week 2 of the hospitalization. The author concluded that carbamazepine may be less effective than lithium or divalproex sodium for the treatment of preadolescent patients with bipolar disorder, but acknowledged numerous limitations of this retrospective study (Davanzo, 2003).

In an open trial, Kowatch et al. (2000) studied 42 outpatients with bipolar disorder who were randomized to receive divalproate, lithium, or carbamazepine for 6 weeks in a nonblind manner. Response rates were calculated at 53% for divalproate and 38% for both lithium and carbamazepine. All had large effect sizes (1.63 for divalproex sodium, 1.06 for lithium, and 1.00 for carbamazepine) (Kowatch et al., 2000). This study is summarized in the section on valproic acid.

Joshi et al. (2010) conducted an 8-week prospective open-label trial of extended-release carbamazepine (CBZ-ER) for the treatment of 27 youth with bipolar disorder (9.1 ± 1.9 years of age). CBZ-ER doses averaged 788 ± 252 mg/day. Three subjects continued their long-standing stimulant medication for comorbid ADHD. The YMRS, CGI-I, CDRS, and BPRS were used to assess response to treatment. Response was identified as having a >30% reduction in YMRS scores or by being rated "improved" or "very much improved" on the CGI-I for mania. At the end of the study, 52% of subjects had a 30% reduction in YMRS scores and 44% had a 50% reduction in YMRS scores. Thirty-three percent of subjects were judged to be "improved" or "very much improved" on CGI-I scores. On the basis of the defined response criteria (either a 30% reduction on YMRS or CGI-Mania Improvement score of ≤2), the rate of antimanic response was 63%. Investigators concluded that CBZ-ER treatment resulted in statistically significant, but modest, improvements in YMRS scores, and resulted in significant improvement in symptoms of depression, ADHD, and psychotic symptoms. CBZ-ER was deemed well tolerated during the trial. Two subjects had to discontinue the medication because of rash, although in both cases the rash was nonprogressive and resolved within 1 week of discontinuing

CBZ-ER. The most common adverse effects reported were headache (23%), gastrointestinal complaints (18%), cold symptoms (15%), dizziness (8%), aches and pains (8%), and insomnia (4%). No laboratory abnormalities were detected. Study authors concluded that depending on this open study, CBZ-ER may be effective for the treatment of PBD, but acknowledged modest response rates compared with atypical antipsychotic medication (Joshi et al., 2010).

Carbamazepine in the Treatment of Children Diagnosed with Conduct Disorder

Kafantaris et al. (1992) reported an open pilot study in which 10 children (9 male and 1 female; age range, 5.25 to 10.92 years; mean, 8.27 years), diagnosed with CD and hospitalized for symptoms of explosive aggressiveness, were treated with carbamazepine. Five of the subjects previously failed to respond to lithium. One week after enrollment, carbamazepine was administered in three divided doses, beginning with 200 mg/day and titrated over 3 to 5 weeks to a maximum of 800 mg/day, or a serum level of 12 µg/mL. Optimal dose range was 600 to 800 mg/day (mean, 630 mg/day) with serum levels from 4.8 to 10.4 µg/mL (mean, 6.2 µg/mL). Target symptoms of aggressiveness and explosiveness declined significantly on all measures compared with baseline ratings. On the Global Clinical Consensus Ratings, four subjects were rated as markedly improved, four as moderately improved, one as slightly improved, and one as not improved. Three of the lithium nonresponders showed marked improvement, and one showed moderate improvement; the fifth did not respond to either drug. Untoward effects during regulation and at optimal dose included fatigue (2 of 10 cases), blurred vision (2 of 10), and dizziness (1 of 10). Untoward effects above optimal dose included diplopia (2 of 10), mild ataxia (2 of 10), mild dysarthria (1 of 10), headache (2 of 10), and lethargy (1 of 10). One child experienced worsening of preexisting behavioral symptoms and loosening of associations, which were thought to be manifestations of behavioral toxicity. Overall, the untoward effects were transient and were decreased or eliminated by carbamazepine dose reduction. WBC counts remained within normal limits, although four children had reductions from baseline determinations.

Cueva et al. (1996) reported a 9-week, double-blind, placebo-controlled study comparing carbamazepine and placebo in 22 children (20 males and 2 females; mean age, 8.97 years; age range, 5.33 to 11.7 years) who were diagnosed with CD, solitary aggressive type by *DSM-III-R* (APA, 1987) criteria and who required hospitalization for treatment-resistant aggressiveness and explosiveness. Thirty-eight children who met protocol criteria entered the initial 2-week placebo washout period. At the end of this period, 14 were eliminated because they no longer met study or aggression criteria. Of the 24 subjects who entered the treatment phase of the study, 13 were assigned to carbamazepine and 11 to placebo; 22 subjects completed the study. Efficacy was measured using the CPRS, the National Institute of Mental Health CGI-S and, CGI-I Scales, the OAS, and the GCJCS, with a blind rating by all clinical staff occurring just before the code is broken. Medication was dispensed in two capsules given three times daily throughout the study. Carbamazepine was initiated at a dose of 200 mg/day and increased over a 2-week period in predetermined steps of 200 mg/dose to a maximum of 1,000 mg/day or until therapeutic effects were observed or untoward effects prevented further increase. For the 11 subjects for whom values were available, the mean optimal dose of carbamazepine was 683 mg/day (range, 400 to 800 mg/day), and the mean serum carbamazepine level was 6.81 µg/mL (range, 4.98 to 9.1 µg/mL).

The results showed no significant differences in the clinical improvement of aggression between carbamazepine and placebo on any of the rating scales. Both groups improved on the aggression factor of the CPRS over time and both improved similarly on the GCJCS as rated by clinical staff. Carbamazepine treatment resulted in significantly more untoward effects than did placebo. About 12 of the 13 subjects on carbamazepine reported a total of 57 untoward effects, whereas only 6 of 11 subjects on placebo reported six untoward effects. Two subjects on carbamazepine developed marked leukopenia (2,000 to 3,000 WBC/mm^3), and four developed moderate leukopenia (3,000 to 3,500 WBC/mm^3); one subject on placebo also developed moderate leukopenia. Leukopenia was transient in all seven cases. Other untoward effects experienced by the treatment group subjects included dizziness ($N = 7, 54\%$), rash ($N = 6, 46\%$), headache (46%), diplopia ($N = 5, 38\%$), drowsiness ($N = 4$, 31%), nausea (31%), ataxia ($N = 3, 23\%$), and vomiting (23%) (Cueva et al., 1996).

Carbamazepine in the Treatment of Children and Adolescents with Symptoms of Attention-Deficit/Hyperactivity Disorder

Silva et al. (1996) searched the world literature for reports in which carbamazepine was used to treat children and adolescents with behavioral problems and hyperactivity. Twenty-nine such reports were located; 10 of them provided information suitable for a meta-analysis. Seven studies, with a total of 189 patients, were open; 70% of subjects experienced at least a marked improvement in target symptoms (significance ranged from $P < .001$ to $P = .05$). There was a significant correlation between longer treatment and positive outcome. In the three double-blind studies, 53 subjects were assigned to carbamazepine and 52 to placebo. Thirty-eight (72%) subjects on carbamazepine and 14 (27%) subjects on placebo were rated as moderately to markedly improved. Meta-analysis of these three studies found carbamazepine significantly ($P = .018$) more efficacious than placebo in diminishing target symptoms. The most common untoward effects in the studies reviewed were sedation and rash. The authors concluded that carbamazepine merited further study as a possible second-line treatment for children and adolescents with ADHD that is not responsive to stimulant medication or when stimulant medication cannot be tolerated.

Note: The FDA has directed that black box warnings be added to the labeling of carbamazepine products indicating *cardiovascular risk with rapid iv infusion.*

Oxcarbazepine (Trileptal)

Note: In 2008, the FDA also issued an alert advising providers to monitor patients who are taking or starting antiepileptic medication for any changes in behavior that could indicate the emergence of depression or worsening suicidal thoughts or behavior (*PDR*.net, 2008).

Pharmacokinetics of Oxcarbazepine

Oxcarbazepine is an antiepileptic drug and a 10 keto-analog of carbamazepine; pharmacologic activity is exerted primarily through its 10-monohydroxy metabolite (MHD). Its mechanism of action is unknown; however, *in vitro* studies have indicated that oxcarbazepine and MHD produce blockade of voltage-sensitive sodium channels, resulting in stabilization of hyperexcited neural membranes. Oxcarbazepine taken orally is completely absorbed and extensively metabolized to MHD. The half-life of oxcarbazepine is approximately 2 hours, and the half-life of MHD is approximately 9 hours. Food does not appear to affect the bioavailability of either oxcarbazepine or MHD. The median peak plasma level is 4.5 hours (range, 3 to 13 hours) for film-coated tablets and 6 hours for the oral suspension preparation; both preparations have similar bioavailability. Steady-state plasma concentrations are achieved in 2 to 3 days when a given dose is administered twice daily. Clearance of oxcarbazepine and its metabolites is primarily (above 95%) through the kidneys. Clearance in children below 8 years of age is 30% to 40% greater than in older children and adults; and in a controlled clinical trial, such patients had the highest maintenance doses.

Contraindications for the Administration of Oxcarbazepine

Hypersensitivity to oxcarbazepine or its components is a contraindication to the administration of oxcarbazepine. Approximately 25% to 30% of patients who had hypersensitivity reactions to carbamazepine are likely to do so with oxcarbazepine; hence, they should be asked about any such prior exposure.

Interactions of Oxcarbazepine with Other Drugs

Oxcarbazepine can inhibit CYP2C19 and induce CYP3A4 and CYP3A5, which can potentially significantly affect plasma concentrations of other drugs. Drugs that induce cytochrome P450, including some other antiepileptic drugs, can result in decreases in plasma levels of oxcarbazepine and MHD. Plasma levels of phenytoin increased by up to 40% when oxcarbazepine was given in doses >1,200 mg/day; however, phenobarbital levels increased by only 15%. Carbamazepine, phenytoin, and phenobarbital, which are all strong inducers of cytochrome P450 enzymes, decreased the plasma level of MHD by 29% to 40%.

Coadministration of oxcarbazepine with an oral hormonal contraceptive decreased plasma concentrations of ethinylestradiol and levonorgestrel, which may decrease the effectiveness of the contraceptive.

Untoward Effects of Oxcarbazepine

The most common untoward effects reported in pediatric patients being treated for a partial seizure disorder include fatigue, vomiting, nausea, headache, somnolence, dizziness, ataxia, nystagmus, diplopia, vision abnormalities, and emotional liability. One manufacturer noted that approximately 9.2% (14) of 152 pediatric patients who were treated with oxcarbazepine, but had not been treated previously with antiepileptic drugs, discontinued the drug because of untoward effects. Although relatively infrequent (<1%), "rash" was responsible for 5.3% (8) and "maculopapular rash" for 1.3% (2) of those discontinuing. In a second group of 456 pediatric patients who were being treated with oxcarbazepine as monotherapy or adjunctive therapy, and who were previously treated with antiepileptic drugs, 11% (50) discontinued the drug because of untoward effects. Patients discontinued for the following reasons: somnolence 2.4% (11), vomiting 2.0% (9), ataxia 1.8% (8), diplopia 1.3% (6), dizziness 1.3% (6), fatigue 1.1% (5), and nystagmus 1.1% (5).

Oxcarbazepine has a reduced risk for leukopenia, rashes, drug interactions, and enzyme autoinduction compared with carbamazepine (see references cited by Teitelbaum, 2001).

Hyponatremia

Clinically significant hyponatremia (sodium < 125 mmol/L) may occur during treatment with oxcarbazepine. This usually occurs within 3 months of initiation of therapy, but may also occur after over a year of treatment. In 14 studies with a total of 1,524 patients, 38 (2.5%) developed a sodium level of <125 mmol/L sometime during treatment compared with no patients on placebo or active control (other antiepileptic drugs). Symptoms that may reflect hyponatremia such as nausea, malaise, headache, lethargy, confusion, obtundation, or increase in seizure frequency or severity should prompt checking of sodium plasma levels. Periodic monitoring of sodium levels during treatment should be considered. Precaution should be taken when prescribing oxcarbazepine along with other medications known to reduce sodium levels.

Indications for Oxcarbazepine

Oxcarbazepine is indicated as monotherapy or adjunctive therapy in the treatment of partial seizures in adults, as monotherapy in youth aged ≥4 years with epilepsy, and as adjunctive therapy in children ≥2 years with partial seizures. There are no definitive child and adolescent psychiatric indications for oxcarbazepine.

Oxcarbazepine Dosage Schedule Initiation of Monotherapy

- Total daily dose should always be administered in two divided doses (bid) for immediate-release tablets.
- *Children 4 years of age through adolescents 16 years of age (not taking other antiepileptic drugs):* An initial daily dose of 4 to 5 mg/kg bid is recommended. The dose should be increased by 5 mg/kg every

Indications for Oxcarbazepine (*continued*)

third day to reach recommended weight-specific maintenance doses (see the package insert for complete dosing guidelines).

- *Adults and adolescents 17 years of age and older (not taking other antiepileptic drugs):* An initial dose of 300 mg twice daily (600 mg/day) is recommended. Dose may be increased by 300 mg/day every third day to a dose of 1,200 mg/day. Many patients are unable to tolerate doses of 2,400 mg/day.

Oxcarbazepine Dosage Schedule as Adjunctive Treatment or to Convert to Monotherapy

- See the package insert or the current *PDR* for guidelines.

Dosage Forms Available (Oxcarbazepine)

- *Immediate-release tablets:* 150, 300, and 600 mg
- *Extended release (Oxtellar XR) tablets:* 150, 300, 600 mg
- *Oral suspension:* 300 mg/5 mL (store in original container; shake well before using). The oral suspension preparation and film-coated tablets are interchangeable at equal doses.

Reports of Interest

Oxcarbazepine for the Treatment of Pediatric Bipolar Disorder and Aggression

Staller et al. (2005) conducted a retrospective chart review of 14 outpatients (ages 6 to 17 years; 6 males and 8 females) who were prescribed oxcarbazepine to address moderate-to-severe problems with anger, irritability, and aggression. Many subjects had additional symptoms including depression, mania, anxiety, disruptiveness, oppositionality, and psychosis. Subjects were rated as moderately ill (6), markedly ill (7), and severely ill (1) on the CGI-S Scale. Subjects' Axis I diagnoses, including multiple diagnoses in 11, included bipolar disorder (5); other mood disorders (3); ADHD (4); disruptive behavior disorder (3); and PDD spectrum disorders (2). Ten (71.4%) of the subjects failed to respond adequately to prior drug trials. During treatment, 70% of subjects received oxcarbazepine in combination with other medication, including atypical antipsychotics (7), selective serotonin reuptake inhibitors (4), stimulants (2), alpha agonists (2), antihistamines (2), beta blocker (1), and VPA (1). The average daily dose of oxcarbazepine was 878 mg (ranged from 600 to 1,800 mg/day). Duration of oxcarbazepine treatment averaged 9.8 months (ranged from 0.5 to 30 months). Clinical improvement was rated on the CGI-I Scale. Moderate clinical global improvement was reported in 50% of patients treated with oxcarbazepine. Mild AEs including dizziness, muscle aches, and tremors resulted in discontinuation of only two (14%) of the subjects studied, and oxcarbazepine was generally considered well tolerated.

Wagner et al. (2006) completed a double-blind, randomized, placebo-controlled trial of oxcarbazepine as monotherapy in the treatment of PBD and concluded that oxcarbazepine is not significantly superior to placebo. In this trial, 116 pediatric outpatients, aged 7 to 18 years of age, with bipolar-I disorder, manic or mixed, were randomized to receive flexibly dosed oxcarbazepine ($N = 59$) or placebo ($N = 57$) for 7 weeks. The mean dose of oxcarbazepine used in the trial was 1,515 mg/day and the median duration of treatment was 48 days. Subjects aged 7 to 12 years averaged 1,200 mg/day, whereas those aged 13 to 18 years averaged 2,040 mg/day. The dose titration was fairly rapid during this trial, with subjects receiving 300 mg increment increases every 2 days, until a maximum weight-based dose of 900 to 2,400 mg/day was reached by week 2 of the study. The primary outcome measure included the change in YMRS scores from start to endpoint. Adverse effects that occurred at least twice as often in the oxcarbazepine group as in the placebo group were dizziness, nausea, somnolence, diplopia, fatigue, and rash. Each was reported in at least 5% of patients in the oxcarbazepine group. Six patients in the oxcarbazepine group, versus zero in the placebo group, experienced serious psychiatric adverse events, all of which required hospitalization. These adverse events included exacerbation of bipolar disorder ($N = 3$), aggressive outburst ($N = 1$), suicide attempt ($N = 1$), and inappropriate sexual behavior ($N = 1$). Investigators determined that only three of these adverse events (exacerbation of bipolar disorder, aggressive behavior, and suicide attempt) were related to the study medication itself. The study authors ultimately concluded that oxcarbazepine did not separate from placebo during this trial, and they noted a higher incidence of psychiatric adverse events for both the oxcarbazepine group and placebo group than those seen in epilepsy populations (Wagner et al., 2006). Additional controlled studies are needed to support or refute these findings.

Oxcarbazepine for the Treatment of Disruptive Mood Dysregulation Disorder

Matthews et al. (2017) conducted a retrospective chart review of 91 children and adolescents aged 6 to 17 years with disruptive mood dysregulation disorder. The participants were documented to display severe aggression, impulsivity, and mood lability requiring inpatient treatment. They were discharged from inpatient treatment on an oxcarbazepine and amantadine protocol. For children and adolescents who adhered to the protocol with little to no adjustment, 8% (5 of 64) required rehospitalization compared to 26% (7 of 27) of those who discontinued the protocol or switched to another medication regimen. The study provides preliminary support for the selected treatment regimen; although given the study limitations, additional research is needed before definitive conclusions can be drawn (Matthews et al., 2017).

Oxcarbazepine for the Treatment of Youth with Autistic Disorder

Kapetanovic (2007) reported three cases of patients with autistic disorder who responded favorably to treatment with oxcarbazepine. In the first case, a 13-year-old Hispanic male with poor sleep and frequent aggression, who failed prior trials of risperidone and olanzapine, responded positively to oxcarbazepine 300 mg in the morning and 600 mg at night (titrated up over 7 days). His mother reported improved compliance, school reports, sleep, aggression, and attention after 2 weeks of treatment with oxcarbazepine, and he remained stable for 4 months. In the second case, a 19-year-old Caucasian female with dysfunctional compulsive routines, head banging, and violence, whose compulsive symptoms improved with fluoxetine 20 mg daily over 2 months, but whose aggressive and self-injurious symptoms persisted despite a trial of risperidone, was started on oxcarbazepine and titrated to 600 mg bid. Two months later, her tantrums and head banging were notably reduced and her level of cooperation improved. She remained stable on fluoxetine and oxcarbazepine for 6 months. In the third case, a 4½-year-old Hispanic child with problematic head banging, property destruction, aggression, hyperactivity, and irregular sleep, who failed prior trials of methylphenidate and amphetamine salts (increased agitation), risperidone, and guanfacine, was started on oxcarbazepine, which was titrated to 150 mg every morning and 300 mg every night over a 2½-month period. The addition of oxcarbazepine resulted in improved sleep, reduced aggression, and improved cooperation, which maintained for 3½ months. None of the three patients developed hyponatremia or other adverse effects, and the author expressed hope that these preliminary positive findings would encourage future research into the efficacy of oxcarbazepine for the treatment of autistic disorder (Kapetanovic, 2007).

Phenytoin, Diphenylhydantoin (Dilantin)

Note: The FDA has directed that black box warnings be added to the labeling of phenytoin warning of cardiovascular risk including death with rapid infusion. The risk is greater when underlying cardiac disease is present such as atrioventricular block, bundle branch block, or cardiac arrhythmias.

Note: In 2008, the FDA issued an alert advising providers to monitor patients who are taking or starting antiepileptic medication for any changes in behavior that could indicate the emergence of depression or worsening suicidal thoughts or behavior (*PDR*.net, 2008).

Contraindications for Phenytoin Administration

Known hypersensitivity to the phenytoin or a related drug is a contraindication.

Phenytoin is classified as pregnancy category D and is not for use in nursing.

Interactions of Phenytoin with Other Drugs

Acute alcohol intake may increase serum phenytoin levels, whereas chronic alcohol use may decrease levels.

Tricyclic antidepressants may precipitate seizures in susceptible patients, necessitating increased phenytoin doses.

Specific drugs have been reported to increase, decrease, or either increase or decrease phenytoin levels. Obtaining serum phenytoin levels may help clarify the situation when necessary. Some drugs that increase phenytoin levels are alcohol (when acutely ingested), benzodiazepines, phenothiazines, salicylates, and methylphenidate. Some drugs that decrease phenytoin levels are carbamazepine, alcohol (with chronic abuse), and molindone.

Interactions of phenytoin and phenobarbital, valproic acid, and sodium valproate are unpredictable, and serum levels of the drugs involved may either increase or decrease.

Reports of Interest (Phenytoin)

Three double-blind, placebo-controlled studies that treated children and adolescents with phenytoin (diphenylhydantoin) for psychiatric disorders reported that it was not significantly better than placebo.

Lefkowitz (1969) reviewed some of the earlier literature in which phenytoin was administered, primarily on an open basis, to nonepileptic children with psychiatric disorders with discrepant results. Lefkowitz compared the efficacy of placebo and phenytoin in treating disruptive behavior in male juvenile delinquents (mean age, 14 years, 11 months; range, 13 to 16 years, 3 months) in a residential treatment center. Each group contained 25 subjects. Phenytoin or placebo was administered in doses of 100 mg twice daily for 76 days. Both groups showed marked reductions in disruptive behavior. Phenytoin, however, was not significantly better than placebo on any of the 11 behavioral measures. In fact, placebo was significantly more efficacious than phenytoin in diminishing distress, unhappiness, negativism, and aggressiveness. The author suggested that mild toxic effects of phenytoin, such as insomnia, irritability, quarrelsomeness, ataxia, and gastric distress, may have accounted for the superiority of placebo.

Conners et al. (1971) treated 43 particularly aggressive or disturbed delinquent males (mean age, 12 years; range, 9 to 14 years) living in a residential training school with phenytoin (200 mg/day), methylphenidate (20 mg/day), or placebo administered for 2 weeks in a double-blind protocol. Although the authors noted some limitations in their study, they found no significant difference between drugs and placebo on ratings by cottage parents, teachers, clinicians, and scores on the Rosenzweig Picture Frustration Test and Porteus Maze Test.

Overall, although there are individual patients without seizure disorder who appear to benefit from phenytoin, as yet there is no convincing evidence for the effectiveness of phenytoin prescribed for psychiatric symptoms.

Gabapentin (Neurontin)

Note: In 2008, the FDA issued an alert advising providers to monitor patients who are taking or starting antiepileptic medication for any changes in behavior that could indicate the emergence of depression or worsening suicidal thoughts or behavior (*PDR*.net, 2008).

Pharmacokinetics of Gabapentin

Gabapentin is not significantly metabolized in humans. It is eliminated unchanged by renal secretion, which is directly proportional to creatinine clearance. Half-life is 5 to 7 hours, and food has no effect on its absorption or excretion. Bioavailability of gabapentin decreases with dose, with a greater percentage of lower doses being available; at doses of approximately 600 mg/day and higher, it stabilizes at approximately 60% of the dose being available.

Contraindications for the Administration of Gabapentin

Gabapentin is contraindicated for patients with known hypersensitivity to the drug.

Interactions of Gabapentin with Other Drugs

Antacids, calcium carbonate, iron, magnesium, and ginkgo may decrease gabapentin's efficacy. Naproxen sodium may increase gabapentin levels. Gabapentin may decrease levels of hydrocodone in a dose-dependent manner.

Untoward Effects of Gabapentin

The most common untoward effects reported somnolence, dizziness, ataxia, fatigue, and nystagmus. Many other effects have been reported.

Gabapentin Mechanism and Indications

Gabapentin is an anticonvulsant whose mechanism of action is unknown. Gabapentin is indicated as adjunctive therapy in the treatment of partial seizures with and without secondary generalization in persons 3 years and older, and for management of postherpetic neuralgia and moderate-to-severe primary restless legs syndrome in adults. Gabapentin is not approved for any psychiatric indication at this time. The manufacturer notes that it is not necessary to monitor serum levels to optimize therapy (*PDR*.net, 2017).

Dosage Schedule

- Because of its short serum half-life, gabapentin should be given three times daily, with the time interval between any two doses no longer than 12 hours.
- *Dose reduction/substitution/withdrawal:* Gradually over a minimum of 1 week.
- *Children < 3 years of age:* Not recommended. Safety and efficacy have not been evaluated in this age group.
- *Children 3 through 12 years of age:* A starting dose of 10 to 15 mg/kg/day in three divided doses is recommended. Increase to an effective dose over 3 days. The recommended effective dose for 3- and 4-year-old patients is 40 mg/kg/day divided tid, whereas for patients ages 5 years and older, the typical effective dose is between 25 and 35 mg/kg/day, divided tid. The maximum daily dose for children ages 3 to 12 years is 50 mg/kg/day.
- *Adolescents > 12 years of age and adults:* An initial daily dose of 900 mg (300 mg tid) is recommended. The usual effective dose is between 900 and 1,800 mg/day. On the basis of clinical response, the dose may be titrated upward to 2,400 mg/day. Higher doses have been tolerated by some patients with epilepsy. Doses as high as 3,600 mg/day were used in adult populations for short durations.

Gabapentin Dose Forms Available

- *Capsules:* 100, 300, and 400 mg
- *Immediate-release tablets (scored):* 600 and 800 mg
- *Extended-release tablets (Gralise; Horizant):* 300 and 600 mg
- *Oral solution:* 250 mg/5 mL dispensed in 470-mL bottles.

Reports of Interest (Gabapentin)

Gabapentin Use for Pediatric Mania

Controlled trials of gabapentin use in adults with mania have failed to demonstrate efficacy, and data supporting its use for pediatric mania are considerably limited.

Soutullo et al. (1998) reported on a 13-year-old boy with bipolar-I disorder, manic episode, and comorbid ADHD, who was treated with gabapentin 1,500 mg/day as an add-on medication to carbamazepine. Within 1 month of adding gabapentin, he experienced a marked improvement and subsequently remained stable for 7 months. This patient had previously failed a trial of divalproex and was unable to tolerate lithium. Monotherapy with carbamazepine was not adequate to control his symptoms (Soutullo et al., 1998).

Gabapentin Use for Pediatric Sleep Disruption

Robinson et al. (2013) reviewed the medical records of 23 children with insomnia treated with gabapentin. Of these, 87% were diagnosed with neurodevelopmental or neuropsychiatric disorders, and 70% had both sleep onset and maintenance insomnia. Gabapentin was started at an average dose of 5 mg/kg (max dose of 15 mg/kg at bedtime) and was given 30 to 45 minutes before bedtime. Follow-up visits were completed every 3 to 6 months. The study authors determined that 78% of the children experienced improved sleep at follow-up. One child experienced agitated awakenings at 15 mg/kg/night, which resolved with a dose decrease to 10 mg/kg/night. Five children had a paradoxical "wired" reaction resulting in worsened sleep onset, which resolved when gabapentin was discontinued. No other adverse effects were recorded. Investigators concluded that gabapentin was generally safe and well tolerated. The retrospective nature of the study, small sample size, lack of placebo group for comparison, and reliance on parent report were limitations. Although the results are encouraging, randomized placebo-controlled trials are needed to definitively determine gabapentin's efficacy in treating pediatric insomnia (Robinson et al., 2013).

Lamotrigine (Lamictal)

Note: The FDA has directed that a black box warning be added to the labeling of lamotrigine indicating that *serious rashes* including SJS, toxic epidermal necrolysis, and/or rash-related death. Serious rashes may require hospitalization or discontinuing of the medication. The incidence of these rashes is approximately 8/1,000 (0.8%) in pediatric patients aged 2 to 16 years old (vs. 0.3% incidence in adults), who receive lamotrigine as adjunctive therapy for epilepsy. The incidence of serious rash may be increased by coadministration of VPA, exceeding the recommended dose, or exceeding the recommended dose escalation for lamotrigine. Lamotrigine should be discontinued at the first sign of rash, unless the rash is clearly not drug related. Discontinuing lamotrigine may not prevent a rash from becoming life threatening or permanently disabling or disfiguring. (This is a summary; see the package insert or current *PDR* for the complete warning.)

In 2008, the FDA also issued an alert advising providers to monitor patients who are taking or starting antiepileptic medication for any changes in behavior that could indicate the emergence of depression or worsening suicidal thoughts or behavior (*PDR.net*, 2017).

Pharmacokinetics of Lamotrigine

Lamotrigine is absorbed quickly, has an absolute bioavailability of 98%, and is not affected by food intake. Time to peak plasma concentrations is between 1.4 and 4.8 hours. The elimination half-life for adults when prescribed alone is 32.8 hours for single-dose lamotrigine and 25.4 hours for multiple-dose lamotrigine. Lamotrigine's elimination half-life varies when certain other medication are taken concurrently and are summarized in the package insert. Population pharmacokinetic analyses reveal that lamotrigine's clearance is predominantly influenced by total body weight and concurrent antiepileptic therapy. The oral clearance of lamotrigine is higher in youth than in adults, depending on body weight. Patients weighing <30 kg may need a 50% increase in maintenance lamotrigine doses to maintain therapeutic levels. Lamictal clearance does not appear to be altered by age.

Contraindications for the Administration of Lamotrigine

Lamotrigine is contraindicated when patients have a hypersensitivity to lamotrigine or its ingredients.

Lamotrigine use may cause false-positive readings on rapid urine drug screens, particularly for phencyclidine, requiring additional laboratory analyses to confirm positive results (*PDR.net*, 2017).

Interactions of Lamotrigine with Other Drugs

The clearance of lamotrigine is affected by coadministration of several medications. VPA, for example, increases lamotrigine levels by approximately twofold. Oral estrogen-containing contraceptives, oxcarbazepine, and carbamazepine, by contrast, reduce lamotrigine levels. Oral progestin-only contraceptives may not protect as well against pregnancy when used concurrently with lamotrigine, which patients should be made aware of. Many other drug interactions are summarized in the package insert and should be considered before prescribing lamotrigine. In some instances, dose adjustments will need to be made.

Untoward Effects of Lamotrigine

See the summary of the black box warning for information regarding the risk of serious rash with lamotrigine. Common side effects of lamotrigine include nausea/vomiting, somnolence, headache, dizziness, and tremor. There have been reports of blood dyscrasias, and suicidal ideation and behavior should be monitored for, as is the case with all antiepileptic medication.

Lamotrigine is classified as pregnancy category C. It is present in breast milk, so caution must be taken if prescribing lamotrigine to a nursing patient.

Indications for Lamotrigine

Lamotrigine is an antiepileptic drug of the phenyltriazine class and is chemically unrelated to antiepileptic drugs currently in use. Its mechanism of action is unknown. Lamotrigine is approved for use in the adjunctive treatment of partial seizures, primary generalized tonic-clonic seizures, and generalized seizures of Lennox–Gastaut syndrome, in patients ≥2 years old. Lamotrigine is also approved for use in adults with partial seizures who are being treated with a single hepatic enzyme-inducing antiepileptic drug (e.g., carbamazepine, phenytoin, phenobarbital, primidone, or VPA) to convert them to monotherapy with lamotrigine. Lamotrigine is further indicated for the maintenance treatment of bipolar-I disorder to decrease the frequency of mood episodes (depression, mania, hypomania, mixed episodes) in patients at least 18 years old who are being treated for an acute mood episode with standard therapy. Lamotrigine has not been proved effective in treating acute mood episodes. There are no definitive indications or conclusive empiric support for lamotrigine in child and adolescent psychiatry.

Dosage Schedule

- *Children <2 years old:* Not recommended.
- *Children ≥2 years old, adolescents, and adults:* The initial, titration, and target doses for lamotrigine vary considerably according to age and which other medications the patient is taking. The package insert or current *PDR* should be consulted for the appropriate medication protocol.

Dosage Forms Available (Lamotrigine)

- *Immediate-release tablets:* 25, 100, 150, and 200 mg
- *Extended-release tablets:* 25, 50, 100, 200, 250, and 300 mg
- *Chewable dispersible tablets:* 2, 5, and 25 mg
- *Orally disintegrating tablets:* 25, 50, 100, and 200 mg

Reports of Interest

Lamotrigine for Youth with Bipolar Disorder

Carandang et al. (2003) reported a retrospective study of nine adolescents with mood disorders refractory to previous pharmacotherapy who responded positively to lamotrigine. Six of the youth had bipolar depression, two had unipolar depression, and one was diagnosed with mood disorder NOS. Three patients received lamotrigine as monotherapy, whereas the others received lamotrigine in conjunction with concurrent pharmacotherapy (antidepressants, antipsychotics, a second mood stabilizer, anxiolytics, or sedative-hypnotics). The mean age of subjects was 16.4 years, and the mean lamotrigine dose was 141.7 mg (ranging from 25 to 250 mg/day). Eight of nine subjects demonstrated improvement as measured by the Clinical Global Impressions–Bipolar Version overall illness rating. Seven were deemed "much improved," and one was judged to be "very much improved." One subject had to discontinue lamotrigine after developing an erythematous rash, which resolved a few days after stopping lamotrigine. Although the findings were positive, the study authors emphasized the need for additional trials to support or refute findings (Carandang et al., 2003).

Soutullo et al. (2006) published a small open retrospective review of five adolescent patients diagnosed with bipolar disorder, who were treated with adjunctive lamotrigine in their outpatient clinic. Three of the patients were diagnosed with bipolar disorder NOS, one with bipolar-I disorder, and one with bipolar II disorder. All five were depressed at baseline, and failed to demonstrate an adequate treatment response to their current medication regimen. The average lamotrigine dose was 100 $\pm$ 87.5 mg/day and the mean treatment duration was 28 $\pm$ 28 weeks. Treatment response was rated using the CGI-I Scale. The study authors reported a marked or moderate improvement in four patients (80%) and minimal improvement in one patient (20%). No skin rashes were reported, although one patient complained of dizziness. Lamotrigine was determined to be well tolerated in this small sample; however, given numerous inherent methodological limitations, definitive conclusions regarding lamotrogine's efficacy were unable to be determined. Regardless, the findings were regarded as provisional positive results for adjunctive use of lamotrigine in adolescents with bipolar depression (Soutullo et al., 2006).

In an 8-week open-label trial, Chang et al. (2006) prospectively studied the efficacy of lamotrigine as adjunctive or monotherapy for 20 adolescents with bipolar depression. The subjects were between 12 and 17 years (mean 15.8 years) and were diagnosed with bipolar-I disorder, bipolar II disorder, or bipolar NOS. Subjects who were taking antidepressant medication were tapered and discontinued off the medication over 2 to 4 weeks, after which time they were reassessed for entry criteria. Lamotrigine was started at 12.5 to 25 mg daily and was gradually titrated to a mean dose of 131.6 mg/day. Primary response criteria was a 1 or 2 on the CGI-I Scale by the end of the study. At least a 50% reduction in CDRS-R ratings served as a secondary response criteria. Seven subjects were on other psychotropic medication during the trial (mood stabilizers, antipsychotics, stimulants, strattera), although they could enter the trial only if no changes were made to these medications within 1 month of enrolling. A total of 18 subjects completed the study. Eighty-four percent of subjects responded by primary response criteria and 63% by secondary response criteria. Scores on the YMRS and OAS–Modified also significantly decreased. By the end of the study, 58% of subjects were judged to be in remission (score of 28 or less on the CDRS-R and a CGI-S score of 1 or 2). Lamotrigine was weight-neutral during the trial, and no rash or other adverse effects were noted. The authors concluded that lamotrigine may decrease depression, mania, and aggression in adolescents with bipolar depression, although they acknowledged that larger placebo-controlled studies are needed to confirm this (Chang et al., 2006).

Pavuluri et al. (2009) studied lamotrigine's efficacy and tolerability for the maintenance treatment of PBD in a 14-week open-label trial with 46 subjects who presented with mania or hypomania (ages 8 to 18 years, mean age 13.3 years). Before the start of the study, all subjects underwent a 1- to 4-week washout period of their previous medications. This was followed by acute stabilization with a second-generation antipsychotic (SGA) and concurrent gradual titration of lamotrigine over an 8-week period. It was planned to have all subjects achieve an endpoint Lamictal dose of 150 mg if ≤30 kg body weight, or 200 mg if >30 kg body weight by week 6 of the 8-week titration phase. The SGA was tapered off over 2 to 4 weeks between weeks 4 and 8, such that all subjects were on lamotrigine monotherapy by the end of the 8-week dosing period of the trial. Subjects were then maintained on Lamictal monotherapy for an additional 6 weeks. By the end of the 14-week trial, the depression response rate on the CDRS-R was 82%, the YMRS response rate was 71%, and the remission rate was 56%. Authors noted that depressive symptoms continued to improve over the 14-week period and that aggression and irritability (measured via the OAS) declined over the initial 8-week period and maintained during the additional 6 weeks with lamotrigine monotherapy. Lamotrigine was determined to be well tolerated in this trial, with the most common side effects being sedation (23.8%), stomachache (19.6%), increased urination (10.9%), and increased appetite (10.9%). There was no significant weight gain, no cases of serious skin rashes, and no increase in suicidal ideation. The dropout rate due to adverse effects was 6.4%, all due to benign skin rashes that ultimately resolved without incident. Two cases of rashes were treated with prednisone to assist in their resolution. Investigators concluded that lamotrigine was overall well tolerated and appeared effective as a monotherapy agent in maintaining control of manic, hypomanic, and depressive symptoms, for 6 weeks following acute stabilization with an SGA (Pavuluri et al., 2009).

Biederman et al. (2010) studied the use of lamotrigine as monotherapy for youth with bipolar disorder in a 12-week, open-label, prospective trial. Thirty-nine youth with bipolar disorder were enrolled, and 56% completed the trial. Several participants stopped the trial because of skin rash, although in all cases the rash resolved once lamotrigine was discontinued. During this trial, lamotrigine was titrated to 160.7 ± 128.3 mg in the 22 children younger than 12 years of age, and to 219.1 ± 172.2 mg/day for the 17 children aged 12 to 17 years. The study authors reported statistically significant improvements in YMRS scores associated with lamotrigine treatment and concluded that lamotrigine was well tolerated and may be efficacious for youth with bipolar disorder. An improvement in symptoms of depression, ADHD, and psychosis were also reported in this small trial (Biederman et al., 2010).

During the same year, Pavuluri et al. (2010) studied the impact of lamotrigine treatment on the neurocognitive profile of youth with bipolar disorder. Twenty-four healthy controls and 34 matched and unmedicated youth with manic, mixed, or hypomanic episodes were administered a neurocognitive battery at baseline. The youth with bipolar disorder were then treated for 14 weeks with lamotrigine, after which time both groups were readministered a neurocognitive battery. Although overall cognitive performance in the PBD group remained impaired relative to healthy controls, the study authors noted that global neurocognitive function improved with lamotrigine treatment over time. Working and verbal memory were most prominently improved in patients treated with lamotrigine, such that these cognitive domains were no longer significantly impaired relative to healthy controls. Improvements in executive functioning were noted in the lamotrigine-treated group, but continued to lag behind the performance of healthy controls. Attention did not improve in the lamotrigine-treated group, and comorbid ADHD was an exclusionary criterion for this study. Authors reported that no significant results ($P > .05$) were found to be related to improvements seen in the YMRS and CDRS-R scores, supporting that the cognitive improvements seen in this study were not solely due to symptomatic improvement. Ultimately, the investigators concluded that lamotrigine may reduce some of the cognitive deficits associated with PBD (Pavuluri et al., 2010).

Lamotrigine for Youth with Depression

Shon et al. (2014) completed a 12-week retrospective chart review of 37 adolescents (15 with bipolar and 22 with unipolar depression) treated with lamotrigine (65.4 ± 37.5 mg/day) for 199.9 ± 217.4 days. Depressive symptoms were retrospectively scored using the CGI-S and CGI-I Scales at 4, 8, and 12 weeks of treatment. Encouragingly, study authors reported a 45.9% treatment response (defined as a CGI-I score ≤ 2). Efficacy did not differ between adolescents with unipolar and bipolar depression. Five subjects experienced a benign skin rash that resolved after lamotrigine was discontinued. Although this study provides preliminary support for lamotrigine's safety and efficacy in treating adolescent depression, randomized placebo-controlled trials are needed to support or refute these findings (Shon et al., 2014).

Lamotrigine for Youth with Autism Spectrum Disorder

Belsito (2001) reported a negative double-blind placebo-controlled trial of lamotrigine for treatment of autistic disorder. Twenty-eight youth aged 3 to 11 years with a diagnosis of autistic disorder received either placebo or lamotrigine. Lamotrigine was gradually titrated upward over 8 weeks to a mean maintenance dose of 5.0 mg/kg/day and was dosed twice daily for an additional 4 weeks. Outcome measures included the Autism Behavior Checklist, the ABC, and the Vineland Adaptive Behavior scales. The study demonstrated no significant difference between lamotrigine and placebo on the outcome measures used (Belsito, 2001). However, a more recent case report suggested a positive treatment response to lamotrigine in an adolescent patient with autistic disorder and comorbid bipolar disorder (Howell et al., 2011). Additional studies are needed before firm conclusions can be drawn.

Topiramate (Topamax)

Note: In 2008, the FDA issued an alert advising providers to monitor patients who are taking or starting antiepileptic medication for any changes in behavior that could indicate the emergence of depression or worsening suicidal thoughts or behavior (*PDR*.net, 2017).

Topiramate, an antiepileptic drug, is a sulfamate-substituted monosaccharide. The mechanisms responsible for its antiepileptic and migraine prophylaxis effects have not been elucidated; however, preclinical studies suggest that at clinically effective concentrations, topiramate blocks voltage-dependent sodium channels, augments the activity of the neurotransmitter gamma-aminobutyrate (GABA) at some subtypes of the GABA-A receptor, antagonizes the AMPA/kainate subtype of the glutamate receptor, and inhibits the carbonic anhydrase enzyme, particularly isoenzymes II and IV (package insert).

Pharmacokinetics of Topiramate

The bioavailability of topiramate is not affected by food. Peak plasma concentrations occur in approximately 2 hours. Mean plasma elimination half-life is 21 hours after single or multiple doses and steady state occurs in approximately 4 days at a given dose. Topiramate is not extensively metabolized, and approximately 70% is eliminated unchanged through the kidneys. Pediatric patients, aged 4 to 17 years, have approximately a 50% higher clearance than adults. Consequently, such patients have a shorter elimination half-life than adults, and their plasma concentration of topiramate may be lower than that of adults receiving the same dose.

Contraindications for the Administration of Topiramate

Topiramate is contraindicated in patients with a history of sensitivity to topiramate or any of the components included in the pill. Clearance may be significantly reduced in patients with renal or hepatic impairment.

Interactions of Topiramate with Other Drugs

Hyperammonemia with or without encephalopathy has been associated with the combined use of topiramate and valproic acid in patients who have not developed these symptoms when treated with either drug alone. Patients who develop symptoms such as acute alterations in the level of consciousness or cognitive functioning in combination with lethargy or vomiting, which may be associated with hyperammonemic encephalopathy, should have their serum ammonia levels determined. Oligohydrosis and hyperthermia have been reported, primarily in pediatric patients, and may be more likely to occur when topiramate is used in conjunction with other medications that predispose to heat-related disorders, such as carbonic anhydrase inhibitors or drugs with anticholinergic activity. Decreased sweating and elevated body temperatures need to be monitored for. Topiramate may decrease the efficacy of oral contraceptives. Topiramate can decrease the AUC and maximum serum concentration of lithium by up to 20% and can also reduce levels of warfarin and benzodiazepines. Many other drug interactions are possible (see package insert).

Untoward Effects of Topiramate

Topiramate is associated with hyperchloremic, non–anion gap metabolic acidosis, which if chronic and untreated may cause osteomalacia/rickets and may reduce growth rate and maximal stature in pediatric patients. Treatment-emergent adverse effects in children in the age group 10 through 16 years who were being treated with monotherapy (400 mg/day) for epilepsy that occurred with an incidence of at least 5% and which were more frequent than those at lower doses (50 mg/day) included fever (9%), paresthesias (16%), diarrhea (11%), weight loss (21%), anorexia (14%), mood problems (11%), difficulty with concentration/attention (9%), and alopecia (5%). Topiramate may cause cleft lip or palate in infants when used during pregnancy and is a category D medication for pregnancy. Nephrolithiasis has been reported with the use of topiramate.

Indications for Topiramate

Topiramate is approved for use as monotherapy or adjunct therapy in patients ≥2 years of age with partial-onset or primary generalized tonic-clonic seizures; as an adjunctive therapy in patients ≥2 years of age with partial-onset seizures, primary generalized tonic-clonic seizures, or seizures associated with Lennox–Gastaut syndrome; and for the prophylaxis of migraine headache in adults and children ≥12 years of age.

Topiramate Dosage Schedule for Monotherapy (Epilepsy)

- *Children 2 to <10 years of age:* Maintenance dose is based on weight (see product insert for details). An initial dose of 25 mg/day in the evening is recommended. After 1 week, increase to 25 mg twice daily as tolerated. May increase by 25 to 50 mg/day each week as tolerated. Titrate to the minimum weight-based maintenance dose over a total of 5 to 7 weeks.
- *Children ≥ 10 years of age, adolescents, and adults:* An initial dose of 25 mg, twice daily is recommended. Dose should be increased as tolerated by 50 mg weekly to reach a recommended target dose of 200 mg, twice daily (total dose, 400 mg/day).

Topiramate Dosage Schedule for Prophylaxis (Migraine Headache)

- *Children <12 years of age:* Not recommended.
- *Children and adolescents ≥ 12 years of age and adults:* An initial evening dose of 25 mg is recommended. Dose should be increased as tolerated by 25 mg weekly (week 2, 25 mg bid, week 3, 25 mg in the morning and 50 mg in the evening to a recommended target dose of 50 mg bid during week 4; total dose, 100 mg/day).

Topiramate Adjunct Dosage Schedule for Treating Partial-Onset Seizures, Primary Generalized Tonic-Clonic Seizures or Lennox–Gastaut Syndrome

- See package insert.

Indications for Topiramate (*continued*)

Dosage Forms Available (Topiramate)

- *Tablets:* 25, 50, 100, and 200 mg
- *Extended-release capsules (Qudexy XR; Trokendi XR):* 25, 50, 100, 150, and 200 mg
- *Sprinkle capsules:* 15- and 25-mg sprinkle capsules may be swallowed whole or opened and put on a small amount of soft food, which should be swallowed without chewing immediately and not stored for future use.

Reports of Interest

Topiramate for the Treatment of Pediatric Bipolar Disorder

Two small retrospective chart reviews provided preliminary evidence that adjunctive topiramate may be beneficial for the treatment of PBD (Barzman et al., 2005; DelBello et al., 2002). DelBello et al. (2002) looked at outpatient medical charts of 26 youth diagnosed with bipolar disorder, type I or II, who were treated with adjunctive topiramate. The CGI and CGAS were used to rate response to treatment. The mean duration of topiramate treatment was 4.1 ± 6.1 months, and the average daily dose was 104 ± 77 mg/day. The authors concluded that the response rate (defined as a CGI-I score of ≤2 at endpoint) was 73% for mania and 62% for overall illness. CGAS scores were significantly improved, and no adverse effects were reported. Barzman et al. (2005) completed a record review of 25 hospitalized children and adolescents with bipolar-I disorder who were treated with adjunctive topiramate at a mean dose of 126 mg/day. The CGI-S score was used as the primary outcome measure. The authors concluded that 64% of patients responded positively to adjunctive topiramate, based on significantly improved CGI-S scores. No adverse effects were recorded (Barzman et al., 2005).

DelBello et al. (2005) reported a 4-week, multicenter, randomized, double-blind, placebo-controlled, parallel-group trial of topiramate monotherapy in treating mania in 56 children and adolescent mean age 13.8 ± 2.56 years (range 6 to 17 years), who were diagnosed with bipolar disorder type I; 33 subjects (58.9%) had codiagnoses of ADHD. This study was originally designed to enroll approximately 230 subjects, but was curtailed early after learning of negative studies of topiramate for the treatment of acute mania in adults. The primary outcome measure was the YMRS scores at baseline and 4, 7, 14, 21, and 28 days of treatment. Secondary outcome measures included baseline and weekly scores on the CGI-I Scale, the BPRS-C, the CGAS, and the CDRS.

The baseline YMRS score for the topiramate group ($N = 29$) was 31.7 ± 5.53, and it was decreased by −9.7 ± 9.65 at endpoint. The baseline YMRS score for the placebo group ($N = 27$) was 29.9 ± 6.01, and it was decreased by −4.7 ± 9.79 at endpoint, less than one-half the improvement seen in the topiramate group. However, there was no significant group difference at any visit for the change in YMRS score, the total BPRS-C score, total CDRS score, or CGAS score. Treatment-emergent adverse effects occurring in >10% of subjects and greater for topiramate than for placebo included decreased appetite (27.6% vs. 0%), nausea (24.1% vs. 0%), diarrhea (13.8% vs. 7.4%), paresthesia (13.8% vs. 3.7%), somnolence (13.8% vs. 3.7%), insomnia (10.3% vs. 3.7%), and rash (10.3% vs. 3.7%). Mean change in body weight from baseline to endpoint was significantly different, with the topiramate group losing a mean of −1.76 ± 2.03 kg and the placebo group gaining a mean of 0.95 ± 1.45 kg ($P < .001$). No subject experienced a serious adverse event. This study was ultimately deemed inconclusive because of inadequate sample sizes stemming from the early discontinuation of the study.

Wozniak et al. (2009) studied 40 outpatients, aged 6 to 17 years, who were diagnosed with bipolar disorder, in two partially concurrent 8-week open-label trials of either olanzapine monotherapy ($N = 17$) or olanzapine augmented with topiramate

($N = 23$). Olanzapine was initiated at 2.5 mg/day and increased by 2.5 to 5 mg weekly as indicated, to a maximum dose of 20 mg daily. Topiramate was started at 25 mg/day and increased by 25 mg/day each week as tolerated, to the maximum dose of 100 mg daily. Primary outcome measures included the YMRS and the CGI-I mania scales. Investigators discovered that both groups showed a clinically and statistically significant reduction in YMRS scores. Weight gain in the olanzapine plus topiramate group, however, was statistically significantly lower (2.6 ± 3.6 kg) than in the olanzapine monotherapy group. Investigators concluded that although topiramate as augmentation of olanzapine did not lead to improved mania over olanzapine alone, it did lead to reduced weight gain in this trial (Wozniak et al., 2009).

Topiramate for the Treatment of Weight Gain Associated with Psychotropic Medication

Shapiro et al. (2016) completed a retrospective chart review of youth (mean age 13.4 years, mean baseline BMI 30.2) first prescribed zonisamide or topiramate. Ninety-eight youth met inclusion criteria but only 47 also met exclusion criteria, which consisted of (1) treatment with other medication known to cause weight loss, (2) eating disorder diagnosis, (3) medical illness with negative effects on weight, (4) medications prescribed in other departments or sites, and (5) only 1 documented visit. Of subjects taking psychotropic medication in addition to zonisamide and topiramate (76.6%), 91.7% were prescribed an antipsychotic. The majority (91%) of patients were prescribed topiramate instead of zonisamide, which study authors attributed to topiramate's favorable side-effect profile and FDA indication for adjunct therapy in pediatric populations. The average length of medication treatment was 199.8 days and 6.7 appointments. Excluding patients whose baseline weight was healthy or underweight, investigators determined that statistically significant weight loss was seen during all dosing levels of zonisamide and topiramate, with the exception of doses greater than 200 mg daily (mean BMI reduction of 6.1 for doses below 50 mg and 3.2 for doses above 200 mg). Despite promising results, authors cautioned that additional studies are needed to definitively determine the safety and efficacy of topiramate or zonisamide to target weight gain in youth taking psychotropic medication (Shapiro et al., 2016).

Topiramate for the Treatment of Prader–Willi Syndrome

Smathers et al. (2003) completed an open-label study in which topiramate was used to treat youth with a diagnosis of Prader–Willi syndrome (PWS). Eight patients between the ages of 10 and 19 years were titrated, as indicated and tolerated, to a dose of topiramate 100 to 600 mg/day. Mood and behavior were assessed by parental questionnaires and phone surveys. Three patients experienced somnolence, which resolved with continued treatment or dose reduction. Seven patients completed the trial (one discontinued after 3 months due to perceived lack of benefit), all of whom were reported to have a positive change in mood, evidenced by increased interactions with others and improved self-esteem. All seven were reported to have decreased aggressiveness, violence, and acting out. Two patients stopped self-injurious skin picking after 2 months of treatment, and most had reduced obsessive behaviors such as hair brushing or hair washing. One patient had worsened skin picking and hair pulling, which necessitated the use of another medication. Parents reported reduced food foraging and hoarding, and all patients who completed the study either maintained or lost weight. Study authors opined that although this small and unblinded study provides preliminary positive support for efficacy of topiramate in treating problematic features of PWS, larger and controlled trials are needed to further support or refute this finding (Smathers et al., 2003).

Topiramate for the Treatment of Autistic Disorder

Mazzone et al. (2006) described five boys with autistic disorder (ages 9 to 13 years), who were referred for severe behavioral problems (mean IQ 54 ± 27.2).

Two previously failed a trial of at least one typical antipsychotic medication. Topiramate was started at 0.5 mg/kg/day for 2 weeks, after which time it was increased by 0.5 mg/kg/day at 2-week intervals to a maximum of 2.5 mg/kg/day. The average topiramate dose was 2.1 mg/kg/day, and the mean duration of treatment was 22 ± 8.33 weeks. Treatment response was assessed by CGI-I and Child Behavior Checklist scores. Two patients were judged to be responders, defined as receiving a 1 or 2 on the CGI-I, and three patients showed no improvement. The authors concluded that clinical response to topiramate in severely impaired autistic disorder appears variable and that additional studies are needed (Mazzone et al., 2006).

Topiramate for the Treatment of Tourette Syndrome

Jankovic et al. (2010) completed a randomized, double-blind, placebo-controlled, parallel-group study of topiramate for the treatment of Tourette syndrome. Twenty-nine patients (mean age 16.5 years; range 7 to 65 years) with moderate-to-severe symptoms, based on a Yale Global Tic Severity Scale of ≥19, were randomized to receive either topiramate (mean dose 118 mg/day) or placebo. The primary endpoint was the Total Tic Score, which improved 14.29 points by day 70 in the topiramate-treated group, compared with an improvement of only 5 points by day 70 in the placebo group. Secondary measures, including the CGI and premonitory urge CGI, also showed improvements in the treatment group. Adverse effects between groups did not differ. The study authors concluded that this study provides evidence that topiramate may be efficacious in the treatment of moderate-to-severe Tourette syndrome (Jankovic et al., 2010).

Non-SSRI/SNRI Anxiety Medication

JULIA C. JACKSON AND NATOSHA S. OSANSANYA

BENZODIAZEPINES

Benzodiazepines, introduced into clinical practice in the early 1960s, were the most frequently prescribed drugs in the United States between 1968 and 1980. In 1978 alone, 68 million prescriptions for benzodiazepines were written for approximately 10 million individuals; more than half of these were for diazepam (Ayd, 1980). Greenblatt et al. (1983) noted that by 1980, however, the trend toward increasing use of benzodiazepines reversed, perhaps because of negative publicity regarding the potential for abuse and dependency with these medications. In 1989, in response to these concerns, New York State mandated that all benzodiazepine prescriptions be written on triplicate forms, as was required for other controlled drugs. Many experts at the time, however, felt the dangers of benzodiazepines were "greatly exaggerated" (Simeon & Ferguson, 1985). In a summary statement, the American Psychiatric Association (APA) Task Force opined that "benzodiazepines, when prescribed appropriately, are therapeutic drugs with relatively mild toxic profiles and low tendency for abuse" (Salzman, 1990, p. 62). An exception to this occurs among substance abusers, however. Benzodiazepine abuse is very frequent among alcoholics and cocaine, narcotic, and methadone abusers, who use benzodiazepines to "augment the euphoria (narcotics and methadone users), decrease anxiety and withdrawal symptoms (alcoholics), or to ease the 'crash' from cocaine-induced euphoria" (Salzman, 1990, p. 62).

Little was known at the time about the efficacy of benzodiazepine medications for child and adolescent psychiatric disorders. In a 1974 monograph, after reviewing the use of benzodiazepines in youth, Greenblatt and Shader stated, "At present it is doubtful that the benzodiazepines have a role in the pharmacotherapy of psychoses or in the treatment of emotional disorders in children" (p. 88). Werry concluded that if pharmacotherapy is necessary for certain childhood sleep disturbances, including insomnia, night waking, night terrors, and somnambulism, benzodiazepines are "probably" indicated, and for some kinds of anxiety they are "possibly" indicated (Rapoport et al., 1978b).

In 1983, Coffey et al. reported that benzodiazepines appeared to be prescribed to both older adolescents and adults for relief of anxiety and tension, muscle relaxation, sleep disorders, and seizures. In children, however, they were used primarily for treatment of sleep and seizure disorders and were used much less commonly for their anxiolytic and muscle-relaxant qualities.

The literature concerning benzodiazepine use in children was reviewed by both Campbell et al. (1985) and Simeon and Ferguson (1985). Most published reports appeared in the 1960s, involved open studies composed of diagnostically heterogeneous subjects, and resulted in discrepant findings. The most common drugs studied were diazepam and chlordiazepoxide.

At present, the childhood psychiatric conditions that have the most convincing rationale for the use of a benzodiazepine as the drug of choice are sleep terror disorder (pavor nocturnus) and sleepwalking disorder (somnambulism). These conditions are not usually treated with pharmacotherapy; however, unless they are unusually frequent or severe. Both sleep terror disorder and sleepwalking disorder typically occur "during the first third of the major sleep period (the interval of nonrapid eye movement [NREM] sleep that typically contains EEG delta activity, sleep stages 3 and 4)" (APA, 1987, pp. 310–311). Because benzodiazepines decrease stage 4 sleep, they are thought to be of value in these conditions. Reite et al. (1990) suggested that either 2 mg of diazepam or 0.125 mg of triazolam at bedtime may decrease the frequency of night terrors or somnambulism in children with severe cases. Conversely, benzodiazepines were hypothesized to be contraindicated in treating sleep disturbance associated with psychosocial dwarfism (psychosocially determined short stature) because of concern that they may further compromise nocturnal secretion of growth hormone, which occurs maximally during sleep stages 3 and 4, slow-wave sleep (Green, 1986).

It is well known that if a benzodiazepine is used as a hypnotic, consideration of the serum half-life of the drug is important. Flurazepam (Dalmane), temazepam (Restoril), and triazolam (Halcion) can all be used for treating sleep disorders. Flurazepam is a long-acting benzodiazepine with a half-life (for it and its metabolites) of 47 to 100 hours. The manufacturer notes that this pharmacokinetic profile may explain the clinical observation that flurazepam is increasingly effective on the second or third night of use and that after discontinuing the drug, both sleep latency and total wake time may still be decreased. Because of flurazepam's long half-life, it appears to be most useful in persons with both insomnia and significant daytime anxiety. Temazepam and triazolam, by contrast, are short-acting benzodiazepines, with a relatively rapid onset of action and half-lives of only 9.5 to 12.4 hours (temazepam) and 1.5 to 5.5 hours (triazolam). Triazolam's notably short half-life renders it a drug of choice for sleep-onset insomnia and for times when daytime sedation is of concern.

Klein et al. (1980) suggested that a low dose of a benzodiazepine (e.g., diazepam 5 mg) might be useful in treating residual anticipatory anxiety in school-phobic youngsters whose separation anxiety had been alleviated by treatment with imipramine. Simeon and Ferguson (1985) reported that some overly inhibited children may show lasting behavioral improvement following brief (not exceeding 4 to 6 weeks) treatment with a benzodiazepine. They attributed the improvement to an interaction between disinhibition facilitated by the medication and social learning. Consistent with this finding, they noted that children and adolescents with impulsivity and aggression, who were under significant environmental stress, should not be treated with benzodiazepines because the disinhibition could result in a worsening of behavior (Simeon & Ferguson, 1985).

Most of the literature suggests that benzodiazepines worsen symptoms in psychotic children and provide little benefit for hyperactive youth. In studies comparing dextroamphetamine, placebo, and chlordiazepoxide or diazepam in treating hyperactive children, both chlordiazepoxide and diazepam were less effective than dextroamphetamine, and placebo was rated better than diazepam (Zrull et al., 1963, 1964).

Contraindications and Cautions for Benzodiazepine Administration

Known hypersensitivity to benzodiazepines and acute narrow-angle glaucoma are usually considered absolute contraindications.

Persons predisposed to substance abuse or alcoholism should not be prescribed benzodiazepines unless the benefits clearly outweigh the increased risk for physical and psychological dependence in this patient population. Benzodiazepines should not be abruptly discontinued after extended therapy, as this may result in withdrawal symptoms.

Adolescents who are likely to become pregnant or who are known to be pregnant should not be prescribed benzodiazepines, because there is a risk of congenital malformations particularly during the first trimester of pregnancy. Maternal abuse of benzodiazepines may cause a withdrawal syndrome in the newborn (Rall, 1990). Simeon and Ferguson (1985) concluded that benzodiazepines are relatively contraindicated in children and adolescents with significant impulsivity, aggressiveness, and environmental stress, because negative disinhibiting drug effects may occur.

Interactions of Benzodiazepines with Other Drugs

Additive effects, when combined with other sedative or hypnotic drugs, including alcohol (ethanol), are clinically important drug interactions to consider when prescribing benzodiazepine medication. Phenothiazines, narcotics, barbiturates, monoamine oxidase inhibitors (MAOIs), tricyclic antidepressants, and cimetidine (Tagamet) may potentiate benzodiazepines. Both the rate of absorption of benzodiazepines and the resulting central nervous system depression are increased by ethanol (Rall, 1990). CYP3A inhibitors, such as oral antifungals, may increase benzodiazepine levels. Benzodiazepines are relatively safe drugs, and even large overdoses are infrequently fatal unless taken in combination with other drugs (Rall, 1990).

Flumazenil (Romazicon) is a benzodiazepine receptor antagonist that reverses the sedative effects of benzodiazepines. Flumazenil does not reverse hypoventilation or respiratory suppression caused by benzodiazepines, however. In pediatric patients, flumazenil is indicated for the reversal of benzodiazepine-induced conscious sedation (ages 1 to 17 years). It is also indicated for the management of benzodiazepine overdose in adults. In cases of benzodiazepine overdose in adults, flumazenil is administered intravenously in doses of 0.2 mg (2 mL) over a 30-second period. A second dose of 0.3 mg may be administered over 30 seconds, and additional doses of 0.5 mg over 30 seconds, at 1-minute intervals to a maximum of 3 mg, may be given until the desired level of consciousness is obtained. Only rarely do patients benefit from higher doses. In view of its relatively short half-life, resedation may occur. In such cases, additional flumazenil may be given at 20-minute intervals (max of 1 mg/dose and 3 mg/hour).

Untoward Effects of Benzodiazepines

Note: The U.S. Food and Drug Administration (FDA) directed manufacturers of benzodiazepine medication to label their products with the following black box warning: Concomitant use of benzodiazepine and opioids may result in profound respiratory depression, sedation, coma, and death. This treatment combination should be limited to patients for whom alternative options are not adequate. If these medications are prescribed together, the dose and duration of treatment should be for the minimum amount and duration needed to achieve the desired clinical effect.

In 2017, the FDA urged caution about withholding buprenorphine or methadone treatment when patients concurrently take benzodiazepines, because the harm inherent in withholding opioid addiction medication may outweigh the potential harm of taking these medications concurrently. In these scenarios, providers are advised to prescribe cautiously, to include educating patients on risks, tapering and discontinuing benzodiazepine medication when able, considering nonbenzodiazepine treatment options for anxiety or insomnia, monitoring for illicit drug use, and coordinating care with other treating providers.

Benzodiazepine medication should be used with extreme caution in patients with sleep apnea, bronchitis, pneumonia, asthma, or any other respiratory disease, as this class of medication may worsen respiratory depression.

Given that benzodiazepines are central nervous system depressants, the most common untoward effects are oversedation, fatigue, drowsiness, and ataxia. Confusion progressing to coma may occur at high doses. When daytime symptoms such as anxiety are targeted, benzodiazepines should be administered in divided doses to minimize sedation.

"Paradoxical reactions," or episodes of marked dyscontrol and disinhibition, have been reported in children and adolescents. Symptoms have included acute excitation, increased anxiety, increased aggression and hostility, rage reactions, loss of all control, hallucinations, insomnia, and nightmares.

Psychiatric and behavioral disturbances, including suicidality, have also been attributed to clonazepam use. For example, Kandemir et al. (2008) reported that a 9-year-old boy with no personal or family psychiatric history experienced excessive anger, irritability, and suicidal thinking and behavior after being prescribed clonazepam 1.5 mg/day by his neurologist to treat blepharospasm. On the fourth day of treatment with clonazepam, he developed suicidal thoughts and admitted to cutting his arms and chest with a razor in response to these thoughts. His parents reported he had no history of like behavior prior to treatment with clonazepam and stated he was taking no other medication. They described him as a "calm, well adjusted, and happy" child at baseline. A complete medical workup, including head imaging, was negative. After clonazepam was decreased and stopped over a 3-day period, his psychiatric symptoms resolved entirely. At follow-up 6 months later, he had no recurrence of symptoms (Kandemir et al., 2008).

Use of Benzodiazepines in Child and Adolescent Psychiatry

In general psychiatry, benzodiazepines are indicated for the management of anxiety disorders or for short-term relief of anxiety and/or sleep disorders. They are also used to treat acute symptoms of alcohol withdrawal. The effectiveness of benzodiazepines for chronic treatment (lasting >4 months) has not been assessed in systematic clinical studies.

At present, randomized controlled trials do not suggest efficacy of benzodiazepine medication for the treatment of childhood anxiety disorders. In clinical practice, benzodiazepines are used at times in youth, however, to acutely reduce severe anxiety until more effective medications, such as selective serotonin reuptake inhibitors (SSRIs), achieve therapeutic effect. If used, manufacturers' clinical recommendations for children should not be exceeded. Table 10.1 gives usual daily dosages for some representative benzodiazepines, an estimate of the serum half-life of the parent compound and/or its significant active metabolites, the youngest age for which the FDA has approved their use for any purpose, and, when applicable, suggested dosages for their use in child and adolescent psychiatric disorders.

The need for benzodiazepines should be reassessed frequently, and long-term, chronic use should be avoided.

As previously mentioned, there is a relative paucity of studies examining the use of benzodiazepines in youth. The few studies done are reviewed in what follows, although many entail older, uncontrolled studies or case reports.

TABLE 10.1 » Some Representative Benzodiazepines

Benzodiazepine (Trade Name) (Estimated Serum Half-life)	Minimum Age Approved for Any Use	Usual Daily Dosage
Alprazolam (Xanax) (12–15 h)	18 y	0.25–0.5 mg PO TID, maximum 4 mg/d in divided doses
Chlordiazepoxide (Librium) (24–48 h)	6 y	5 mg 2–4 times/d, maximum 30 mg/d
Clonazepam (Klonopin) (18–50 h)	Infants and children ≤ 10 y	Initially 0.01–0.03 mg/kg/d divided t.i.d; Increase by not more than 0.25–0.5 mg every third day to a maximum maintenance dose of 0.1–0.2 mg/kg/d, divided t.i.d.
Clorazepate (Tranxene) (approximately 48 h)	9 y	For children 9–12 y old, maximum initial dose of 7.5 mg twice daily. Maximum weekly increase, 7.5 mg. Maximum daily dose, 60 mg
Diazepam (Valium) (30–60 h)	6 mo	1–2.5 mg PO t.i.d.–q.i.d.
Estazolam (ProSom) (10–24 h)	18 y	1–2 mg at bedtime
Flurazepam (Dalmane) (47–100 h)	15 y	15–30 mg at bedtime
Lorazepam (Ativan) (12–18 h)	12 y	2–3 mg/d PO, divided b.i.d.–t.i.d.
Oxazepam (Serax) (5.7–0.9 h)	12 y	10–15 mg t.i.d.–q.i.d., max 30 mg t.i.d.–q.i.d.
Quazepam (Doral) (73 h)	18 y	7.5–15 mg at bedtime
Temazepam (Restoril) (9.5–12.4 h)	18 y	15–30 mg at bedtime
Triazolam (Halcion) (1.5–5.5 h)	18 y	0.125–0.25 mg at bedtime

Chlordiazepoxide (Librium)

Reports of Interest

Chlordiazepoxide in the Treatment of Behaviorally Disordered Children and Adolescents of Various Diagnoses

Kraft et al. (1965) prescribed chlordiazepoxide to 130 patients (99 males and 31 females) who ranged in age from 2 to 17 years (112 were between 7 and 14 years of age). The most common diagnoses were primary behavior disorder (50), school phobia (18), adjustment reaction of adolescence (17), and chronic brain damage (14). Most subjects had marked hyperactivity and neurotic traits. Doses ranged from 20 to 130 mg/day and were administered in divided doses; 94 subjects (72%) received 40 mg or more daily. Moderate or marked improvement occurred in 53 subjects (40.8%). Forty subjects (30.8%) had either no or insignificant improvement, and 37 (28.5%) worsened. The diagnostic group showing the greatest improvement was school phobia (77%). Only 38% of the primary behavior disorder subjects and 41.2% of the adolescent adjustment disorder subjects improved to a moderate or marked degree. Of those with organic brain damage, 50% worsened, 28.6% showed minimal or no benefit, and none had an excellent response. Across diagnoses, symptoms of hyperactivity, fear, night terrors, enuresis, reading and speech problems, truancy, and disturbed or bizarre behavior were moderately or markedly improved in 40.8% of the 130 subjects. The authors concluded that chlordiazepoxide was effective in decreasing anxiety and "emotional overload" (Kraft et al., 1965). The authors also reported that 22 of the 130 had untoward effects of sufficient severity to interfere with treatment results and that 14 other subjects had milder untoward effects that were transient or responded to a lowering of the dose.

Breitner (1962) administered chlordiazepoxide, 20 to 50 mg/day, to more than 50 juvenile delinquents between 8.5 and 24 years of age. He reported that the drug produced cooperativeness, released tension, created a feeling of well-being, and made the subjects more accessible to psychotherapy.

D'Amato (1962) treated nine children 8 to 11 years of age, who were diagnosed with school phobia, with 10 to 30 mg/day of chlordiazepoxide for 5 to 30 days. The children were also seen in psychotherapy. Only one child did not attend school regularly after the second week of treatment. The author compared these 9 children with 11 others, aged 5 to 12 years, also diagnosed with school phobia, who were treated over the six preceding years with psychotherapy only. Only 2 of these 11 children returned to school within 2 weeks, and 9 remained out of school for 1 month or longer. The author thought that this strongly suggested that chlordiazepoxide was an effective adjunct to psychotherapy in mobilizing children with school phobia to return to school.

Petti et al. (1982) treated nine boys (7 to 11 years of age) with chlordiazepoxide who failed to respond to 3 weeks of hospitalization and treatment with placebo. The subjects' diagnoses were conduct disorder (five, three of whom had borderline features), personality disorder (three, one of whom had borderline features), and schizophrenia (one). Verbal IQs on the Wechsler Intelligence Scale for Children (WISC) ranged from 71 to 110. Target symptoms were anxiety, depression, impulsivity, and explosiveness. The initial dose of chlordiazepoxide was 15 mg, administered in divided doses. The optimal dose was determined by individual titration and ranged from 15 to 120 mg/day (0.58 to 5.28 mg/kg/day). Children's ratings on optimal dose were compared with baseline ratings. Marked improvement was noted in two boys, improvement in four, and no change or worsening in three. The major improvements were increased verbal production, increased rapidity of thought associations, and a shift from blunted affect or depressed mood to a more animated appearance and feeling subjectively better. The authors noted that chlordiazepoxide had the most positive effect on children who were withdrawn, inhibited, anergic, depressed, or anxious. The child with schizophrenia had a worsening of psychotic symptoms, and two children with severe impulsive aggressiveness experienced a worsening of behavior. The authors suggest that chlordiazepoxide's use may be contraindicated in such children (Petti et al., 1982).

Diazepam (Valium)

Reports of Interest

Diazepam in the Treatment of Children and Adolescents with Various Psychiatric Diagnoses

Lucas and Pasley (1969), in one of the few double-blind, placebo-controlled studies of benzodiazepines in this age group, administered diazepam to 12 subjects, 7 to 17 years of age (mean, 12.3 years), who were diagnosed as psychoneurotic ($N = 10$) or schizophrenic ($N = 2$). All subjects were inpatients or in a daycare program. Target symptoms included moderate to high anxiety levels, highly oppositional behavior, poor peer relationships, and aggression. The initial dose of diazepam was 2.5 mg twice daily. The drug was increased until a satisfactory therapeutic response or untoward effects occurred. The maximum dose achieved was 20 mg/day. The study lasted 16 weeks, during which subjects were assigned randomly to four different sequences of drug and placebo. Subjects were rated on 10 items: hyperactivity, anxiety and tension, oppositional behavior, aggressiveness, impulsivity, relationship to peers, relationship to adults, need for limit setting, response to limit setting, and participation in program. There was no significant difference between diazepam and placebo on any item for the nine patients who completed the study. (The two patients with schizophrenia and one other patient dropped out.) However, when scores on all 10 items were combined, diazepam scored significantly better than placebo ($P < .05$), although clinically the difference was not very apparent. Eleven of the 12 children who participated in the study long enough were rated on a global rating scale. Five subjects showed no change, two were somewhat more anxious, and four were definitely worse, with increased anxiety and deterioration in their behavior on diazepam compared with placebo. From this study and their clinical experience with diazepam, the authors concluded that diazepam was not clinically effective in reducing anxiety or acting-out behavior in children and young adolescents. Older adolescents appeared to react similarly to adults, and diazepam was thought to be useful in treating their anxiety.

Diazepam in the Treatment of Sleep Disorder

In an open study, three children with somnambulism and night terrors (pavor nocturnus), and four children with insomnia were treated with 2 to 5 mg of diazepam near bedtime, and all seven responded favorably (Glick et al., 1971).

Alprazolam (Xanax)

Glue et al. (2006) studied the effects of Alprazolam XR in 12 adolescents and 12 adults in a randomized, open-label, single dose (1 or 3 mg), two-period crossover trial and discovered that parent-metabolite ratios were similar in both age groups, the medication was well tolerated by both groups, and the most common side effect was dose-related somnolence. In this trial, blood samples were obtained predose and 48 hours postdose. Because of similar pharmacokinetic profiles noted in this study, the authors concluded that Alprazolam XR should be dosed similarly in adult and adolescent patients (Glue et al., 2006).

Reports of Interest

Alprazolam in the Treatment of Night Terrors (Pavor Nocturnus)

Cameron and Thyer (1985) successfully treated night terrors in a 10-year-old girl with alprazolam. She was initially prescribed 0.5 mg of alprazolam at bedtime for 1 week. The dose was increased to 0.75 mg nightly for the next 4 weeks, after which alprazolam was tapered off. Night terrors ceased on the first night and at follow-up 9 months later had not recurred.

Alprazolam in the Treatment of Anxiety Disorders

Pfefferbaum et al. (1987) used alprazolam to treat anticipatory and acute situational anxiety and panic in 13 patients, aged 7 to 14 years, who were being treated with stressful procedures for concomitant cancer. Alprazolam treatment was initiated 3 days before and continued through the day of the stressful procedures. This study was conducted under an Investigational New Drug permit, and the maximum dose allowed was 0.02 mg/kg/dose or 0.06 mg/kg/day, with the exception of one child for whom the FDA granted approval to receive a total of 0.05 mg/kg/dose, or 0.15 mg/kg/day. In this study, alprazolam was initiated at 0.005 mg/kg or lower and was titrated upward based on efficacy and tolerability. Typical total daily doses ranged from 0.375 to 3 mg (0.003 to 0.075 mg/kg/day). Subjects were rated on four scales measuring anxiety, distress, and panic. The subjects' improvement was statistically significant ($P < .05$) on three scales and reached borderline significance on the fourth scale. Mild drowsiness was the most frequently reported adverse effect. Overall, untoward effects were minimal in this small study.

Klein and Last (1989) reported Klein's unpublished data from a clinical trial of alprazolam in children and adolescents whose separation anxiety disorder did not respond to psychotherapy. Alprazolam was clinically effective when administered to 18 subjects (ages 6 to 17 years) for 6 weeks in daily doses of 0.5 to 6 mg/day (mean dose 1.9 mg/day). Parents and the psychiatrist judged that >80% of the subjects improved significantly, whereas only 65% of the subjects rated themselves as improved.

Simeon and Ferguson (1987) administered alprazolam openly to 12 children and adolescents (8.8 to 16.5 years of age; mean, 11.5 years) diagnosed with overanxious and/or avoidant disorder. After 1 week of treatment with placebo, to which none of the subjects responded, alprazolam was titrated individually over a subsequent 2-week period to maximum daily doses of 0.50 to 1.5 mg. The total period of active treatment was 4 weeks. Seven of the 12 youth showed at least a moderate improvement on several rating scales, and no child worsened. Clinician ratings showed significant improvement of anxiety, depression, and psychomotor excitation; parents reported significant improvement of anxiety and hyperactivity on questionnaires, and teachers reported significant improvement on an anxious–passive factor. Parents frequently reported improvement in the subjects' sleep problems. Simeon and Ferguson (1987) observed that subjects with good premorbid personalities and prominent symptoms of inhibitions, shyness, and nervousness responded best to alprazolam and showed continued improvement after the medication was discontinued. By contrast, patients with poor premorbid personalities and poor family backgrounds were more commonly observed to develop undesirable symptoms of disinhibition, such as increased aggressiveness and impulsivity, especially at higher doses, and were more apt to relapse following drug withdrawal. The few untoward effects noted in this small study were mild and transient. Ferguson and Simeon (1984) reported no adverse effects of alprazolam on cognition or learning when used at therapeutically effective doses.

Simeon et al. (1992) reported a double-blind placebo-controlled study of alprazolam in 30 children and adolescents (23 males and 7 females; aged 8.4 to 16.9 years; mean age 12.6 years) who had primary diagnoses of overanxious disorder ($N = 21$) or avoidant disorder ($N = 9$). Clinical impairment ranged from moderate to severe. Placebo was administered for 1 week and was followed by random assignment to a 4-week period of either placebo or alprazolam. Medication was tapered with placebo substitution during the fifth week. During the sixth week, all subjects received only placebo. Patients who weighed <40 kg received an initial dose of 0.25 mg of alprazolam, whereas heavier patients received an initial dose of 0.5 mg. The maximum daily dosage permitted was 0.04 mg/kg. Alprazolam was increased at 2-day intervals until an optimal dose was achieved. At completion of the active drug phase, the average daily dose of alprazolam was 1.57 mg (range 0.5 to 3.5 mg). Untoward effects were few and minor (e.g., dry mouth and feeling tired) and did not appear to interfere with academic performance.

Simeon et al. (1992) noted a strong treatment effect in both placebo and alprazolam groups during this trial. Overall, alprazolam was judged to be superior to placebo based on clinical global ratings, but the differences were not statistically significant. There were strong individual responders in both groups. At study completion, there was a slight relapse of original symptoms among subjects receiving alprazolam, whereas subjects who took placebo showed no change in symptoms and/or continued to improve. The authors commented that doses employed in this study were relatively low and were administered for only 4 weeks. They suggested that higher doses and longer trials be investigated in the future and recommended that alprazolam be tapered more gradually over a period of several weeks in the future (Simeon et al., 1992).

Bernstein et al. (1990) similarly discovered that alprazolam did not separate from placebo (or imipramine) in a small placebo-controlled double-blind study of youth with anxiety disorders. In their study, 24 youth (aged 7 to 18 years old) with diagnoses of school refusal and separation anxiety disorder were randomized to receive either placebo, imipramine (50 to 175 mg/day), or alprazolam (0.75 to 4.0 mg/day). The authors concluded that there was no significant difference between the three treatment groups by the end of the study (Bernstein et al., 1990).

Clonazepam (Klonopin)

Clonazepam is approved for the treatment of seizure disorders in pediatrics.

■ *Reports of Interest*

Clonazepam in the Treatment of Panic Disorder

In an open clinical trial, Kutcher and MacKenzie (1988) treated four adolescents (three females and one male; average age 17.2 years; range 16 to 19 years) diagnosed with panic disorder by DSM-III criteria, with a fixed dose of clonazepam (0.5 mg twice daily). Average ratings on the Hamilton Anxiety Rating Scale fell from 32 at baseline to 7.5 at week 1 and 5.7 at week 2. The number of panic attacks fell from an average of 3 to 0.5 per week after 1 week to 0.25 per week after 2 weeks. One adolescent complained of initial drowsiness that resolved within 4 days, and no other untoward effects were reported. At follow-up examinations 3 to 6 months later, all four patients continued to take clonazepam and appeared to maintain improved functioning in school and interpersonal relations.

Clonazepam in the Treatment of Childhood Anxiety Disorders

Graae et al. (1994) treated 15 subjects (8 males and 7 females; age range 7 to 13 years; mean 9.8 ± 2.1 years) diagnosed with various anxiety and comorbid disorders with clonazepam in an 8-week, double-blind, placebo-controlled crossover study. Diagnoses included separation anxiety disorder ($N = 14$), overanxious disorder ($N = 6$), social phobia ($N = 5$), oppositional disorder ($N = 3$), avoidant disorder ($N = 2$), conduct disorder ($N = 1$), and attention-deficit/hyperactivity disorder (ADHD) ($N = 1$). Clonazepam was initiated with a 0.25-mg dose at breakfast and increased by 0.25 mg every third day to a total dose of 1.0 mg/day. Subsequent increments of 0.25 mg were made every other day until a dose of 2 mg/day was reached or until untoward effects or compliance issues prevented it. After receiving clonazepam at a maximum of 2 mg/day for 4 days, subjects' clonazepam was gradually tapered off by the end of the 4-week period.

Three boys dropped out while on active medication, two because of serious disinhibition, including marked irritability, tantrums, aggressivity, and self-injurious behavior and the other because of noncompliance. Nine children were rated as clinically improved (five had good/marked improvement, and four had some/moderate improvement), and three children showed no improvement of anxiety or overall functioning while on clonazepam. Although there was no statistically significant difference between clonazepam and placebo for the 12 subjects, the authors thought that individual patients made significant clinical improvements while on clonazepam. The most common untoward effects were drowsiness, irritability, lability, and oppositional behavior. Overall, 10 (83%) children had untoward effects on clonazepam compared with 7 (53%) on placebo. The difference was not statistically significant, however. Disinhibition was not seen in the placebo-treated group, and the two boys taking clonazepam who dropped out because of this effect were not included in the data analysis. Study authors suggested that a slower upward dose titration might reduce the untoward effects seen with clonazepam, including disinhibition (Graae et al., 1994).

Clonazepam in the Treatment of Obsessive-Compulsive Disorder

Ross and Piggott (1993) treated a 14-year-old male with clonazepam who was hospitalized with severely disabling obsessive-compulsive disorder. The patient did not respond adequately to prior trials of clomipramine, thioridazine, alprazolam, fluoxetine, or diazepam, either alone or in various combinations. Clonazepam was administered at an initial dose of 0.5 mg twice daily and increased to 1.0 mg twice daily after 1 week. Behavioral improvement was noted by week 2 on the medication, and he was able to be discharged home after taking clonazepam for 11 weeks.

Leonard et al. (1994) reported the use of clonazepam as an augmenting agent in a 20-year-old who had severely disabling obsessive-compulsive disorder with onset at age 7. He was treatment-resistant to prior trials of clomipramine, desipramine, fluoxetine, fluvoxamine, and buspirone augmentation, either alone or in various combinations. He experienced marked clinical improvement with at least 75% reduction in symptom severity on a combination of 60 mg/day of fluoxetine and 4 mg/day of clonazepam, which was maintained for approximately 1 year. The authors suggested that clonazepam might be efficacious and safe when used to augment specific serotonin reuptake inhibitors in treating obsessive-compulsive disorder in children and adolescents.

AZASPIRODECANEDIONES

Buspirone Hydrochloride (Buspar)

Buspirone hydrochloride is a drug with anxiolytic properties that is chemically distinct from benzodiazepines, barbiturates, or other sedative or anxiolytic medication. It has a high affinity for $5-HT_{1A}$ serotonin receptors, an affinity associated with clinical anxiolytic properties and anticonflict activity in animals (Sussman, 1994b). Buspirone has moderate affinity for brain D_2-dopamine receptors. It does not have significant affinity for benzodiazepine receptors, nor does it affect gamma-aminobutyric acid (GABA) binding. Furthermore, buspirone has no cross-tolerance with benzodiazepines, will not suppress panic attacks, and lacks anticonvulsant activity (Sussman, 1994b); hence, it does not block the withdrawal syndrome that may occur when benzodiazepines and other common sedative hypnotic drugs are abruptly discontinued. At therapeutic doses, buspirone is less sedating than benzodiazepines. It does not result in physical or psychological dependence or notable withdrawal when discontinued, and because of its low abuse potential it is not classified as a controlled (Schedule II) substance.

Buspirone is approved by the FDA for the management of anxiety disorders, including short-term relief of the anxiety symptoms. However, unlike benzodiazepines, which have an immediate anxiolytic effect, buspirone may take 3 to 6 weeks for its antianxiety effect to develop fully.

Pharmacokinetics of Buspirone Hydrochloride

Buspirone is rapidly absorbed, with peak plasma levels occurring between 40 and 90 minutes after an acute oral dose of buspirone. Average elimination half-life after single doses of 10 to 40 mg of buspirone is usually between 2 and 3 hours. In a 21-day open-label, multisite, dose-escalation study comparing buspirone pharmacokinetics in children ($N = 13$, ages 6 to 12 years), adolescents ($N = 12$, ages 13 to 17 years), and adults ($N = 14$, ages 18 to 45 years), Salazar et al. (2001) demonstrated that mean plasma concentrations of buspirone are equal to or higher in youth compared with adults. Furthermore, 1-pyrimidinylpiperazine (1-PP), buspirone's primary metabolite, was significantly higher in children than in both adolescents and adults in all four dosing arms (5, 7.5, 15, and 30 mg b.i.d.) (Salazar et al., 2001).

Contraindications for Buspirone Hydrochloride Administration

A known hypersensitivity to buspirone hydrochloride is a contraindication for its use.

Interactions of Buspirone Hydrochloride with Other Drugs

Buspirone should not be used concomitantly with MAOIs, as this may result in hypertension. Buspirone is a CYP450 3A4 substrate, and hence CYP450 3A4 inducers (phenytoin, carbamazepine, modafinil, etc.) may decrease buspirone concentrations. Similarly, CYP450 3A4 inhibitors (ketoconazole, ritonavir, etc.) may increase buspirone concentrations. On account of additive effects, buspirone may increase the risk of serotonin syndrome when used concomitantly with other serotonergic medications (SSRIs, tramadol, triptans, etc.).

Untoward Effects of Buspirone Hydrochloride

The untoward effects most frequently reported by adults taking buspirone include dizziness (12%), drowsiness (10%), nausea (8%), headache (6%), insomnia (3%), and lightheadedness (3%). It may be noted, however, that drowsiness and insomnia were reported to occur with approximately equal frequency in subjects taking placebo; hence, these effects may not have been related to buspirone *per se* (PDR, 2000). In a 3-week dose-escalation study, Salazar et al. (2001) discovered that the most commonly reported adverse effects in youth (ages 6 to 17 years) were lightheadedness (67% of subjects), headache (50% of subjects), and dyspepsia (21% of subjects), whereas in adults (ages 18 to 45 years) the most commonly reported adverse effects were somnolence (21.4% of subjects), and lightheadedness, nausea, vomiting, and diarrhea (all 14.3% of subjects). In this particular study, buspirone was dosed as follows for all study participants: buspirone 5 mg b.i.d. (days 1 to 3), 7.5 mg b.i.d. (days 4 to 7), 15 mg b.i.d. (days 8 to 14), and 30 mg b.i.d. (days 15 to 21) (Salazar et al., 2001).

Indications for Buspirone Hydrochloride in Child and Adolescent Psychiatry

Buspirone is approved only for treatment of anxiety disorders and the short-term relief of anxiety in individuals at least 18 years of age. There are no definitive child and adolescent psychiatric indications for this medication, and its use in youth is necessarily "off-label."

Buspirone Dosage Schedule

- *Children and adolescents up to 17 years of age:* Not approved. Coffey (1990), however, suggested the following doses if a clinician elects to use buspirone in this age group:

  Prepubescent children: An initial total daily dose of 2.5 to 5 mg with increases of 2.5 mg every 3 to 4 days to a maximum of 20 mg/day.

  Younger adolescents: An initial total daily dose of 5 to 10 mg with increases of 5 to 10 mg every 3 to 4 days to a maximum of 60 mg/day. In a small dose-escalation study, Salazar et al. (2001) discovered that buspirone was generally safe and well tolerated in doses up to 30 mg b.i.d. in adolescents ($N = 12$, ages 13 to 17 years) and adults ($N = 14$, ages 18 to 45 years), although it was less well tolerated in children (ages 6 to 12 years) when used at doses higher than 7.5 mg b.i.d. Specifically, 2 of the 13 children withdrew from the study because of mild or moderate adverse effects when taking buspirone at the higher doses (15 and 30 mg b.i.d.). Study authors hence concluded that buspirone appeared well tolerated in youth ages 6 to 12 years at doses up to 7.5 mg b.i.d. (Salazar et al., 2001).

- *Adolescents at least 18 years of age and adults:* Initiate treatment with 7.5 mg twice daily. Titrate to optimal therapeutic response by increases of 5 mg every 2 to 3 days to a maximum daily dose of 60 mg. Usual optimal doses in clinical trials were 20 to 30 mg/day in divided doses.

Buspirone Hydrochloride Dose Forms Available

- *Tablets:* 5, 7.5, 10, 15, 30 mg

Reports of Interest

Buspirone Hydrochloride in the Treatment of Anxiety Disorders in Children and Adolescents

Kranzler (1988) reported a single case study in which a 13-year-old adolescent diagnosed with overanxious disorder (now defined as DSM-5 GAD), school refusal, and intermittent enuresis was administered buspirone. A previous trial of desipramine yielded some improvement but was discontinued at the patient's request because of untoward effects. Buspirone was initially administered at 2.5 mg three times daily. At doses of 5 mg three times daily, she experienced morning drowsiness, so buspirone was decreased to 5 mg twice daily. Scores on the Hamilton Anxiety Rating Scale dropped from 26 to 15, and improvements were noted in phobic anxiety, insomnia, depressed mood, cardiovascular symptoms, and anxious behavior, although enuresis did not improve.

Simeon et al. (1994) treated 15 children (10 males and 5 females; age range: 6 to 14 years; mean age, 10 years) diagnosed with separation anxiety disorder (5), overanxious disorder (2), comorbid separation anxiety and overanxious disorders (4), separation, overanxious, and avoidant disorders (1), separation, overanxious, and obsessive-compulsive disorders (1), and overanxious disorder and ADHD (2). Subjects were rated moderately to severely impaired on the Clinical Global Impressions Scale (CGI). A single-blind placebo was administered for the first 2 weeks, which was followed by 4 weeks of treatment with buspirone, administered initially at 5 mg daily and increased weekly by 5 mg increments as needed to a maximum of 20 mg/day (mean dose 18.6 mg/day). No subjects improved significantly on placebo. After 4 weeks on buspirone, subjects' ratings on the CGI showed marked improvement (3), moderate improvement (10), and minimal improvement (2). Repeated measures of multivariate analysis of variance (MANOVA) showed a statistically significant treatment effect after 2 weeks on medication ($P < .016$), which increased in significance to $P < .001$ after both 3 and 4 weeks on medication. Significant improvements were also seen on several rating scales as reported by parents, teachers, and subjects themselves. Untoward effects, which were mild and appeared to follow dose increases, included nausea or stomach pain ($N = 5$), headache ($N = 4$), occasional sleepwalking, sleep talking, or nightmares, and daytime tiredness ($N = 8$).

Zwier and Rao (1994) reported treating a hospitalized 16-year-old male with social phobia and schizotypal personality disorder using buspirone, initially at 5 mg/day, followed by 5-mg dose increases every 3 days, to a total daily dose of 20 mg. At 12 days of buspirone treatment, scores on the Hamilton Anxiety Rating Scale dropped from 5 to 0, at which time the patient was discharged. Over the subsequent year, buspirone was tapered to 5 mg/day, the patient's mild psychotic symptoms resolved, and he was reported to have maintained his treatment gains.

Buspirone Hydrochloride in the Treatment of Autism Spectrum Disorder

Realmuto et al. (1989) treated four autistic children, 9 to 10 years of age, with buspirone 5 mg administered three times daily for 4 weeks, followed by a week-long washout period and 4 weeks of 10 mg twice daily of either fenfluramine or methylphenidate. Two of the four children showed decreased hyperactivity while on buspirone. None of the children experienced adverse untoward effects from buspirone.

In a 3-week, double-blind, placebo-controlled crossover study, McCormick (1997) studied the safety and efficacy of buspirone for the treatment of hyperactivity in a patient with autistic disorder. The child received placebo for 3 weeks, followed by buspirone treatment for 3 weeks. The Conners abbreviated parent and teacher questionnaires, as well as the number of daily performance tasks completed by the child at school, were used as primary outcome measures. Buspirone was ultimately determined to be safe and efficacious for reducing hyperactivity and increasing school-based performance tasks. The author concluded that buspirone may be a beneficial medication for autistic patients, but cautioned that further study is needed (McCormick, 1997).

Buitelaar et al. (1998) evaluated the efficacy and safety of buspirone in a 6- to 8-week, open-label study treating chronic manifest pervasive anxiety, irritability, and/or affect dysregulation in 22 inpatients (20 males and 2 females; age range, 6 to 16 years), 20 of whom were diagnosed with pervasive developmental disorder not otherwise specified (PDDNOS) and 2 of whom were diagnosed with autistic disorder by DSM-III-R criteria (APA, 1987). Target symptoms were anxiety in 14 patients, irritability in 1, and both anxiety and irritability in 7. Efficacy was determined by ratings on the CGI Scale, using subscales CGI–Anxiety and CGI–Irritability, and the CGI–Severity (CGI-S) and the CGI–Improvement (CGI-I) Scales. Buspirone was initiated at a dose of 5 mg three times daily and individually titrated based on clinical response, to a maximum dose of 45 mg/day, which could be achieved within 3 weeks. Eighteen subjects received buspirone only, and four subjects continued to receive one additional drug. Twenty-one subjects completed 6 to 8 weeks on buspirone, whereas one subject dropped out earlier because of a lack of clinical response. Therapeutic improvement was apparent after 2 to 3 weeks of treatment in many subjects (mean daily dose was 29.3 mg/day). Overall on the CGI-I, 16 (76%) of 21 patients were responders (9 "marked" improvement and 7 "moderate" improvement) with clinically significant reductions of overwhelming anxiety, irritability, and temper tantrums. Six subjects did not experience therapeutic benefit. Of the 21 patients with targeted anxiety, 16 were responders (9 "marked" and 7 "moderate"), and of the 8 patients with "irritability" 5 were responders (2 "marked" and 3 "moderate"). Mild untoward effects were reported in 5 subjects and included initial sedation (N = 2), mild agitation (N = 2), and initial nausea (N = 1). All 16 responders continued to receive buspirone, were followed for 2 to 12 months, and maintained all therapeutic gains. One child, however, developed abnormal involuntary movement of the mouth, cheeks, and tongue after receiving 20 mg/day of buspirone for 10 months. The authors considered this a buspirone-associated orofacial-lingual dyskinesia and discontinued medication. The abnormal movements completely remitted within 2 weeks. This study suggests buspirone may be therapeutically useful in treating anxiety and irritability in some children and adolescents with pervasive developmental disorders.

Chugani et al. (2016) conducted a randomized placebo-controlled trial to investigate the efficacy of low-dose buspirone for restricted and repetitive behavior in 166 young children (2 to 6 years of age) with autism spectrum disorder. Participants were randomized to placebo, 2.5 mg twice daily, or 5.0 mg twice daily of buspirone for 24 weeks. Study authors aimed to determine the effect of 24 weeks of buspirone treatment on the Autism Diagnostic Observation Schedule (ADOS) Composite Total Score. Secondary objectives consisted of evaluating for tolerability of buspirone, along with efficacy for social competence, repetitive behaviors, language, sensory dysfunction, and anxiety. Study authors found no difference in the ADOS Composite Total Score between baseline and 24 weeks among the three treatment groups ($P = .400$), although the ADOS Restricted and Repetitive Behavior score showed significant improvement in the 2.5-mg buspirone group ($P = .003$), whereas placebo and the 5.0-mg buspirone groups showed no change (Chugani et al., 2016).

Buspirone Hydrochloride in the Treatment of Aggression

Quiason et al. (1991) treated a hospitalized 8-year-old boy exhibiting conduct symptoms and ADHD with buspirone hydrochloride. Buspirone was initially administered at 5 mg three times per day and titrated gradually to 15 mg three times a day. By day 10, there was a notable decrease in aggressive and assaultive behavior, and the need for timeouts or seclusion ceased altogether.

Pfeffer et al. (1997) treated 25 anxious and moderately aggressive prepubertal inpatients (19 males and 6 females; ages 5 to 11 years, mean age, 8.0 ± 1.8 years) with buspirone. Subjects' DSM-III-R (APA, 1987) diagnoses included mood disorder (N = 9), disruptive behavior disorder (N = 21), anxiety disorders (N = 8), and specific developmental disorders (N = 9). This 11-week study began with a 2-week baseline evaluation phase that was followed by 3 weeks of active buspirone treatment. Buspirone was dosed initially at 5 mg/day and was increased by 5 to 10 mg every 3 days to a maximum of 50 mg/day. Subjects were then maintained at their optimal dose of buspirone for an additional 6 weeks. Efficacy was determined by analysis of ratings on the Child Depression Inventory (CDI); the Revised Children's Manifest Anxiety Scale (RCMAS); the Measure of Aggression, Violence, and Rage in Children (MAVRIC); the Suicidal and Assaultive Behavior Scales (SABS); the Overt Aggression Scale (OAS); the Children's Global Assessment Scale (CGAS); and the Udvalg for Kliniske Undersogelser (UKU) Side Effects Rating Scale (Lingjaerde et al., 1987).

During the second week of titration, four children developed behavioral toxicity (agitation and increased aggressivity) and were terminated from the study. Of the 21 subjects who entered the maintenance phase, 2 were terminated because they developed severe euphoric symptoms, increased impulsivity, and maladaptive behavior. Thus, only 19 (76%) subjects completed the 11-week study. The mean dose for completers was 28 mg/day, administered in two divided doses. For the 19 completers, there was a significant decrease ($P = .001$) in CDI scores from baseline (19 ± 8.2) to end point (9.2 ± 7.5). This level of improvement was achieved during the sixth week on buspirone. Seven of the 10 completers with clinically significant depression at baseline (CDI score > 18) had a CDI score of <12 (i.e., below the cutoff for non-clinically significant depression). There was a significant reduction in the number of restraints and/or seclusions used ($P = .01$), and the duration of time children spent restrained and/or secluded decreased significantly ($P = .02$). Although there was a significant decrease ($P = .02$) in the MAVRIC at endpoint, subjects continued to exhibit clinically significant levels of aggression. Similarly, CGAS scores, reflecting clinical global functioning, improved from 40.68 ± 10.49 at baseline to 54.47 ± 14.18 at endpoint ($P = .01$), and significant clinical impairments persisted. Three children improved sufficiently to continue on buspirone following completion of the study. Overall, although significant, the therapeutic efficacy on aggression and anxiety was limited, and clinically significant aggression, anxiety, and global impairment remained. Furthermore, six patients terminated prematurely from the study because of significant untoward effects. The study authors concluded that, overall, the results of this study were not very promising (Pfeffer et al., 1997).

Buspirone Hydrochloride in the Treatment of ADHD

McCormick et al. (1994) conducted a 4-week, double-blind, placebo-controlled, crossover study in which buspirone hydrochloride was administered to 10 males ranging in age from 11 years, 3 months to 16 years, 10 months (mean age, 13 years, 7 months) who were diagnosed with ADHD by DSM-III-R criteria (APA, 1987). The only comorbid diagnoses were learning disorders, which occurred in four (40%) of the subjects. Each subject was randomly assigned to *receive* buspirone or placebo for 2 weeks, after which the conditions were reversed for an additional 2 weeks. On school days only, subjects received either buspirone 5 mg (at 8:00 and 11:00 AM) or placebo. During weekly telephone interviews with subjects' families, the 10-item Conners' Abbreviated Teacher Rating Scale was completed. Analysis showed no significant carryover effect between the two conditions.

The mean Conners' baseline score of 20.2 decreased to 19.3 during the second week of placebo therapy and decreased to 14.8 during the second week of buspirone therapy. Nine of the 10 subjects improved on buspirone compared with placebo, which was a significant treatment effect ($P < .025$). The only reported untoward effect for buspirone was 3 days of nausea experienced by one subject.

In a 6-week open-label trial, Malhotra and Santosh (1998) treated 12 outpatients (10 males and 2 females; mean age, 8.2 years; age range, 6 to 12 years) diagnosed with ADHD with buspirone. The Conners' Parent Abbreviated 10-item index (CPAI) and the CGAS at baseline, and 1, 2, 4, 6, and 8 weeks (i.e., after 2 weeks off medication) were used to assess efficacy. Subjects were administered an initial buspirone dose of 0.5 mg/kg/day (dose range, 15 to 30 mg/day) divided into two doses, which was continued for 6 weeks. No other medication was administered during the study. The mean CPAI improvement at day 7 was significant ($P < .001$). Clinical improvement continued over the 6-week period, and at the end of the study, at day 42, all four domains of the CPAI (inattention, hyperactivity, impulsivity, and behavior) improved significantly ($P < .0001$ for each domain). Based on reduced symptom severity of >50% and significant clinical improvement, all 12 patients were deemed responders. The CGAS scores improved significantly from baseline by day 7 ($P < .0001$) and by day 42 ($P < .0001$). All 12 subjects experienced symptom relapse within 2 weeks of discontinuing buspirone (the mean CPAI score returned nearly to baseline), and all families elected to restart their children on buspirone. Only two subjects reported untoward effects, with both experiencing mild transient dizziness during the first week of treatment. The authors concluded that buspirone was safe and effective in reducing the symptoms of ADHD in this group of subjects.

In a double-blind and randomized trial, Davari-Ashtiani et al. (2010) studied buspirone versus methylphenidate for the treatment of ADHD. Thirty-four youth were randomized to receive buspirone (0.5 mg/kg/day) or methylphenidate (0.3 to 1 mg/kg/day) for 6 weeks. The principal outcome measures were the parent and teacher ADHD Rating Scale scores. At week 6, both groups' parent and teacher ADHD Rating Scale scores significantly declined from baseline ($P < .001$), which correlated with significant improvements in ADHD symptoms. No significant differences between total scores occurred between groups, although methylphenidate was found to be superior to buspirone for inattentive symptoms. The author noted that buspirone had a more favorable side-effect profile than methylphenidate and opined that while these preliminary findings are positive, larger trials are needed before definitive conclusions can be drawn (Davari-Ashtiani et al., 2010).

Because of inconsistent findings from prior studies, Mohammadi et al. (2012) conducted a 6-week randomized double-blind study that aimed to discover whether buspirone could compare to methylphenidate for treatment of ADHD in children. Forty drug-naïve children between the ages of 6 and 14 with a DSM-IV-TR diagnosis of ADHD were recruited from an outpatient child and adolescent clinic. The children were randomly assigned to receive treatment using buspirone 20 to 30 mg/day (20 mg/day for <30 kg and 30 mg/day for >30 kg) or methylphenidate 20 to 30 mg/day. Patients were assessed at baseline, at 21 and 42 days after treatment was initiated. The principal measure of outcome was the Teacher and Parent ADHD Rating Scale IV. In this study, buspirone was shown to be less effective than methylphenidate in the treatment of ADHD. The incidence of side effects between the two treatment groups was not significant with the exception of decreased appetite, headache, and insomnia which were more frequent in the methylphenidate group (Mohammadi et al., 2012).

Buspirone Hydrochloride for the Treatment of Bruxism

Sabuncuoglu et al. (2009) reported a case of an adolescent with fluoxetine-induced bruxism that was successfully treated with buspirone. The authors hypothesized that buspirone, as a 5-HT_{1A} agonist, reduces serotonergic activity and increases dopaminergic activity, which may help with the theorized SSRI-led dopamine depletion that manifests as nocturnal bruxism (Sabuncuoglu et al., 2009).

Orsagh-Yentis et al. (2011) reported a case of a 7-year-old boy with PDD-NOS and moderate mental retardation, who presented with significant bruxism, predominantly diurnal, but also nocturnal. His severe bruxism led to his teeth being ground flush with his gum-line. Due to concern that his bruxism may represent internal distress, he was started on buspirone 2.5 mg daily for 1 week, which was then increased to 2.5 mg twice daily. After 2 weeks on this dose, he showed no improvement in symptoms, so buspirone was increased to 5 mg twice daily. Due to only brief improvement over the subsequent 2 months, an additional dose increase to 5 mg three times daily was made. On this dose, his parents reported that his bruxism ceased during both days and nights. At follow-up 9 months after starting buspirone, he remained overall improved, although his afternoon bruxism recurred, which prompted a final buspirone dose increase to 7.5 mg three times daily. Within weeks, his bruxism again remitted. Although buspirone was considered overall effective for bruxism in this patient, it was associated with daytime sedation and sleep disturbance, which did not respond to melatonin and only partially responded to trazodone (Orsagh-Yentis et al., 2011). Future studies are warranted.

CHAPTER 11

Medications Used to Treat Substance Use Disorders in Adolescents

CHRISTINA G. WESTON, JAMIE L. SNYDER, AND KARI S. HARPER

Substance use disorders (SUDs) have been a significant problem for adolescents and young adults for many years. Most recently the opioid epidemic has led to an increased emphasis on medication-assisted treatment (MAT) to help treat SUDs. The use of MAT for adult opioid addicts has become the treatment standard, whereas its use in adolescents is less commonplace. This chapter departs from the book's organization by medication class, and instead groups all medications frequently used to treat SUDs.

MEDICATIONS USED TO TREAT OPIOID USE DISORDERS

Methadone and buprenorphine are the two primary methods of MAT available to treat patients with opioid addictions. Methadone is highly regulated and is only available to patients over the age of 18 in the United States. Buprenorphine/ naloxone is approved for use in patients who are at least 16 years old and can be considered in the treatment plan for adolescents with opioid addictions. In a recent policy statement on the use of MAT for adolescents with opioid use disorders, the American Academy of Pediatrics Committee on Substance Use and Prevention (2016) recommended that resources for MAT be improved. They recommend that pediatricians have access to buprenorphine waiver training and consider offering MAT to adolescents in their practice or provide appropriate referrals.

BUPRENORPHINE/NALOXONE (SUBOXONE) AND BUPRENORPHINE (SUBUTEX)

Buprenorphine is a schedule III drug. It requires additional training to prescribe it. Health care providers must meet certain requirements and have notified the Secretary of Health and Human Services of their intent to prescribe this product for the treatment of opioid dependence. They are assigned a unique identification number that must be included on every prescription. Buprenorphine is a mu-opioid partial agonist with a greater margin of safety than full agonists and a less intensive withdrawal. It is approved by the U.S. Food and Drug Administration (FDA) for treatment of individuals aged 16 or older; however, it was studied primarily in adults who were addicted for 5 to 10 years or longer. It is often combined with naloxone, an antagonist, in a ratio of 4:1 in an attempt to decrease abuse potential when injected. Alho et al. (2007) found that this combination reduced "street" value and most likely decreased abuse potential.

DOSAGE AND ADMINISTRATION

Induction

Before induction, consideration should be given to the type of opioid dependence, the time since last use, and the degree or level of opioid dependence. To avoid precipitating an opioid withdrawal syndrome, the first dose should be started only when objective signs of moderate withdrawal are present generally 48 hours after last opioid use. For patients who are dependent on short-acting opioid products who are in opioid withdrawal, on day 1 administer an initial dose of 5 mg/0.5 mg buprenorphine/naloxone and titrate upward in 2 or 4 mg increments of buprenorphine at 2-hour intervals under supervision up to 8 mg/2 mg buprenorphine/naloxone film (or tablets) depending on control of acute withdrawal symptoms. On day 2, administer up to 16 mg/4 mg buprenorphine/naloxone as a single dose. The absorption of the naloxone is somewhat higher after buccal than after sublingual administration; it is necessary that the sublingual site of administration be used during induction to minimize exposure to naloxone, to reduce the risk of precipitate withdrawal. It is recommended that an adequate maintenance dose, titrated to clinical effectiveness, be achieved as soon as possible.

Maintenance

For maintenance, buprenorphine/naloxone film may be administered buccally or sublingually. The dosage of buprenorphine/naloxone film from day 3 onward should be progressively adjusted in increments/decrements of 2 mg/0.5 mg or 4 mg/1 mg buprenorphine/naloxone to a level that holds the patient in treatment and suppresses opioid withdrawal signs and symptoms. After treatment induction and stabilization, the maintenance dose of buprenorphine/naloxone is generally in the range of 4 mg/1 mg to 24 mg/6 mg per day depending on the individual patient and clinical response. The recommended target dose during maintenance is 16 mg/4 mg buprenorphine/naloxone per day as a single dose. Dosages higher that 24 mg/6 mg per day have not been demonstrated to provide a clinical advantage compared with lower dosages. Doses of 24 mg/6 mg per day should only be given in conjunction with a consultation with an addiction specialist. Once in maintenance, the prescription quantity for unsupervised administration needs to be considered with the patient's level of stability, the security of their home situation, and other factors likely to affect the patient's ability to manage supplies of take-home administration.

Method of Administration

Buprenorphine/naloxone is available in dissolvable tablets or in a dissolvable film. For sublingual administration, the film or tablet is placed under the tongue, close to the base on the left or right side. It must be kept under the tongue until completely dissolved. The tablet takes slightly longer than the film to dissolve. For buccal administration, place one film on the inside of the right or left cheek. Keep the film/pill inside the cheek until completely dissolved, usually in about 10 minutes. During this time, no food or beverages should be taken; nor should smoking occur. Oral ingestion of buprenorphine/naloxone has very poor absorption; however, it is more likely to cause gastrointestinal disturbances than sublingual administration does.

Clinical Supervision

Ideally, treatment is provided as part of a comprehensive treatment setting which includes therapy and should be initiated with supervised administration, progressing to unsupervised administration as the patients' clinical stability permits. Buprenorphine/naloxone is subject to diversion and abuse. Patients should be seen by the prescriber at reasonable intervals (i.e., at least weekly during the first month of treatment) depending on their individual circumstances. At no point should the patient be seen less frequently than once a month. Medication should be prescribed in consideration of the frequency of visits. Once a stable dosage has been found and patient urine drug screening does not indicate illicit drug use, less frequent follow-up visits may be appropriate. A once-monthly visit schedule may be reasonable in patients who are stable and making treatment progress.

Warnings and Precautions

Buprenorphine can be abused in a manner similar to other opioids. Significant respiratory depression and death have occurred in association with buprenorphine, particularly when taken by the intravenous route in combination with benzodiazepines or other central nervous system (CNS) depressants including alcohol. Consider dose reduction and avoid prescription of both CNS depressants and buprenorphine/naloxone. Buprenorphine needs to be stored safely out of the sight and reach of children because it can cause severe, possibly fatal respiratory depression in children. Neonatal opioid withdrawal syndrome is an expected and treatable outcome of prolonged use of opioids during pregnancy. Adrenal insufficiency has been reported with opioid use greater than 1 month. If diagnosed, treat with physiologic replacement of corticosteroids and wean patient off the opioid. Chronic administration produces opioid-type physical dependence. Abrupt discontinuation or rapid dose taper may result in opioid withdrawal syndrome. Liver function tests need to be monitored before initiation and during treatment to evaluate suspected hepatic events. Buprenorphine/naloxone should not be administered to patients with known hypersensitivity to buprenorphine/naloxone. An opioid withdrawal syndrome is likely to occur with parenteral misuse of buprenorphine/naloxone by individuals physically dependent on full opioid agonists, or by sublingual or buccal administration before the agonist effects of other opioids have subsided. Buprenorphine is not an appropriate analgesic; there have been reported deaths of opioid naïve individuals who received a 2-mg sublingual dose. Buprenorphine/naloxone products are not recommended in patients with severe hepatic impairment and may not be appropriate for patients with moderate hepatic impairment. Caution patients about the risk of driving or operating hazardous machinery.

Adverse Reactions

Adverse events commonly observed with the sublingual/buccal administration of buprenorphine/naloxone were oral hypoesthesia, glossodynia, oral mucosal erythema, headache, nausea, vomiting, hyperhidrosis, constipation, signs and symptoms of withdrawal, insomnia, pain, and peripheral edema.

Drug Interactions

Use caution in prescribing buprenorphine/naloxone for patients receiving benzodiazepines or other CNS depressants and warn patients against concomitant self-administration/misuse. Monitor patients starting or ending CYP3A4 inhibitors or inducers for potential over- or underdosing. Patients who are on chronic buprenorphine treatment should have their dose monitored if nucleoside reverse transcriptase inhibitors are added to their regimen. Monitor patients taking buprenorphine and atazanavir with and without ritonavir, and dose reduction of buprenorphine may be warranted. Concomitant use with serotonergic drugs may result in serotonin syndrome; discontinue buprenorphine/naloxone if serotonin syndrome is suspected.

REPORTS OF INTEREST

Buprenorphine in the Detoxification of Adolescents with Opioid Use Disorder

Marsch et al. (2005) conducted one of the first studies to use buprenorphine in opioid-dependent adolescents. Their study compared two groups of randomly assigned adolescents to receive a 28-day outpatient, medication-assisted withdrawal treatment with either buprenorphine or clonidine. Both treatment arms received medications (and placebo of other medication) along with participation in thrice-weekly behavioral counseling and incentives contingent on opiate abstinence. Participants who successfully completed detoxification were offered continued treatment with the opiate antagonist, naltrexone hydrochloride. The study had 36 youth aged 13 to 18 who were randomized to receive either buprenorphine or clonidine detoxification. Subjects in the buprenorphine arm received a flexible dose of either 6 mg or 8 mg of buprenorphine depending on their weight and opiate use history. Buprenorphine was then decreased by 2 mg every week. The clonidine group received transdermal clonidine patches 0.1 to 0.3 mg depending on withdrawal symptoms for the first 7 days. Patches were decreased weekly by day 21 and were replaced with a placebo clonidine patch. Urine specimens were collected 3 days a week and were tested for methadone, opiates, propoxyphene, cocaine, marijuana, and benzodiazepines. Blood alcohol levels were analyzed via a breathalyzer. At conclusion of the study, a significantly greater percentage of adolescents who received buprenorphine were retained in treatment (72%) than those treated with clonidine (39%; $P < .05$). Those in the buprenorphine group had a significantly higher percentage of scheduled urine drug test results that were opiate negative (64% vs. 32%; $P = .01$). All participants had relief of withdrawal-related symptoms and reduction in risky drug-related behaviors. Participants in the buprenorphine group reported more positive effects from the medication. At the conclusion of the study, 61% of those in the buprenorphine arm compared with only 5% of the clonidine arm initiated treatment with naltrexone.

Buprenorphine/Naloxone in the Treatment of Adolescents with Opioid Use Disorder

Woody et al. (2008) conducted a multicenter outpatient comparison trial of buprenorphine-naloxone used for extended 12-week treatment compared with short-term detoxification. The study was conducted at six sites worldwide. It was open to youth 14 to 21 years old, but was only able to enroll one 15-year-old and only 16% of the total number of participants (156) were under the age of 18. Participants were randomized to two treatment arms. The detox treatment arm received a maximum amount of 14 mg of buprenorphine per day, which was tapered off by day 14 of the study. Patients in the 12-week group received up to a maximum of 24 mg of buprenorphine per day. They began a taper at week 9 that ended at week 12. Patients were also enrolled in one individual and one group counseling session weekly. Primary outcome measures were opioid-positive urine drug tests at weeks 4, 8, and 12. Secondary outcomes were dropout from the assigned condition, self-reported use, injecting, other drug use, and enrollment in another treatment outside of the assigned condition. Follow-up visits were also conducted at months 6, 9, and 12, which assessed self-reported opioid use, alcohol, marijuana, and cocaine and injecting in the past month as well as determining whether participants were in other treatments. The study did not include enough patients younger than 18 to analyze separately. Overall, the patients in the detox group had higher proportions of opioid-positive urine test results. Sixty-one percent of the detox patients had positive results at week 4 compared with 26% of the buprenorphine-naloxone group.

At week 8, 54% of detox patients had opioid-positive urines compared with 23% of the buprenorphine-naloxone patients. At week 12, 51% of the detox patients had positive urines compared with 43% of the buprenorphine-naloxone group. The buprenorphine-naloxone group had significantly better treatment retention 70% compared with 20.5% in the detox group ($P < .001$). They reported less opioid use, less injecting, and less non-study addiction treatment. High levels of opioid use occurred in both groups at follow-up. Four of 83 patients who tested negative for hepatitis C at baseline were positive for hepatitis C at week 12; 6, 9 and 12 months' follow-up showed that the patients in the detox group had higher proportions of positive urine test results than in patients in the 12-week buprenorphine-naloxone group. Unfortunately, high rates of use were seen in both groups—83% of the detox group and 71% of the 12-week buprenorphine-naloxone group. The authors propose that this study shows the benefit of outpatient buprenorphine-naloxone treatment as a treatment option for opioid addicted adolescents.

Warden et al. (2012) did an analysis of the data set from Woody et al. (2008) to find predictors of attrition in opioid-dependent youth. They found that in the detox group, 36% left between weeks 2 and 4 at the end of their dose taper off buprenorphine, whereas the buprenorphine 12-week group lost only 8% by week 4. Retention in the buprenorphine 12-week group was associated with early adherence to buprenorphine/naloxone, early opioid-negative urines, use of any medication in the month before treatment entry, and lifetime non-heroin opioid use. Prior 30-day hallucinogen use was associated with attrition in this group. In the detox group, only use of sleep medications was associated with retention; but it was not an independent predictor. This suggests that patients with early nonadherence to medication or early opioid-positive urine in the first 2 weeks of treatment are groups in need of additional interventions to be retained in treatment.

Use of Buprenorphine/Naloxone for Long-term Outpatient Treatment in Adolescents

A retrospective case review was conducted by Matson et al. (2014) to examine treatment outcomes in young adults in an outpatient buprenorphine/naloxone clinic. The charts of 103 opioid-dependent adolescents were examined. Their opioid abstinence and compliance with buprenorphine/naloxone were assessed by urine drug screen at each visit. The mean age of the group was 19.2 years; 50.5% male and 98.1% White non-Hispanic. In this group, 31.9% were prescription opioid dependent. They found that overall rates of opioid abstinence and buprenorphine/naloxone were high (85.2% and 86.6%, respectively). They had 75% of patients return for a second visit. Patient retention was fairly poor, with only 45% still in treatment at 60 days and 9% in treatment at 1 year. They found that female sex ($P < .05$), negative UDS for opioids ($P < .001$) or tetrahydrocannabinol ($P < .001$), and positive UDS for buprenorphine/naloxone ($P < .001$) were associated with longer retention in treatment. This small study of one treatment center highlights difficulty in retaining patients in an outpatient buprenorphine/naloxone treatment program.

Mutlu et al. (2016) completed a retrospective case review of the outcomes of adolescents who were treated in a program that started with an 8-week inpatient treatment program where buprenorphine/naloxone was started followed by an outpatient treatment program where patients were monitored for a year. In contrast to Matson et al. (2014), in this study the addition of an inpatient treatment program had improved retention at 1 year, 24% compared with 9%. At the end of a year of treatment with buprenorphine/naloxone, only 9% had achieved abstinence.

Extended-Release Naltrexone/Vivitrol

Given that adolescents generally do not have a history of several years of chronic opioid dependence as adults do, many providers are hesitant to initiate use of buprenorphine. Hammond and Gray (2016) noted that opioid agonists are not considered the primary intervention in youths because of the stigma associated with medications that promote a prolonged state of physical dependence and concerns about the impact long-term maintenance of these medications may have on neuro-development. This may make the injectable extended-release naltrexone (XR-NTX) a more acceptable option for adolescents. In addition, XR-NTX does not require a special Drug Enforcement Administration which requires registration with the secretary of health. Any prescriber can write for it. XR-NTX is FDA approved for adults 18 years and over for alcohol and opioid use disorders. Oral naltrexone has been available for treatment for alcohol and opioid use disorders for years; however, in clinical practice, patients rarely adhere to taking their naltrexone daily and frequently relapse. XR-NTX has been developed as a monthly injection to improve patient adherence.

Dosage and Administration

It is recommended that patients be off all opioid-containing medicines (including tramadol, methadone, or buprenorphine) for 7 to 10 days before initiation of XR-NTX to diminish the likelihood of precipitation of opioid withdrawal. Patients transitioning from buprenorphine or methadone may be vulnerable to precipitated withdrawal for as long as 2 weeks.

Because the absence of an opioid drug in the urine is often not definitive proof that a patient is opioid-free, if there are concerns regarding occult opioid use, a naloxone challenge test can be performed.

A naloxone challenge test, administered by subcutaneous (SC) injection or an oral naltrexone challenge can be performed to assess physical dependence on opioids. These tests should not be performed on a patient showing clinical signs or symptoms of opioid withdrawal or on a patient whose urine drug screen tests positive for opioids. To perform an SC naloxone challenge test, administer 0.8 mg of naloxone. Observe for 20 minutes for signs or symptoms of opioid withdrawal (symptoms usually last 30 to 60 minutes if they occur). Monitor vital signs and observe the patient for signs or symptoms (usually lasting 30 to 60 minutes) of opioid withdrawal such as irritability, anxiety, agitation, runny nose, teary eyes, hot and cold sweats, goose bumps, yawning, muscle aches and pains, abdominal cramping, nausea, vomiting, and diarrhea. Be aware that in some patients taking buprenorphine, the naloxone challenge test may not be sufficient to detect occult buprenorphine use. In addition, urine drug screens may not be adequate to detect buprenorphine without a special requisition for this agent. In other settings, an oral naltrexone challenge can be completed. Initiate a test dose of 25 to 50 mg of oral naltrexone for 1 to 3 days. If on reassessment no withdrawal reaction has occurred, the clinician may then initiate the XR-NTX injection per protocol. In some clinical settings such as youth who are in juvenile justice facilities, there are no concerns regarding occult opioid use. The clinician may proceed to initiate the XR-NTX 380 mg intramuscular injection per manufacturer prescribing instructions.

Reports of Interest

Fishman et al. (2010) performed a retrospective case report of a series of 16 adolescents and young adults they treated for opioid use disorder with XR-NTX in an outpatient setting. Their group had an average age of 18.5 years, were 50% female and 94% Caucasian. The majority 12 of 16 used heroin and 11 of the 16 injected opioids. They had two patients drop out after the first injection, and 63% were retained in treatment for 4 months. The mean number of doses of XR-NTX received during the 4 months after initiation was 2.5. Besides, 75% received at least two doses. At the time of data analysis, 69% of the patients were abstinent or had substantial reductions in opioid use and 56% met criteria for a good outcome at

4 months. They had no reports of overdoses. This report suggests that XR-NTX is well tolerated in adolescents and has good outcomes in a community-based treatment setting.

MEDICATIONS USED TO TREAT CANNABIS USE DISORDER

Cannabis is the most commonly used illicit drug by adolescents in the United States. Its recent legalization in several states and approval for medicinal use has contributed to a perception among adolescents that it is safe. There are currently no medications FDA approved to treat cannabis use disorders (CUDs).

Reports of Interest

N-Acetylcysteine

N-Acetylcysteine (NAC) is a prodrug that is available as an over-the-counter supplement. Gray et al. (2012a) completed a double-blind trial of NAC in cannabis-dependent adolescents on the basis of its role as a modulator of intracellular and extracellular glutamate by way of the cysteine-glutamate exchanger. In their study, adolescents with CUD were randomized to receive a double-blind, 8-week course of NAC or placebo along with contingency management (CM) and brief weekly cessation counseling. Follow-up was conducted at 4 weeks and after the end of treatment, and urine cannabinoid testing was completed at all visits. They enrolled 116 subjects aged 15 to 21 years. The NAC was dosed at 1,200 mg twice daily. They found that participants receiving NAC had more than twice the odds when compared with those receiving placebo of having negative urine cannabinoid test results during treatment (odds ratio = 2.4, 95% CI = 1.1 to 5.2) Negative urine cannabinoid tests were achieved at 41% of the visits in the NAC group compared with 27% of the visits in the placebo group. End-of-treatment abstinence was achieved by 36% of the NAC participants and 21% of the placebo participants. Posttreatment follow-up abstinence rates were not statistically different, but the authors point out that the study was not adequately powered to evaluate this outcome. NAC was well tolerated with minimal adverse events. This study suggests that NAC may be safely and effectively used to increase cannabis cessation in adolescents enrolled in CM and a brief counseling intervention.

MEDICATIONS USED TO TREAT ALCOHOL USE DISORDERS

Alcohol remains a commonly used psychoactive substance by adolescents and adults in the United States. There are several medications approved for the treatment of adults with alcohol use disorders (AUDs) following detoxification from alcohol. Fortunately, adolescents who abuse alcohol often do not have enough years of use to have a need for medically assisted detoxification from alcohol. Readers are referred to adult literature on ways to manage alcohol detoxification when needed. There are no FDA-approved medications for the treatment of AUDs in children and adolescents.

Naltrexone (see Chapter 12, Other Useful Medications For Specific Conditions of Interest for detailed prescribing and pharmacokinetic information)

Reports of Interest

Naltrexone is an opiate receptor agonist that has shown efficacy in adults with AUD and is FDA approved for that use. It is not FDA approved for use in children. It has been evaluated in adolescent populations. Deas et al. (2005) conducted a 6-week open-label clinical trial of naltrexone in five adolescents seeking treatment for their AUD. Naltrexone was dosed in a flexible manner 25 or 50 mg daily depending on whether side effects occurred. Youth were assessed with the Adolescent Obsessive Compulsive Drinking Scale. Patients were monitored with liver function tests as naltrexone is metabolized by the liver. At the end of the 6 weeks, the average drinks per day decreased from baseline to the end of week 6 by 7.61 standard drinks. Subjects had a significant reduction in alcohol-related thoughts and obsessions. The authors are conducting a 12-week randomized placebo-controlled trial of naltrexone, the results of which have not been published. Another study examined the effect of naltrexone on adolescent alcohol cue reactivity and sensitivity in adolescents with AUD. Miranda et al. (2014) examined 28 adolescents who were heavy drinkers who were not seeking treatment for their AUD. They used a double-blind, placebo-controlled crossover design with randomization into a naltrexone condition and a placebo condition for 8 to 10 days with a washout period between conditions. Adolescents aged 15 to 19 were given 50 mg of naltrexone or placebo a day. Results showed that naltrexone use reduced the likelihood of drinking and heavy drinking ($P < .04$) and changed subjective responses to alcohol consumptions ($P < .01$). In this study, naltrexone was well tolerated by participants, blunted alcohol cravings in laboratory and natural settings, and was associated with a decreased likelihood of drinking on a study day and drinking heavily.

Disulfiram (Antabuse)

Disulfiram is an FDA-approved agent for the treatment of AUD in adults. It is not FDA approved for use in children or adolescents. It is known as an alcohol-sensitizing/aversive agent. It works by inhibiting alcohol dehydrogenase; this leads to a rapid increase in acetaldehyde when alcohol is consumed, resulting in aversive symptoms such as skin flushing, hypotension, reflex tachycardia, tachypnea, palpitations, anxiety, headache, nausea, and vomiting. Niederhofer and Staffen (2003a) completed a randomized double-blind, placebo-controlled study of the use of disulfiram in treatment-seeking adolescents aged 16 to 19 years. They enrolled 49 patients, and 26 completed the 90-day double-blind treatment. Participants underwent detoxification for alcohol withdrawal and were randomized to either disulfiram (200 mg/day) or placebo after 5 days of alcohol abstinence and then followed up weekly for 90 days. The mean cumulative abstinence duration was significantly greater in the disulfiram group than in the placebo group (68.5 vs. 29.7 days). Most of the patients who withdrew from the study did so because they relapsed. This occurred within the first 30 days of treatment. On day 90, two of the placebo-treated patients compared with seven of the disulfiram-treated patients had been abstinent continuously ($P = .0063$). Subjects tolerated disulfiram and reported few side effects.

Acamprosate (Campral)

Acamprosate is FDA approved for use in adults with AUD. It is not FDA approved for use in children or adolescents. It is an N-methyl-D-aspartate glutamate antagonist and reduces craving through mesolimbic dopaminergic effects. It is absorbed through the gastrointestinal tract and is not metabolized by the liver. The kidney is the route of excretion. Steady state is reached after 7 days. Only one study has investigated its use in adolescents. Niederhofer and Staffen (2003b) investigated it in a double-blind, placebo-controlled trial of 26 patients aged 16 to 19 years. In this trial, patients were randomly treated with acamprosate dosed at 1,332 mg daily or placebo for 90 days. Acamprosate was dosed two tablets in the morning, one at midday and one in the evening. Subjects were assessed at start and on days 30 and 90 by interview, self-report, questionnaire, and laboratory screening. At the end of treatment, the authors found that seven in the acamprosate group and two placebo-treated patients had been continuously abstinent ($P = .0076$). The mean cumulative abstinence duration was significantly greater in the acamprosate group than in the placebo group (79.8 vs. 32.8 days; $P = .012$).

MEDICATION-ASSISTED TREATMENT FOR ADOLESCENT SMOKING CESSATION

Smoking among adolescents is a considerable public health issue. Johnston et al. (2016), in monitoring the future national survey on drug use, reported that in 2015 about one of every three high school seniors reported ever having smoked a cigarette. Six percent (or almost 1 in 17 seniors) were regular daily smokers. Although this is a significant decrease over the past 20 years (from 28%), the Surgeon General in 2014 estimated that 5.6 million children alive in 2014 would eventually die early from smoking unless more is done to further reduce smoking rates among youth. These statistics make it clear that smoking-cessation interventions remain critical.

There are three FDA-approved categories of medications used to assist with tobacco cessation in adults: (1) various forms of nicotine replacement therapies, (2) buproprion SR, and (3) varenicline. The evidence for the use of these agents in adolescents is less clear.

Nicotine Replacement Therapies

Nicotine replacement therapy (NRT) provides the nicotine that would otherwise be delivered by smoking to reduce craving and withdrawal symptoms. It is available in different forms and dosages depending on the number of cigarettes smoked. Several products are approved for use in adults: nicotine patch (NP), nicotine gum (NG), nicotine lozenges, nicotine nasal spray (NNS), and nicotine inhaler. NP delivers nicotine through the skin in a steady dose and is available in 7-, 14-, and 21-mg doses worn over 24 hours or in 5-, 10-, and 15-mg doses in a 16-hour patch. NG and nicotine lozenges deliver nicotine through the oral mucosa at doses of 2 or 4 mg; smokers are advised to chew 1 piece every 1 to 2 hours, depending on the number of cigarettes smoked daily (maximum 24 pieces per day). NNS delivers nicotine through the mucous membrane of the nose. One dose is two sprays (one in each nostril), is equivalent to 1 mg of nicotine and one to two doses are recommended per hour (do not exceed 5 doses per hour or 40 doses per day). The nicotine inhaler comes in 10 mg per cartridge, dosing is 6 to 16 cartridges per day; it is inhaled using short puffing or sipping actions (Bailey, 2012).

Although each cigarette may contain between 8 and 20 mg of nicotine, the amount inhaled or absorbed is typically less than 1 mg per cigarette. It is recommended that if you smoke more than 11 cigarettes per day, the initial NP should be 21 mg and should be used for 4 to 6 weeks before tapering to the 14-mg patch for 2 to 4 weeks, then the 7-mg patch for 2 to 4 weeks. If you smoke 6 to 10 cigarettes per day, then start with the 14-mg patch for 4 to 6 weeks, then the 7 mg for 2 to 4 weeks. If you use the NG or nicotine lozenges and you smoke 20 or more cigarettes per day, start with the 4-mg product, and taper as comfortable. The NP, NG, and nicotine lozenges are available over the counter. The NNS and inhaler are available by prescription only.

Warnings/Precautions

Tobacco use must be stopped when initiating NRT to avoid nicotine toxicity. Product labeling instructs using caution with these products if a person is pregnant; if a person has an unstable coronary syndrome such as ischemia, arrhythmia, or angina; if the person has a peptic ulcer (using the gum or lozenges), or use under 18 years of age. Each type of NRT has some specific contraindications as well: for the NP, do not use if there is severe eczema or other extensive skin condition, for the NG do not use if there is temperomandibular joint or other jaw problems, dentures or other dental appliances, or if toothless. Lozenges are contraindicated with oral thrush or other oral lesions. NNS is contraindicated with rhinitis, nasal polyps, or sinusitis. Nicotine inhalers should not be used with asthma or allergy to menthol. Instructions are to stop using these products if a person experiences any of the following: nausea, dizziness, weakness, vomiting, and fast or irregular heartbeat.

Drug Interactions

Tobacco smoke contains polycyclic aromatic hydrocarbons, which are potent inducers of cytochrome P450 isoenzymes 1A1, 1A2, and, possibly, 2E1. Many drugs are substrates for these cytochromes and smoking results in clinically significant decreases in pharmacologic effects. Thus, active smokers may require higher doses of these drugs to achieve the same effects. After a person quits smoking, it is important to consider how quickly the induction dissipates, but drug doses that were raised to compensate for smoking will need to be decreased. Kroon (2007) described the drug interactions with smoking. There are pharmaco*kinetic* interactions that lead to reduced blood levels. The most common drugs affected by this process are caffeine, clozapine, fluvoxamine, olanzapine, tacrine, thiothixene, thioridazine, selegiline, duloxetine, clomipramine, chlorpromazine, asenapine, mirtazapine, and theophylline. Insulin peaks faster and reaches higher concentrations in smokers than in nonsmokers. There are also pharmaco*dynamic* drug interactions with smoking, primarily with hormonal contraceptives and inhaled corticosteroids. For women 35 and over who smoke 15 or more cigarettes daily, hormonal contraceptives are considered contraindicated because of the increased risk of serious cardiovascular adverse effects. The efficacy of inhaled corticosteroids may be reduced in patients with asthma who smoke. It is important to recognize that the pharmaco*kinetic* drug interactions are caused by the tobacco smoke and not by the nicotine. NRT does not contribute to these drug interactions. Pharmaco*dynamic* drug interactions are largely due to nicotine. Because it activates the sympathetic nervous system, nicotine can counteract the pharmacologic actions of certain drugs.

Faber and Fuhr (2004) studied CYP1A2 activity using caffeine clearance in 12 subjects who smoked 20 or more cigarettes daily. At steady-state reduction, CYP1A2 activity was 36.1%. The half-life of CYP1A2 activity after smoking cessation was 38.6 hours. The authors recommended a 10% daily dose reduction of CYP1A2 substrates until the fourth day following smoking cessation. This could be especially important if a smoker were hospitalized and abruptly quit smoking, or for drugs with narrow therapeutic windows such as theophylline. Although the study was done with heavy smokers, it is not known how the number of cigarettes smoked daily or interindividual variation might affect CYP1A2 induction.

Reports of Interest

There have been numerous small open trials of NRT in adolescent smokers, the earliest conducted by Smith et al. (1996) using NP. Rates of abstinence are typically quite low (<10%), but decrease in withdrawal symptoms and reduction in daily smoking was observed. Adverse effects reported were most commonly related to skin reactions.

The first randomized, double-blind, placebo-controlled study of NRT in adolescents was conducted by Hanson et al. (2003). Hundred participants received 10 weeks of NP or placebo patch, along with cognitive behavioral therapy (CBT) and a CM procedure. There were no significant differences between groups in biologically verified point-prevalence abstinence at 7 days or 30 days. The active NP group did report a lower craving score and a lower overall withdrawal symptom score.

Moolchan et al. (2005) completed a study that was a double-blind, double-dummy, randomized three-arm trial. There were 120 adolescent participants who reported smoking 10 or more cigarettes daily for more than a year and were motivated to quit smoking. Of these, 75% had at least one current psychiatric diagnosis. They were randomized to an NP with placebo gum, an NG with placebo patch, or a placebo NP and NG, with all participants receiving CBT. Abstinence was assessed through self-report and verified with exhaled carbon monoxide (CO) levels. Smoking reduction was assessed using thiocyanate concentrations. Intent-to-treat analyses showed CO-confirmed prolonged abstinence rates of 18% for the active NP group, 6.5% for the active NG group, and 2.5% for the placebo group. The difference between the active NP and the placebo group was statistically significant. Reductions in cigarette consumption were not statistically associated with treatment group assignment. At the follow-up 3 months after the study ended, there was sustained abstinence but not significantly associated with treatment group. Both the NP and the NG were well tolerated with adverse events similar to those reported in adult trials.

Rubinstein et al. (2008) conducted a pilot randomized trial of NNS in 40 adolescent smokers. Participants were assigned to either weekly group therapy for 8 weeks ($N = 17$) or 8 weeks of therapy plus 6 weeks of NNS. They were advised to use the spray whenever they had strong cravings (not to exceed 40 doses per day). There was no significant difference in biologically verified continuous abstinence (at least 7 days) between groups at the end of treatment (8 weeks). NNS use was low, with only 26% of participants reporting daily use of NNS during the first week, and only 46% still using it by the end of treatment. The most common side effects were nasal irritation and burning (35%), and complaints about taste and smell (13%).

Scherphof et al. (2014a) conducted a double-blind, randomized controlled trial of NRT with 257 adolescents. The initial study focused on the short-term efficacy of NP compared with placebo at 2, 6, or 9 weeks after their quit date. A continuation study that Scherphof et al. (2014b) later completed examined 6- and 12-month quit rates. One of the initial goals was to look at whether abstinence is moderated by compliance with the NRT. The initial study found that independent of NRT compliance at the 2-week point use of the NP predicted abstinence, but at the end of treatment this was true only in the high-compliance group. As with other studies, NRT was deemed safe and well tolerated in adolescence.

Bupropion Slow Release/Zyban

Buproprion is an antidepressant of the aminoketone class. It is chemically unrelated to tricyclic, tetracyclic, selective serotonin reuptake inhibitors, or other known antidepressant agents, often called an atypical antidepressant. It was approved in 1997 under the name Zyban as the first non-nicotine medication to aid in smoking cessation in adults. Bupropion is believed to inhibit the reuptake of dopamine, serotonin, and norepinephrine in the CNS and may also function as a nicotinic acetylcholine-receptor antagonist (Bailey, 2012).

Bupropion is available as an immediate-release, slow-release (12-hour), or an extended-release (24-hour) format. It is approved for treatment of major depressive disorder and seasonal affective disorder in adults.

See Chapter 8 Antidepressant Medications for detailed prescription information. Only Zyban is approved for smoking cessation in adults. It is available in 150-mg tablets. It is to be initiated 1 week before a chosen "target quit day" at 150 mg daily and increased after 3 days to 300 mg given as 150 mg twice daily. It should be continued for 7 to 12 weeks. Discuss discontinuing Zyban after 12 weeks if the patient feels ready, but consider whether the patient might benefit from ongoing treatment. Combination treatment in conjunction with NP may be prescribed.

Reports of Interest

Early studies of Zyban use for adolescents were open-label pilot studies and were underpowered. Upadhyahya et al. (2004) used Zyban in 16 adolescent smokers, 11 of which also had attention-deficit/hyperactivity disorder. They received bupropion SR for 6 weeks along with two smoking cessation counseling sessions. Analyses were conducted on participants who took at least one dose of Zyban during the study ($N = 15$). Of these, 31.3% were described as abstinent at 4 weeks, but end-of-study cessation at 6 weeks and biologic confirmation of abstinence were not well specified.

Niederhofer and Huber (2004) randomized 22 participants to receive 150 mg of immediate-release bupropion or placebo for 90 days. These participants underwent inpatient nicotine withdrawal treatment using NRT before the study. Those who achieved at least 5 days of abstinence were then randomized to one of the two study groups. All participants received psychotherapy. At 90-day assessment, continuous abstinence rates were higher in the bupropion group (55%) than in the placebo group (18%), and mean cumulative abstinence duration was higher in the treatment group versus the placebo group (78 ± 40 vs. 30 ±19 days, respectively). Interpretation of these results is difficult because the definition of relapse is not comparable to other study protocols and the level of CO used to confirm abstinence was not specified.

Killen et al. (2004) examined bupropion SR use in combination with NP. Adolescent smokers were randomized to receive 8 weeks on NP therapy and either 9 weeks of bupropion SR at 150 mg daily or placebo. All participants ($N = 211$) received group skills training sessions on a weekly basis. No statistically significant differences were found between treatment groups at the end of 10 weeks of treatment or at the 26-week follow-up; at 10 weeks, 28% of the NP + placebo group and 23% of the NP + bupropion SR group were abstinent. At 26 weeks, abstinence rates were 7% and 8%, respectively. The author noted that although abstinence rates were not significantly different, participants in the bupropion group who had a detectable level of bupropion metabolite at week 5 had significantly lower levels of smoking during treatment than did participants without a detectable level, suggesting that compliance may have had a significant effect on outcomes.

Muramoto et al. (2007) recruited 312 adolescents aged 14 to 17 who smoked six or more cigarettes per day, had an exhaled CO level of 10 ppm or greater, had at least two prior quit attempts, and no other current major psychiatric diagnosis. Participants were randomized in a double-blinded manner into three groups who received either bupropion SR 150 mg daily, 300 mg daily, or placebo for 6 weeks, plus weekly brief individual counseling. The main outcome measure was 7-day point-prevalence abstinence at 6 weeks and 30-day prolonged abstinence. CO levels were checked at every visit and abstinence was defined as <10 ppm. Urinary cotinine levels were obtained at weeks 2 and 6, with abstinence defined as ≤50 µg/L. Seven-day point-prevalence abstinence rates at week 6 were placebo 5.6%; 150 mg, 10.7%; 300 mg, 14.5% ($P = .03$, 300 mg vs. placebo). At 26 weeks, confirmed point-prevalence abstinence rates were placebo 10.3%; 150 mg, 3.1%; and 300 mg, 13.9% ($P = .049$). Confirmed point-prevalence rates were significantly higher for 300 mg than placebo at every week during treatment except week 4. Abstinence rates are lower than those for adults, with rapid relapse seen after medication discontinuation.

In 2011, Gray et al. studied bupropion SR and concomitant CM. In a double-blind, placebo-controlled design, 134 smokers aged 12 to 21 years who smoked at least five cigarettes per day, had urine cotinine levels ≥100 ng/mL, were not pregnant and willing to take birth control, lacked other substance abuse or dependence, had no history of serious psychiatric or medical illness, had no suicide attempts in the past year and no suicidal ideation in the past month, had no history of seizures or eating disorders, and were not taking any other pharmacotherapy for smoking cessation were randomized to receive a 6-week course of bupropion SR + CM, bupropion SR+ non-CM, placebo + CM, or placebo + non-CM, with final follow-up at 12 weeks. The 7-day point-prevalence self-report abstinence rates were confirmed with urine cotinine levels ≤100 ng/mL at weekly treatment visits starting at week 3 (following a 2-week grace period) and at the posttreatment follow-up visit. Combined bupropion SR + CM treatment yielded significantly superior abstinence rates during active treatment when compared with placebo + non-CM treatment ($P < .05$). This combination treatment appears to be efficacious in the short term for adolescent smoking cessation and may be superior to either intervention alone.

Varenicline (Chantix)

In 2006, the FDA approved varenicline as a prescription-only MAT for adult smoking cessation. It is a selective nicotinic acetylcholine-receptor partial antagonist that is thought to reduce the reinforcing effects of nicotine. Owing to its mixed agonist–antagonist properties, it is effective in relieving craving and withdrawal during abstinence, and blocking the reinforcing effects of smoking. Adult studies show that it has superior efficacy when compared with bupropion SR and NP, all of which are FDA approved for MAT for smoking cessation in adults. Although several studies have looked at NRT and bupropion use in adolescents, only two studies so far have looked at varenicline use in adolescents.

Varenicline is a biconvex capsular tablet: it is available in 0.5 and 1 mg. It should be taken orally after eating and with a full glass of water. Smokers begin varenicline 1 week before their quit date, titrating from 0.5 mg on days 1 to 3 to 0.5 mg twice daily on days 4 to 7. After the titration week, the recommended dose is 1 mg twice a day for 12 weeks. It is recommended that successful quitters continue taking varenicline for an additional 12 weeks to increase the likelihood of long-term abstinence. Patients who have trouble setting a quit date may begin taking varenicline and then quit smoking between 8 and 35 days after starting treatment.

Alternatively, those who are sure that they are not willing or able to stop smoking abruptly can start varenicline and reduce smoking by 50% in the first 4 weeks, then reduce by another 50% in the next 4 weeks, then continue reducing until they reach abstinence by 12 weeks. Continue treatment for another 12 weeks, for a total of 24 weeks. Patients who are motivated to quit but have been unsuccessful in the first course of treatment, or who have relapsed after treatment should be encouraged to make another attempt at treatment once factors that contributed to the failed attempt have been identified and addressed. If patients have significant adverse effects of varenicline, consider a temporary or permanent dose reduction.

Warnings/Precautions

Serious neuropsychiatric adverse events have been reported in patients being treated with varenicline, including changes in mood, psychosis, hallucinations, paranoia, delusions, homicidal ideation, aggression, hostility, agitation, anxiety, and panic, as well as suicidal ideation, suicide attempt, and completed suicide. These adverse events occurred in patients with and without preexisting psychiatric disease; some patients experienced worsening of their psychiatric illness. Some of these adverse events may have been worsened by concomitant use of alcohol. Patients should be instructed to stop varenicline and contact their health care provider immediately if agitation, depressed mood, or changes in behavior or thinking that are unusual for the patient are observed, or if the patient develops suicidal ideation or suicidal behavior. The health care provider should evaluate the severity of the symptoms and the extent to which the patient is benefiting from treatment and consider options including dose reduction, continued treatment with closer monitoring, or discontinuing treatment.

Although the FDA placed a black box warning on varenicline in 2009 on the basis of reports regarding neuropsychiatric adverse events, the warning was removed in 2016 following the outcomes in the EAGLES (Evaluating Adverse Events in a Global Smoking Cessation Study), completed by Anthenelli et al.

Along with neuropsychiatric warnings, caution should be used in patients with serious renal impairment, women who are pregnant or breastfeeding, and in persons under the age of 18. Seizures have been reported with varenicline treatment. Some patients had no history of seizures, whereas others had a history of seizures that was remote or well controlled. In most cases, the seizure occurred within the first month of therapy. There have been reports of patients experiencing a heightened effect of alcohol while taking varenicline, and was often accompanied by amnesia for the events. Patients should be warned to be cautious while driving or operating machinery because there have been reports of somnolence, dizziness, and loss of consciousness that resulted in impairment. Cases of sleepwalking have been reported. Hypersensitivity including angioedema has occurred. Serious skin reactions occur rarely, including Stevens-Johnson syndrome and erythema multiforme.

For patients with stable cardiovascular disease, there has been concern regarding the risks of varenicline causing cardiovascular serious adverse events (SAEs) such as myocardial infarction, stroke, sudden death, arrhythmia, congestive heart failure, and unstable angina. A number of studies have been done to attempt to clarify the issue: an initial meta-analysis by Singh et al. (2011) found that varenicline increased risk, but subsequent studies and further meta-analyses with larger populations have found either no significant difference in risk, or decreased risk with varenicline.

Adverse Events

In placebo-controlled premarketing studies, the most common adverse events associated with varenicline (>5% and twice the rate seen in placebo-treated patients) were nausea, abnormal dreams (vivid, unusual, or strange), constipation, flatulence, and vomiting.

Drug Interactions

On the basis of varenicline characteristics and clinical experience, varenicline has no clinically meaningful pharmacokinetic drug interactions. Specifically looking at the use of varenicline with other medication-assisted therapies for smoking cessation, varenicline did not alter the steady-state pharmacokinetics of bupropion or nicotine. Smoking cessation, however, with or without varenicline, may impact metabolism of certain drugs (theophylline, warfarin, insulin) for which dosage adjustment may be necessary (see more extensive discussion earlier).

Reports of Interest

Faessel et al. (2009) conducted a study to characterize pharmacokinetics, safety, and tolerability of varenicline in a multicenter, randomized, double-blind, placebo-controlled, parallel-group study. They enrolled 12- to 16-year-old smokers (≥3 cigarettes daily) into high-body-weight (≥55 kg) and low-body-weight (≤55 kg) groups. Subjects were randomized to receive 14 days of treatment with a high dose of varenicline (0.5 or 1 mg bid), a low dose of varenicline (0.5 mg BID or once daily), or placebo. Apparent renal clearance and volume of distribution were calculated. Adverse effects were monitored. The most common adverse effects were nausea, headache, vomiting, and dizziness. Adverse effect rates were significantly higher in the treatment groups than in the placebo group, but 92% were mild in intensity, and no subject discontinued the study because of adverse effects. Varenicline steady-state exposure in the high-body-weight group was similar to that observed previously in adults. The body-weight effect on varenicline pharmacokinetics, which resulted in higher exposure in the low-body-weight group, was adequately offset by administration of half the varenicline dose recommended in adults. The study did not examine varenicline's efficacy in helping adolescents become abstinent from nicotine.

Gray et al. (2012b) examined the use of varenicline and bupropion XL for smoking cessation in older adolescent smokers (ages 15 to 20). Treatment-seeking youth were randomized (double-blind) to varenicline (N = 15) or bupropion XL (N = 14), with 1-week titration and active treatment for 7 weeks. Structured safety, tolerability, and efficacy assessments (cotinine-confirmed 7-day point-prevalence abstinence) were conducted weekly. There were no SAEs; two participants discontinued bupropion XL due to adverse effects, and none discontinued varenicline. Over the course of treatment, participants receiving varenicline reduced from 14 ± 6 to 1 ± 2 cigarettes per day (four achieved abstinence). Those taking bupropion XL reduced from 16 ± 4 to 3 ± 4 cigarettes per day (two achieved abstinence). The difference between the two groups was not statistically significant.

Results of these preliminary studies support the feasibility and safety of conducting larger and adequately powered adolescent smoking cessation trials with varenicline.

CHAPTER 12

Other Useful Medications for Specific Conditions of Interest

RICK T. BOWERS AND ROBERT P. CUSSER

ANTIHISTAMINES

Diphenhydramine (Benadryl) and hydroxyzine (Atarax, Vistaril) are the antihistamines most frequently used in treating children and adolescents with emotional disorders. Chronologically, they were also among the earliest medications used in child and adolescent psychopharmacotherapy, and they remain among the safest medications ever employed.

Contraindications for Antihistamine Administration

Known hypersensitivity to antihistamines is a contraindication for their prescription.

Infants born prematurely and infants are especially sensitive to the stimulating effects of antihistamines, and overdose may cause hallucinations, convulsions, or death. Because antihistamines may be secreted in breast milk, nursing mothers should also avoid taking antihistamines.

Narrow-angle glaucoma, stenosing peptic ulcer, pyloroduodenal obstruction, and symptomatic prostatic hypertrophy or bladder-neck obstruction are relative contraindications. The anticholinergic effects of antihistamines and the additional atropine-like effect of diphenhydramine hydrochloride may cause drying and thickening of bronchial secretions; hence, they should be used with caution in patients with clinical symptoms of asthma or poorly controlled asthma.

Interactions of Antihistamines with Other Medications

Diphenhydramine and hydroxyzine have potentiating effects when used in conjunction with other central nervous system (CNS) depressants, such as alcohol, narcotics, nonnarcotic analgesics, barbiturates, hypnotics, antipsychotics, and anxiolytics.

Monoamine oxidase inhibitors prolong and intensify the drying effect (an anticholinergic action) of antihistamines.

Diphenhydramine Hydrochloride (Benadryl)

Diphenhydramine hydrochloride has been used for more than 50 years to treat psychiatrically disturbed children (Effron & Freedman, 1953). Although such use is still not approved for advertising by the U.S. Food and Drug Administration (FDA), it is reviewed here because some child psychiatrists continue to find it clinically effective.

Fish (1960) reported that diphenhydramine is most effective in behavioral disorders associated with anxiety and hyperactivity, but that it could also be useful in moderately (not severely) disturbed children with organic or schizophrenic (including autistic) disorders. A later study of 15 children, however, found no significant difference in behavioral improvement between diphenhydramine in doses of 200 to 800 mg/day and placebo (Korein et al., 1971).

Diphenhydramine is also effective as an anxiolytic, reducing anxiety before producing drowsiness or lethargy, in children up to approximately 10 years of age. However, it shows a marked decrease in efficacy when administered to older children; their response is similar to that of adults, with untoward effects of malaise or drowsiness. Therefore, for older children, diphenhydramine is useful primarily as a bedtime sedative for insomnia and/or nighttime anxiety (Fish, 1960).

Diphenhydramine has also been used to treat children with insomnia and/or children who wake up after falling asleep and have marked difficulty falling asleep again. Russo et al. (1976) compared diphenhydramine and placebo administered to 50 children, aged 2 to 12 years, who had difficulty falling asleep or problems with night awakenings. Diphenhydramine 1 mg/kg was significantly better than placebo in decreasing sleep-onset latency and decreasing the number of awakenings over a 7-day trial period. Total sleeping time, however, was not significantly increased. Side effects (SEs) were minimal.

Contraindications for the Administration of Diphenhydramine Hydrochloride

The administration of diphenhydramine is contraindicated in premature infants and infants.

Untoward Effects of Diphenhydramine Hydrochloride

The most frequent untoward effects are anticholinergic effects and sedation. Children do seem more tolerant of the sedative effects of diphenhydramine, but the clinician should still be alert to any cognitive dulling that may interfere with learning. Young children may sometimes be excited rather than sedated by diphenhydramine. It is cautioned that overdose may cause hallucinations, convulsions, or death, particularly in infants and young children.

Diphenhydramine Hydrochloride Dosage Schedule for Treatment of Children and Adolescents

- *Premature infants and infants below 20 lb:* The use of diphenhydramine is contraindicated.
- *Infants >20 lb (9.1 kg) and older children:* Administer initially a 12.5- or 25-mg dose and titrate upward with 12.5- or 25-mg increases for optimal response. A maximum dose of 300 mg/day or 5 mg/kg/day, whichever is less, is recommended. Maximum activity occurs in about 1 hour, and the effects last about 4 to 6 hours; therefore, the medication is usually administered three to four times daily. Young children appear to tolerate a higher dose per unit of weight than do adolescents and adults. Fish (1960) found a dose range from 2 to 10 mg/kg/day, with an average daily dose of 4 mg/kg, to be most effective in treating behaviorally disturbed youngsters.

Diphenhydramine Hydrochloride Dose Forms Available

- *Capsules:* 25 and 50 mg
- *Elixir:* 12.5 mg/5 mL
- *Injectable preparations:* 10 and 50 mg/mL

Hydroxyzine Hydrochloride (Atarax), Hydroxyzine Pamoate (Vistaril)

Hydroxyzine is an antihistamine that is absorbed rapidly from the gastrointestinal (GI) tract. Its clinical effects usually become evident within 15 to 30 minutes of oral administration. It has been used widely as a preanesthetic medication in children and adolescents because it produces significant sedation with minimal circulatory and respiratory depression. It also produces bronchodilation; decreases salivation; has antiemetic, antiarrhythmic, and analgesic effects; and produces a calming, tranquilizing effect (Smith & Wollman, 1985).

Use in Child and Adolescent Psychiatry

One manufacturer stated that "hydroxyzine has been shown clinically to be a rapid-acting, true ataraxic with a wide margin of safety. It induces a calming effect in anxious, tense, psychoneurotic adults, and also in anxious, hyperkinetic children without impairing mental alertness" (*Physicians' Desk Reference [PDR]*, 1990, p. 1858); this statement has been deleted from the more recent *PDRs* (PDR, 1995, 2000, 2006). Hydroxyzine is approved for the symptomatic relief of anxiety and tension associated with psychoneurosis and as an adjunct in organic disease states in which anxiety is manifested. Its efficacy for periods longer than 4 months has not been demonstrated by systematic clinical studies.

Although not specifically indicated in the manufacturer's labeling, the sedation caused by hydroxyzine (as with diphenhydramine) has been utilized in the short-term treatment of insomnia and frequent night awakening in children.

Untoward Effects of Hydroxyzine

The most common untoward effects of hydroxyzine are sedation and dry mouth.

Hydroxyzine Hydrochloride Dosage Schedule for Treating Children and Adolescents

- *Children below 6 years of age:* Medication should be titrated individually and administered four times daily to a maximum of 50 mg/day.
- *Children 6 years of age and older and adolescents:* Medication should be titrated individually and administered three to four times daily to a maximum of 100 mg/day.

Hydroxyzine Dose Forms Available

- *Tablets (hydroxyzine hydrochloride):* 10, 25, 50, and 100 mg
- *Capsules (hydroxyzine pamoate):* 25, 50, and 100 mg
- *Syrup (hydroxyzine hydrochloride):* 10 mg/5 mL
- *Oral suspension (hydroxyzine pamoate):* 25 mg/5 mL
- *Intramuscular injection (hydroxyzine hydrochloride):* 25 and 50 mg/mL

OPIATE ANTAGONISTS

Opiate antagonists have been investigated in the treatment of mentally retarded persons with self-injurious behavior (for review, see Sokol & Campbell, 1988) and in the treatment of autistic disorder. Deutsch (1986) has given a theoretic rationale for the use of opiate antagonists in the treatment of autistic disorder.

Naltrexone Hydrochloride (Trexan, Revia) and Monthly Injectable Naltrexone (Vivitrol)

Naltrexone hydrochloride is a pure opioid antagonist. It is a synthetic congener of oxymorphone without any opioid agonist properties and completely blocks or markedly attenuates the subjective effects of intravenous opioids and precipitates withdrawal symptoms in subjects with physical tolerance to opioids.

Pharmacokinetics of Naltrexone Hydrochloride

Naltrexone is almost completely absorbed from the GI tract and undergoes substantial first-pass metabolism by the liver to 6-beta-naltrexol. Peak plasma levels of naltrexone and 6-beta-naltrexol occur within 1 hour of an oral dose. Both compounds are biologically active and are excreted primarily by the kidneys. Serum half-life of naltrexone is approximately 4 hours and that of 6-beta-naltrexol is approximately 13 hours.

Contraindications for Naltrexone Hydrochloride Administration

The main contraindications are hypersensitivity, any liver abnormalities, and the concomitant use of any opiate-containing substances, legal or illegal.

Interactions of Naltrexone Hydrochloride with Other Medications

Serious adverse effects (e.g., a severe, precipitous withdrawal syndrome) may occur if naltrexone is administered to individuals taking opioids.

Indications for Naltrexone Hydrochloride in Child and Adolescent Psychiatry

Naltrexone hydrochloride is approved for the treatment of alcoholism and for the blockade of the effects of exogenously administered opiates. The safety and efficacy of injectable naltrexone have not been established in the pediatric population. The pharmacokinetics of injectable naltrexone have not been evaluated in a pediatric population.

Naltrexone Dosage Schedule

- *Children and adolescents up to 17 years of age:* Not recommended. Safety and efficacy have not been determined for this age group.
- *Adolescents at least 18 years of age and adults:* Usual recommended dose in the treatment of alcoholism or opioid dependency is 50 mg/day. (Read package insert carefully before using.)

Naltrexone Hydrochloride Dose Forms Available

- *Tablets:* 25 and 50 mg.
- *Injectable suspension:* 380 mg of naltrexone in an extended-release microsphere formulation for monthly injections.

Reports of Interest

Naltrexone in the Treatment of Alcohol and Opiate Substance Abuse Disorders

Refer to Chapter 11 on the off-label pharmacologic management of injectable naltrexone in adolescents with severe substance use disorders.

Naltrexone in the Treatment of Autistic Disorder

Campbell et al. (1989) administered naltrexone on an open basis to 10 hospitalized children aged 3.42 to 6.5 years (mean age, 5.04 years). The study lasted 6 weeks. Following a 2-week baseline, single doses of 0.5, 1, and 2 mg/kg/day were administered at 1-week intervals. Ratings were made 1, 3, 5, 7, and 24 hours after each dose and 1 week after the last dose. Subjects showed diminished withdrawal at all three dose levels. Verbal production increased at 0.5 mg/kg/day, and stereotypies decreased following the 2 mg/kg/day dose. Symptoms such as aggressiveness and "self-aggressiveness" showed little improvement. The major untoward effect was mild sedation, which occurred in 70% of the subjects. Laboratory measurements, including liver function tests and electrocardiograms (ECGs), showed no significant change from baseline. Overall, raters considered 80% of the children to be positive responders for some symptoms (Campbell et al., 1989).

Campbell et al. (1990) subsequently conducted a double-blind, placebo-controlled study of naltrexone in 18 children, aged 3 to 8 years, diagnosed with autistic disorder. The study consisted of a 2-week placebo baseline phase, random assignment to placebo or naltrexone for 3 weeks, and a posttreatment 1-week placebo phase. The initial naltrexone dose was 0.5 mg/kg/day; this was increased to 1 mg/kg/day, if no adverse effects occurred. Nine children received naltrexone; the optimal dose was 1 mg/kg/day. Six subjects receiving naltrexone were rated moderate (five) or marked (one) in improvement on Clinical Global Consensus Ratings, whereas only one child on placebo achieved a moderate rating and none was markedly improved. The difference was significant ($P = .026$). In contrast, no reduction in symptoms occurred on the Children's Psychiatric Rating Scale or Clinical Global Impressions (CGI) Scale. Naltrexone did not appear to affect discrimination learning in an automated laboratory. The authors also reported that overall symptom reduction seemed better in older autistic children than in younger ones.

Although there are case studies and open studies with some encouraging data, the 1993 report of Campbell et al.—an 8-week double-blind study in which 41 hospitalized children (2.9 to 7.8 years of age; mean, 4.9 years) diagnosed with autistic disorder were treated with naltrexone or placebo—did not support the efficacy of naltrexone in this population. All their subjects received placebo during the first 2 weeks while baseline data were obtained. Following this phase, subjects were randomly assigned to naltrexone or placebo for the next 3 weeks. During the final week, all subjects again received placebo. Twenty-three patients were assigned to the naltrexone group and 18 to the placebo group. The initial dose was 0.5 mg/kg/day of either placebo or active medication given in the morning; the dose was increased to 1.0 mg/kg/day after 1 week and maintained at that level because untoward effects were minimal and did not require a reduction in dose. Naltrexone did not improve the core symptoms of autism. The only significant finding was a modest decrease in hyperactivity on three different measures. It did not improve discrimination learning significantly more than placebo did. Naltrexone was no better than placebo in reducing self-injurious behavior, but six of eight subjects who had a severity rating of mild or above on the Aggression Rating Scale who received naltrexone experienced rebound (increase) in symptoms during the final placebo period; only one child in the placebo group exhibited worsening of self-injurious behavior during that time. The authors concluded that it remains to be determined whether naltrexone is efficacious in treating moderate-to-severe self-injurious behavior and that its use cannot be recommended as a first-line treatment for patients diagnosed with either autistic disorder or self-injurious behavior (Campbell et al., 1993).

In a 7-week, double-blind, placebo-controlled, crossover study, Feldman et al. (1999) evaluated the efficacy of naltrexone in improving communication skills, a core deficit, in 24 children (mean age, 5.1 years; range, 3 to 8.3 years) diagnosed with autistic disorder by *Diagnostic and Statistical Manual of Mental Disorders, Third Edition–Revised* (DSM-III-R) criteria (American Psychiatric Association [APA], 1987) who had previously shown modest behavioral improvement on naltrexone in previous studies by the authors (Kolman et al., 1995, 1997). Communication skills of the subjects at baseline ranged from preverbal to nearly normal for age. During the active medication phase, 1 mg/day of naltrexone was administered.

There was no significant improvement in communication skills with naltrexone treatment, including number of utterances, total number of words, number of different words, or reduction in echolalia in these subjects who had shown some behavioral improvement on naltrexone. Also, the authors reported that use of parental language with the patient did not change according to whether the child was receiving naltrexone. The authors suggested that medications that improve core deficits and target symptoms of autistic disorder should be preferred over those that improve only associated symptoms.

De Sousa (2008) conducted an open pilot study to evaluate the safety and efficacy of naltrexone in the management of 14 patients with childhood-onset trichotillomania. The mean age of the children was 9 years, and the mean age of onset of symptoms in the group was around 7 years. The children in the study were initially started on naltrexone at 25 mg/day for 1 week, and if tolerated well were increased to a maximum of 100 mg on the basis of symptom evaluation and response over a period of 2 weeks. Once enrolled into the study, the children were evaluated clinically using the CGI–Severity (CGI-S) for improvement every 2 weeks. Liver function was evaluated monthly for the first 2 months and every 2 months thereafter. A mean dose of 66.07 ± 22 mg/day naltrexone was well tolerated; 11 out of 14 (78.6%) subjects showed a positive response ($P < .0001$), and 3 of those responders reported no hair pulling at all. No abnormality in liver function was noted in the study. No adverse effects were reported by the children in the study.

BETA-ADRENERGIC BLOCKERS

Propranolol Hydrochloride (Inderal)

Although initially used primarily in controlling hypertension, angina pectoris, various cardiac arrhythmias, migraine prophylaxis, and other medical disorders, there has been considerable interest in the use of propranolol in general psychiatry.

Propranolol is a nonselective beta-adrenergic receptor-blocking agent with no other autonomic nervous system activity. Propranolol and other beta-adrenergic blocking agents reduce peripheral autonomic tone, thereby lessening somatic symptoms of anxiety such as palpitations, tremulousness, perspiration, and blushing. There is some evidence that the beta-adrenergic blocking agents significantly reduce these peripheral, autonomic, and physical manifestations of anxiety, but may not affect the psychological (emotional) symptoms of anxiety (Noyes, 1988). Noyes (1988) concludes from his review of the literature that beta-blockers are relatively weak anxiolytics compared with benzodiazepines and should be used for generalized anxiety disorder, primarily in patients for whom the use of benzodiazepines is contraindicated.

In adults, propranolol has been investigated in treating anxiety disorders, including generalized anxiety, performance anxiety (stage fright), social phobia, post-traumatic stress disorder (PTSD), panic disorder and agoraphobia, and episodic dyscontrol and rage outbursts (Hayes & Schulz, 1987; Noyes, 1988). It has also been used in treating schizophrenia. Propranolol is effective in the treatment of some antipsychotic-induced akathisias (Adler et al., 1986).

Pharmacokinetics of Propranolol Hydrochloride

Propranolol is almost completely absorbed from the GI tract. Peak serum values occur within 60 to 90 minutes; serum half-life is approximately 4 hours.

The manufacturer recommends using weight to determine propranolol doses for children, because this usually results in plasma levels comparable to those in the therapeutic range for adults.

The manufacturer notes that higher-than-expected serum levels of propranolol have occurred in patients diagnosed with Down syndrome (trisomy 21), suggesting that its bioavailability may be increased in such patients.

Contraindications for Propranolol Administration

Known hypersensitivity to propranolol is a contraindication.

Patients with bronchospastic diseases (bronchial asthma), cardiovascular conditions, diabetes, hyperthyroidism, or other medical disorders should have their medical status carefully reviewed (consultation with the physician providing care for the medical condition is recommended) before prescribing propranolol. Gualtieri et al. (1983)

have cautioned that propranolol is contraindicated in children and adolescents with a history of cardiac or respiratory disease, those who have hypoglycemia, or those who are being medicated with a monoamine oxidase inhibitor. Because significant depression has been reported as an untoward effect, propranolol is not recommended for children and adolescents who are already depressed.

Interactions of Propranolol with Other Medications

Propranolol may interact with many medications. Three interactions among those most likely to be seen in child and adolescent psychiatric practice are (a) if used concomitantly with chlorpromazine, plasma levels of both medications are increased over what they would be if used separately; (b) alcohol slows the rate of absorption of propranolol; and (c) phenytoin, phenobarbital, and rifampin accelerate propranolol clearance.

Untoward Effects of Propranolol

There are few reports of untoward effects in children or adolescents who received propranolol for psychiatric indications. Of greatest concern have been cardiovascular effects, which are detailed in the subsequent text. Propranolol has also been reported to cause significant depression of mood, manifested by insomnia, lethargy, weakness, and fatigue. Vivid dreams, nightmares, and GI symptoms have also been reported.

Indications for Propranolol Hydrochloride in Child and Adolescent Psychiatry

There are no approved uses of propranolol in psychiatrically disturbed children and adolescents.

Propranolol Dosage Schedule

- *Children and adolescents up to 17 years of age:* Manufacturer's recommendations for treating hypertension in this age group are an initial twice daily (bid) dose of 0.5 mg/kg followed by individual titration based on clinical response. Usual dose range is 2 to 4 mg/kg/day in two divided doses. Doses of >16 mg/kg/day should not be used.
- *Adolescents at least 18 years of age and adults:* Manufacturer's recommendations for treating hypertension are an initial dose of 80 mg daily in two divided doses followed by individual titration based on clinical response. The usual dose range is 120 to 240 mg/day. Some patients may require higher doses and some will need three-times-daily dosing.

Propranolol Discontinuation/Treatment Withdrawal

Because of the possibility of rebound in blood pressure, the dose of propranolol should be gradually tapered over 7 to 14 days when discontinued.

Propranolol Hydrochloride Dosage Forms Available

- *Tablets:* 10, 20, 40, 60, and 80 mg
- *Long-acting capsules (Inderal LA):* 60, 80, 120, and 160 mg

---

Reports of Interest

Propranolol in the Treatment of Children and Adolescents with Brain Dysfunction, Uncontrolled Rage Outbursts, and/or Aggressiveness

Williams et al. (1982) administered propranolol to 30 subjects (11 children, 15 adolescents, and 4 adults) with organic brain dysfunction and uncontrolled rage outbursts who had not responded to other treatments. The subjects had various psychiatric diagnoses, including 15 with diagnoses of both conduct disorder (CD), unsocialized, aggressive type, and attention-deficit disorder with hyperactivity; 7 with comorbid diagnoses of CD, unsocialized, aggressive type, and attention-deficit disorder without hyperactivity; 3 with CD only; 3 with intermittent explosive disorders; and 2 with pervasive developmental disorders. Thirteen had intelligence quotients (IQs) in the retarded range, and 8 had borderline IQs. The authors reported that 80% of their subjects demonstrated moderate to marked improvement on follow-up examination between 2 and 30 months (mean, 8 months) later. Optimal dosages of propranolol ranged from 50 to 960 mg/day (mean, 160 mg/day). All untoward effects were transient and reversible with dosage reduction. Most of the patients were additionally treated with other medication: 13 subjects received anticonvulsants; 6, antipsychotics; and 3, stimulants. Twenty-one had ongoing psychotherapy (Williams et al., 1982).

Kuperman and Stewart (1987) treated openly with propranolol 16 subjects whose mean age was 13.4 years (8 patients were 4 to 14 years old, 4 were between 14 and 17, and 4 were 18 to 24 years old). Seven subjects were diagnosed with CD, undersocialized aggressive type, five had infantile autism with varying degrees of mental retardation (MR), two had moderate MR only, one had borderline intellectual functioning, and one had attention-deficit disorder. All subjects exhibited significant physically aggressive behavior that had not responded adequately to behavior therapy and/or psychotropic medication. Propranolol was administered initially at 20 mg twice daily and increased by 40 mg every fourth day until symptom improvement occurred or standing systolic blood pressure fell below 90 mm Hg, diastolic blood pressure fell below 60 mm Hg, or resting pulse fell below 60 beats per minute. The average dose of propranolol was 164 ± 55 mg/day. Ten patients (62.5%) were rated moderately or much improved, depending on concurrence of ratings by parents, teachers, and clinicians. Responders and nonresponders did not differ significantly regarding age, sex, IQ, vital signs, or dosage. The authors noted that, although not significant, six of their eight patients who were mentally retarded responded favorably, which is consistent with earlier findings in adults that suggest that aggressive patients with suspected CNS damage respond best. Nonresponders as a group tended to develop bradycardia, which may have prevented them from reaching potentially therapeutic doses of propranolol. The authors additionally noted that before considering propranolol as a therapeutic failure, a patient should receive the maximum therapeutic dose tolerated for at least 1 month. When propranolol is discontinued, it should be tapered gradually over a 2-week period to avoid rebound tachycardia (Kuperman & Stewart, 1987).

Two 12-year-old boys treated with propranolol for episodic dyscontrol and aggressive behavior showed marked improvement (Grizenko & Vida, 1988). Dosage was initiated at 10 mg three times daily and was gradually increased to 50 mg three times daily.

Propranolol in the Treatment of Children Diagnosed with PTSD

Famularo et al. (1988) reported that 11 children (mean age, 8.5 years old) diagnosed with PTSD, acute type, had significantly lower scores on an inventory of PTSD symptoms during the period when they were receiving propranolol, compared with scores before and after the medication. Dosage was initiated at 0.8 mg/kg/day and administered in three divided doses; it was increased gradually over 2 weeks to approximately 2.5 mg/kg/day. Untoward effects prevented raising the dosage to this level in only three cases. Propranolol was maintained at this level for 2 weeks and then tapered and discontinued over the fifth week. The authors emphasized that their subjects had presented in agitated, hyperaroused states and that propranolol might be useful during this particular stage of the disorder (Famularo et al., 1988).

At present, although there are some encouraging initial data, the use of propranolol and the beta-blockers in children and adolescents must be further investigated. In particular, the use of propranolol in anxiety disorders remains to be elucidated.

Pindolol (Visken)

Pindolol is a synthetic, nonselective beta-adrenergic receptor-blocking agent that has sympathomimetic activity at therapeutic doses but does not possess quinidine-like membrane-stabilizing activity (package insert).

It is approved for use in treating hypertension, but its safety and effectiveness have not been established in children.

Report of Interest

Buitelaar et al. (1994a) conducted a double-blind, placebo-controlled comparison of pindolol and methylphenidate in 52 subjects (age range, 6 to 13 years) diagnosed with attention-deficit/hyperactivity disorder (ADHD). Treatment periods were of 4 weeks' duration. For the first 3 days, a morning dose of 10 mg of methylphenidate or 20 mg of pindolol or placebo was given. This was increased to 10 mg twice daily of methylphenidate or 20 mg twice daily of pindolol or placebo for the remainder of the period. Subjects were rated on various Conners' Scales by parents and teachers. After 4 weeks, teachers rated students receiving methylphenidate as significantly better on impulsivity/hyperactivity, inattentiveness, and conduct than subjects receiving either pindolol or placebo. Parental ratings did not show a significant difference between pindolol and methylphenidate on improvements in impulsivity/hyperactivity or conduct, although both were better than placebo. The authors thought that the main effect of pindolol was to improve behavioral symptoms and conduct and that the medication was only modestly effective in treating ADHD.

Untoward effects of pindolol were of particular concern and limit the potential usefulness of this medication in children. Paresthesias were reported in 10% of children during treatment with pindolol and none while receiving placebo or methylphenidate ($P < .05$). Although hallucinations and nightmares were not significantly more frequent in children on pindolol, they were of significantly greater intensity ($P < .01$) and caused so much distress that the children's daily functioning was affected adversely. These adverse effects totally remitted within 1 day of discontinuation of pindolol. The authors note that some children may be particularly sensitive to these distressing untoward effects, further limiting the usefulness of pindolol in ADHD and requiring the clinician to be very cautious whenever prescribing pindolol to children (Buitelaar et al., 1994a, 1994b).

BARBITURATES AND HYPNOTICS

At present, the barbiturates and hypnotics have little, if any, place in treating psychiatric disorders in children and adolescents. Today barbiturates, especially phenobarbital, are used in children and adolescents primarily for their antiepileptic properties. Behaviorally disordered children frequently may worsen when given barbiturates. As long ago as 1939, Cutts and Jasper administered phenobarbital to 12 children with behavior problems with abnormal electroencephalograms. Behavior worsened in nine (75%), with increased irritability, impulsivity, destructiveness, and temper tantrums. The authors concluded that phenobarbital was contraindicated in the treatment of such children. For sleep disorders, diphenhydramine and benzodiazepines, which are much safer to use, are now the medications of choice.

Clinically, barbiturates have a disinhibiting and disorganizing effect on many psychiatrically disturbed children, including the psychotic. Cognitive dulling, an untoward effect of barbiturates, is also of major concern in children and adolescents. In adults, phenobarbital was found to decrease speed of access to information in short-term memory, and short-term memory itself was highly sensitive to phenobarbital levels (MacLeod et al., 1978). The authors noted that this effect could impair the ability of children and adolescents to maintain attention in the classroom and interfere with their learning new information.

Clinically, it is also important for the child and adolescent psychiatrist to remember that phenobarbital may contribute to disturbed behavior in some patients with seizure disorder in whom it is being used to control seizures. This is also the case in some younger children when phenobarbital is being used prophylactically (e.g., after febrile seizures). Some such children may show behavioral and cognitive improvement when they are switched to other anticpileptic medications or when they are gradually tapered off medication after a sufficiently long seizure-free period.

SLEEP AGENTS

Many clinicians typically think of adults when discussing sleep disorders, but clinicians in the field of child psychiatry can attest that early, middle, and late sleep complaints from parents about their children is a common and often very concerning complaint that is presented in sessions. Indeed, pediatric sleep study programs are now common in pediatric hospitals. Owing to limited data regarding the use of FDA-approved adult sleep hypnotics in children, many pediatric clinicians initially utilize "natural" agents such as 3 to 9 mg of melatonin 45 minutes before bedtime or over-the-counter agents such as diphenylhydramine. Although these agents may be clinically useful for some, for many others the sleep complaints continue to be problematic and other agents are trialed. Clinical experience has led to the use of select antidepressants by clinicians in an attempt to address these sleep issues. Antidepressants are known to work through the modulation of monoamine neurotransmitters (NTs) including dopamine, norepinephrine, and serotonin (SER) as well as other NTs such as muscarinic acetylcholine (ACh), alpha-1-adrenergic, and histamine which are all known to effect sleep regulation, wakefulness, and sleep architecture. Norepinephrine and SER are involved in suppressing rapid eye movement (REM) sleep, whereas ACh has a role in the initiation of REM sleep.

Melatonin

Melatonin is an inexpensive and safe supplement for treating insomnia. Endogenously produced in the pineal gland, melatonin inhibits the ascending arousal system of the hypothalamus, the suprachiasmatic nucleus (SCN) "the master clock." Melatonin release from the pineal gland increases in the evening, reaches a maximum between 2 and 4 AM, and then slowly declines to lower daytime levels. Mouse models demonstrate that exogenous melatonin supplementation normalizes melatonin levels, whose production varies among individuals and decrease with age. Research by Rasmussen et al. (2003) indicated that melatonin restores serum leptin and insulin levels and suppresses intra-abdominal fat storage. Furthermore, it was found that the effects of melatonin on the SCN help minimize weight gain associated with second-generation antipsychotic (SGA) use by regulating body weight, energy balance, and metabolism. It was proposed that that with an elimination half-life of about 45 minutes, the lowest effective dosages would be in the range of 0.5 to 10 mg, taken 15 to 45 minutes before bedtime, although there is also evidence supporting that lower doses (0.3 mg) taken up to 3 to 4 hours before bedtime will be effective in entraining the sleep cycle.

Insomnia contributes to chronic health problems, including cardiovascular, metabolic, immunologic, reproductive, and psychiatric illness. Achieving insufficient sleep can increase the amount of the hormone *ghrelin* (appetite) relative to *leptin* (satiety), leading to increased hunger than when fully rested, which leads to higher peaks in blood glucose level, resulting in insulin insensitivity. Sleep deficiency impedes learning, growth, regulation of emotions and behavior and increases the risk for depression and suicide. If optimizing a child's sleep behaviors, for example, maintaining a consistent sleep time and stimulus control, is insufficient to improve rest, adjunctive pharmacologic interventions may be needed.

Clinical Fast Facts:
- Indications: early insomnia, jet lag, ↓SGA/lithium-related weight gain/triglycerides, suppresses intra-abdominal fat storage, anti-inflammatory, prolonged-release formulation (indicated >55 years old) may reduce HbA_{1c} in DM II.
- Take 0.5 to 10 mg 15 to 45 minutes before bedtime.

- Equilibrates ghrelin (appetite), leptin (satiety), and insulin levels
- Accumulative effect, no withdrawal phenomenon; not curative
- Prolonged-release melatonin minitablets seeking approval in 2018 for insomnia in autism

Hoebert et al. (2009) conducted a controlled, double-blind, 30-day crossover trial of placebo versus melatonin in 27 stimulant-treated children with ADHD. Melatonin 5 mg dosed 20 minutes before bedtime reduced sleep-onset latency by 16 minutes versus placebo (effect size 0.6), which increased at 90 days posttrial to 60 minutes (effect size 1.7). In a separate study, Weiss et al. (2006) concluded that the best results were apparent when melatonin was combined with improved sleep hygiene. Although the Hoebert et al. (2009) study supported the cumulative effectiveness of melatonin, a long-term ($\leq$3.7 years) follow-up study of 94 children with ADHD and chronic sleep-onset insomnia found that several years of melatonin treatment was not curative. Melatonin 3 to 6 mg was effective for sleep-onset insomnia in 88% and improved behavior and mood in 71% and 61%, respectively, with no serious adverse effect reported (Hoebert et al., 2009), but discontinuation often led to a relapse of sleep-onset insomnia and resuming melatonin treatment.

Wright et al. (2011) completed a double-blind, randomized, controlled crossover trial of 17 autistic children with severe dyssomnias refractory to supportive behavioral management, in which children were treated for 3 months with placebo versus 3 months of melatonin (10 mg maximum dose). The clinicians found that all the children treated with melatonin had significantly improved sleep latency and total sleep time compared to placebo, but melatonin did not influence the number of night awakenings.

Modabbernia et al. (2014) conducted an 8-week, double-blind, placebo-controlled study of 48 patients with first-episode schizophrenia, who were randomized to take either olanzapine with melatonin 3 mg or olanzapine with placebo. Interestingly, the melatonin group had significantly less weight gain, smaller increases in abdominal obesity, lower triglycerides, and a significantly greater reduction in Positive and Negative Syndrome Scale (PANSS) score, compared to that in the placebo group.

Romo-Nava et al. (2014) completed an 8-week, double-blind, placebo-controlled trial of patients diagnosed with schizophrenia ($N = 24$) or bipolar disorder ($N = 20$) that were treated with clozapine, quetiapine, risperidone, or olanzapine and then randomized to receive adjunctive melatonin 5 mg or placebo. The melatonin group had significantly less weight gain and reduced diastolic blood pressure. Wang et al. (2016) conducted a systematic review of melatonin, finding, in addition to preventing SGA-related metabolic adverse effects, that melatonin reduced weight gain associated with lithium usage. The review also detailed that melatonin has been found effective; in treating migraine headaches, jet lag, nicotine withdrawal, chronic fatigue, sleep rhythm disorders in the blind; and in enhancing cytokine release.

As a scavenger of both oxygen- and nitrogen-based radical species, melatonin is an attractive treatment option as well in diabetic insomniacs. A randomized, double-blind, crossover study by Garfinkel et al. (2011) of 29 adults with type 2 diabetes and insomnia, treated with 2 mg/day of prolonged-release melatonin for 5 months, demonstrated a significant reduction in HbA_{1c} of 0.66% $\pm$ 1.15%

Prolonged-release melatonin "Circadin" was introduced in Europe in 2007 for treatment of middle and late insomnia in adults 55 years and older, in whom melatonin production has diminished. Wade et al. (2010) observed its effect actually accumulated over time, with an increased effect and an additional 10% of responders at 90 days, with no withdrawal phenomenon.

Gringras et al. (2017) reported on prolonged-release melatonin minitablets (Ped-PRM) that were studied in 95 autistic children (96.8% autism spectrum disorders, 3.2% Smith–Magenis syndrome) in a 13-week double-blinded, placebo-controlled trial. PedPRM increased total sleep by 32 minutes, and decreased sleep latency by 25 minutes on average, over placebo, without causing an earlier wakeup time (number needed to treat [NNT] = 3.38). PedPRM successfully completed a phase 3 clinical trial; and a long-term, 78-week efficacy and safety trial will be completed in 2018, with regulatory submissions currently under way—stay tuned.

Trazodone

Although not FDA approved as a sleep hypnotic for pediatrics or adults, low-dose trazodone used as a hypnotic may be the most common off-label use of any psychotropic. Trazodone is an example of what psychopharmacologists refer to as a dose-dependent "multifunctional medication"—a medication that has more than one therapeutic mechanism. Trazodone at low dosages of 25 to 150 mg has hypnotic actions due to total blockade of $5\text{-}HT_{2A}$ receptors as well as alpha-1-adrenergic receptors and H_1 receptors to a significant but lesser degree. Low-dose trazodone seems to not only promote sleep onset but also aid sleep maintenance. Trazodone was compared with the sedating tricyclic antidepressant trimipramine in a small, double-blind crossover study in six healthy young men. Only trazodone significantly increased deep sleep without otherwise altering the normal architecture of sleep (Ware & Pittard, 1990).

At high dosages of 300 to 450 mg, trazodone is a strong SER transporter inhibitor in addition to the aforementioned SER receptor blocker activity resulting in unique antidepressant actions.

The immediate-release formulation at low dosages is the preferred trazodone agent for hypnotic usage. A new controlled-release formulation, Trazodone ER (Oleptro), is designed to avoid sedation and improve tolerability when used as an antidepressant would theoretically be less useful as a hypnotic. There are surprisingly few controlled studies on the efficacy of trazodone for improving sleep onset and sleep architecture, and potential bothersome SEs include sedation, dizziness, and psychomotor impairment. A well-known but rare SE associated with trazodone is priapism, which should be discussed with patients for early identification. There is some evidence of tolerance associated with chronic usage. Although at times one hears of street abuse of trazodone, typically trazodone does not cause dependence and its relatively short half-life makes it attractive as a sleep hypnotic.

Prazosin

As stated, alpha-1-adrenergic antagonist agents are known to affect sleep regulation, wakefulness, and sleep architecture. Clinical experience has led to the use of these agents in alleviating nightmares, a feature of REM disruption, and other sleep disruptions associated with trauma and PTSD. More recent clinical research into the use of the antihypertensive agent prazosin to alleviate nightmares and sleep disruptions such as insomnia in U.S. military personnel deployed in Afghanistan and Iraq has been ongoing and supports the prior clinical usage of such agents for sleep complaints in patients undergoing trauma. In a small study of 34 veterans, prazosin corrected dream characteristics typical of trauma-related nightmares to those more typical of normal dreams (Raskind et al., 2007). In animal models, prazosin protects REM sleep from disruption by adrenergic agonists, which has clinical relevance in PTSD models and in regard to medications used in psychiatry.

Typically, clinicians may start with 0.5 mg for smaller children or 1 mg for larger children 1 hour before bedtime. Positive efficacy is usually evident in the first night or two. In most cases, an increase in dosage will be needed, but the majority of patients respond to 5 mg or less. Rare cases may require dosing up to 10 mg in the evening. Prazosin has a fairly short half-life of 2 to 3 hours, but daytime flashbacks may be significantly reduced even when bedtime-only dosing is implemented. Occasionally, these persistent flashbacks may require an additional morning dose. Prazosin is an antihypertensive, and thus a baseline blood pressure (BP) and heart rate is recommended as well as follow-up assessments at each visit. If dosing is gradual, SEs such as hypotension and lightheadedness should be minimal. Baseline ECG monitoring may be indicated because polypharmacy is not uncommon in such a patient population.

Doxazosin

Because patients undergoing trauma and PTSD often have symptoms during the day as well as at night, investigators and clinicians have begun to utilize other longer acting formulations of alpha-1 antagonists to address these issues as well as minimize the need for slower titration and SEs of drowsiness or dizziness that may occur when initiating agents such as prazosin with its short half-life. A controlled extended release (XL) formulation of the selective alpha-1 antagonist antihypertensive medication doxazosin (Cardura XL) has a half-life of 16 to 30 hours. In a small open-label study utilizing subjective sleep measures, 12 adult patients with PTSD initiated at 4 mg for 4 weeks and increased to 8 mg thereafter showed statistically significant benefit in PTSD scale symptoms of recurrent distressing dreams and difficulty falling or staying asleep (de Jong et al., 2008). Placebo-controlled trials will need to be conducted to confirm the efficacy of this agent in PTSD.

OBESITY IS A HUGE PROBLEM IN PSYCHIATRY

Obesity in our current culture is occurring at an alarming rate, with some estimates that more than 50% of the American population is overweight or obese. In fact, obesity in the pediatric population is at such a staggering level that this generation will reportedly be the first generation to not outlive the lifespan of their parents. A poor diet coupled with a sedentary lifestyle often associated with excessive TV watching and video game watching is far too common for many teenagers, especially males. Given this scenario, it is understandable that the utilization of atypical antipsychotics for the treatment of mental health conditions in the present pediatric population is fraught with potential health-related perils. Most SGA and third-generation antipsychotics/mood stabilizers (TGAs) as well as the first-generation antipsychotics (FGAs) can cause weight gain. Weight gain can lead to decreased adherence to treatment and consequently increase the risk of psychotic or mood stability relapse in addition to the associated increased risks of diabetes and cardiovascular disease. Antipsychotics exhibit variability in the amount of weight gain and diabetic/metabolic risk they may impose on a given patient (see Table "Risk of Weight Gain/Metabolic/Diabetes/Prolactin/QTc Issues with Atypical Antipsychotic/Mood Stabilizer Medications on page 153 in Chapter 7). Olanzapine and clozapine definitely increase the risk for diabetes. The association of diabetes with risperidone and quetiapine is probable, whereas the experience with aripiprazole and ziprasidone thus far does not indicate an increased risk of diabetes (Newcomer, 2007). The more recently released SGAs (paliperidone, asenapine, iloperidone, and lurasidone) and the TGA (cariprazine) appear to fall in the area between aripiprazole and ziprasidone in regard to their risk for weight gain and metabolic issues. The following is a summary representation and approximation of the risk of weight gain for the currently available SGAs and TGAs in the United States.

Weight gain risk: (high) clozapine/olanzapine > (moderate) quetiapine/risperidone > (low to moderate) paliperidone/aripiprazole/asenapine/iloperidone > (low) lurasidone/cariprazine > (none to low) ziprasidone.

Although it is clear that there is no "magic potion" or pill that produces long-term weight loss, it is much more accepted now that there are medical interventions in addition to lifestyle changes involving diet and exercise that may have potential in maintaining a healthy weight; and the most promising options are discussed.

Weight-Control Agents

Topiramate

Topiramate was approved by the FDA in 1996 as an add-on treatment for treatment-resistant partial seizures in adults and pediatric seizures in children above the age of 2 years, and more recently for migraine headache prophylaxis in adults. In fact, it is presently the most prescribed medication for migraines in adults because of its efficacy and overall very tolerable side-effect profile. Topiramate does have potential noteworthy SEs, however. The anorectic and cognitive-blunting SEs of topiramate in particular have been well known for years to neurologists prescribing this medication in the pediatric population for seizure control. It was a logical corollary, therefore, for clinicians to trial topiramate in overweight patients, but this intervention in isolation has found limited success (Faulkner et al., 2007). In July 2012, the FDA approved three different formulations of a combination agent of topiramate combined with an extended-release formulation of the stimulant appetite-suppressant phentermine (called Qsymia) as an addition to a reduced-calorie diet and exercise for chronic weight management in adults. The patients must qualify to meet criteria for obesity with either a body mass index (BMI) of at least 30 kg/m^2 or a BMI of 27 plus a comorbid condition such as type 2 diabetes. At 56 weeks, 39% of patients taking the upper strength (phentermine 15 mg/topiramate 92 mg) of (Qsymia) + lifestyle modification achieved the composite goal of a >5% weight loss from baseline, an HbA$_{1c}$ level lower than 6.5%, and a systolic BP lower than 130 mm Hg versus 12% of patients on lifestyle modification + placebo. When looking at a goal of >10% weight loss, 31% of patients on the upper strength dose achieved this goal versus only 4% of controls—medication + lifestyle modification was approximately eightfold more effective than lifestyle modification alone.

Although the combination agent of topiramate and an extended-release formulation of phentermine is currently approved only for adults, there is an extensive history of topiramate usage in pediatrics with much relevant data available about its SE profile in the pediatric population. The use of topiramate for weight loss in pediatrics is an off-label use; but given the problem of childhood obesity and the propensity of most atypical and antiepileptic mood stabilizers to cause weight gain, topiramate is popular in child psychiatry as an add-on medication for weight loss in dosages typically in a range of 100 to 400 mg/day. Topiramate has mild CNS SEs overall, such as fatigue, somnolence, dizziness, ataxia, irritability, altered taste sensation, renal stones, glaucoma, and mental slowing that appear to be titration and dose related. This mental-slowing SE actually only occurs infrequently, but is well known to clinicians and is often referred to as "topadope" or "topadumb," because when present can be quite impairing to the patient. Sometimes, this bothersome SE can be alleviated by dose lowering or by its own resolution over a period of weeks to months if manageable. Many of these SEs are minimized by slow weekly titration. Monotherapy of topiramate should be titrated rather slowly, starting at 25 to 50 mg/day for the first week and increasing 50 mg/week utilizing bid dosing up to 100 to 200 mg/day depending on effect and tolerability. For larger children/adolescents who are not experiencing benefit and without SEs, subsequent 50-mg increases per week up to an efficacious dosage of 400 mg/day are reasonable. A bid dosing may be utilized, and most patients respond to dosages of 400 mg/day or less for weight loss (dosages as high as 1,600 mg have been used in adults for seizures). There are other potential concerning psychiatric SEs such as depression and psychosis, which may occur early or after years of treatment. If the overweight patient has ADHD and is treated with a stimulant, one can expect an augmenting anorectic effect to topiramate when used in combination. The medication did poorly in trials as a mood stabilizer, but is still used occasionally as a mood stabilizer in refractory affective disorders. It has also been proposed for use in bulimia nervosa and in chronic pain syndromes, but studies are very limited.

Metformin

Metformin (MFN) is another medication that may be utilized in the battle to combat weight gain with psychotropics and the subsequent development of metabolic syndromes.

MFN is indicated as an adjunct to diet and exercise to improve glycemic control in adults and children with type 2 diabetes mellitus. Promising evidence indicates that

MFN alone and in combination with lifestyle changes is superior to lifestyle changes alone or placebo. MFN has been effective in reducing weight in youth taking SGAs.

MFN is an oral type 2 diabetes medication that decreases intestinal absorption of glucose, reduces glucose production in the liver, and increases insulin receptor sensitivity in muscle and adipose tissue, which leads to decreased appetite, increased glucose uptake by muscles, and less lipolysis. Obese individuals with type 2 diabetes may also expect weight loss. There is some evidence that MFN reduces cholesterol, low-density lipoprotein (LDL), triglycerides, and increases in high-density lipoprotein (HDL), although not until insulin sensitivity increases (up to 6 months after initiating MFN). MFN's lipid lowering effect is less robust than that of diet, plant stanols/sterols, and statins.

MFN is a first-line treatment for type 2 diabetes in children $\geq$10 years and adults. It is manufactured in tablet and liquid forms; and as Handen et al. (2017) concluded, it may be relatively safe to use in children as young as 6 years old. Unlike other anti-hypoglycemics, MFN does not induce hypoglycemia and may have fewer adverse effects than does fluoxetine, bupropion, topiramate, and fenfluramine used for weight loss. Per the Endocrine Society Pediatric Obesity Guidelines, MFN is not indicated for weight loss in those not taking an SGA.

Metabolic derangement in those treated with antipsychotics is postulated to result either from diets with an excessive caloric intake (positive feedback of decreasing insulin sensitivity, decreasing lipid metabolism causing weight gain), or a diet of foods with elevated glycemic index (carbohydrates that rapidly metabolize causing serum sugar spike). Compounding poor diet and low exercise, there are other risk factors for diabetes that are present in the general population. Some of these additional risk factors may include patients treated with antipsychotics, specific food preferences such as a diet of only macaroni-and-cheese and an avoidance of activity in autism, amotivation in depression, pretreatment genetic vulnerability for insulin resistance in schizophrenia, and natural vulnerability of adolescence to insulin resistance and weight gain. Antipsychotics may further enhance appetite and sedation, as well as directly dysregulate hormonal control of insulin. A family history of type 2 diabetes, polycystic ovarian syndrome, male-pattern baldness, and obesity are additional risk factors.

It is recommended to start MFN to prevent weight gain in patients who are treated with antipsychotics in whom behavioral modifications have failed, and consider starting MFN at time of initiating antipsychotic treatment in patients at high risk of metabolic syndrome. Baseline health screening for diabetes in pediatric population in psychiatric clinics includes complete blood count (CBC) with differential, electrolytes and fasting glucose, lipids, insulin level (poor prognosis with early elevations), HbA$_{1c}$, pregnancy testing, and renal function testing with blood urea nitrogen (BUN)/creatinine (Cr) and urinalysis (UA).

An effective dosing strategy utilized by Walkup et al. (2017) for antipsychotic-related obesity in 6- to 9-year-old children is to start MFN 250 mg at dinner for 1 week, then 250 mg bid for 1 week, and then 500 mg bid thereafter. For youth 10 to 17 years old, clinicians may increase to 850 mg at week 4, with peak dose ~1,000 mg bid. MFN is FDA approved in 10- to 18-year-olds, starting at 500 mg once-a-day, and then increasing to 500 mg/day every 1 to 2 weeks as tolerated. The recommended maximum dose is 2,000 mg/day.

Twenty percent of patients will not tolerate the initial SEs of MFN, but the adverse effects can resolve with time; so rechallenge MFN if possible. There is an 18% absolute risk of nausea and diarrhea; also flatulence, metallic taste, and very rarely lactic acidosis. One can improve tolerance by titrating slowly, using generic metformin ER (Glucophage XR), dosing with meals, and beginning the first dose in the evening. In a well-known study by Knowler et al. (2002), "Reduction in the Incidence of Type II Diabetes with Lifestyle Intervention or Metformin," the incidence of diabetes was reduced by 58% with an intense lifestyle intervention of diet, exercise, and weight loss alone versus 31% with MFN, as compared with placebo. Compared to placebo, MFN treatment caused a 37.1% increase in GI symptoms, whereas lifestyle modification resulted in a 17.8% decrease in GI symptoms. This appears to be strong evidence that the combination of MFN with lifestyle changes is superior to either treatment in isolation. It is recommended to discontinue MFN only when the patient is able to address dietary and lifestyle factors and to expect rebound weight gain upon discontinuation.

Clinical Fast Facts of Metformin:
   Indications: DM II; weight gain from SGAs if failed exercise/diet
   ↓Glucose absorption in GI, ↓hepatic gluconeogenesis, ↑insulin sensitivity

   May improve lipid profile after 6 months

   Does not cause hypoglycemia

   CBC, fasting glucose/lipids, electrolytes, insulin level, HbA_{1c}, hCG, BUN/Cr, UA
   Start 250 mg q dinner × 1 week → 250 mg bid × 1 week → 500 mg bid; 10- to 17-year-olds at week 4 ↑850 mg, maximum 1,000 mg bid

   Adverse effects are time limited: nausea, diarrhea; flatulence, metallic taste, lactic acidosis very rare.

   Improve tolerance: titrate slowly, use MFN ER, dose w/meals, first dose in evening.

   MFN + dietary changes + exercise = most effective for weight loss.

The dosages used in these predominantly adult studies for weight loss vary across the adult FDA-recommended dosage range of 500 to 2,550 mg in two or three divided doses. In children aged 10 to 16 years, the maximal dosage is 2,000 mg in divided dosages. There are no clear established dosing recommendations thus far for the purpose of weight loss in adults or pediatrics.

After reviewing the literature, Schumann and Ewigman (2008) recommend initiating MFN 250 mg three times a day, along with lifestyle modifications, to promote weight loss and decrease insulin resistance in patients who gain more than 10% of their pretreatment body weight on antipsychotic medications.

The Klein et al. (2006) pediatric study initiated MFN 500 mg with the evening meal for 1 week, and then increased to 500 mg bid with meals for a week before titrating to a target dosage of MFN 850 mg bid dosed with meals at week 3. It would appear to be a safe strategy to initiate low dosing in a bid or tid manner and titrate to effect in weekly increments of no more than 500 mg/week.

Contraindications

MFN should not be prescribed to patients with serum creatinine concentrations of more than 1.5 mg/dL or those with unstable heart failure, because of the risk of lactic acidosis.

An early review of the literature by Faulkner et al. (2007) looking at interventions such as MFN to reduce weight gain in schizophrenics was disappointing in outcome measures. However, a more recent study from China by Wu et al. (2008), which was a well-designed, randomized controlled trial (RCT) conducted in 128 adults aged 18 to 45 with a first psychotic episode of schizophrenia, is more encouraging. To enter the study, patients had to have gained more than 10% of their pretreatment body weight during the first year of treatment with an antipsychotic medication (clozapine, olanzapine, risperidone, or sulpiride [not approved for use in the United States]). Unfortunately, patients with diabetes, cardiovascular disease, liver or renal dysfunction, substance abuse, or psychiatric diagnoses other than schizophrenia were excluded. This patient group was then randomized to one of four groups for the 12 weeks of the study:

   MFN alone, 250 mg three times daily
   Placebo alone
   Lifestyle intervention plus MFN
   Lifestyle intervention plus placebo

Interested readers can read the full details, but the summary results evidenced that participants in all three intervention groups showed significant decreases in the mean fasting glucose, insulin levels, and insulin resistance index. Compared with baseline, weight decreased by 4.9% in the MFN-only group and by 2.2% in the lifestyle-only group. The best result was observed in the lifestyle changes plus MFN cohort, where weight decreased by 7.3%. In the placebo group, weight increased by 4.8%.

In an actual pediatric study, Klein et al. (2006) conducted a randomized placebo-controlled trial of MFN titrated weekly up to 850 mg/day dosed with meals in 39 children aged 10 to 17 whose weight had increased more than 10% on atypical antipsychotic therapy. The children treated with placebo gained a mean of 4 kg and increased their mean BMI by 1.12 kg/m^2 during 16 weeks of treatment, whereas those in the MFN group did not gain weight and decreased their mean BMI by 0.43 kg/m^2.

Shin et al. (2009) conducted a 12-week, open-label trial to evaluate MFN's effectiveness and safety for weight management as monotherapy. Eleven subjects, aged 10 to 18 years, participated in the study. Patients were instructed not to change their baseline diet or activity level during the study. Each subject was initiated with MFN at 500 mg/day for 1 week and then titrated in increments of 500 mg/week as tolerated up to a target dose of 2,000 mg/day. Primary outcome measures included weight, BMI, and waist circumference, with secondary outcome measures assessing serum glucose, insulin, and fasting lipid profile. The authors were disappointed that the mean reduction in weight, waist, BMI, serum glucose, and serum insulin was not statistically significant. However, 5 out of 11 patients lost weight (mean, -2.82 kg $\pm$ 7.25), and overall the sample did not continue to gain weight. Notably, MFN did not improve insulin sensitivity and showed a trend toward increasing both LDL and cholesterol. Triglyceride levels did improve. MFN was fairly well tolerated with the following SEs reported in order of decreasing frequency: decreased appetite, irritability, constipation, decreased attention, drowsiness, anxiety, abnormal taste, and musculoskeletal pain. This study requested subjects not to change their diets or energy levels, which may have accounted for subpar results. This med-only intervention with MFN supports the need for a comprehensive approach to significant weight loss.

Handen et al. (2017) studied a modest sample of 6- to 17-year-old children diagnosed with autism, treated with antipsychotics ($\geq$85th percentile BMI for age, >5% annual weight increase since starting antipsychotics), who were randomized in a 16-week trial to MFN versus placebo. There was also a 16-week open-label extension to assess metabolic, weight, and tolerability of MFN. Results showed that patients on MFN during the closed-label trial lost weight, but there were no changes in metabolic parameters. In the 16-week open extension, participants initially on MFN maintained their weight loss, whereas those transitioned from placebo to MFN experienced weight loss and had a lowering of their HbA$_{1c}$, with otherwise unchanged metabolic parameters. It appears that a combination of MFN, dietary changes, and an exercise regimen for patients treated with antipsychotics will be the most effective means of effecting and maintaining weight loss.

The short story about MFN is that as monotherapy it may help minimize the trajectory of weight gain, but the weight loss is usually less than that with topiramate. However, before adding topiramate or MFN to help with weight loss, clinicians may consider switching from a medication with a higher risk for weight gain, such as olanzapine, risperidone, or quetiapine to one with a lower risk, such as aripiprazole or ziprasidone, because Weiden (2007) demonstrated that this strategy can result in significant weight loss. Some clinicians who specialize in the treatment of diabetes at times utilize MFN with topiramate, especially in prediabetic conditions. For both medications, unless lifestyle changes are enacted, weight loss efforts will be disappointing.

Since the release of phentermine/topiramate ER (Qsymia), two additional agents have been approved for weight loss in adults and one long-acting formulation of melatonin is expected to get approval in 2018. One of the new agents is another two-medication combination of naltrexone/bupropion (Contrave) that is approved in adults. An additional medicine approved in adults is the novel SER 2C receptor agonist agent Lorcaserin HCL (Belviq & Belviq XR) which has been released in a short- and long-acting formulation. The final agent pending approval in 2018 is the investigational long-acting formulation of melatonin discussed earlier. For a comparison summary of all of these agents as well as information on dosing, SEs, and relevant clinical facts, refer to the tables in the Appendix on Recommendations for Children versus Adult FDA-Approved Weight Loss Medications as an Adjunct to Comprehensive Weight Loss Interventions.

REVERSIBLE VESICULAR MONOAMINE TRANSPORTER 2 INHIBITORS AGENTS FOR TARDIVE DYSKINESIA

It is cause for celebration when a novel treatment is made available for clinicians to address a serious condition in psychiatry. In 2017, two pharmaceutical agents received the first-ever FDA approval for the treatment of tardive dyskinesia (TD).

TD in its most severe form can be a functionally disabling condition, and in milder forms it is still cosmetically and socially stigmatizing for those effected whether in the pediatric population or in adults. SGAs and TGAs are commonly used as first-line agents in schizophrenia and mood spectrum disorders. Early consensus was that SGA and TGA caused less extrapyramidal side effects (EPSs), such as parkinsonism and akathisia, than did FGAs. Although there was less evidence for a decreased risk with SGAs for abnormal involuntary movements, particularly TD, it was speculated that this reduction was also the case for TD (Caroff et al., 2002; Casey, 1999; Dolder & Jeste, 2003; Jeste et al., 1999a, 1999b; Marder et al., 2002; Kane et al., 1993).

More recent studies, such as the naturalistic study by de Leon (2007), continue to demonstrate a beneficial SE profile with SGAs for EPS and TD, but the separation in incidence between FGAs and SGAs/TGAs is not as great as once thought.

There is limited data on TD in the pediatric population, but a study by Correll and Kane (2007) reviewed 10 studies in youth ($N = 783$, mean age: 9.7 years) treated mainly with risperidone (94%) and found a low annualized average TD incidence rate of only 0.42% using SGAs.

Unfortunately, TD persists in 66% to 80% of patients even when the FGAs/SGAs/TGAs are stopped, which in most cases is not even an option. TD remains one of the most feared medication SEs to child and adolescent psychiatrists. The treatment of TD has been frustrating, with no clear established treatments, although in 2013, an evidence-based guideline by the American Academy of Neurology proposed there was some clinical support to using clonazepam and ginkgo biloba, followed by amantadine and tetrabenazine (TBZ).

TBZ, which was only made available in the United States in 2008 to treat movement disorders related to Huntington disease, was used off-label by clinicians to treat TD. TBZ was the prototype of a new class of medications labeled "reversible vesicular monoamine transporter 2 (VMAT-2) inhibitors." VMAT-2 is a transport protein located almost exclusively in the CNS, whereas vesicular monoamine transport type 1 (VMAT-1) is located in the peripheral nervous system, which when active can lead to orthostasis.

Intracellular transporter proteins are essential to package various monoamine NTs (dopamine, SER, norepinephrine, and histamine) into synaptic vesicles enclosed within presynaptic neurons. Blocking these transporters decreases the uptake of these NTs into synaptic vesicles, which when released from the cell membrane will be reduced in quantity. The reduced quantities of NTs released from the nerve terminals, specifically dopamine, theoretically lower the suspected postsynaptic receptor upregulation and dopaminergic supersensitivity in conditions such as Huntington disease, TD, and Tourette syndrome. However, Marder et al. (2016) relates that this theory may better explain withdrawal dyskinesias because this process of postsynaptic receptor upregulation and dopaminergic supersensitivity is often rapidly reversible in animal models and that the low remission rates after discontinuing antipsychotics may indicate a problem with neuroplasticity, with environmental stressors such as oxidative distress, and genetic predispositions. TBZ has many SEs because its (−) enantiomer metabolites are not selective; and as inhibitors of SER and dopamine neurons, this may result in depression and parkinsonism, respectively. TBZ's short half-life, at times requiring tid dosing, as well as its SE issues greatly hindered its usability.

Trials to develop VMAT-2 inhibitors that are more tolerable and safer than TBZ were successful, resulting in the release of valbenazine (Ingrezza) in April of 2017, for the treatment of adults with TD. Later in 2017, a second VMAT-2 inhibitor, deutetrabenazine (Austedo) was also given approval for the treatment of adults with TD. Although these agents only have adult FDA approval, it is probable that these agents will be utilized cautiously in the pediatric population, particularly in adolescents, given the social and physical impairment associated with TD, the modest SE profile of these agents, and the lack of other treatment options. It is not known whether these agents are safe and effective in children and adolescents, but as two phase 2 clinical trials with valbenazine (see subsequent text) are under way for adults in addition to children and adolescents (ages 6 to 17) with Tourette syndrome, it is hopeful that additional efficacy and safety data will be available in the next few years.

Valbenazine (Ingrezza)

Valbenazine approval was based on positive results from several studies, including the Kinect 3 phase 3 trial of valbenazine versus placebo, which included 234 patients with moderate-to-severe TD plus schizophrenia, schizoaffective disorder, or a mood disorder. Hauser et al. (2017) presented findings demonstrating that although patients in the placebo group had a nonsignificant change in the Abnormal Involuntary Movement Scale (AIMS) of 0.1 points, patients who received 80 mg/day of the active treatment valbenazine had a significant decrease in TD symptoms on the AIMS of 3.2 at 6 weeks, and patients who received 40 mg/day had a decrease in AIMS of −1.9.

Freudenriech and Remington (2017) explain that valbenazine is basically a prodrug that is metabolized into two metabolites, both of which are active but the (+)-alpha-dihydrotetrabenazine metabolite is the most potent metabolite in terms of inhibition of VMAT-2 with a half-life in the 15- to 22-hour range, allowing once-a-day dosing. Valbenazine and its one major (+) metabolite have a preferable SE profile because they act more selectively on centrally located VMAT-2 and not on peripheral VMAT-2 systems, which produce many of the problematic SEs such as early orthostatic hypotension that is seen with TBZ. Valbenazine also has very low off-target binding to SER and dopaminergic sites, which may explain why in 234 randomized patients studied there were no safety concerns depending on changes in depression/suicidality, parkinsonism, akathisia, and changes in schizophrenia symptoms. In addition, prolactin elevation was only mild. For valbenazine, somnolence was the only consistent SE across studies at 10.9% versus 4.2 % for placebo, which was not statistically different between the 40- and 80-mg dosages. The package insert (PI) indicates other SEs may include changes in balance, headache, feelings of restlessness, dry mouth, constipation, and blurred vision. The PI also notes the possibility of QTc interval prolongation if used with CYP3A4 inhibitors (ketoconazole) or CYP2D6 inhibitors (e.g., paroxetine, fluoxetine, bupropion); and in these instances, it is recommended to remain at the starting dose of 40 mg/day. It is not recommended to use valbenazine with strong 3A4 inducers (carbamazepine) because the active metabolite is reduced by 75%. Valbenazine should not be prescribed to patients with congenital long QT syndrome or with arrhythmias related to prolonged QT interval. For any patients at increased risk of a prolonged QT interval, it is important to assess the QT interval before increasing the dosage.

Prescribing labeling in adults recommends starting at 40 mg/day in the morning with or without food for 1 week and then increasing to 80 mg/day thereafter, which is the more therapeutic dosage with no increase in SEs noted. Valbenazine at the 80-mg dosage resulted in a 3.2 point decrease on the AIMS score, which equated to a large effect size of 0.90 (Cohen's d), whereas the 40-mg dose only reduced the AIMS score 1.9 points. Initially, valbenazine was only prescribed and distributed through a specialty pharmacy that shipped valbenazine directly to patients' homes, but it is now available in local retail pharmacies. Presently, it is not known whether valbenazine is safe and effective in children and adolescents, but studies are planned as given subsequently.

Valbenazine

Reports of Interest

Neurocrine Biosciences, the manufacturer of valbenazine, has initiated a phase 2b clinical trial (T-Force GOLD) in children and adolescents with Tourette syndrome. The T-Force GOLD study is a multicenter, randomized, double-blind, placebo-controlled, parallel group phase 2b study evaluating the safety, tolerability, efficacy, and optimal dose of valbenazine in up to 120 pediatric patients with moderate-to-severe Tourette syndrome. Patients will receive either valbenazine or placebo for 12 weeks followed by 2 weeks off medication. The primary endpoint of the study is the change from baseline of the Yale Global Tic Severity Scale between placebo and active treatment groups at the end of week 12. Tourette syndrome symptoms will also be evaluated using the Premonitory Urge for Tics Scale as well as the CGI Scales. Top-line data from this study is expected in late 2018.

Deutetrabenazine

Deutetrabenazine (Austedo) was the second agent given approval for the treatment of adults with TD. It is a VMAT-2 inhibitor indicated for the treatment of chorea associated with Huntington disease and TD in adults. Deutetrabenazine is related to the older agent TBZ, discussed earlier; but through "deuterization" (replacing hydrogen atoms with the nontoxic isotope deuterium), a much stronger carbon covalent bond to break is created, which essentially extends the half-life of the various metabolites. The deuterated form of TBZ is metabolized to deutetrabenazine, which has a longer half-life and lower peaks in concentration, allowing less frequent dosing and greater tolerability.

The efficacy of deutetrabenazine in the treatment of TD was established in two 12-week, randomized, double-blind, placebo-controlled, multicenter trials conducted in 335 adult ambulatory patients with TD caused by the use of dopamine receptor antagonists. Concurrent diagnoses included schizophrenia/schizoaffective disorder (62%) and mood disorder (33%). With respect to concurrent antipsychotic use, 64% of patients were receiving atypical antipsychotics, 12% were receiving typical or combination antipsychotics, and 24% were not receiving antipsychotics. The AIMS was the primary efficacy measure for the assessment of TD severity.

Study 1 was a 12-week, placebo-controlled, fixed-dose trial; adults with TD (AIMS score of 6 or more) were randomized 1:1:1:1 to 12 mg deutetrabenazine, 24 mg deutetrabenazine, 36 mg deutetrabenazine, or placebo. Treatment duration included a 4-week dose escalation period and an 8-week maintenance period followed by a 1-week washout. The dose of deutetrabenazine was started at 12 mg/day and increased at weekly intervals in 6 mg/day increments to a dose target of 12, 24, or 36 mg/day. The population ($N = 222$) was 21 to 81 years old (mean 57 years), 48% male, and 79% Caucasian.

In Study 1, the AIMS total score for patients receiving deutetrabenazine demonstrated statistically significant improvement, from baseline to week 12. Compared with a change of −1.4 points in the placebo group, the least-squares mean AIMS score improved by −3.3 points in the deutetrabenazine 36 mg/day group, by −3.2 points in the 24 mg/day group, and by −2.1 points in the 12 mg/day group. The proportion of patients who showed an improvement of 50% or more in AIMS total score was significantly greater in the deutetrabenazine 24 mg/day (35%) and 36 mg/day (33%) groups than in the placebo group (12%). AIMS total score data over the course of the study did not suggest substantial differences in efficacy across various demographic groups.

Study 2 was a more real-world assessment because it was a 2-week, placebo-controlled, flexible-dose trial in adults with TD ($N = 113$) who received daily doses of placebo or deutetrabenazine, starting at 12 mg/day with increases allowed in 6-mg increments at 1-week intervals until satisfactory control of dyskinesia was achieved, until intolerable SEs occurred, or until a maximal dose of 48 mg/day was reached. Treatment duration included a 6-week dose titration period and a 6-week maintenance period followed by a 1-week washout. The population was 25 to 75 years old (mean 55 years), 48% male, and 70% Caucasian. Patients were titrated to an optimal dose over 6 weeks. The average dose of deutetrabenazine after treatment was 38.3 mg/day. Once again, there was no evidence suggesting substantial differences in efficacy across various demographic groups. In Study 2, the AIMS total score for patients receiving deutetrabenazine demonstrated statistically significant improvement by 3.0 units from baseline to endpoint (week 12), compared with 1.6 units in the placebo group with a treatment effect of −1.4 units.

Deutetrabenazine comes in 6-, 9-, and 12-mg tablets. The initial dose recommended for TD is 12 mg/day with titration at weekly intervals by 6 mg/day depending on reduction of TD, and tolerability, up to a maximum recommended daily dosage of 48 mg (24 mg twice daily). The PI recommends that total daily dosages of 12 mg or above be administered in two divided equal doses. It is recommended that deutetrabenazine tablets be swallowed whole with water and taken with food. Treatment with deutetrabenazine can be discontinued without tapering. Following treatment interruption of greater than 1 week, deutetrabenazine therapy should be re-titrated when resumed. For treatment interruption of less than 1 week, treatment can be resumed at the previous maintenance dose without titration. It is advised not to take deutetrabenazine if one is taking valbenazine (Ingrezza).

Sedation (sleepiness) is a common dose-limiting adverse reaction of deutetrabenazine. The most common SEs of deutetrabenazine in people with TD include inflammation of the nose and throat (nasopharyngitis) and problems sleeping (insomnia). Depression/dysthymic disorder and akathisia/agitation/restlessness were reported in 2% of patients on deutetrabenazine and 1% of patients on placebo.

Because deutetrabenazine is related to TBZ, a closely related VMAT2 inhibitor, many of the potential SEs of TBZ may also be a concern with deutetrabenazine. These potential SEs may include an increase in the corrected QT (QTc) interval, especially in combination with other medications known to prolong QTc. For patients requiring deutetrabenazine doses greater than 24 mg/day who are using deutetrabenazine with other medications known to prolong QTc, assess the QTc interval before and after increasing the dose of deutetrabenazine or the other medications. Medications known to prolong QTc include antipsychotic medications (e.g., chlorpromazine, haloperidol, thioridazine, ziprasidone), antibiotics (e.g., moxifloxacin), or when used with strong CYP2D6 inhibitors (e.g., paroxetine, fluoxetine, quinidine, bupropion) that have been shown to increase the systemic exposure to the active dihydro-metabolites of deutetrabenazine by approximately threefold. Deutetrabenazine should be avoided in patients with congenital long QT syndrome and in patients with a history of cardiac arrhythmias.

It is not known whether deutetrabenazine is safe and effective in children. It is noteworthy that deutetrabenazine carries a black box warning for patients with untreated or inadequately treated depression or for patients who are suicidal. This warning, however, is directed at patients with Huntington chorea. Because valbenazine is not approved for Huntington chorea, no such warning is present in the valbenazine PI. Nonetheless, this labeling may give some clinicians pause about using deutetrabenazine as a first-line medication. Although it is often difficult to compare SEs across studies, it appears that deutetrabenazine had lower sedation rates in the TD trials than did valbenazine, but these were not long-term trials.

Dosage and Administration in Tardive Dyskinesia in Adults					
	Pill size	Initial dose	Recommended Dose	Titration Rate	Dosing Frequency
Valbenazine	40 mg, 80 mg	40 mg	80 mg	Weekly	Once daily
Deutetrabenazine	6-, 9-, and 12-mg tablets	12 mg/d	12–48 mg/d; the average dose after treatment in a flexible dose study was 38.3 mg/d	6 mg/d/wk	Administer total daily dosages of 12 mg or above in two divided doses

DISRUPTIVE MOOD DYSREGULATION DISORDER

The Development of a New Diagnostic Category in *DSM-5*

In the past two decades, the misuse or the misapplication of the diagnosis of bipolar disorder and especially the diagnosis of bipolar disorder not otherwise specified occurred in increasing manner because there was a strong movement in the clinical research arena to accept the view that pediatric bipolar affective disorder (PBAD) existed with a presentation alternative to that in adults. This proposed pediatric presentation was typified by chronic severe irritability without cycling (that met accepted duration criteria) and the absence of manic phases with true euphoria, the later manifestation being key to diagnosing true bipolar disorder. This symptomology in youth was referred to in the literature as temper dysregulation disorder with dysphoria, or severe mood dysregulation (SMD) in research settings such as the National Institute of Mental Health (NIMH). Longitudinal studies conducted by Leibenluft et al. (2003) at the NIMH and field studies by epidemiologists Costello et al. (2006) followed up youth diagnosed with this "alternative" bipolar criteria into young adulthood and reported that the vast majority never progressed to true bipolar disorder but rather continued to experience depression symptoms, meeting criteria for major depression and or anxiety conditions in later life. Another clinically relevant finding uncovered by Brotman et al. (2007) is that youth with actual bipolar disorder were more likely to have parents with bipolar disorder compared to youth with SMD.

These findings were a strong impetus to develop the new diagnosis of disruptive mood dysregulation disorder (DMDD) in the *DSM-5* (APA, 2013). The review committee assessing the new proposed condition elected not to incorporate all of the criteria of SMD into the final *DSM-5* criteria for DMDD. The hyperarousal criterion of the SMD diagnosis (with symptoms such as insomnia, agitation, distractibility, racing thoughts/flight of ideas, pressured speech, and intrusiveness) were not included in the DMDD diagnosis criteria. In addition, the age of onset criterion was 12 years or earlier for SMD; this was reduced to 10 for DMDD.

The outcome findings from the longitudinal studies have also led to some troubling realizations. The lifetime prevalence of 3.2% for DMDD is much higher than the reported prevalence for PBAD of 0.1% and the functional impairment is as great as that found in children with actual bipolar disorder in terms of difficulties in areas of academics, family function, and legal aspects. As stated, the longitudinal studies reveal that by early adulthood, symptom complexes that are more consistent with major depression and anxiety disorders persist. This outcome may be one positive aspect for youth with DMDD in that although second-generation mood stabilizers as discussed appear to be the most effective medical interventions for the most troubling symptoms of severe irritability and aggression, the need for chronic mood stabilizers should not be a lifelong requisite. During the phase of life when this SMD is present, however, aggressive interventions need to be utilized on par with those for a youth who has formal bipolar disorder. This will likely include comprehensive treatments such as child- and family-focused cognitive-behavioral therapy (rainbow therapy), which was developed by researchers West et al. (2014) and has been shown to be effective for bipolar disorder. Perepletchikova et al. (2017) conducted an innovative trial using dialectical behavior therapy that may also hold promise as an effective treatment specifically for DMDD.

It appears that the field of psychiatry is some years away from formal treatment guidelines being available to guide clinicians in the treatment of DMDD. Until that time, it is highly probable that the pharmacologic management of DMDD will be based on treating individual key symptoms that make up this disorder. Tourian et al. (2015) chose to address this lacking knowledge base by conducting a review of published treatment options for temper, rage, and chronic irritability—the cardinal symptoms of DMDD as they refer to them.

The authors conducted a very informative and clinically useful review of medication options in the treatment of DMDD. Because DMDD is a new diagnosis, the authors could not find any clinical trials reporting on the treatment of this disorder. Thus, their review looked at the findings of 57 open studies and 28 RCTs investigating various compounds, and three meta-analyses of clinical studies involving the treatment of some key individual symptoms such as irritability and aggression that partially constitute the diagnosis of DMDD. They also reported on a few select studies that looked at the pharmacotherapy of SMD, a phenotype close to DMDD.

First discussed are the three treatment studies of patients with a diagnosis of SMD. The first study conducted by Waxmonsky and colleagues in 2008 was a randomized crossover study of children aged 5 to 12 years with ADHD, which indicated that treatment with methylphenidate (0.15, 0.3, and 0.6 mg/kg tid) combined with behavior modification therapy led to a decrease in symptoms associated with SMD.

Dickstein and colleagues in 2009 conducted an inpatient RCT of lithium in the treatment of young patients aged 7 to 17 years with SMD. These inpatients received a 2-week period of placement on placebo after which nearly half of the patients showed significant improvement. The remaining 25 patients diagnosed with severe SMD who were nonresponders to placebo were randomized and showed no observable superiority for lithium at therapeutic serum levels over placebo.

The last reviewed study investigating the treatment of SMD was conducted by Krieger and colleagues in 2011 as an open-label trial of 21 SMD adolescents, which evidenced that risperidone (3 mg/day) is potentially an effective treatment for SMD given that it was associated with a significant reduction of the Aberrant Behavior Checklist–Irritability scores after 2, 4, 6, and 8 weeks of treatment. Interestingly, improvements in symptoms of ADHD, depression, and global functioning were also observed.

Summary Recommendations for Prescribing to Treat Symptoms Associated with Severe Mood Dysregulation

Tourian et al. (2015) also looked at studies that addressed the issue of aggression in youth because this is an element of DMDD that must be addressed clinically. They concluded that their review suggests that methylphenidate is very efficacious in decreasing aggression in subjects with ADHD. In addition, if aggression does not respond to methylphenidate, adjunctive risperidone or divalproex has been shown to successfully decrease aggressive behavior. Risperidone is efficacious in decreasing aggression in patients with CD, autism, and MR/intellectual disability (ID). Lithium, anticonvulsants, selective serotonin reuptake inhibitors (SSRI), serotonin and nor-epinephrine reuptake inhibitors (SNRI), norepinephrine reuptake inhibitors (NRIs), and alpha-2 agonists have been shown to decrease aggression; however, their effect has been found to be low to mild at best, and some compounds show secondary effect profiles that prevent their use as a first option.

On the basis of writings by Sadock (2007), reviewing studies that address the treatment of aggression is clinically relevant because aggression is believed to be the single most common reason for referrals to child and adolescent mental health clinics reaching as high as 50% to 60%. The following studies address the benefit of traditional mood stabilizers in reducing the symptom of aggression in youth.

Lithium is FDA approved for the treatment of acute pediatric mania and the maintenance treatment of mania in bipolar youth (12 years of age or older). Review-ing the five double-blind, RCTs of children and adolescents with CD using lithium (Campbell et al., 1984; Campbell et al., 1995; Carlson et al., 1984; Carlson et al., 1992; Malone et al., 2000; Rifkin et al., 1997), it was noted that four out of the five studies concluded that lithium significantly reduced aggression when compared to placebo. The remaining study failed to find any difference between lithium and placebo, but was only a 2-week study. One is also referred to Chapter 9 on page 309 in the section discussing lithium in the treatment of youth with SMD that references a small study ($N = 25$) conducted by Dickstein et al. (2009) in which the authors concluded that lithium provided only a small degree of improvement in the youth aged 7 to 17 years treated.

Anticonvulsant mood stabilizers, such as valproic acid (divalproex), carbamazepine, and lamotrigine are FDA indicated in the treatment of bipolar disorder in adults, and although not approved in children and adolescents are frequently used in the youth population for mood stability and temper. Donovan et al. (2000) completed a cross-over study with placebo investigating aggression in children and adolescents with CD associated with chronic explosive temper and mood lability. The superior efficacy of divalproex compared to that of placebo was noted, but unfortunately the study was underpowered to allow confident conclusions. The two other RCT studies by Hellings et al. (2005) and Hollander et al. (2009) investigating the efficacy of valproate in aggressive behavior associated with autism concluded with contradictory results.

Cueva et al. (1996) completed one RCT investigating the impact of carbamazepine on aggression, but carbamazepine was not superior to placebo in reducing aggression and explosiveness.

Lamotrigine is approved for adults for the maintenance treatment of bipolar I disorder, but no such indication exists for youth populations. Belsito et al. (2001) completed a study of autistic youth treated with lamotrigine, which did not demon-strate that lamotrigine was efficacious in decreasing behavioral disturbance features commonly associated with autism.

Psychostimulants are first-line treatments for ADHD. Impulsive aggression frequently co-occurs with ADHD with or without comorbid oppositional defiant disorder (ODD) or CD. Pappadopulos et al. (2006) published a review of eight RCTs utilizing psychostimulants (predominantly methylphenidate) in the treatment of aggression in youth with ADHD with or without comorbid ODD, CD, and MR. The impact of psychostimulants on decreasing aggression was very significant with an impressive effect size of 0.78.

SGAs such as olanzapine, risperidone, quetiapine, aripiprazole, asenapine, and lurasidone are FDA approved for the acute treatment of type I bipolar disorder in youth. Risperidone and aripiprazole are FDA approved for the treatment of irrita-bility (including aggression, temper tantrums, self-injurious behavior, and quickly changing moods) in autistic disorder in children and adolescents.

Pappadopulos and colleagues (2006) identified nine RCTs of aggressive children and adolescents being treated with risperidone. All nine studies showed greater re-ductions in aggression with risperidone compared to those with placebo in subjects with CD, ODD, ADHD, autism, and MR/ID. The overall effect size of risperidone was quite high at 0.9.

Two studies completed by Aman et al. (2004) and Correia Filho et al. (2005) demonstrated that for children and adolescents with MR and ADHD symptoms, risperidone, independent of psychostimulant usage, was an effective treatment for disruptive behavior disorders and comorbid ADHD. Connor et al. (2008) in a small study of 19 patients found that for adolescents with CD, quetiapine at 200 to 600 mg/day was effective in decreasing overt aggression.

Antidepressants of the SSRI, SNRI, and NRI classes have all been trialed in studies to address the symptom of aggression. DMDD is placed in the Depression Disorders section of *DSM-5*, and as a logical corollary one would assume that trials of antidepressants might be beneficial.

Pappadopulous and colleagues (2016) identified two RCTs utilizing fluoxetine 0.5 mg/kg for aggression in youth with depression or selective mutism, but the effect sizes were disappointing ranging from 0 to 0.3. Atomoxetine is an NRI that is FDA approved for the treatment of ADHD in children and adolescents, but it is also known to have antidepressant properties. Four RCTs of atomoxetine also reported very low effect sizes of 0.18 on aggression, indicating that it would not be the treatment of choice in youth with ADHD having marked aggression. Other antidepressants utilized in their review included three RCTs with bupropion reporting an effect size ranging from 0 to 0.55 and one RTC with desipramine that resulted in an effect size of 0.85. The authors noted that this significant effect size with desipramine represented global improvement of ADHD symptoms, not only aggression.

Alpha-2 agonists such as clonidine have been shown to reduce symptoms of disruptive disorders in children and adolescents. Conner and colleagues (2003) published a meta-analysis of 11 double-blind RCTs published in the 1980s and 1990s demonstrating that the alpha-2 agonist clonidine exerts a moderate effect on symptoms of ADHD and may help diminish impulsive aggression. Jaselskis et al. (1992) presented additional findings that clonidine significantly decreases aggressive behavior compared to placebo. Scahill et al. (2001) demonstrated that guanfacine, another alpha-2 agonist also used to treat ADHD, decreases aggressive behavior compared to placebo. Note that clonidine ER and guanfacine ER are the only forms of these agents FDA approved for the treatment of ADHD as a sole treatment and as an augmentation strategy in the treatment of ADHD.

Beta-blockers, primarily propranolol, were well studied in the 1980s by Kuperman and Stewart (1987), Luchins and Dojka (1989), and Williams et al. (1982) in non-RCT studies that supported the use of the beta-blocker to decrease aggression in youth populations even if diagnosed with MR or organic brain dysfunction. In their review study, Tourian et al. (2015) was unable to locate any RCTs showing the use of beta-blockers in children or adolescents with aggression.

Summary Recommendations to Treat the Symptom of Aggression and Possibly DMDD

The results of the Tourian et al. (2015) review summary would suggest that stimulants or second-generation mood stabilizers would be first-line treatments depending on efficacy alone and ignoring SE profiles. Stimulants (methylphenidate more commonly used than amphetamine) are very efficacious with an effect size of 0.78 in decreasing aggression in subjects with ADHD and generally have less SE burden than do SGAs, making them likely first-line agents. If aggression does not respond to methylphenidate or amphetamine, the most efficacious agents actually appear to be SGAs such as risperidone (by far the most common agent used in the past studies) with a very high overall effect size of 0.9. How other second-generation mood stabilizers compare to risperidone is not known because there are no large RTCs that have compared these agents against one another, so one is left to compare effect sizes or NNT across studies, which is not ideal. Lithium, anticonvulsants, SSRIs, SNRIs, NRIs, and alpha-2 agonists have been shown to decrease aggression; however, their effect size has been found to be low to mild at best, and some compounds such as beta-blockers that have shown moderate efficacy may demonstrate SE profiles that prevent their use as a first-line option.

Irritability

Another key core symptom that is targeted in DMDD treatment is irritability. Risperidone and aripiprazole are the only FDA-approved medications to treat irritability associated with autism, which does not prove efficacy with DMDD; but the irritability component is a troubling symptom in both conditions. These agents appear to have similar efficacy in their respective RTC trials that supported their FDA approvals in autism for irritability; and as discussed previously, risperidone has shown impressive efficacy for the treatment of aggression in multiple trials.

DMDD most often co-occurs with depressive disorders and ODD, which has its own irritability dimension criterion. Kim and Boylan (2016) note that the consistent association between ODD irritability and later in life mood and anxiety disorders provides the strongest theoretic rationale for antidepressants having a role in treating irritability. Irritability is included as a core diagnostic symptom of unipolar depression in youth, and the presence of irritability is a very poor prognostic factor for a child. Holtmann et al. (2010) in their study reported that irritable youth are disproportionately affected by suicidality, substance use, and lower goal attainment; whereas Carlson et al. (2009) noted that they require higher acuity mental health services, especially inpatient services. As discussed previously, SMD, with its chronic irritability component, is a distinct condition separate from bipolar disorder but the authors astutely note that it is still unknown, given the lack of RTC trials, what the specific effects of antidepressant exposure on chronically or episodically irritable youth will be, acutely or long term. This uncertainty as well as the FDA black box warnings on the risk of "suicidality" in youth on antidepressants should give clinicians caution when prescribing antidepressants in this population, especially if one suspects the youth has been misdiagnosed and are actually in the bipolar spectrum.

Kim and Boylan (2016) identified 99 studies assessing the effect of antidepressants in improving irritability, aggression, or oppositional symptoms as secondary outcomes. Only two studies specifically measured the outcome of irritability, but they were uncontrolled studies. Studies reporting the effect of antidepressant exposure on disruptive behavior symptom outcome utilized medications from several classes. The SSRIs included fluoxetine, sertraline, paroxetine, and citalopram. The SNRI included venlafaxine. The non-SSRI studied was trazodone. The NRIs studied were desipramine, clomipramine, and imipramine.

These numerous studies, in aggregate, suggest that antidepressant medications are associated with small reductions in irritability, aggression, and behavioral symptoms in youth with depression as a primary diagnosis, as well as for youth with primarily behavioral diagnoses. It is disappointing to find that systematic reviews of the literature involving the use of antidepressants for the treatment of irritability have only demonstrated small effect sizes, with many studies showing effect sizes less than 0.25. Treatment response and ODD symptoms seemed to be linked in some youth with depression. Other studies in this review suggested that there is some effect of antidepressants on irritability and ODD symptoms that is likely independent of depression. The authors note that because only randomized studies included youth with a diagnosis of MDD, it is important that future trials examine this question in controlled studies on youth who do not have depression. Clearly, more RCTs addressing which symptoms mediate the irritability response are needed.

In summary, this review of utilizing antidepressants to treat irritability that overall resulted in low effect sizes was comparable to the studies utilizing antidepressants to treat aggressive symptoms, which also reflected low effect sizes. At this time, antidepressants may be beneficial for some patients with DMDD, but in general seem relegated to a role as an augmentation strategy or as an option when other more efficacious medications agents have failed.

References

Abilify [package insert]. Tokyo, Japan: Otsuka Pharmaceutical Co, Ltd; 2012.

Abilify [package insert]. Tokyo, Japan: Otsuka Pharmaceutical Co, Ltd; 2017.

Adler L, Angrist B, Peselow E, et al. A controlled assessment of propranolol in the treatment of neuroleptic-induced akathisia. *Br J Psychiatry*. 1986;149:42–45.

Adler LA, Rotrosen J, Edson R, et al. Vitamin E treatment of tardive dyskinesia. *Arch Gen Psychiatry*. 1999;56:836–841.

Alaghband-Rad J, Hakimshooshtary M. A randomized controlled clinical trial of citalopram versus fluoxetine in children and adolescents with obsessive-compulsive disorder (OCD). *Eur Child Adolesc Psychiatry*. 2009;18(3):131–135.

Alderman J, Wolkow R, Chung M, et al. Sertraline treatment of children and adolescents with obsessive-compulsive disorder or depression: pharmacokinetics, tolerability, and efficacy. *J Am Acad Child Adolesc Psychiatry*. 1998;37:386–394.

Alderman J, Wolkow R, Fogel I. Drug concentration monitoring with tolerability and efficacy assessments during open-label sertraline treatment of children and adolescents. *J Child Adolesc Psychopharmacol*. 2006;16(1–2):117–129.

Alfaro CL, Wudarsky M, Nicolson R, et al. Correlation of antipsychotic and prolactin concentration in children and adolescents acutely treated with haloperidol, clozapine, or olanzapine. *J Child Adolesc Psychopharmacol*. 2002;12:83–91.

Alho H, Sinclair D, Vuori E, et al. Abuse liability of buprenorphine-naloxone tablets in untreated IV drug users. *Drug Alcohol Depend*. 2007;88(1):75–78.

Allen RP, Safer D, Covi L. Effects of psychostimulants on aggression. *J Nerv Ment Dis*. 1975;160:138–145.

Altamura AC, Montgomery SA, Wernicke JF. The evidence for 20 mg a day of fluoxetine as the optimal dose in the treatment of depression. *Br J Psychiatry*. 1988;153(suppl 3):109–112.

Althaus M, Vink HJF, Minderaa RB, et al. Lack of effect of clonidine on stuttering in children. *Am J Psychiatry*. 1995;152:1087–1089.

Alvir JM, Lieberman JA, Safferman AZ, et al. Clozapine-induced agranulocytosis. Incidence and risk factors in the United States. *N Engl J Med*. 1993;329:162–167.

Alwan S, Friedman JM, Chambers C. Safety of selective serotonin reuptake inhibitors in pregnancy: a review of current evidence. *CNS Drugs*. 2016;30:499–515. doi:10.1007/s40263-016-0338-3.

Aman M, Binder C, Turgay A. Risperidone effects in the presence/absence of psychostimulant medicine in children with ADHD, other disruptive behavior disorders, and subaverage IQ. *J Child Adolesc Psychopharmacol*. 2004;14(2):243–254.

Aman MG, Arnold LE, McDougle CJ, et al. Acute and long-term safety and tolerability of risperidone in children with autism. *J Child Adolesc Psychopharmacol*. 2005;15:869–884.

Aman MG, Bukstein OG, Gadow KD, et al. What does risperidone add to parent training and stimulant for severe aggression in child attention-deficit/hyperactivity disorder? *J Am Acad Child Adolesc Psychiatry*. 2014;53(1):47.e1–60.e1.

Aman MG, Findling RL, Derivan A, et al. Risperidone versus placebo for severe conduct disorder in children with mental retardation. (Abstract, 40th Annual NCDEU meeting). *J Child Adolesc Psychopharmacol*. 2000;10:253.

Aman MG, Singh NN. Preface. In: Aman MG, Singh NN, eds. *Psychopharmacology of the Developmental Disabilities*. New York, NY: Springer-Verlag; 1988:v–ix.

Ambrosini PJ, Bianchi MD, Rabinovich H, et al. Antidepressant treatments in children and adolescents: I, affective disorders. *J Am Acad Child Adolesc Psychiatry*. 1993;32:1–6.

Ambrosini PJ, Sheikh RM. Increased plasma valproate concentrations when coadministered with guanfacine. *J Child Adolesc Psychopharmacol*. 1998;8:143–147.

Ambrosini PJ, Wagner KD, Biederman J, et al. Multicenter open-label sertraline study in adolescent outpatients with major depression. *J Am Acad Child Adolesc Psychiatry*. 1999;38:566–572.

American Academy of Child and Adolescent Psychiatry. Desipramine and sudden death. Ad hoc committee on DMI [desipramine] and sudden death (J. Biederman, chair). 1992 Member Forum. Washington, DC: AACAP Program; 1992:8.

American Academy of Child and Adolescent Psychiatry. Rating scales. The American Academy of Child and Adolescent Psychiatry website. 2010. http://www.aacap.org/cs/clinical_care_quality_improvement/rating_scales. Accessed March 2, 2013.

American Academy of Child and Adolescent Psychiatry. A guide for public child serving agencies on psychotropic medications for children and adolescents. Washington, DC: AACAP; 2012:8. http://www.aacap.org/App_Themes/AACAP/docs/press/guide_for_community_child_serving_agencies_on_psychotropic_medications_for_children_and_adolescents_2012.pdf. Accessed July 7, 2018.

American Academy of Child and Adolescent Psychiatry. Practice parameter on the use of psychotropic medication in children and adolescents. *J Am Acad Child Adolesc Psychiatry*. 2009;48:961.

American Academy of Child and Adolescent Psychiatry. Recommendations about the use of psychotropic medications for children and adolescents involved in child-serving systems. Washington, DC:AACAP; 2015. https://www.aacap.org/App_Themes/AACAP/docs/clinical_practice_center/systems_of_care/AACAP_Psychotropic_Medication_Recommendations_2015_FINAL.pdf. Accessed July 7, 2018.

American Academy of Pediatrics Committee on Substance Use and Prevention. Medication-assisted treatment of adolescents with opioid use disorders. *Pediatrics*. 2016;138(3). doi:10.1542/peds.2016-1893.

American Diabetes Association and American Psychiatric Association. Consensus development conference on antipsychotic drugs and obesity and diabetes. *Diabetes Care*. 2004;27:596–601.

American Medical Association. *Drug Evaluations Annual 1994*. Chicago, IL: American Medical Association; 1993.

American Medical Association. *Drug Evaluations*. 6th ed. Chicago, IL: American Medical Association; 1986.

American Medical Association. *Informed consent. Code of Medical Ethics Opinion 2.1.1*. Chicago, IL: The American Medical Association; 2016. https://www.ama-assn.org/delivering-care/informed-consent. Accessed November 20, 2017.

American Psychiatric Association. *Diagnostic and Statistical Manual of Mental Disorders*. 2nd ed. Washington, DC: American Psychiatric Association; 1968.

American Psychiatric Association. *Diagnostic and Statistical Manual of Mental Disorders*. 3rd ed. Washington, DC: American Psychiatric Association; 1980a.

American Psychiatric Association. *Tardive Dyskinesia: Task Force Report 18*. Washington, DC: American Psychiatric Association; 1980b.

American Psychiatric Association. *Diagnostic and Statistical Manual of Mental Disorders*. 3rd ed. rev. Washington, DC: American Psychiatric Association; 1987.

American Psychiatric Association. *Diagnostic and Statistical Manual of Mental Disorders*. 4th ed. Washington, DC: American Psychiatric Association; 1994.

American Psychiatric Association. *Diagnostic and Statistical Manual of Mental Disorders*. 4th ed. Text Revision. Washington, DC: American Psychiatric Association; 2000.

American Psychiatric Association. *Diagnostic and Statistical Manual of Mental Disorders (DSM-5)*. 5th ed. Washington, DC: American Psychiatric Association; 2013.

American Psychiatric Association. Task force on tardive dyskinesia. *Tardive Dyskinesia: a Task Force Report of the American Psychiatric Association*. Washington, DC: American Psychiatric Association; 1992.

Amery B, Minichiello MD, Brown GL. Aggression in hyperactive boys: response to d-amphetamine. *J Am Acad Child Psychiatry*. 1984;23:291–294.

Amitai M, Sachs E, Zivony A, et al. Effects of long-term valproic acid treatment on hematological and biochemical parameters in adolescent psychiatric inpatients: a retrospective naturalistic study. *Int Clin Psychopharmacol*. 2015;30:241–248.

Amitai M, Zivony A, Kronenberg S, et al. Short-term effects of lithium on white blood cell counts and on levels of serum thyroid-stimulating hormone and creatinine in adolescent inpatients: a retrospective naturalistic study. *J Child Adolesc Psychopharmacol*. 2014;24(9):494–500.

Amitai Y, Frischer H. Excess fatality from desipramine in children and adolescents. *J Am Acad Child Adolesc Psychiatry*. 2006;45:54–60.

Amstutz U, Ross CJ, Castro-Pastrana LI, et al. HLA-A 31:01 and HLA-B 15:02 as genetic markers for carbamazepine hypersensitivity in children. *Clin Pharmacol Ther*. 2013;94(1):142–149.

Anderson LT, Campbell M, Grega DM, et al. Haloperidol in the treatment of infantile autism: effects on learning and behavioral symptoms. *Am J Psychiatry*. 1984;141:1195–1202.

Anthenelli RM, Benowitz NL, West R, et al. Neuropsychiatric safety and efficacy of varenicline, bupropion, and nicotine patch in smokers with and without psychiatric disorders (EAGLES): a double-blind, randomised, placebo-controlled clinical trial. *Lancet*. 2016;387(10037):2507–2520.

Apter A, Lipschitz A, Fong R, et al. Evaluation of suicidal thoughts and behaviors in children and adolescents taking paroxetine. *J Child Adolesc Psychopharmacol*. 2006;16(1–2):77–90.

Apter A, Ratzone G, King RA, et al. Fluvoxamine open-label treatment of adolescent in patients with obsessive-compulsive disorder or depression. *J Am Acad Child Adolesc Psychiatry*. 1994;33:342–348.

Armenteros JL, Whitaker AH, Welilson M, et al. Risperidone in adolescents with schizophrenia: an open pilot study. *J Am Acad Child Adolesc Psychiatry*. 1997;36:694–700.

Arnold LE, Huestis RD, Smeltzer DJ, et al. Levoamphetamine vs dextroamphetamine in minimal brain dysfunction. *Arch Gen Psychiatry*. 1976;33:292–301.

Arnold LE, Lindsay RL, Conners K, et al. A double-blind, placebo-controlled withdrawal trial of dexmethylphenidate hydrochloride in children with attention deficit hyperactivity disorder. *J Child Adolesc Psychopharmacol*. 2004;14:542–554.

Arnsten AF, Scahill L, Findling RL. Alpha-2 adrenoreceptors agonists for the treatment of attention-deficit/hyperactivity disorder: emerging concepts from new data. *J Child Adolesc Psychopharmacol*. 2007;17(4):393–406.

Atkinson S, Lubaczewski S, Ramaker S. Desvenlafaxine versus placebo in the treatment of children and adolescents with major depressive disorder. *J Child Adolesc Psychopharmacol*. 2018;28(1):55–65.

Atkinson SD, Prakash A, Zhang Q. A double-blind efficacy and safety study of duloxetine flexible dosing in children and adolescents with major depressive disorder. *J Child Adolesc Psychopharmacol*. 2014;24(4):180–189.

Atomoxetine [package insert]. Indianapolis, IN: Eli Lilly and Company; 2012.

Avari JM. Paradoxical agitation in adolescent male on valproate. *J Child Adolesc Psychopharmcol*. 2016;26(1):78–79.

Axelson DA, Perel JM, Birmaher B, et al. Sertraline pharmacokinetics and dynamics in adolescents. *J Am Acad Child Adolesc Psychiatry*. 2002;41:1037–1044.

Ayd FJ Jr. *Lexicon of Psychiatry, Neurology and the Neurosciences*. Baltimore, MD: Lippincott Williams & Wilkins; 1995.

Ayd FJ Jr. *Lexicon of Psychiatry, Neurology, and the Neurosciences*. 2nd ed. Baltimore, MD: Lippincott Williams & Wilkins; 2000.

Ayd FJ Jr. Social issues: misuse and abuse. In: Benzodiazepines 1980: current update. *Psychosomatics*. 1980;21(suppl):21–25.

Bailey SR, Crew EE, Riske EC, et al. Efficacy and tolerability of pharmacotherapies to aid smoking cessation in adolescents. *Paediatr Drugs*. 2012;14(2):91–108.

Baker M, Bellonci C, Huefner JC, et al. Polypharmacy and the pursuit of appropriate prescribing for children and adolescents. *Child Adolesc Psychopharmacol*. 2017;1(22):1.

Baldessarini RJ. Drugs and the treatment of psychiatric disorders. In: Gilman AG, Rall TW, Nies AS, et al, eds. *Goodman and Gilman's The Pharmacological Basis of Therapeutics*. 8th ed. New York, NY: Pergamon Press; 1990:383–435.

Baldessarini RJ, Stephens JH. Clinical pharmacology and toxicology of lithium salts. *Arch Gen Psychiatry*. 1970;22:72–77.

Balogh S, Hendricks SE, Kang J. Treatment of fluoxetine-induced anorgasmia with amantadine. *J Clin Psych*. 1992;53(6):212–213.

Ban TA, ed. *An Oral History of Neuropsychopharmacology: The First Fifty Years, Peer Interviews*. Brentwood, CA: ACNP; 2011.

Bangs ME, Petti TA, Janus MD. Fluoxetine-induced memory impairment in an adolescent. *J Am Acad Child Adolesc Psychiatry*. 1994;33:1303–1306.

Bangs ME, Tauscher-Wisniewski S, Polzer J, et al. Meta-analysis of suicide-related behavior events in patients treated with atomoxetine. *J Am Acad Child Adolesc Psychiatry*. 2008;47(2):209–218.

Bard DE, Wolraich ML, Neas B, et al. The psychometric properties of the Vanderbilt attention-deficit hyperactivity disorder diagnostic parent rating scale in a community population. *J Dev Behav Pediatr*. 2013;34(2):72–82. doi:10.1097/DBP.0b013e31827a3a22.

Barrickman LL, Perry PJ, Allen AJ, et al. Bupropion versus methylphenidate in the treatment of attention-deficit hyperactivity disorder. *J Am Acad Child Adolesc Psychiatry*. 1995;34:649–657.

Barzman DH, DelBello MP, Adler CM, et al. The efficacy and tolerability of quetiapine versus divalproex for the treatment of impulsivity and reactive aggression in adolescents with co-occurring bipolar disorder and disruptive behavior disorder. *J Child Adolesc Psychopharmacol.* 2006;16(6):665–670.

Barzman DH, DelBello MP, Kowatch RA, et al. Adjunctive topiramate in hospitalized children and adolescents with bipolar disorders. *J Child Adolesc Psychopharmacol.* 2005;15(6):931–937.

Beck AT, Steer RA, Brown GK. *Beck Depression Inventory—Second Edition Manual.* San Antonia, TX: The Psychological Corporation; 1996.

Bellonci C, Baker M, Huefner JC, et al. Deprescribing and its application to child psychiatry. *Child Adolesc Psychopharmacol.* 2016;22(1):1.

Belsito K, Law P, Kirk K, et al. Lamotrigine therapy for autistic disorder: a randomized, double-blind, placebo-controlled trial. *J Autism Dev Disord.* 2001;31(2):175–181.

Benedek EP, Ash P, Scott CL, eds. *Principles and Practice of Child and Adolescent Forensic Mental Health.* Washington, DC: American Psychiatric Press Inc; 2010.

Benfield P, Heel RC, Lewis SP. Fluoxetine: a review of its pharmacodynamic and pharmacokinetic properties, and therapeutic efficacy in depressive illness. *Drugs.* 1986;32:481–508.

Berard R, Fong R, Carpenter DJ, et al. An international, multicenter, placebo-controlled trial of paroxetine in adolescents with major depressive disorder. *J Child Adolesc Psychopharmacol.* 2006;16:59–75.

Berg I, Hullin R, Allsopp M, et al. Bipolar manic-depressive psychosis in early adolescence, a case report. *Br J Psychiatry.* 1974;125:416–417.

Bergstrom RF, Lemberger L, Farid NA, et al. Clinical pharmacology and pharmacokinetics of fluoxetine: a review. *Br J Psychiatry.* 1988;153(suppl 3):47–50.

Berney T, Kolvin I, Bhate SR, et al. School phobia: a therapeutic trial with clomipramine and short-term outcome. *Br J Psychiatry.* 1981;138:110–118.

Bernstein GA, Borchardt CM, Perwien AR. Imipramine plus cognitive-behavioral therapy in the treatment of school refusal. *J Am Acad Child Adolesc Psychiatry.* 2000;39:276–283.

Bernstein GA, Carroll ME, Crosby RD, et al. Caffeine effects on learning, performance, and anxiety in normal school-age children. *J Am Acad Child Adolesc Psychiatry.* 1994;33:407–415.

Bernstein GA, Garfinkel BD, Borchardt CM. Comparative studies of pharmacotherapy for school refusal. *J Am Acad Child Adolesc Psychiatry.* 1990;29(5):773–778.

Bevan P, Cools AR, Archer T. *Behavioural Pharmacology of 5-HT.* Hillsdale, NJ: Lawrence Erlbaum; 1989.

Bezchlibnyk-Butler KZ, Virani AS, eds. *Clinical Handbook of Psychotropic Drugs for Children and Adolescents.* Cambridge, MA: Hogrefe & Huber Publishers; 2004.

Biederman J, Baldessarini RJ, Goldblatt A, et al. A naturalistic study of 24-hour electrocardiographic recordings and echocardiographic findings in children and adolescents treated with desipramine. *J Am Acad Child Adolesc Psychiatry.* 1993;32:805–813.

Biederman J, Baldessarini RJ, Wright V. A double-blind placebo controlled study of desipramine in the treatment of ADD: I, efficacy. *J Am Acad Child Adolesc Psychiatry.* 1989a;28:777–784.

Biederman J, Baldessarini RJ, Wright V, et al. A double-blind placebo controlled study of desipramine in the treatment of ADD: II, serum drug levels and cardiovascular findings. *J Am Acad Child Adolesc Psychiatry.* 1989b;28:903–911.

Biederman J, Gastfriend DR, Jellinek MS. Desipramine in the treatment of children with attention deficit disorder. *J Clin Psychopharmacol.* 1986;6:359–363.

Biederman J, Joshi G, Mick E, et al. A prospective open-label trial of lamotrigine monotherapy in children and adolescents with bipolar disorder. *CNS Neurosci Ther.* 2010;16(2):91–102.

Biederman J, Lopez FA, Boellner SW, et al. A randomized, double-blind, placebo controlled, parallel-group study of SLI381 (Adderall XR) in children with attention-deficit/hyperactivity disorder. *Pediatrics.* 2002;110:258–266.

Biederman J, Mick E, Hammerness P, et al. Open-label, 8 week trial of olanzapine and risperidone for the treatment of bipolar disorder in preschool-age children. *Biol Psychiatry.* 2005a;58(7):589–594.

Biederman J, Mick E, Wozniak J, et al. An open-label trial of risperidone in children and adolescents with bipolar disorder. *J Child Adolesc Psychopharmacol.* 2005b;15:311–317.

Biederman J, Monuteaux M, Spencer T, et al. Stimulant therapy and risk for subsequent substance use disorders in male adults with ADHD: a naturalistic controlled 10-year follow-up study. *Am J Psychiatry.* 2008;165:597–603.

Birchwood M, Todd P, Jackson C. Early intervention in psychosis. The critical period hypothesis. *Br J Psychiatry.* 1998;172:53–59.

Birmaher B, Axelson DA, Monk K, et al. Fluoxetine for the treatment of childhood anxiety disorders. *J Am Acad Child Adolesc Psychiatry.* 2003;42:415–423.

Birmaher B, Baker R, Kapur S, et al. Clozapine for the treatment of adolescents with schizophrenia. *J Am Acad Child Adolesc Psychiatry.* 1992;31:160–164.

Birmaher B, Brent DA, Chiappetta L, et al. Psychometric properties of the Screen for Child Anxiety Related Emotional Disorders (SCARED): a replication study. *J Am Acad Child Adolesc Psychiatry.* 1999;38:1230–1236.

Birmaher B, Greenhill LL, Cooper TB, et al. Sustained release methylphenidate: pharmacokinetic studies in ADDH males. *J Am Acad Child Adolesc Psychiatry.* 1989;28:768–772.

Birmaher B, Khetarpal S, Brent DA, et al. The Screen for Child Anxiety Related Emotional Disorders (SCARED): scale construction and psychometric characteristics. *J Am Acad Child Adolesc Psychiatry.* 1997;36:545–553.

Birmaher B, Quintana H, Greenhill LL. Methylphenidate treatment of hyperactive autistic children. *J Am Acad Child Adolesc Psychiatry.* 1988;27:248–251.

Birmaher B, Waterman GS, Ryan N, et al. Fluoxetine for childhood anxiety disorders. *J Am Acad Child Adolesc Psychiatry.* 1994;33:993–999.

Birmaher B, Waterman GS, Ryan ND, et al. Randomized, controlled trial of amitriptyline versus placebo for adolescents with "treatment resistant" major depression. *J Am Acad Child Adolesc Psychiatry.* 1998;37:527–535.

Black B, Uhde TW. Treatment of elective mutism with fluoxetine: a double-blind, placebo-controlled study. *J Am Acad Child Adolesc Psychiatry.* 1994;33:1000–1006.

Blader JC. Not just another antipsychotic-for-conduct-problems trial. *J Am Acad Child Adolesc Psychiatry.* 2014;53(1):17–20.

Blader JC, Schooler NR, Jensen PS, et al. Adjunctive divalproex versus placebo for children with ADHD and aggression refractory to stimulant monotherapy. *Am J Psychiatry.* 2009;166(12): 1392–1401.

Blanz B, Schmidt MH. Clozapine for schizophrenia [letter]. *J Am Acad Child Adolesc Psychiatry.* 1993;32:223–224.

Boarati M, Wang YP, Ferreira-Maia A, et al. Six month open-label follow up of risperidone long-acting injection use in pediatric bipolar disorder. *Prim Care Companion CNS Disord.* 2013;15. doi:10.4088/PCC.12m01368.

Bonate PL, Howard DR. *Pharmacokinetics in Drug Development: Clinical Study Design and Analysis.* Vol 1 (Google eBook). Heidelberg, Germany: Springer; 2005.

Borison RL, Pathiraja AP, Diamond BI, et al. Risperidone: clinical safety and efficacy in schizophrenia. *Psychopharmacol Bull.* 1992;28:213–218.

Boulos C, Kutcher S, Gardner D, et al. An open naturalistic trial of fluoxetine in adolescents and young adults with treatment-resistant major depression. *J Child Adolesc Psychopharmacol.* 1992;2:103–111.

Boulos C, Kutcher S, Marton P, et al. Response to desipramine treatment in adolescent major depression. *Psychopharmacol Bull.* 1991;27:59–65.

Bowers R, Weston C, Jackson J. Child and adolescent affective disorders and their treatment. In: Klykylo WM, Kay J, eds. *Clinical Child Psychiatry.* 3rd ed. Pennsylvania, PA: John Wiley & Sons Inc; 2012.

Bradley C. The behavior of children receiving Benzedrine. *Am J Psychiatry.* 1937;94:577–585.

Braña-Berríos M, Lam K. In discussion of: Coffey B. Dysphoria associated with neuroleptic withdrawal in an adolescent with Tourette's disorder. *J Child Adolesc Psychopharmacol.* 2011;21(4):371–374.

Breitner C. An approach to the treatment of juvenile delinquency. *Ariz Med.* 1962;19:82–87.

Brent D, Emslie G, Clarke G, et al. Switching to another SSRI or to venlafaxine with or without cognitive behavioral therapy for adolescents with SSRI-resistant depression: the TORDIA randomized controlled trial. *JAMA.* 2008;299(8):901–913.

Bridge JA, Iyengar S, Salary CB, et al. Clinical response and risk for reported suicidal ideation and suicide attempts in pediatric antidepressant treatment: a meta-analysis of randomized controlled trials. *JAMA.* 2007;297(15):1683–1696.

Brotman M, Kassem L, Reising M, et al. Parental diagnoses in youth with narrow phenotype bipolar disorder or severe mood dysregulation. *Am J Psychiatry.* 2007;164(8):1238–1241.

Brown SL, van Praag HM, eds. *The Role of Serotonin in Psychiatric Disorders.* New York, NY: Brunner/Mazel; 1991.

Bruun R. TSA medical update: treatment with clonidine. *Tourette Syndrome Association Newsletter.* Spring. 1983.

Buitelaar JK, van der Gaag RJ, Swaab-Barneveld H, et al. A placebo-controlled comparison of methylphenidate and pindolol in ADHD. In: American Academy of Child and Adolescent Psychiatry: Scientific Proceedings of the 41st Annual Meeting; October 25–30, 1994; New York, NY. New Research NR-6. 1994a;X:43.

Buitelaar JK, van der Gaag RJ, Swaab-Barneveld H, et al. Side effects of pindolol, a beta-blocker, in ADHD. In: American Academy of Child and Adolescent Psychiatry: Scientific Proceedings of the 41st Annual Meeting; October 25–30, 1994; New York, NY. New Research NR-7. 1994b;X:43.

Buitelaar JK, van der Gaag RJ, van der Hoeven J. Buspirone in the management of anxiety and irritability in children with pervasive developmental disorders: results of an open-label study. *J Clin Psychiatry*. 1998;59:56–59.

Burchfield RW, ed. *Oxford English Dictionary Supplement*. Vol 3: O-Scz. Oxford, England: Clarendon Press; 1982.

Burcu M, Safer DJ, Zito JM. Antipsychotic prescribing for behavioral disorders in US youth: physician specialty, insurance coverage, and complex regimens. *Pharmacoepidemiol Drug Saf*. 2015;25(1):26–34.

Burke P, Puig-Antich J. Psychobiology of childhood depression. In: Lewis M, Miller SM, eds. *Handbook of Developmental Psychopathology*. New York, NY: Plenum Press; 1990:327–339.

Burke RE, Fahn S, Jankovic J, et al. Tardive dystonia: late-onset and persistent dystonia caused by antipsychotic drugs. *Neurology*. 1982;32:1335–1346.

Caldwell PH, Sureshkumar P, Wong WC, et al. Tricyclic and related drugs for nocturnal enuresis in children. *Cochrane Database Syst Rev*. 2016;(1):CD002117.

Cameron OG, Thyer BA. Treatment of pavor nocturnus with alprazolam. *J Clin Psychiatry*. 1985;46:504.

Campbell M, Adams PB, Small AM, et al. Lithium in hospitalized aggressive children with conduct disorder: a double-blind and placebo-controlled study. *J Am Acad Child Adolesc Psychiatry*. 1995;34:445–453.

Campbell M, Anderson LT, Small AM, et al. Naltrexone in autistic children: a double-blind and placebo-controlled study. *Psychopharmacol Bull*. 1990;26:130–135.

Campbell M, Anderson LT, Small AM, et al. Naltrexone in autistic children: behavioral symptoms and attentional learning. *J Am Acad Child Adolesc Psychiatry*. 1993;32:1283–1291.

Campbell M, Green WH, Deutsch SI. *Child and Adolescent Psychopharmacology*. Beverly Hills, CA: SAGE; 1985.

Campbell M, Overall JE, Small AM, et al. Naltrexone in autistic children: an acute open dose range tolerance trial. *J Am Acad Child Adolesc Psychiatry*. 1989;28:200–206.

Campbell M, Perry R, Green WH. The use of lithium in children and adolescents. *Psychosomatics*. 1984a;25:95–106.

Campbell M, Silva RR, Kafantars V, et al. Predictors of side effects associated with lithium administration in children. *Psychopharmacol Bull*. 1991;27(3):373–380.

Campbell M, Small AM, Green WH, et al. Behavioral efficacy of haloperidol and lithium carbonate: a comparison in hospitalized aggressive children with conduct disorder. *Arch Gen Psychiatry*. 1984b;41:650–656.

Cantwell DP, Swanson J, Connor DF. Case study: adverse response to clonidine. *J Am Acad Child Adolesc Psychiatry*. 1997;36:539–544.

Carandang CG, Maxwell DJ, Robbins D. Lamotrigine in adolescent mood disorders. *J Am Acad Child Adolesc Psychiatry*. 2003;42(7):750–751.

Carlson G, Glovinsky I. The concept of bipolar disorder in children. A history of the bipolar controversy. *Child Adolesc Psychiatric Clin N Am*. 2009;18:257–271.

Carlson GA. Classification issues of bipolar disorders in childhood. *Psychiatr Dev*. 1984;2(4):273–285.

Carlson JS, Kratochwill TR, Johnston HF. Sertraline treatment of 5 children diagnosed with selective mutism: a single-case research trial. *J Child Adolesc Psychopharmacol*. 1999;9:293–306.

Caroff S, Mann S, Campbell E, et al. Movement disorders associated with atypical antipsychotic drugs. *J Clin Psychiatry*. 2002;63(suppl 4):12–19.

Casat CD, Pleasants DZ, Schroeder DH, et al. Bupropion in children with attention deficit disorder. *Psychopharmacol Bull*. 1989;25:198–201.

Casey D. Tardive dyskinesia and atypical antipsychotic drugs. *Schizophrenia Res*. 1999;35:61–66.

Castellanos FX, Giedd JN, Elia J, et al. Controlled stimulant treatment of ADHD and comorbid Tourette's syndrome: efficacy of stimulant and dose. *J Am Acad Child Adolesc Psychiatry*. 1997;36:589–596.

Centers for Disease Control Growth Charts. National Center for Health Statistics. Growth Charts. https://www.cdc.gov/growthcharts. Published May 30, 2000. Modified November 11, 2000. Accessed December 6, 2017.

Chakos MH, Lieberman JA, Alvil J, et al. Caudate nuclei volumes in schizophrenic patients treated with typical antipsychotics or clozapine. *Lancet*. 1995;345(8947):456–457.

Chang K, Saxena K, Howe M. An open-label study of lamotrigine adjunct or monotherapy for the treatment of adolescents with bipolar depression. *J Am Acad Child Adolesc Psychiatry*. 2006;45(3):298–304.

Chang S, Himle MB, Tucker BPT, et al. Initial psychometric properties of a brief parent-report instrument for assessing tic severity in children with chronic tic disorders. *Child Fam Behav Ther.* 2009;31(3):181–191. doi:10.1080/07317100903099100.

Chappell PB, Riddle MA, Scahill L, et al. Guanfacine treatment of comorbid attention deficit hyperactivity disorder and Tourette's syndrome: preliminary clinical experience. *J Am Acad Child Adolesc Psychiatry.* 1995;34:1140–1146.

Charach A, Figueroa M, Chen S, et al. Stimulant treatment over 5 years: effects on growth. *J Am Acad Child Adolesc Psychiatry.* 2006;45:415–421.

Chatoor I, Wells KC, Conners CK, et al. The effects of nocturnally administered stimulant medication on EEG sleep and behavior in hyperactive children. *J Am Acad Child Psychiatry.* 1983;22:337–342.

Chen H, Patel A, Sherer J, et al. The definition and prevalence of pediatric psychotropic polypharmacy. *Psychiatr Serv.* 2011;62(12):1450.

Chouinard G, Jones B, Remington G, et al. A Canadian multicenter placebo-controlled study of fixed doses of risperidone and haloperidol in the treatment of chronic schizophrenic patients. *J Clin Psychopharmacol.* 1993;13:25–40.

Chue P, Emsley R. Long-acting formulations of atypical antipsychotics: time to reconsider when to introduce depot antipsychotics. *CNS Drugs.* 2007;21:441–448.

Chugani DC, Chugani HT, Wiznitzer M, et al; Autism Center of Excellence Network. Efficacy of low-dose buspirone for restricted and repetitive behavior in young children with autism spectrum disorder: a randomized trial. *J Pediatr.* 2016;170(45):45–53.e1–e4.

Cioli V, Corradino C, Piccinelli D, et al. A comparative pharmacological study of trazodone, etoperidone, and 1-(m-chlorophenyl) piperazine. *Pharmacol Res Commun.* 1984;16:85–100.

Cipriani A, Zhou X, Del Giovane C, et al. Comparative efficacy and tolerability of antidepressants for major depressive disorder in children and adolescents: a network meta-analysis. *Lancet.* 2016;388(10047):881–890.

Ciraulo DA, Shader RI, Greenblatt DJ, et al, eds. *Drug Interactions in Psychiatry.* Baltimore, MD: Williams & Wilkins; 1989.

Ciraulo DA, Shader RI, Greenblatt DJ, et al, eds. *Drug Interactions in Psychiatry.* 3rd ed. Baltimore, MD: Williams & Wilkins; 2006.

Clark DB, Birmaher B, Axelson D, et al. Fluoxetine for the treatment of childhood anxiety disorders: open-label, long-term extension to a controlled trial. *J Am Acad Child Adolesc Psychiatry.* 2005;44:1263–1270.

Clarke G, Dickerson J, Gullion CM, et al. Trends in youth antidepressant dispensing and refill limits, 2000 through 2009. *J Child Adolesc Psychopharmacol.* 2012;22(1):11–20.

Clay TH, Gualtieri CT, Evans RW, et al. Clinical and neuropsychological effects of the novel antidepressant bupropion. *Psychopharmacol Bull.* 1988;24:143–148.

Coccaro EF, Murphy DL, eds. *Serotonin in Psychiatric Disorders.* Washington, DC: American Psychiatric Press; 1990.

Coffey BJ. Anxiolytics for children and adolescents: traditional and new drugs. *J Child Adolesc Psychopharmacol.* 1990;1:57–83.

Coffey B, Shader RI, Greenblatt DJ. Pharmacokinetics of benzodiazepines and psychostimulants in children. *J Clin Psychopharmacol.* 1983;3:217–225.

Cohen DJ, Detlor J, Young JG, et al. Clonidine ameliorates Gilles de la Tourette syndrome. *Arch Gen Psychiatry.* 1980;37:1350–1357.

Cohen JA, Mannarino AP, Perel JM, et al. A pilot randomized controlled trial of combined trauma-focused CBT and sertraline for childhood PTSD symptoms. *J Am Acad Child Adolesc Psychiatry.* 2007;46(7):811–819.

Comings DE. *Tourette Syndrome and Human Behavior.* Duarte, CA: Hope Press; 1990.

Comings DE, Comings BG. Tourette's syndrome and attention deficit disorder with hyperactivity: are they genetically related? *J Am Acad Child Psychiatry.* 1984;23:138–146.

Conners C, Sitarenios G, Parker JD, et al. The revised Conners' Parent Rating Scale (CPRS-R): factor structure, reliability, and criterion validity. *J Abnorm Child Psychol.* 1998a;26:257–268.

Conners C, Sitarenios G, Parker JD, et al. Revision and restandardization of the Conners Teacher Rating Scale (CTRS-R): factor structure, reliability, and criterion validity. *J Abnorm Child Psychol.* 1998b;26:279–291.

Conners C, Wells KC, Parker JD, et al. A new self-report scale for assessment of adolescent psychopathology: factor structure, reliability, validity, and diagnostic sensitivity. *J Abnorm Child Psychol.* 1997;25:487–497.

Conners CK. Recent drug studies with hyperkinetic children. *J Learn Disabil.* 1971;4:476–483.

Conners CK, Casat CD, Gualtieri CT, et al. Bupropion hydrochloride in attention deficit disorder with hyperactivity. *J Am Acad Child Adolesc Psychiatry.* 1996;34:1314–1321.

Conners CK, Kramer R, Rothschild GH, et al. Treatment of young delinquent boys with diphenyl-hydantoin sodium and methylphenidate. *Arch Gen Psychiatry.* 1971;24:156–160.

Connor D, Glatt S, Lopez I, et al. Psychopharmacology and Aggression II. A meta-analysis of non-stimulant medication effects on overt aggression-related behaviors in youth with SED. *J Emot Behav Disord.* 2003;11(3):157–168.

Connor DF, Fletcher KE, Swanson JM. A meta-analysis of clonidine for symptoms of attention-deficit hyperactivity disorder. *J Am Acad Child Adolesc Psychiatry.* 1999;38:1551–1559.

Connor DF, McLaughlin TJ, Jeffers-Terry M. Randomized controlled pilot study of quetiapine in the treatment of adolescent conduct disorder. *J Child Adolesc Psychopharmacol.* 2008;18(2):140–156.

Connor DF, Ozbayrak KR, Kusiak KA, et al. Combined pharmacotherapy in children and adolescents in a residential treatment center. *J Am Acad Child Adolesc Psychiatry.* 1997;36(2):248.

Cooper GL. The safety of fluoxetine: an update. *Br J Psychiatry.* 1988;153(suppl 3):77–86.

Cooper TB, Bergner PE, Simpson GM. The 24-hour lithium level as a prognosticator of dosage requirements. *Am J Psychiatry.* 1973;130:601–603.

Correia Filho A, Bodanese R, Silva T, et al. Comparison of risperidone and methylphenidate for reducing ADHD symptoms in children and adolescents with moderate mental retardation. *J Am Acad Child Adolesc Psychiatry.* 2005;44(8):748–755.

Correll C, Kane J. One-year incidence rates of tardive dyskinesia in children and adolescents treated with second generation antipsychotics: a systematic review. *J Child Adolesc Psychopharmacol.* 2007;17:647–656.

Correll CU. Effect of hyperprolactinemia during development in children and adolescents. *J Clin Psychiatry.* 2008;69(8):e24.

Correll CU, Carlson HE. Endocrine and metabolic adverse effects of psychotropic medications in children and adolescents. *J Am Acad Child Adolesc Psychiatry.* 2006;45:771–791.

Correll CU, Manu P, Olshanskiy V, et al. Cardiometabolic risk of second-generation antipsychotic medications during first-time use in children and adolescents. *JAMA.* 2009;302(16):1765–1773.

Corson P, Nopoulos P, Miller D, et al. Change in basal ganglia volume over 2 years in patients with schizophrenia: typical versus atypical neuroleptics. *Am J Psychiatry.* 1999;156:1200–1204.

Costello E, Foley D, Angold A. A 10-year research update review: the epidemiology of child and adolescent psychiatric disorders, II: developmental epidemiology. *J Am Acad Child Adolesc Psychiatry.* 2006;45:8–25.

Craven C, Murphy M. Carbamazepine treatment of bipolar disorder in an adolescent with cerebral palsy. *J Am Acad Child Adolesc Psychiatry.* 2000;39(6):680–681.

Crismon ML, Trivedi MJ, Pigott TA, et al. The Texas Medication Algorithm Project: report of the Texas consensus conference panel on medication treatment of major depressive disorder. *J Clin Psychiatry.* 1999;60:142–156.

Croarkin PE, Emslie GJ, Mayes TL. Neuroleptic malignant syndrome associated with atypical antipsychotics in pediatric patients: a review of published cases. *J Clin Psychiatry.* 2008;69(7):1157–1165.

Croonenberghs J, Fegert JM, Findling RL, et al; and the Risperidone Disruptive Behavior Study Group. Risperidone in children with disruptive behavior disorders and subaverage intelligence: a 1-year, open-label study of 504 patients. *J Am Acad Child Adolesc Psychiatry.* 2005; 44:64–72.

Cross-Disorder Group of the Psychiatric Genomics Consortium. Identification of risk loci with shared effects on five major psychiatric disorders: a genome-wide analysis. *Lancet.* 2013;381(9875):1371–1379. doi:10.1016/S0140-6736(12)62129-1.

Crumlish N, Whitty P, Clarke M, et al. Beyond the critical period: longitudinal study of 8-year outcome in first episode non-affective psychosis. *Br J Psychiatry.* 2009;194:18–24.

Crumrine PK, Feldman HM, Teodori J, et al. The use of methylphenidate in children with seizures and attention deficit disorder. *Ann Neurol.* 1987;22:441–442.

Cueva JE, Overall JE, Small AM, et al. Carbamazepine in aggressive children with conduct disorder: a double-blind and placebo-controlled study. *J Am Acad Child Adolesc Psychiatry.* 1996;35:480–490.

Cutler A, Mokliatchouk O, Laszlovszky I, et al. Cariprazine in acute schizophrenia: a fixed-dose phase III, randomized, double-blind, placebo-and active-controlled trial. Abstract presented at: 166th Annual Meeting of the American Psychiatric Association; May 18–22, 2013; San Francisco, CA.

Cutts KK, Jasper HH. Effect of benzedrine sulfate and phenobarbital on behavior problem children with abnormal electroencephalograms. *Arch Neurol Psychiatry.* 1939;411:1138–1145.

D'Amato G. Chlordiazepoxide in management of school phobia. *Dis Nerv Sys.* 1962;23:292–295.

da Costa CZ, de Morais RM, Zanetta DM, et al. Comparison among clomipramine, fluoxetine, and placebo for the treatment of anxiety disorders in children and adolescents. *J Child Adolesc Psychopharmacol.* 2013;23(10):687–692.

Davanzo P. Mood stabilizers in hospitalized children with bipolar disorder: a retrospective review. *Psychiatry Clin Neurosci.* 2003;57(3):504–510.

Davari-Ashtiani R, Shahrbabaki ME, Razjouyan K, et al. Buspirone versus methylphenidate in the treatment of attention deficit hyperactivity disorder: a doubleblind and randomized trial. *Child Psychiatry Hum Dev.* 2010;41(6):641–648.

Davis KL, Charney D, Coyle JT, et al, eds. *Neuropsychopharmacology: The Fifth Generation of Progress.* Philadelphia, PA: Lippincott Williams & Wilkins; 2002.

Daviss WB, Bentivoglio P, Racusin R, et al. Bupropion sustained release in adolescents with comorbid attention-deficit/hyperactivity disorder and depression. *J Am Acad Child Adolesc Psychiatry.* 2001;40(3):307–314.

Daviss WB, Perel JM, Rudolph GR, et al. Steady-state pharmacokinetics of bupropion SR in juvenile patients. *J Am Acad Child Adolesc Psychiatry.* 2005;44:349–357.

Dean AJ, Hendy A, McGuire T. Antidepressants in children and adolescents—changes in utilisation after safety warnings. *Pharmacoepidemiol Drug Saf.* 2007;16(9):1048–1053.

Deas D, May K, Randall C, et al. Naltrexone treatment of adolescent alcoholics: an open-label pilot study. *J Child Adolesc Psychopharmacol.* 2005;15(5):723–728.

DeGatta MF, Garcia MJ, Acosta A, et al. Monitoring of serum levels of imipramine and desipramine and individuation of dose in enuretic children. *Ther Drug Monit.* 1984;6:438–443.

De Jong J, Wauben P, Oolders H. Doxazosine, an alpha1-adrenergic antagonist, has positive effects on posttraumatic stress disorder. Poster presented at: The 25th Annual Meeting of The International Society for Traumatic Stress Studies; November 2008; Chicago, IL. Poster # T-208.

DelBello M, Chang K, Welge J, et al. A double-blind, placebo-controlled pilot study of quetiapine for depressed adolescents with bipolar disorder. *Bipolar Disord.* 2009;11:483–493.

DelBello M, Goldman R, Phillips D, et al. Efficacy and safety of lurasidone in children and adolescents with bipolar I depression: a double-blind, placebo-controlled study. *J Am Acad Child Adolesc Psychiatry.* 2017;56(12):1015–1025.

DelBello MP, Findling RL, Kushner S, et al. A pilot controlled study of topiramate for mania in children and adolescents with bipolar disorder. *J Am Acad Child Adolesc Psychiatry.* 2005;44:539–547.

DelBello MP, Hochadel TJ, Portland KB, et al. A double-blind, placebo-controlled study of selegiline transdermal system in depressed adolescents. *J Child Adolesc Psychopharmacol.* 2014;24(6): 311–317.

DelBello MP, Kowatch RA, Adler CM, et al. A double-blind randomized pilot study comparing quetiapine and divalproex for adolescent mania. *J Am Acad Child Adolesc Psychiatry.* 2006;45(3):305–313.

DelBello MP, Kowatch RA, Warner J, et al. Adjunctive topiramate treatment for pediatric bipolar disorder: a retrospective chart review. *J Child Adolesc Psychopharmacol.* 2002;12(4):323–330.

de Leon J. The effect of atypical *vs* typical antipsychotics on tardive dyskinesia: a naturalistic study. *Eur Arch Psychiatry Clin Neurosci.* 2007;257:169–172.

DeLong GR, Aldershof AL. Long-term experience with lithium treatment in childhood: correlation with clinical diagnosis. *J Am Acad Child Adolesc Psychiatry.* 1987;26:389–394.

De Sousa A. An open-label pilot study of naltrexone in childhood-onset trichotillomania. *J Child Adolesc Psychopharmacol.* 2008;1:30–33.

Denckla MB, Bemporad JR, MacKay MC. Tics following methylphenidate administration: a report of 20 cases. *JAMA.* 1976;235:1349–1351.

Detke H, DelBello M, Landry J, et al. Olanzapine/fluoxetine combination in children and adolescents with bipolar I depression: a randomized, double-blind, placebo-controlled trial. *J Am Acad Child Adolesc Psychiatry.* 2015;54:217–224.

Deutsch SI. Rationale for the administration of opiate antagonists in treating infantile autism. *Am J Ment Defic.* 1986;90:631–635.

Devane CL, Nemeroff CB. Clinical pharmacokinetics of quetiapine: an atypical antipsychotic. *Clin Pharmacokinet.* 2001;40:509–522.

DeVeaugh-Geiss MD, Moroz G, Biederman J, et al. Clomipramine hydrochloride in childhood and adolescent obsessive-compulsive disorder—a multicenter trial. *J Am Acad Child Adolesc Psychiatry.* 1992;31:45–49.

Dickstein D, Towbin K, Van Der Veen J, et al. Randomized double-blind placebo-controlled trial of lithium in youths with severe mood dysregulation. *J Child Adolesc Psychopharmacol.* 2009;19(1):61–73.

Diler RS, Avci A. Selective serotonin reuptake inhibitor discontinuation syndrome in children: six case reports. *Curr Ther Res.* 2002;63(3):188–197.

Dockett S, Perry B. Researching with young children: seeking assent. *Child Indicators Res.* 2011;4(2):231–247.

Dolder C, Jeste D. Incidence of tardive dyskinesia with typical *vs* atypical antipsychotics in very high risk patients. *Biol Psychiatry.* 2003;53:142–1145.

Dolle K, Schulte-Körne G, O'Leary AM, et al. The Beck Depression Inventory-II in adolescent mental health patients: cut-off scores for detecting depression and rating severity. *Psychiatry Res.* 2012;200(2):843–848.

Dolle K, Schulte-Korne G. The treatment of depressive disorders in children and adolescents. *Dtsch Arztebl Int.* 2013;110(50):854–860.

Donnelly M, Zametkin AJ, Rapoport JL, et al. Treatment of childhood hyperactivity with desipramine: plasma drug concentration, cardiovascular effects, plasma and urinary catecholamine levels, and clinical response. *Clin Pharmacol Ther.* 1986;39:72–81.

Donovan SJ, Stewart JW, Nunes EV, et al. Divalproex treatment for youth with explosive temper and mood lability: a double-blind, placebo-controlled crossover design (Published errata appear in *Am J Psychiatry* 157:1038 and *Am J Psychiatry* 157:1192). *Am J Psychiatry.* 2000;157:818–820.

Donovan SJ, Susser ES, Nunes Stewart JW, et al. Divalproex treatment of disruptive adolescents: a report of 10 cases. *J Clin Psychiatry.* 1997;58:12–15.

Dostal T. Antiaggressive effect of lithium salts in mentally retarded adolescents. In: Annell A-L, ed. *Depressive States in Childhood and Adolescence.* Stockholm, Sweden: Almqvist & Wiksell; 1972:491–498.

Driver D, Gogtay N, Rapoport J. Childhood onset schizophrenia and early onset schizophrenia spectrum disorders. *Child Adolesc Psychiatric Clin N Am.* 2013;22:539–555.

Drug Facts and Comparisons. 49th ed. St Louis, MO: Facts and Comparisons; 1995.

Dubovsky SL. Severe nortriptyline intoxication due to change from a generic to a trade preparation. *J Nerv Ment Dis.* 1987;175:115–117.

Duff G. Safety of Seroxat (paroxetine) in children and adolescents under 18 years–contraindication in the treatment of depressive illness. Epinet message from Professor G. Duff, Chairman of Committee on Safety of Medicines. 2003. http://www.mhra.gov.uk/Safetyinformation/Safetywarningsalertsandrecalls/Safetywarningsandmessagesformedicines/CON2015704. Accessed July 16, 2018.

Duffy FF, Narrow WE, Rae DS, et al. Concomitant pharmacotherapy among youths treated in routine psychiatric practice. *J Child Adolesc Psychopharmacol.* 2005;15(1):12.

Dugas M, Zarifian E, Leheuzey M-F, et al. Preliminary observations of the significance of monitoring tricyclic antidepressant plasma levels in the pediatric patient. *Ther Drug Monit.* 1980;2:307–314.

Dummit ES III, Klein RG, Tancer NK, et al. Fluoxetine treatment of children with selective mutism: an open trial. *J Am Acad Child Adolesc Psychiatry.* 1996;35:615–621.

Duncan MK. Using psychostimulants to treat behavioral disorders of children and adolescents. *J Child Adolesc Psychopharmacol.* 1990;1:7–20.

DuPaul GJ, Barkley RA, McMurray MB. Response of children with ADHD to methylphenidate: interaction with internalizing symptoms. *J Am Acad Child Adolesc Psychiatry.* 1994;33:894–903.

DuPaul GJ, Power TJ, McGoey KE, et al. Reliability and validity of parent and teacher ratings of attention-deficit/hyperactivity disorder symptoms. *J Psychoeduc Assess.* 1998;16:55–68.

Durgam S, Starace A, Li D, et al. An evaluation of the safety and efficacy of cariprazine in patients with acute exacerbation of schizophrenia: a phase II, randomized clinical trial. *Schizophr Res.* 2014;152(2–3):450–457.

Effron AS, Freedman AM. The treatment of behavioral disorders in children with benadryl. *J Pediatr.* 1953;42:261–266.

Elia J, Borcherding BG, Rapoport JL, et al. Methylphenidate and dextroamphetamine treatments of hyperactivity: are there true nonresponders? *Psychiatry Res.* 1991;36:141–155.

Elliott GR, Popper CW. Tricyclic antidepressants: the QT interval and other cardiovascular parameters [editorial]. *J Child Adolesc Psychopharmacol.* 1990/1991;1:187–189.

Emsley R, Chiliza B, Asmal L. The evidence for illness progression after relapse in schizophrenia. *Schizophr Res.* 2013;148:117–121.

Emslie GJ, Findling RL, Yeung PP, et al. Venlafaxine ER for the treatment of pediatric subjects with depression: results of two placebo-controlled trials. *J Am Acad Child Adolesc Psychiatry.* 2007;46(4):479–488.

Emslie GJ, Heiligenstein JH, Wagner KD, et al. Fluoxetine for acute treatment of depression in children and adolescents: a placebo-controlled, randomized clinical trial. *J Am Acad Child Adolesc Psychiatry.* 2002;41(10):1205–1215.

Emslie GJ, Mayes T, Porta G, et al. Treatment of resistant depression in adolescents (TORDIA): week 24 outcomes. *Am J Psychiatry.* 2010;167(7):782–791.

Emslie GJ, Prakash A, Zhang Q, et al. A double-blind efficacy and safety study of duloxetine fixed doses in children and adolescents with major depressive disorder. *J Child Adolesc Psychopharmacol.* 2014;24(4):170–179.

Emslie GJ, Rush AJ, Weinberg WA, et al. A double-blind, randomized, placebocontrolled trial of fluoxetine in children and adolescents with depression. *Arch Gen Psychiatry*. 1997;54:1031–1037.

Emslie GJ, Ventura D, Korotzer A, et al. Escitalopram in the treatment of adolescent depression: a randomized placebo-controlled multisite trial. *J Am Acad Child Adolesc Psychiatry*. 2009;48:721–729.

Emslie GJ, Wagner KD, Kutcher S, et al. Paroxetine treatment in children and adolescents with major depressive disorder: a randomized, multicenter, double-blind, placebo-controlled trial. *J Am Acad Child Adolesc Psychiatry*. 2006;45(6):709–719.

Emslie GJ, Wells TG, Prakash A. Acute and longer-term safety results from a pooled analysis of duloxetine studies for the treatment of children and adolescents with major depressive disorder. *J Child Adolesc Psychopharmacol*. 2015;25(4):293–305.

ESKALITH [prescribing information] EL:L50. Greenville, NC: GlaxoSmithKline; 2003.

Esposito S, Prange AJ Jr, Golden RN. The thyroid axis and mood disorders: overview and future prospects. *Psychopharmacol Bull*. 1997;33:205–217.

Evans RW, Clay TH, Gualtieri CT. Carbamazepine in pediatric psychiatry. *J Am Acad Child Adolesc Psychiatry*. 1987;26:2–8.

Faber MS, Fuhr U. Time response of cytochrome P450 1A2 activity on cessation of heavy smoking. *Clin Pharmacol Ther*. 2004;76(2):178–184.

Fabrega M, Sugranyes G, Baeza I. Two cases of long-acting paliperidone in adolescence. *Ther Adv Psychopharmacol*. 2015;5:304–306.

Faessel H, Ravva P, Williams K. Pharmacokinetics, safety, and tolerability of varenicline in healthy adolescent smokers: a multicenter, randomized, double-blind, placebo-controlled, parallel-group study. *Clin Ther*. 2009;31(1):177–189.

Fairbanks JM, Pine DS, Tancer NK, et al. Open fluoxetine treatment of mixed anxiety disorders in children and adolescents. *J Child Adolesc Psychopharmacol*. 1997;7:17–29.

Famularo R, Kinscherff R, Fenton T. Propranolol treatment for childhood posttraumatic stress disorder, acute type. *Am J Dis Child*. 1988;142:1244–1247.

Fanapt [package insert]. East Hanover, NJ: Novartis Pharmaceuticals Co; 2012.

Faraone SV, Biederman J, Monuteaux M, et al. Long-term effects of extended release mixed amphetamine salts treatment of attention-deficit/hyperactivity disorder. *J Child Adolesc Psychopharmacol*. 2005;15:191–202.

Faulkner G, Cohn T, Remington G. Interventions to reduce weight gain in schizophrenia. *Cochrane Database Syst Rev*. 2007;(1):CD005148.

Feeney DJ, Klykylo W. TD from Risperidone? *J Am Acad Child Adolesc Psychiatry*. 1997;36(7):867.

Feighner JP, Cohen JB. Analysis of individual symptoms in generalized anxiety: a pooled, multi-study double-blind evaluation of buspirone. *Neuropsychobiology*. 1989;21:124–130.

Feldman HM, Kolman BK, Gonzaga AM. Naltrexone and communication skills in young children with autism. *J Am Acad Child Adolesc Psychiatry*. 1999;38:587–593.

Fenichel RR. Combining methylphenidate and clonidine: the role of post-marketing surveillance. *J Child Adolesc Psychopharmacol*. 1995;5:155–156.

Ferguson HB, Simeon JG. Evaluating drug effects on children's cognitive functioning. *Prog Neuropsychopharmacol Biol Psychiatry*. 1984;8:683–686.

Fernándes-Alcantara AL, Caldwell SW, Stoltzfus E. Child Welfare: Oversight of Psychotropic Medication for Children in Foster Care. Washington, DC: Congressional Research Service; 2015. CRS Report R43466.

Fernández-Jaén A, Fernández-Mayoralas DM, Calleja Pérez B, et al. Atomoxetine for attention deficit hyperactivity disorder in mental retardation. *Pediatr Neurol*. 2010;43(5):341–347.

Findling R, McNamara N, Stansbrey R, et al. Combination lithium and divalproex sodium in pediatric bipolar symptom restabilization. *J Am Acad Child Adolesc Psychiatry*. 2006a;45(2):142–148.

Findling R, Pathak S, Earley W, et al. Efficacy and safety of extended-release quetiapine fumarate in youth with bipolar depression: an 8 week, double-blind, placebo-controlled trial. *J Child Adolesc Psychopharmacol*. 2014;24:325–335.

Findling RL, Frazier TW, Youngstrom EA, et al. Double-blind placebo-controlled trial of divalproex monotherapy in the treatment of symptomatic youth at high risk for developing bipolar disorder. *J Clin Psychiatry*. 2007a;68(5):781–788.

Findling RL, Greenhill LL, McNamara NK, et al. Venlafaxine in the treatment of children and adolescents with attention-deficit/hyperactivity disorder. *J Child Adolesc Psychopharmacol*. 2007b;17(4):433–445.

Findling RL, Groark J, Chiles D, et al. Safety and tolerability of desvenlafaxine in children and adolescents with major depressive disorder. *J Child Adolesc Psychopharmacol*. 2014;24(4):201–209.

Findling RL, Kafantaris V, Pavuluri M, et al. Dosing strategies for lithium monotherapy in children and adolescents with bipolar I disorder. *J Child Adolesc Psychopharmacol.* 2011;21(3):195–205.

Findling RL, Kauffman R, Sallee FR, et al. An open-label study of aripiprazole: pharmacokinetics, tolerability, and effectiveness in children and adolescents with conduct disorder. *J Child Adolesc Psychopharmacol.* 2009;19:431–439.

Findling RL, Landersdorfer CB, Kafantaris V, et al. First-dose pharmacokinetics of lithium carbonate in children and adolescents. *J Clin Psychopharmacol.* 2010;30(4):404–410.

Findling RL, McNamara NK, Branicky LA. A double-blind pilot study of risperidone in the treatment of conduct disorder. *J Am Acad Child Adolesc Psychiatry.* 2000;39:509–516.

Findling RL, McNamara NK, Gracious BL, et al. Quetiapine in nine youths with autistic disorder. *J Child Adolesc Psychopharmacol.* 2004;14:287–294.

Findling RL, McNamara NK, Youngstrom EA, et al. Double-blind 18-month trial of lithium versus divalproex maintenance treatment in pediatric bipolar disorder. *J Am Acad Child Adolesc Psychiatry.* 2005;44:409–417.

Findling RL, Reed MD, Myers C, et al. Paroxetine pharmacokinetics in depressed children and adolescents. *J Am Acad Child Adolesc Psychiatry.* 1999;38:952–959.

Findling RL, Reed MD, O'Riordan MA, et al. Effectiveness, safety, and pharmacokinetics of quetiapine in aggressive children with conduct disorder. *J Am Acad Child Adolesc Psychiatry.* 2006b;45:792–798.

Findling RL, Robb A, Bose A, et al. Escitalopram in the treatment of adolescent depression: a randomized, double-blind, placebo-controlled extension trial. *J Child Adolesc Psychopharmacol.* 2013;23(7):468–480.

Findling RL, Robb AS, DelBello M, et al. Pharmacokinetics and safety of vortioxetine in pediatric patients. *J Child Adolesc Psychopharmacol.* 2017;27(6)526–534.

Findling RL, Robb AS, DelBello M, et al. A 6-month open-label extension study of vortioxetine in pediatric patients with depressive or anxiety disorders. *J Child Adolesc Psychopharmacol.* 2018;28(1):47–54.

Findling RL, Robb A, McNamara NK, et al. Lithium in the acute treatment of bipolar i disorder: a double-blind, placebo-controlled study. *Pediatrics.* 2015;136(5):885–894.

Finnerty M, Neese-Todd S, Pritam R, et al. Access to psychosocial services prior to starting antipsychotic treatment among Medicaid-insured youth. *J Am Acad Child Adolesc Psychiatry.* 2016;55(1):69.

Finniss DG, Kaptchuk TJ, Miller F, et al. Biological, clinical, and ethical advances of placebo effects. *Lancet.* 2010;375(9715):686–695.

Fish B. Drug therapy in child psychiatry: pharmacological aspects. *Compr Psychiatry.* 1960;1:212–227.

Fish B. The "one child, one drug" myth of stimulants in hyperkinesis. *Arch Gen Psychiatry.* 1971;25:193–203.

Fisher S. *Child Research in Psychopharmacology.* Springfield, IL: Charles C Thomas; 1959.

Fishman MJ, Winstanley EL, Curran E, et al. Treatment of opioid dependence in adolescents and young adults with extended release naltrexone: preliminary case-series and feasibility. *Addiction.* 2010;105(9):1669–1676.

Fitzpatrick PA, Klorman R, Brumaghim JT, et al. Effects of sustained-release and standard preparations of methylphenidate on attention deficit disorder. *J Am Acad Child Adolesc Psychiatry.* 1992;31:226–234.

Flament MF, Rapoport JL, Berg CJ, et al. Clomipramine treatment of childhood obsessive-compulsive disorder: a double blind controlled study. *Arch Gen Psychiatry.* 1985;42:977–983.

Flament MF, Rapoport JL, Murphy DL, et al. Biochemical changes during clomipramine treatment of childhood obsessive-compulsive disorder. *Arch Gen Psychiatry.* 1987;44:219–225.

Fleischhacker WW, Bergmann KJ, Perovich R, et al. The Hillside Akathisia Scale: a new rating instrument for neuroleptic-induced akathisia. *Psychopharmacol Bull.* 1989;25:222–226.

Fleischhacker WW, Cetkovich-Bakmas M, De Hert M, et al. Comorbid somatic illnesses in patients with severe mental disorders: clinical, policy, and research challenges. *J Clin Psychiatry.* 2008;69(4):514–519.

Foa EB, Johnson KM, Feeny NC, et al. The child PTSD symptom scale: a preliminary examination of its psychometric properties. *J Clin Child Psychol.* 2001;30:376–384. doi:10.1207/S15374424JCCP3003_9.

Fontanella CA, Warner LA, Phillips GS, et al. Trends in psychotropic polypharmacy among youths enrolled in Ohio Medicaid, 2002–2008. *Psychiatr Serv.* 2014;65(11):1332–1340.

Ford K, Sankey J, Crisp J. Development of children's assent documents using a child-centered approach. *J Child Health Care.* 2007;11(1):19–28.

Fox N, Cousens S, Scahill R, et al. Using serial registered brain magnetic resonance imaging to measure disease progression in Alzheimer disease: power calculations and estimates of sample size to detect treatment effects. *Arch Neurol*. 2000;57:339–344.

Franowicz JS, Arnsten AF. Action of α-2 noradrenergic agonists on spatial working memory and blood pressure in rhesus monkeys appear to be mediated by the same receptor subtype. *Psychopharmacology*. 2002;162:304–312.

Fras I. Trazodone and violence [letter]. *J Am Acad Child Adolesc Psychiatry*. 1987;26:453.

Frazier JA, Biederman J, Jacobs TG, et al. Olanzapine in the treatment of bipolar disorder in juveniles. (Abstract 40th Annual NCDEU meeting). *J Child Adolesc Psychopharmacol*. 2000;10:237–238.

Frazier JA, Cohen LG, Jacobsen L, et al. Clozapine pharmacokinetics in children and adolescents with childhood-onset schizophrenia. *J Clin Psychopharmacol*. 2003;23:87–91.

Frazier JA, Gordon CT, McKenna K, et al. An open trial of clozapine in 11 adolescents with child-onset schizophrenia. *J Am Acad Child Adolesc Psychiatry*. 1994;33:658–663.

Frazier JA, Meyer MC, Biederman J, et al. Risperidone treatment for juvenile bipolar disorder: a retrospective chart review. *J Am Acad Child Adolesc Psychiatry*. 1999;38:960–965.

Freudenreich O, Remington G. Valbenazine for Tardive Dyskinesia. *Clin Schizophr Relat Psychoses*. 2017;11:113–119.

Friedman JM, Polifka JE. *The Effects of Neurologic and Psychiatric Drugs on the Fetus and Nursing Infant*. Baltimore, MD: Johns Hopkins University Press; 1998.

Fritz GK, Rockney RM, Yeung AS. Plasma levels and efficacy of imipramine treatment for enuresis. *J Am Acad Child Adolesc Psychiatry*. 1994;33:60–64.

Fu-I L, Boarati M, Stravogiannis A, et al. Use of risperidone long-acting injection to support treatment adherence and mood stabilization in pediatric bipolar patients: a case series. *J Clin Psychiatry*. 2009;70:604–606.

Gadow KD, Nolan EE, Sverd J. Methylphenidate in hyperactive boys with comorbid tic disorder: II, short-term behavioral effects in school settings. *J Am Acad Child Adolesc Psychiatry*. 1992;31:462–471.

Gadow KD, Poling AG. *Pharmacotherapy and Mental Retardation*. Boston, MA: College-Hill Press; 1988.

Gadow KD, Sverd J, Sprafkin J, et al. Efficacy of methylphenidate for attention deficit hyperactivity disorder in children with tic disorder. *Arch Gen Psychiatry*. 1995;52:444–455.

Gadow KD, Sverd J, Sprafkin J, et al. Long-term methylphenidate therapy in children with comorbid attention-deficit hyperactivity disorder and chronic multiple tic disorder. *Arch Gen Psychiatry*. 1999;56:330–336.

Gadow KD. *Children on Medication. Volume I: Hyperactivity, Learning Disabilities, and Mental Retardation*. San Diego, CA: College-Hill Press; 1986a.

Gadow KD. *Children on Medication. Volume II: Epilepsy, Emotional Disturbance, and Adolescent Disorders*. San Diego, CA: College-Hill Press; 1986b.

Gammon GD, Brown TE. Fluoxetine and methylphenidate in combination for treatment of attention deficit disorder and comorbid depressive disorder. *J Child Adolesc Psychopharmacol*. 1993;3:1–10.

Garfinkel BD, Wender PH, Sloman L, et al. Tricyclic antidepressant and methylphenidate treatment of attention deficit disorder in children. *J Am Acad Child Psychiatry*. 1983;22:343–348.

Garfinkel D, Zorin M, Wainstein J, et al. Efficacy and safety of prolonged-release melatonin in insomnia patients with diabetes: a randomized, double-blind, crossover study. *Diab Metabol Synd Obes*. 2011;4:307–313.

Gastfriend DR, Biederman J, Jellinek MS. Desipramine in the treatment of adolescents with attention deficit disorder. *Am J Psychiatry*. 1984;141:906–908.

Gaszner P, Makkos Z. Clozapine maintenance therapy in schizophrenia. *Prog Neuropsychopharmacol Biol Psychiatry*. 2004;28:465–469.

Gaw CE, Spiller HA, Russell JL, et al. Evaluation of dose and outcomes for pediatric vilazodone ingestions. *Clin Toxicol*. 2018;56(2):113–119.

Geller B. Commentary on unexplained deaths of children on Norpramin. *J Am Acad Child Adolesc Psychiatry*. 1991;30:682–684.

Geller B, Carr LG. Similarities and differences between adult and pediatric major depressive disorders. In: Georgotas A, Cancro R, eds. *Depression and Mania*. New York, NY: Elsevier; 1988:565–580.

Geller B, Cooper TB, Carr LG, et al. Prospective study of scheduled withdrawal from nortriptyline in children and adolescents. *J Clin Psychopharmacol*. 1987a;7:252–254.

Geller B, Cooper TB, Chestnut EC, et al. Child and adolescent nortriptyline single dose kinetics predict steady state plasma levels and suggested dose: preliminary data. *J Clin Psychopharmacol*. 1985;5:154–158.

Geller B, Cooper TB, Chestnut EC, et al. Preliminary data on the relationship between nortriptyline plasma level and response in depressed children. *Am J Psychiatry.* 1986;143:1283–1286.

Geller B, Cooper TB, Graham DL, et al. Double-blind placebo-controlled study of nortriptyline in depressed adolescents using a "fixed plasma level" design. *Psychopharmacol Bull.* 1990;26:85–90.

Geller B, Cooper TB, Graham DL, et al. Pharmacokinetically designed double blind placebo-controlled study of nortriptyline in 6- to 12-year-olds with major depressive disorder. *J Am Acad Child Adolesc Psychiatry.* 1992;31:34–44.

Geller B, Cooper TB, McCombs HG, et al. Double-blind placebo-controlled study of nortriptyline in depressed children using a "fixed plasma level" design. *Psychopharmacol Bull.* 1989;25:101–108.

Geller B, Cooper TB, Schluchter MD, et al. Child and adolescent nortriptyline single dose pharmacokinetic parameters: final report. *J Clin Psychopharmacol.* 1987b;7:321–323.

Geller B, Cooper TB, Sun K, et al. Double-blind and placebo-controlled study of lithium for adolescent bipolar disorders with secondary substance dependency. *J Am Acad Child Adolesc Psychiatry.* 1998;37:171–178.

Geller B, Fox LW, Fletcher M. Effect of tricyclic antidepressants on switching to mania and on the onset of bipolarity in depressed 6- to 12-year-olds. *J Am Acad Child Adolesc Psychiatry.* 1993;32:43–50.

Geller B, Guttmacher LB, Bleeg M. Coexistence of childhood onset pervasive developmental disorder and attention deficit disorder with hyperactivity. *Am J Psychiatry.* 1981;138:388–389.

Geller B, Luby JL, Joshi P, et al. A randomized controlled trial of risperidone, lithium, or divalproex sodium for initial treatment of bipolar I disorder, manic or mixed phase, in children and adolescents. *Arch Gen Psychiatry.* 2012;69(5):515–528.

Geller D, Donnelly C, Lopez F, et al. Atomoxetine treatment for pediatric patients with attention-deficit/hyperactivity disorder with comorbid anxiety disorder. *J Am Acad Child Adolesc Psychiatry.* 2007;46(9):1119–1127.

Geller DA, Hoog SL, Heiligenstein JH, et al. Fluoxetine treatment for obsessive compulsive disorder in children and adolescents: a placebo-controlled clinical trial. *J Am Acad Child Adolesc Psychiatry.* 2001;40(7):773–779.

Geller DA, Wagner KD, Emslie G, et al. Paroxetine treatment in children and adolescents with obsessive-compulsive disorder: a randomized, multicenter, double-blind, placebo-controlled trial. *J Am Acad Child Adolesc Psychiatry.* 2004;43:1387–1396.

Gentile S. Efficacy of antidepressant medications in children and adolescents with non-obsessive-compulsive disorder anxiety disorders: a systematic assessment. *Expert Opin Drug Saf.* 2014;13(6):735–744.

Geodon [package insert]. New York, NY: Pfizer Inc; 2012.

Geodon [package insert] (2015). New York, NY: Pfizer Inc; 2015.

Gerbino-Rosen G, Roofeh D, Tompkins DA, et al. Hematological adverse events in clozapine-treated children and adolescents. *J Am Acad Child Adolesc Psychiatry.* 2005;44:1024–1031.

Ghanizadeh A, Freeman RD, Berk M. Efficacy and adverse effects of venlafaxine in children and adolescents with ADHD: a systematic review of non-controlled and controlled trials. *Rev Recent Clin Trials.* 2013;8(1):2–8.

Gharabawi GM, Bossie CA, Lasser RA, et al. Abnormal Involuntary Movement Scale (AIMS) and Extrapyramidal Symptom Rating Scale (ESRS): cross-scale comparison in assessing tardive dyskinesia. *Schizophr Res.* 2005;77(2–3):119–128.

Ghaziuddin N, Alessi NE. An open clinical trial of trazodone in aggressive children. *J Child Adolesc Psychopharmacol.* 1992;2:291–297.

Giacino JT, Whyte J, Bagiella E, et al. Placebo-controlled trial of amantadine for severe traumatic brain injury. *N Engl J Med.* 2012;366:819–826.

Gibbons RD, Brown CH, Hur K, et al. Early evidence on the effects of regulators' suicidality warnings on SSRI prescriptions and suicide in children and adolescents. *Am J Psychiatry.* 2007;164:1356–1363.

Gilbert AR, Moore GJ, Keshavan MS, et al. Decrease in thalamic volumes of pediatric patients with obsessive-compulsive disorder who are taking paroxetine. *Arch Gen Psychiatry.* 2000;57:449–456.

Gillberg C, Melander H, von Knorring A-L, et al. Long-term stimulant treatment of children with attention-deficit hyperactivity disorder symptoms. *Arch Gen Psychiatry.* 1997;54:857–864.

Gilbert DL, Batterson JR, Sethuraman G, et al. Tic reduction with risperidone versus pimozide in a randomized, double-blind, crossover trial. *J Am Acad Child Adolesc Psychiatry.* 2004;43:206–214.

Gilbody S, Richards D, Brealey S, et al. Screening for depression in medical settings with the Patient Health Questionnaire (PHQ): a diagnostic meta-analysis. *J Gen Intern Med.* 2007;22(11):1596–1602.

Gillberg C, Melander H, von Knorring A-L, et al. Long-term stimulant treatment of children with attention-deficit hyperactivity disorder symptoms. *Arch Gen Psychiatry.* 1997;54:857–864.

Ginsburg GS, Kendall PC, Sakolsky D, et al. Remission after acute treatment in children and adolescents with anxiety disorders: findings from the CAMS. *J Consult Clin Psychol.* 2011;79(6):806–813.

Gittelman-Klein R, Klein D. Controlled imipramine treatment of school phobia. *Arch Gen Psychiatry*. 1971;25:204–207.

Gittelman-Klein R, Klein DF, Katz S, et al. Comparative effects of methylphenidate and thioridazine in hyperkinetic children: I, clinical results. *Arch Gen Psychiatry*. 1976;33:1217–1231.

Glick BS, Schulman D, Turecki S. Diazepam (Valium) treatment in childhood sleep disorder. *Dis Nerv Sys*. 1971;32:565–566.

Glue P, Fang A, Gendelman K, Klee B. Pharmacokinetics of an extended release formulation of alprazolam (Xanax XR) in healthy normal adolescent and adult volunteers. *Am J Ther*. 2006;13(5):418–422.

Goldstein BI, Stober M, Axelson D, et al. Predictors of first-onset substance use disorders during the prospective course of bipolar spectrum disorders in adolescents. *J Am Acad Child Adolesc Psychiatry*. 2013;52(10):1026–1037.

Good CR, Feaster CS, Krecko VF. Tolerability of oral loading of divalproex sodium in child psychiatry inpatients. *J Child Adolesc Psychopharmacol*. 2001;11:53–56.

Goodyer I, Dubicka B, Wilkinson P, et al. Selective serotonin reuptake inhibitors (SSRIs) and routine specialist care with and without cognitive behavior therapyin adolescents with major depression: randomised controlled trial. *BMJ*. 2007;335:142–146.

Gordon CT, State RC, Nelson JE, et al. A double-blind comparison of clomipramine, desipramine, and placebo in the treatment of autistic disorder. *Arch Gen Psychiatry*. 1993;50:441–447.

Gorenstein G, Gorenstein C, de Oliveira MC, et al. Child-focused treatment of pediatric OCD affects parental behavior and family environment. *Psychiatry Res*. 2015;229(1–2):161–166.

Graae F, Milner J, Rizzotto L, et al. Clonazepam in childhood anxiety disorders. *J Am Acad Child Adolesc Psychiatry*. 1994;33:372–376.

Gray KM, Carpenter MJ, Baker NL, et al. Bupropion SR and contingency management for adolescent smoking cessation. *J Subst Abuse Treat*. 2011;40(1):77–86.

Gray KM, Carpenter MJ, Baker NL, et al. A double-blind randomized controlled trial of N-acetylcysteine in cannabis-dependent adolescents. *Am J Psychiatry*. 2012a;169(8):805–812.

Gray KM, Carpenter MJ, Lewis AL, et al. Varenicline versus bupropion XL for smoking cessation in older adolescents: a randomized, double-blind pilot trial. *Nicotine Tob Res*. 2012b;14(2):234–239.

Green WH. Psychosocial dwarfism: psychological and etiological considerations. In: Lahey BB, Kazdin AE, eds. *Advances in Clinical Child Psychology*. Vol 9. New York, NY: Plenum Press; 1986:245–278.

Green WH. Pervasive developmental disorders. In: Kestenbaum CJ, Williams DT, eds. *Handbook of Clinical Assessment of Children and Adolescents*. Vol 1. New York, NY: New York University Press; 1988:469–498.

Green WH. Schizophrenia with childhood onset. In: Kaplan HI, Sadock BJ, eds. *Comprehensive Textbook of Psychiatry*. 5th ed. Baltimore, MD: Williams & Wilkins; 1989:1975–1981.

Green WH. The treatment of attention-deficit hyperactivity disorder with nonstimulant medications. *Child Adolesc Psychiatr Clin N Am*. 1995;4:169–195.

Green WH, Campbell M, Hardesty AS, et al. A comparison of schizophrenic and autistic children. *J Am Acad Child Psychiatry*. 1984;23:399–409.

Green WH, Deutsch SI. Biological studies of schizophrenia with childhood onset. In: Deutsch SI, Weizman A, Weizman R, eds. *Application of Basic Neuroscience to Child Psychiatry*. New York, NY: Plenum Medical Book; 1990:217–229.

Green WH, Deutsch SI, Campbell M, et al. Neuropsychopharmacology of the childhood psychoses: a critical review. In: Morgan DW, ed. *Psychopharmacology: Impact on Clinical Psychiatry*. St Louis, MO: Ishiyaku EuroAmerica; 1985:139–173.

Green WH, Padron-Gayol M, Hardesty AS, et al. Schizophrenia with childhood onset: a phenomenological study of 38 cases. *J Am Acad Child Adolesc Psychiatry*. 1992;31:968–976.

Greenblatt DJ, Shader RI, Abernethy DR. Current status of benzodiazepines (first of two parts). *N Engl J Med*. 1983;309:354–358.

Greenblatt DJ, Shader RI. *Benzodiazepines in Clinical Practice*. New York, NY: Raven Press; 1974.

Greenhill LL. Attention-deficit hyperactivity disorder in children. In: Garfinkel BD, Carlson GA, Weller EB, eds. *Psychiatric Disorders in Children and Adolescents*. Philadelphia, PA: WB Saunders; 1990:149–182.

Greenhill LL, Pliszka S, Dulcan MK, et al. Practice parameters for the use of stimulant medications in the treatment of children, adolescents, and adults. *J Am Acad Child Adolesc Psychiatry*. 2002;41(suppl):26S–49S.

Greenhill LL, Solomon M, Pleak R, et al. Molindone hydrochloride treatment of hospitalized children with conduct disorder. *J Clin Psychiatry*. 1985;46:20–25.

Gringras P, Nir T, Breddy J, et al. Efficacy and safety of pediatric prolonged-release melatonin for insomnia in children with autism spectrum disorder. *J Child Adolesc Psychopharmacol.* 2017;56:11:948–957.

Grizenko N, Vida S. Propranolol treatment of episodic dyscontrol and aggressive behavior in children [letter]. *Can J Psychiatry.* 1988;33:776–778.

Groh C. The psychotropic effect of Tegretol in non-epileptic children, with particular reference to the drug's indications. In: Birkmayer W, ed. *Epileptic Seizures-Behaviour-Pain.* Bern, Germany: Hans Huber Publishers; 1976:259–263.

Gross MD. Imipramine in the treatment of minimal brain dysfunction in children. *Psychosomatics.* 1973;14:283–285.

Gross MD, Wilson WC. *Minimal Brain Dysfunction.* New York, NY: Brunner/Mazel; 1974.

Grothe DR, Calis KA, Jacobsen L, et al. Olanzapine pharmacokinetics in pediatric and adolescent inpatients with childhood-onset schizophrenia. *J Clin Psychopharmacol.* 2000;20:220–225.

Gualtieri CT. *Brain Injury and Mental Retardation: Psychopharmacology and Neuropsychiatry.* Philadelphia, PA: Lippincott Williams and Wilkins; 2002:294.

Gualtieri CT, Golden R, Evans RW, et al. Blood level measurement of psychoactive drugs in pediatric psychiatry. *Ther Drug Monit.* 1984a;6:127–141.

Gualtieri CT, Golden RN, Fahs JJ. New developments in pediatric psychopharmacology. *J Dev Behav Pediatr.* 1983;4:202–209.

Gualtieri CT, Johnson LG. Antidepressant side effects in children and adolescents. *J Child Adolesc Psychopharmacol.* 2006;16(1–2):147–157.

Gualtieri CT, Keenan PA, Chandler M. Clinical and neuropsychological effect on desipramine in children with attention deficit hyperactivity disorder. *J Clin Psychopharmacol.* 1991;11:155–159.

Gualtieri CT, Quade D, Hicks RE, et al. Tardive dyskinesia and other clinical consequences of neuroleptic treatment in children and adolescents. *Am J Psychiatry.* 1984b;141:20–23.

Gualtieri CT, Wafgin W, Kanoy R, et al. Clinical studies of methylphenidate serum levels in children and adults. *J Am Acad Child Psychiatry.* 1982;21:19–26.

Gupta S, Cahill JD. A prescription for "deprescribing" in psychiatry. *Psychiatr Serv.* 2016;67(8):904–907.

Gutgesell H, Atkins D, Barst R, et al. AHA scientific statement: cardiovascular monitoring of children and adolescents receiving psychotropic drugs. *J Am Acad Child Adolesc Psychiatry.* 1999;38:1047–1050. Reprinted from *Circulation.* 1999;99:979–982.

Guy W. Dosage Record and Treatment Emergent Symptoms Scale (DOTES). In: *ECDEU Assessment Manual for Psychopharmacology—Revised.* Rockville, MD: US Department of Health, Education, and Welfare, Public Health Service, Alcohol, Drug Abuse, and Mental Health Administration, NIMH Psychopharmacology Research Branch, Division of Extramural Research Programs; 1976a:223–244. DHEW Publ No ADM 76–338.

Guy W. *ECDEU Assessment Manual for Psychopharmacology* (NIMH Publ No 76–338). Washington, DC: DHEW, NIMH; 1976b.

Hack S, Chow B. Pediatric psychotropic medication compliance: a literature review and research-based suggestions for improving treatment compliance. *J Child Adolesc Psychopharmacol.* 2001;11:59–67.

Hallowell EM, Ratey JJ. *Delivered from Distraction: Getting the Most Out of Life with Attention Deficit Disorder.* New York, NY: Random House Publishing Group; 2005:253–255.

Hamill PVV, Drizd TA, Johnson CL, et al. NCHS growth charts, 1976. *Monthly Vital Statistics Reports.* 1976;25(suppl 3):1–22. (Health Examination Survey Data, National Center for Health Statistics Publication [HRA] 76–1120.)

Hammond CJ, Gray KM. Pharmacotherapy for substance use disorders in youths. *J Child Adolesc Subst Abuse.* 2016;25(4):292–316.

Handen BJ, Feldman HM, Lurier A, et al. Efficacy of methylphenidate among preschool children with developmental disabilities and ADHD. *J Am Acad Child Adolesc Psychiatry.* 1999;38:805–812.

Handen BJ, Johnson CR, Lubetsky M. Efficacy of methylphenidate among children with autism and symptoms of attention-deficit hyperactivity disorder. *J Autism Dev Disord.* 2000;30:245–255.

Handen BL, Anagnostou E, Aman MG, et al. A randomized, placebo-controlled trial of metformin for the treatment of overweight induced by antipsychotic medication in young people with autism spectrum disorder: open-label extension. *J Am Acad Child Adolesc Psychiatry.* 2017;56:849–856.

Hanson K, Allen S, Jensen S, et al. Treatment of adolescent smokers with the nicotine patch. *Nicotine Tob Res.* 2003;5(4):515–526.

Hanwella R, Senanayake M, de Silva V. Comparative efficacy and acceptability of methylphenidate and atomoxetine in treatment of attention deficit hyperactivity disorder in children and adolescents: a meta-analysis. *BMC Psychiatry.* 2011;11:176.

Harfterkamp M, van de Loo-Neus G, Minderaa RB, et al. A randomized double-blind study of atomoxetine versus placebo for attention-deficit/hyperactivity disorder symptoms in children with autism spectrum disorder. *J Am Acad Child Adolesc Psychiatry.* 2012;51(7):733–741.

Harrigan E, Miceli J, Anziano R, et al. A randomized evaluation of the effects of six antipsychotic agents on QTc, in the absence and presence of metabolic inhibition. *J Clin Psychopharmacol.* 2004;24:62–69.

Harris M, Henry L, Harrigan S, et al. The relationship between duration of untreated psychosis and outcome: an eight-year prospective study. *Schizophr Res.* 2005;79:85–93.

Hasnain M, Fredrickson SK, Vieweg W, et al. Metabolic syndrome associated with schizophrenia and atypical antipsychotics. *Curr Diab Rep.* 2010;10:209–216.

Hauser R, Factor S, Knesevich M, et al. KINECT 3: a phase 3 randomized, double-blind, placebo-controlled trial for Tardive Dyskinesia. *Am J Psychiatry.* 2017;5:476–484.

Hayes PE, Schulz SC. Beta-blockers in anxiety disorders. *J Affect Disord.* 1987;13:119–130.

Hayes TA, Logan Panitch M, Marker E. Imipramine dosage in children: a comment on "imipramine and electrocardiographic abnormalities in hyperactive children." *Am J Psychiatry.* 1975;132:546–547.

Hellings J, Weckbaugh M, Nickel E, et al. A double-blind, placebo-controlled study of valproate for aggression in youth with pervasive developmental disorders. *J Child Adolesc Psychopharmacol.* 2005;15(4):682–692.

Hersh CB, Sokol MS, Pfeffer CR. Transient psychosis with fluoxetine [letter]. *J Am Acad Child Adolesc Psychiatry.* 1991;31:851.

Herskowitz J. Developmental neurotoxicology. In: Popper C, ed. *Psychiatric Pharmacosciences of Children and Adolescents.* Washington, DC: American Psychiatric Press; 1987:81–123.

Hetrick SE, McKenzie JE, Cox GR, et al. Newer generation antidepressants for depressive disorders in children and adolescents. *Cochrane Database Syst Rev.* 2012;(11):CD004851.

Hoebert M, van der Heijden K, van Geijlswijk I, et al. Long-term follow-up of melatonin treatment in children with ADHD and chronic sleep onset insomnia. *J Pineal Res.* 2009;47(1):1–7.

Hollander E, Chaplin W, Soorya L, et al. Divalproex sodium vs placebo for the treatment of irritability in children and adolescents with autism spectrum disorders. *Neuropsychopharmacology.* 2009;35(4):990–998.

Hollander E, Phillips A, Chaplin W, et al. A placebo controlled crossover trial of liquid fluoxetine on repetitive behaviors in childhood and adolescent autism. *Neuropsychopharmacology.* 2005;30:582–589.

Hollander E, Soorya L, Wasserman S, et al. Divalproex sodium vs. placebo in the treatment of repetitive behaviours in autism spectrum disorder. *Int J Neuropsychopharmacol.* 2006;9(2):209–213.

Holtmann M, Buchmann A, Esser G, et al. The child behavior checklist-dysregulation impairment: a longitudinal analysis. *J Child Psychol Psychiatry.* 2010;52:139–147.

Holzer JF. The process of informed consent. *Bull Am Coll Surg.* 1989;74:10–14.

Horrigan JP, Barnhill LJ. Guanfacine for treatment of attention-deficit hyperactivity disorder in boys. *J Child Adolesc Psychopharmacol.* 1995;5:215–223.

Horrigan JP, Barnhill LJ. Risperidone and explosive aggressive autism. *J Autism Dev Disord.* 1997;27:313–323.

Horrigan JP, Barnhill LJ. Does guanfacine trigger mania in children? [letter]. *J Child Adolesc Psychopharmacol.* 1998;8:149–150.

Hosenbocus S, Chahal R. SSRIs and SNRIs: a review of the discontinuation syndrome in children and adolescents. *J Can Acad Child Adolesc Psychiatry.* 2011;20(1):60–67.

Howell C, Larson J, Coffey B. Treatment of bipolar disorder in an adolescent with autistic disorder: a diagnostic and treatment dilemma. *J Child Adolesc Psychopharmacol.* 2011;21(3):283–286.

Huessy HR, Wright AL. The use of imipramine in children's behavior disorders. *Acta Paedopsychiatr.* 1970;37:194–199.

Hughes CW, Emslie GJ, Crismon ML, et al. The Texas children's medication algorithm project: report of the Texas Consensus Conference Panel on medication treatment of childhood major depressive disorder. *J Am Acad Child Adolesc Psychiatry.* 1999;38:1442–1454.

Hughes CW, Emslie GJ, Crismon ML, et al. Texas children's medication algorithm project: update from Texas Consensus Conference Panel on medication treatment of childhood major depressive disorder. *J Am Acad Child Adolesc Psychiatry.* 2007;46(6):667–686.

Hulvershorn L, Parkhurst S, Jones S, et al. Improved metabolic and psychiatric outcomes with discontinuation of atypical antipsychotics in youth hospitalized in a state psychiatric facility. *J Child Adolesc Psychopharmacol.* 2017;27(10):897–907.

Hunt RD. Treatment effects of oral and transdermal clonidine in relation to methylphenidate: an open pilot study in ADD-H. *Psychopharmacol Bull.* 1987;23:111–114.

Hunt RD, Arnsten AFT, Asbell MD. An open trial of guanfacine in the treatment of attention-deficit hyperactivity disorder. *J Am Acad Child Adolesc Psychiatry.* 1995;34:50–54.

Hunt RD, Capper L, O'Connell P. Clonidine in child and adolescent psychiatry. *J Child Adolesc Psychopharmacol.* 1990;1:87–102.

Hunt RD, Cohen DJ, Shaywitz SE, et al. Strategies for study of the neurochemistry of attention deficit disorder in children. *Schizophr Bull.* 1982;8:236–252.

Hunt RD, Lau S, Ryu J. Alternative therapies for ADHD. In: Greenhill LL, Osman BB, eds. *Ritalin: Theory and Patient Management.* New York, NY: Mary Ann Liebert; 1991:75–95.

Hunt RD, Minderaa RB, Cohen DJ. Clonidine benefits children with attention deficit disorder and hyperactivity: report of a double-blind placebo-crossover therapeutic trial. *J Am Acad Child Psychiatry.* 1985;24:617–629.

Invega Sustenna [package insert]. Titusville, NJ: Janssen Pharmaceuticals Inc; 2012.

Isojarvi JIT, Laatikainen TJ, Pakarinen AJ, et al. Polycystic ovaries and hyperandrogenism in women taking valproate for epilepsy. *N Engl J Med.* 1993;329:1383–1388.

Jafarinia M, Mohammadi MR, Modabbernia A, et al. Bupropion versus methylphenidate in the treatment of children with attention-deficit/hyperactivity disorder: a randomized double-blind study. *Hum Psychopharmacol.* 2012;27(4):411–418.

Jafri AB. Fluoxetine side effects [letter]. *J Am Acad Child Adolesc Psychiatry.* 1991;31:852.

Jankovic J, Jimenez-Shahed J, Brown LW. A randomized, double-blind, placebo-controlled study of topiramate in the treatment of Tourette syndrome. *J Neurol Neurosurg Psychiatry.* 2010;81(1):70–73.

Jann MW. Clozapine. *Pharmacotherapy.* 1991;11:179–195.

Jaselskis CA, Cook EH, Fletcher KE, et al. Clonidine treatment of hyperactive and impulsive children with autistic disorder. *J Clin Psychopharmacol.* 1992;12:322–327.

Jasinski DR, Krishnan S. Abuse liability and safety of oral lisdexamfetamine dimesylate in individuals with a history of stimulant abuse. *J Psychopharmacol.* 2009a;23(4):419–427.

Jasinski DR, Krishnan S. Human pharmacology of intravenous lisdexamfetamine dimesylate: abuse liability in adult stimulant abusers. *J Psychopharmacol.* 2009b;23(4):410–418.

Jatlow PI. Psychotropic drug disposition during development. In: Popper C, ed. *Psychiatric Pharmacosciences of Children and Adolescents.* Washington, DC: American Psychiatric Press; 1987:27–44.

Jefferson JW, Greist JH, Ackerman DL, et al. *Lithium Encyclopedia for Clinical Practice.* 2nd ed. Washington, DC: American Psychiatric Press; 1987.

Jefferson JW, Greist JH, Clagnaz PJ, et al. Effect of strenuous exercise on serum lithium level in man. *Am J Psychiatry.* 1982;139:1593–1595.

Jerome L. Hypomania with fluoxetine [letter]. *J Am Acad Child Adolesc Psychiatry.* 1991;30:850–851.

Jerrell JM, McIntyre RS, Park YM. Correlates of incident bipolar disorder in children and adolescents diagnosed with attention-deficit/hyperactivity disorder. *J Clin Psychiatry.* 2014;75(11):e1278–e1283.

Jeste D, Lacro J, Palmer B, et al. Incidence of tardive dyskinesia in early stages of low-dose treatment with typical neuroleptics in older patients. *Am J Psychiatry.* 1999b;156:309–311.

Jeste D, Rockwell E, Harris M, et al. Conventional vs newer antipsychotics in elderly patients. *Am J Geriatr Psychiatry.* 1999a;7:70–76.

Jeste DV, Wyatt RJ. *Understanding and Treating Tardive Dyskinesia.* New York, NY: Guilford Press; 1982.

Johnston HF. More on valproate and polycystic ovaries [letter]. *J Am Acad Child Adolesc Psychiatry.* 1999;38:354.

Johnson JG, Harris ES, Spitzer RL, et al. The patient health questionnaire for adolescents: validation of an instrument for the assessment of mental disorders among adolescent primary care patients. *J Adolesc Health.* 2002;30:196–204.

Johnston C, Pelham WE, Hoza J, et al. Psychostimulant rebound in attention deficit disordered boys. *J Am Acad Child Adolesc Psychiatry.* 1988;27:806–810.

Johnston L, O'Malley P, Miech RA, et al. *Monitoring the Future National Survey National Results on Drug Use, 1975-2015: Overview, Key Findings on Adolescent Drug Use.* Ann Arbor, MI: Institute for Social Research, The University of Michigan; 2016.

Joshi G, Wozniak J, Mick E, et al. A prospective open-label trial of extended release carbamazepine monotherapy in children with bipolar disorder. *J Child Adolesc Psychopharmacol.* 2010;20(1): 7–14.

Joshi PT, Capozzoli JA, Coyle JT. Low-dose neuroleptic therapy for children with childhood-onset pervasive developmental disorder. *Am J Psychiatry.* 1988;145:335–338.

Joshi PT, Walkup JT, Capozzoli JA, et al. The use of fluoxetine in the treatment of major depressive disorder in children and adolescents. Paper presented at: the 36th Annual Meeting of the American Academy of Child and Adolescent Psychiatry; October 11–15, 1989; New York, NY.

Juul Povlsen U, Noring U, Fog R, et al. Tolerability and therapeutic effect of clozapine. A retrospective investigation of 216 patients treated with clozapine for up to 12 years. *Acta Psychiatr Scand.* 1985;71:176–185.

Kafantaris V, Campbell M, Padron-Gayol MV, et al. Carbamazepine in hospitalized aggressive conduct disorder children: an open pilot study. *Psychopharmacol Bull.* 1992;28:193–199.

Kafantaris V, Coletti D, Dicker R, et al. Lithium treatment of acute mania in adolescents: a large open trial. *J Am Acad Child Adolesc Psychiatry.* 2003;42:1038–1045.

Kafantaris V, Coletti DJ, Dicker R, et al. Lithium treatment of acute mania in adolescents: a placebo-controlled discontinuation study. *J Am Acad Child Adolesc Psychiatry.* 2004;43(8):984–993.

Kallen B, Tandberg A. Lithium and pregnancy. *Acta Psychiatr Scand.* 1983;68:134–139.

Kamps-Hughes N. *Curbing the high rates of psychotropic medication prescriptions among children and youth in foster care.* Oakland, CA: National Center for Youth Law; 2016. http://youthlaw.org/publication/reducing-overmedication-appendices/.

Kandemir H, Yumru M, Kul M, et al. Behavioral disinhibition, suicidal ideation, and self-mutilation related to clonazepam. *J Child Adolesc Psychopharmacol.* 2008;18(4):409–410.

Kane J, Woerner M, Pollack S, et al. Does clozapine cause tardive dyskinesia? *J Clin Psychiatry.* 1993;54:327–330.

Kane JM, Lieberman JA. *Adverse Effects of Psychotropic Drugs.* New York, NY: Guilford Press; 1992.

Kapetanovic S. Oxcarbazepine in youths with autistic disorder and significant disruptive behaviors. *Am J Psychiatry.* 2007;164(5):832–833.

Kaplan SL, Simms RM, Busner J. Prescribing practices of outpatient child psychiatrists. *J Am Acad Child Adolesc Psychiatry.* 1994;33:35–44.

Kashani JH, Shekim WO, Reid JC. Amitriptyline in children with major depressive disorder: a double-blind crossover pilot study. *J Am Acad Child Adolesc Psychiatry.* 1984;23:348–351.

Kastner T, Finesmith R, Walsh K. Long-term administration of valproic acid in the treatment of affective symptoms in people with mental retardation. *J Clin Psychopharmacol.* 1993;13:448–451.

Kastner T, Friedman DL, Plummer AT, et al. Valproic acid for the treatment of children with mental retardation and mood symptomatology. *Pediatrics.* 1990;86:467–472.

Kaufmann CA, Wyatt RJ. Neuroleptic malignant syndrome. In: Meltzer HY, ed. *Psychopharmacology: The Third Generation of Progress.* New York, NY: Raven Press; 1987:1421–1430.

Kemner JE, Starr HL, Ciccone PE, et al. Outcomes of OROS methylphenidate compared with atomoxetine in children with ADHD: a multicenter, randomized prospective study. *Adv Ther.* 2005;22:498–512.

Kemph JP, DeVane CL, Levin GM, et al. Treatment of aggressive children with clonidine: results of an open pilot study. *J Am Acad Child Adolesc Psychiatry.* 1993;32:577–581.

Kennard B, Silva S, Vitiello B, et al. Remission and residual symptoms after short-term treatment in the treatment of adolescents with depression study (TADS). *J Am Acad Child Adolesc Psychiatry.* 2006;45(12):1404–1411.

Kennard B, Silva SG, Tonev S, et al. Remission and recovery in the treatment for adolescents with depression study (TADS): acute and long-term outcomes. *J Am Acad Child Adolesc Psychiatry.* 2009;48(2):186–195.

Kessler R, Amminger P, Aguilar-Gaxiola S, et al. Age of onset of mental disorders: a review of recent literature. *Curr Opin Psychiatry.* 2007;20:359–364.

Killen JD, Robinson TN, Ammerman S, et al. Randomized clinical trial of the efficacy of bupropion combined with nicotine patch in the treatment of adolescent smokers. *J Consult Clin Psychol.* 2004;72(4):729.

Kim S, Boylan K, Effectiveness of antidepressant medications for symptoms of irritability and disruptive behaviors in children and adolescents. *J Child Adolesc Psychopharmacol.* 2016;26(8):694–704.

King BH, Hollander E, Sikich L, et al. Lack of efficacy of citalopram in children with autism spectrum disorders and high levels of repetitive behavior; citalopram ineffective in children with autism. *Arch Gen Psychiatry.* 2009;66(6):583–590.

King RA, Riddle MA, Chappell PB, et al. Emergence of self-destructive phenomena in children and adolescents during fluoxetine treatment. *J Am Acad Child Adolesc Psychiatry.* 1991;30:179–186.

Klein DF, Gittelman R, Quitkin F, et al. *Diagnosis and Drug Treatment of Psychiatric Disorders: Adults and Children.* Baltimore, MD: Williams & Wilkins; 1980.

Klein DJ, Cottingham EM, Sorter M, et al. A randomized, double-blind, placebocontrolled trial of metformin treatment of weight gain associated with initiation of atypical antipsychotic therapy in children and adolescents. *Am J Psychiatry.* 2006;163:2072–2079.

Klein RG. Pharmacotherapy of childhood hyperactivity: an update. In: Meltzer HY, ed. *Psychopharmacology: The Third Generation of Progress.* New York, NY: Raven Press; 1987:1215–1224.

Klein RG. Thioridazine effects on the cognitive performance of children with attention-deficit hyperactivity disorder. *J Child Adolesc Psychopharmacol.* 1990/1991;1:263–270.

Klein RG, Abikoff H, Klass E, et al. Clinical efficacy of methylphenidate in conduct disorder with and without attention deficit hyperactivity disorder. *Arch Gen Psychiatry.* 1997;54:1073–1080.

Klein RG, Koplewicz HS, Kanner A. Imipramine treatment of children with separation anxiety disorder. *J Am Acad Child Adolesc Psychiatry.* 1992;31:21–28.

Klein RG, Landa B, Mattes JA, et al. Methylphenidate and growth in hyperactive children: a controlled withdrawal study. *Arch Gen Psychiatry.* 1988;45:1127–1130.

Klein RG, Last CG. *Anxiety Disorders in Children.* Newbury Park, CA: SAGE; 1989.

Klein RG, Mannuzza S. Hyperactive boys almost grown up: III, methylphenidate effects on ultimate height. *Arch Gen Psychiatry.* 1988;45:1131–1134.

Klein-Schwartz W, Benson BE, Lee SC, et al. Comparison of citalopram and other selective serotonin reuptake inhibitor ingestions in children. *Clin Toxicol.* 2012;50(5):418–423.

Klorman R, Brumaghim JT, Salzman LF, et al. Effects of methylphenidate on attention-deficit hyperactivity disorder with and without aggressive/noncompliant features. *J Abnorm Psychol.* 1988a;97:413–422.

Klorman R, Coons HW, Brumaghim JT, et al. Stimulant treatment for adolescents with attention deficit disorder. *Psychopharmacol Bull.* 1988b;24:88–92.

Knight JR, Sherritt L, Shrier LA, et al. Validity of the CRAFFT substance abuse screening test among adolescent clinic patients. *Arch Pediatr Adolesc Med.* 2002;156(6):607–614.

Knight JR, Shrier LA, Bravender TD, et al. A new brief screen for adolescent substance abuse. *Arch Pediatr Adolesc Med.* 1999;153(6):591–596.

Knowler W, Barrett-Connor E, Fowler S, et al. Reduction in the incidence of type 2 diabetes with lifestyle intervention or metformin. *Engl J Med.* 2002;346(6):393–403.

Koelch M, Pfalzer A, Kliegl K, et al. Therapeutic drug monitoring of children and adolescents treated with fluoxetine. *Pharmacopsychiatry.* 2012;45(2):72–76.

Kofoed L, Tadepalli G, Oesterheld JR, et al. Case series: clonidine has no systematic effects on PR or QTc intervals in children. *J Am Acad Child Adolesc Psychiatry.* 1999;38:1193–1196.

Kolman BK, Feldman HM, Handen BL, et al. Naltrexone in young autistic children: a double-blind, placebo-controlled crossover study. *J Am Acad Child Adolesc Psychiatry.* 1995;34:223–231.

Kolman BK, Feldman HM, Handen BJ, et al. Naltrexone in young autistic children: replication study and learning measures. *J Am Acad Child Adolesc Psychiatry.* 1997;36:1570–1578.

Korein J, Fish B, Shapiro T, et al. EEG and behavioral effects of drug therapy in children: chlorpromazine and diphenhydramine. *Arch Gen Psychiatry.* 1971;24:552–563.

Koren G, Nordeng H. Antidepressant use during pregnancy: the benefit-risk ratio. *Am J Obstet Gynecol.* 2012;207(3):157–163. doi:10.1016/j.ajog.2012.02.009.

Kotler LA, Devlin MJ, Davies M, et al. An open trial of fluoxetine for adolescents with bulimia nervosa. *J Child Adolesc Psychopharmacol.* 2003;13(3):329–335.

Kovacs M. The Children's Depression Inventory (CDI). *Psychopharmacol Bull.* 1985;21:995–998.

Kovacs M. *Children's Depression Inventory Manual.* North Tonawanda, NY: Multi-Health Systems; 1992.

Kowatch RA, DelBello MP. The use of mood stabilizers and atypical antipsychotics in children and adolescents with bipolar disorders. *CNS Spectr.* 2003;8(4):273–280.

Kowatch RA, Scheffer RE, Monroe E, et al. Placebo-controlled trial of valproic acid versus risperidone in children 3-7 years of age with bipolar I disorder. *J Child Adolesc Psychopharmacol.* 2015;25(4):306–313.

Kowatch RA, Suppes T, Carmody TJ, et al. Effect size of lithium, divalproex sodium, and carbamezapine in children and adolescents with bipolar disorder. *J Am Acad Child Adolesc Psychiatry.* 2000;39(6):713–720.

Kraft IA, Ardall C, Duffy JH, et al. A clinical study of chlordiazepoxide used in psychiatric disorders of children. *Int J Neuropsychiatry.* 1965;1:433–437.

Kranzler H, Roofeh D, Gerbino-Rosen G, et al. Clozapine: its impact on aggressive behavior among children and adolescents with schizophrenia. *J Am Acad child Adolesc Psychiatry.* 2005;44:55–63.

Kranzler HR. Use of buspirone in an adolescent with overanxious disorder. *J Am Acad Child Adolesc Psychiatry.* 1988;27:789–790.

Kreider AR, Matone M, Bellonci C, et al. Growth in the concurrent use of antipsychotics with other psychotropic medications in Medicaid-enrolled children. *J Am Acad Child Adolesc Psychiatry.* 2014;53(9):960.

Krener PK, Mancina RA. Informed consent or informed coercion? Decision making in pediatric psychopharmacology. *J Child Adolesc Psychopharmacol.* 1994;4(3):183–200.

Krieger F, Pheula G, Coelho R, et al. An open-label trial of risperidone in children and adolescents with severe mood dysregulation. *J Child Adolesc Psychopharmacol*. 2011;21(3):237–243.

Kroon LA. Drug interactions with smoking. *Am J Health Syst Pharm*. 2007;64(18):1917–1921.

Kumar A, Datta SS, Wright SD, et al. Atypical antipsychotics for psychosis in adolescents. *Cochrane Database Syst Rev*. 2013;(10):CD009582. doi:10.1002/14651858.CD009582.pub2.

Kumra S, Frazier J, Jacobsen L, McKenna K, et al. Childhood-onset schizophrenia. A double-blind clozapine-haloperidol comparison. *Arch Gen Psychiatry*. 1996;53:1090–1097.

Kumra S, Herion D, Jacobsen LK, et al. Case study: risperidone-induced hepatotoxicity in pediatric patients. *J Am Acad Child Adolesc Psychiatry*. 1997;36:701–705.

Kumra S, Jacobson LK, Lenane M, et al. Childhood-onset schizophrenia: an open-label study of olanzapine in adolescents. *J Am Acad Child Adolesc Psychiatry*. 1998;37:377–385.

Kumra S, Kranzler H, Gerbino-Rosen G, et al. Clozapine and "high-dose" olanzapine in refractory early-onset schizophrenia: a 12-week randomized and double-blind comparison. *Biol Psychiatry*. 2008;63:524–529.

Kuperman S, Stewart M. Use of propranolol to decrease aggressive outbursts in younger patients. Open study reveals potentially favorable outcome. *Psychosomatics*. 1987;28(6):315–319.

Kurdyak PA, Juurlink DN, Mamdani MM. The effect of antidepressant warnings on prescribing trends in Ontario, Canada. *Am J Public Health*. 2007;97(4):750–754.

Kurian BT, Ray WA, Arbogast PG, et al. Effect of regulatory warnings on antidepressant prescribing for children and adolescents. *Arch Pediatr Adolesc Med*. 2007;161(7):690–696.

Kutcher S, ed. *Practical Child and Adolescent Psychopharmacology*. Cambridge, UK: Cambridge University Press; 2002.

Kutcher S, Boulos C, Ward B, et al. Response to desipramine treatment in adolescent depression: a fixed-dose, placebo-controlled trial. *J Am Acad Child Adolesc Psychiatry*. 1994;33:686–694.

Kutcher SP. *Child and Adolescent Psychopharmacology*. Philadelphia, PA: WB Saunders; 1997.

Kutcher SP, MacKenzie S. Successful clonazepam treatment of adolescents with panic disorder [letter]. *J Clin Psychopharmacol*. 1988;8:299–301.

Kutcher SP, MacKenzie S, Galarraga W, et al. Clonazepam treatment of adolescents with neuroleptic-induced akathisia. *Am J Psychiatry*. 1987;144:823–824.

Kutz G. Foster children: HHS guidance could help states improve oversight of psychotropic prescriptions. GAO-12-270T. Washington, DC: The Government Accountability Office; 2011. www.gao.gov/assets/590/586570.pdf. Accessed March 2, 2013.

Labellarte M, Biederman J, Emslie G, et al. Multiple-dose pharmacokinetics of fluvoxamine in children and adolescents. *J Am Acad Child Adolesc Psychiatry*. 2004;43:1497–1505.

Lachman A. New developments in diagnosis and treatment update: Schizophrenia/first episode psychosis in children and adolescents. *J Child Adolesc Ment Health*. 2014;26:109–124.

Lader M. Fluoxetine efficacy vs comparative drugs: an overview. *Br J Psychiatry*. 1988:153(suppl 3):51–58.

Latuda [package insert]. Marlborough, MA: Sunovion Pharmaceuticals Inc; 2018.

Latz SR, McCracken JT. Neuroleptic malignant syndrome in children and adolescents: two case reports and a warning. *J Child Adolesc Psychopharmacol*. 1992;2:123–129.

Law SF, Schachar RJ. Do typical clinical doses of methylphenidate cause tics in children treated for attention-deficit hyperactivity disorder? *J Am Acad Child Adolesc Psychiatry*. 1999;38:944–951.

Leckman JF, Cohen DJ, Detlor J, et al. Clonidine in the treatment of Tourette syndrome: a review of data. In: Friedhoff AJ, Chase TN, eds. *Gilles de la Tourette Syndrome*. New York, NY: Raven Press; 1982:391–401.

Leckman JF, Detlor J, Harcherik DF, et al. Short- and long-term treatment of Tourette's syndrome with clonidine: a clinical perspective. *Neurology*. 1985;35:343–351.

Leckman JF, Hardin MT, Riddle MA, et al. Clonidine treatment of Gilles de la Tourette's syndrome. *Arch Gen Psychiatry*. 1991;48:324–328.

Lefkowitz MM. Effects of diphenylhydantoin on disruptive behavior. *Arch Gen Psychiatry*. 1969;20:643–651.

Leibenluft E, Charney D, Towbin K, et al. Defining clinical phenotypes of juvenile mania. *Am J Psychiatry*. 2003;160(3):430–437.

Leischow SJ, Muramoto ML, Matthews E, et al. Adolescent smoking cessation with bupropion: the role of adherence. *Nicotine Tob Res*. 2016;18(5):1202–1205.

Lena B, Surtees SJ, Maggs R. The efficacy of lithium in the treatment of emotional disturbance in children and adolescents. In: Johnson FN, Johnson S, eds. *Lithium in Medical Practice*. Baltimore, MD: University Park Press; 1978:79–83.

Le Noury J, Nardo JM, Healy D, et al. Restoring Study 329: efficacy and harms of paroxetine and imipramine in treatment of major depression in adolescence. *BMJ*. 2015;351:h4320.

Le Noury J, Nardo JM, Healy D, et al. Study 329 continuation phase: safety and efficacy of paroxetine and imipramine in extended treatment of adolescent major depression. *Int J Risk Saf Med.* 2016;28(3):143–161.

Leonard HL, Swedo SE, Lenane MC, et al. A double-blind desipramine substitution during long-term clomipramine treatment in children and adolescents with obsessive-compulsive disorder. *Arch Gen Psychiatry.* 1991;48:922–927.

Leonard HL, Swedo SE, Rapoport JL, et al. Treatment of obsessive-compulsive disorder with clomipramine and desipramine in children and adolescents: a double-blind crossover comparison. *Arch Gen Psychiatry.* 1989;46:1088–1092.

Leonard HL, Topol D, Bukstein O, et al. Clonazepam as an augmenting agent in the treatment of childhood-onset obsessive-compulsive disorder. *J Am Acad Child Adolesc Psychiatry.* 1994;33:692–694.

Leucht S, Cipriani A, Spineli L, et al. Comparative efficacy and tolerability of 15 antipsychotic drugs in schizophrenia: a multiple-treatments meta-analysis. *Lancet.* 2013;382:951–962.

Levin GM, Burton-Teston K, Murphy T. Development of precocious puberty in two children treated with clonidine for aggressive behavior. *J Child Adolesc Psychopharmacol.* 1993;3:127–131.

Levkovitch Y, Kaysar N, Kronnenberg Y, et al. Clozapine for schizophrenia [letter]. *J Am Acad Child Adolesc Psychiatry.* 1994;33:431.

Levy RH. Psychopharmacological interventions. In: Katz SE, Nardacci D, Sabatini A, eds. *Intensive Treatment of the Homeless Mentally Ill.* Washington, DC: American Psychiatric Press; 1993:129–165.

Liebenluft E, Charney DS, Towbin KE, et al. Defining clinical phenotypes of juvenile mania. *Am J Psychiatry.* 2003;160:430–437.

Lindstrom L. The effect of long-term treatment with clozapine in schizophrenia: a retrospective study in 96 patients treated with clozapine for up to 13 years. *Acta Psychiatr Scand.* 1998;77:524–529.

Lingjaerde O, Ahlfors UG, Bech P, et al. The UKU side effect rating scale: a new comprehensive rating scale for psychotropic drugs, and a cross sectional study of side effects in neuroleptic-treated patients. *Acta Psychiatr Scand Suppl.* 1987;76:1–100.

Linnoila M, Dejong J, Virkkunen M. Monoamines, glucose metabolism, and impulse control. *Psychopharmacol Bull.* 1989;25:404–406.

Linnoila M, Gualtieri CT, Jobson K, et al. Characteristics of the therapeutic response to imipramine in hyperactive children. *Am J Psychiatry.* 1979;136:1201–1203.

Lobo ED, Quinlan T, Prakash A, et al. Pharmacokinetics of orally administered duloxetine in children and adolescents with major depressive disorder. *Clin Pharmacokinet.* 2014;53(8):731–740.

Lohoff FW, Ferraro TN. Pharmacogenetic considerations in the treatment of psychiatric disorders. *Expert Opin Pharmacother.* 2010;11(3):423–439.

Lowe TL, Cohen DJ, Detlor J, et al. Stimulant medications precipitate Tourette's syndrome. *JAMA.* 1982;247:1729–1931.

Lucas AR, Pasley FC. Psychoactive drugs in the treatment of emotionally disturbed children: haloperidol and diazepam. *Compr Psychiatry.* 1969;10:376–386.

Luchins D, Dojka D. Lithium and propranolol in aggression and self-injurious behavior in the mentally retarded. *Psychopharmacol Bull.* 1989;25(3):372–375.

Lytle S, McVoy M, Sajatovic M. Long-acting injectable antipsychotics in children and adolescents. *J Child Adolesc Psychopharmacol.* 2017;27(1):2–9.

Ma D, Zhang Z, Zhang X, et al. Comparative efficacy, acceptability, and safety of medicinal, cognitive-behavioral therapy, and placebo treatments for acute major depressive disorder in children and adolescents: a multiple-treatments meta-analysis. *Curr Med Res Opin.* 2014;30(6):971–995.

MacLeod CM, Dekaban AS, Hunt E. Memory impairment in epileptic patients: selective effects of phenobarbital concentration. *Science.* 1978;202:1102–1104.

Maisto SA, Chung TA, Cornelius JR, et al. Factor structure of the SOCRATES in a clinical sample of adolescents. *Psychol Addict Behav.* 2003;17(2):98–107. doi:1037/0893-164X.17.2.98.

Malhotra S, Santosh PR. An open clinical trial of buspirone in children with attention-deficit/hyperactivity disorder. *J Am Acad Child Adolesc Psychiatry.* 1998;37:364–371.

Malhotra S, Subodh BN. Informed consent & ethical issues in paediatric psychopharmacology. *Indian J Med Res.* 2009;129(1):19–32.

Malone RP, Delaney MA, Luebbert JF, et al. The lithium test dose prediction method in aggressive children. *Psychopharmacol Bull.* 1995;31(2):379–382.

Malone RP, Delaney M, Luebbert J, et al. A double-blind placebo-controlled study of lithium in hospitalized aggressive children and adolescents with conduct disorder. *Am J Psychiatry.* 2000;57(7):649–654.

Mandoki M. Clozapine for adolescents with psychosis: literature review and two case reports. *J Child Adolesc Psychopharmacol.* 1993;3:213–221.

Mann JJ, Marzuk PM, Arango V, et al. Neurochemical studies of violent and nonviolent suicide. *Psychopharmacol Bull.* 1989;25:407–413.

Manos MJ, Short EJ, Findling RL. Differential effectiveness of methylphenidate and Adderall in school-age youth with attention-deficit/hyperactivity disorder. *J Am Acad Child Adolesc Psychiatry.* 1999;38:813–819.

March J, Franklin ME, Leonard H, et al. Tics moderate treatment outcome with sertraline but not cognitive-behavior therapy in pediatric obsessive-compulsive disorder. *Biol Psychiatry.* 2007a;61(3):344–347.

March J, Silva S, Curry J, et al; TADS Team. The treatment for adolescents with depression study (TADS): outcomes over 1 year of naturalistic follow-up. *Am J Psychiatry.* 2009;166(10):1141–1149.

March JS, Biederman J, Wolkow R, et al. Sertraline in children and adolescents with obsessive-compulsive disorder: a multicenter randomized controlled trial. *JAMA.* 1998;280:1752–1756.

March JS, Entusah AR, Rynn M, et al. A randomized controlled trial of venlafaxine ER versus placebo in pediatric social anxiety disorder. *Biol Psychiatry.* 2007b;62(10):1149–1154.

March JS, Foa E, Gammon P, et al; The Pediatric OCD Treatment Study (POTS) Team. Cognitive-behavioral therapy, sertraline, and their combination for children and adolescents with obsessive-compulsive disorder. *JAMA.* 2004;292:1969–1976.

March JS, Parker JD, Sullivan K, et al. The Multidimensional Anxiety Scale for Children (MASC): factor structure, reliability, and validity. *J Am Acad Child Adolesc Psychiatry.* 1997;36:554–565.

March JS, Silva S, Petrycki S, et al; Treatment for Adolescents with Depression Study (TADS) Team. Fluoxetine, cognitive-behavioral therapy, and their combination for adolescents with depression: treatment for adolescents with depression study (TADS) randomized controlled trial. *JAMA.* 2004;292:807–820.

Marder S, Essock S, Miller A, et al. The Mount Sinai Conference on the pharmacotherapy of schizophrenia. *Schizophr Bull.* 2002;28:5–16.

Marder S, Knesevich MA, Hauser RA, et al. KINECT 3: a randomized, double-blind, placebo-controlled phase 3 trial of valbenazine (NBI-98854) for tardive dyskinesia. Poster presented at the American Psychiatric Association Annual Meeting; May 14–18, 2016; Atlanta, GA.

Marsch LA, Bickel WK, Badger GJ, et al. Comparison of pharmacological treatments for opioid-dependent adolescents: a randomized controlled trial. *Arch Gen Psychiatry.* 2005;62(10):1157–1164.

Marshall M, Lewis S, Lockwood A, et al. Association between duration of untreated psychosis and outcome in cohorts of first-episode patients. *Arch Gen Psychiatry.* 2005;62:975–983.

Martin A, Koenign K, Scahill L, et al. Open-label quetiapine in the treatment of children and adolescents with autistic disorder. *J Child Adolesc Psychopharmacol.* 1999;9:99–107.

Martin A, Landau J, Leebens P, et al. Risperidone-associated with gain in children and adolescents: a retrospective chart review. *J Child Adolesc Psychopharmacol.* 2000;10:259–268.

Martin A, Scahill L, Charney DS, et al, eds. *Pediatric Psychopharmacology: Principles and Practice.* New York, NY: Oxford University Press; 2003.

Matson SC, Hobson G, Abdel-Rasoul M, et al. A retrospective study of retention of opioid-dependent adolescents and young adults in an outpatient buprenorphine/naloxone clinic. *J Addict Med.* 2014;8(3):176–182.

Mattai A, Fung L, Bakalar J, et al. Adjunctive use of lithium carbonate for the management of neutropenia in clozapine-treated children. *Hum Psychopharmacol.* 2009;24(7):584–589.

Mattes J. Clozapine for refractory schizophrenia: an open study of 14 patients treated up to 2 years. *J Clin Psychiatry.* 1989;50:389–391.

Mattes JA, Gittelman R. Growth of hyperactive children on maintenance regimen of methylphenidate. *Arch Gen Psychiatry.* 1983;40:317–321.

Matthews D, Mathews G. Disruptive mood dysregulation disorder: a unique pediatric neuropsychopharmacological approach. Poster presented at: Psych Congress; September 16–19, 2017; New Orleans, LA.

Mazzone L, Reale L. Topiramate in children with autistic spectrum disorders. *Brain Dev.* 2006;28(10):668.

Mazzone L, Reale L, Mannino V, et al. Lower IQ is associated with decreased clinical response to atomoxetine in children and adolescents with attention-deficit hyperactivity disorder. *CNS Drugs.* 2011;25(6):503–509.

McBride MC, Wang DD, Torres C. Methylphenidate in therapeutic doses does not lower seizure threshold. *Ann Neurol.* 1986;20:428.

McClellan J, Stock S. American Academy of Child and Adolescent Psychiatry Committee on quality issues: practice parameter for the assessment and treatment of children and adolescents with schizophrenia. *J Am Acad Child Adolesc Psychiatry.* 2013;52:976–990.

McConville BJ, Arvanitis LA, Thyrum PT. Pharmacokinetics, tolerability, and clinical effectiveness of quetiapine fumarate: an open-label trial in adolescents with psychotic disorders. *J Clin Psychiatry*. 2000;61:252–260.

McConville BJ, Minnery KL, Sorter MT, et al. An open study of the effects of sertraline on adolescent major depression. *J Child Adolesc Psychopharmacol*. 1996;6:41–51.

McCormick LH. Treatment with buspirone in a patient with autism. *Arch Fam Med*. 1997;6(4):368–370.

McCormick LH, Rizzuto GT, Knuckles HB. A pilot study of buspirone in attention-deficit hyperactivity disorder. *Arch Fam Med*. 1994;3:68–70.

McCracken JT, Biederman J, Greenhill LL, et al. Analog classroom assessment of a once-daily mixed amphetamine formulations, SLI381 (Adderall XR) in children with ADHD. *J Am Acad Child Adolesc Psychiatry*. 2003;42:673–683.

McCracken JT, Martin W. Clonidine side effect [letter]. *J Am Acad Child Adolesc Psychiatry*. 1997;36:160–161.

McCracken JT, McGough J, Shah B, et al; Research Units on Pediatric Psychopharmacology Autism Network. Risperidone in children with autism and serious behavioral problems. *N Engl J Med*. 2002;347:314–321.

McDonagh M, Peterson K, Carson S, et al. *Drug Class Review: Atypical Antipsychotic Drugs: Final Update 3 Report*. Portland, OR: Oregon Health & Science University; 2010.

McDougle CJ, Kem DL, Posey DJ. Case series: use of ziprasidone for maladaptive symptoms in youths with autism. *J Am Acad Child Adolesc Psychiatry*. 2002;41:921–927.

McGough J, Faraone S. Estimating the size of treatment effects: moving beyond p-values. *Psychiatry (Edgmont)*. 2009;6:21–29.

McGough JJ, Biederman J, Wigal SB, et al. Long-term tolerability and effectiveness of once-daily mixed amphetamine salts (Adderall XR) in children with ADHD. *J Am Acad Child Adolesc Psychiatry*. 2005;44:539–547.

McGuire JF, Piacentini J, Lewin AB, et al. A meta-analysis of cognitive behavior therapy and medication for child obsessive–compulsive disorder: moderators of treatment efficacy, response, and remission. *Depression and Anxiety*. 2015;32:580–593.

McNally P, McNicholas F, Oslizlok P. The QT interval and psychotropic medications in children. *Eur Child Adolesc Psychiatry*. 2007;16:33–47.

McVoy M, eds. *Clinical Manual of Child and Adolescent Psychopharmacology*. 2nd ed. Washington, DC: American Psychiatric Press Inc; 2012.

Medeiros G, Senco S, Lafer B, et al. Association between duration of untreated bipolar disorder and clinical outcome: data from a Brazilian sample. *Rev Bras Psiquiatr*. 2016;38:6–10.

Meltzer H, Bastani B, Kwon K, et al. A prospective study of clozapine in treatment-resistant schizophrenic patients. I. Preliminary report. *Psychopharmacology (Berl)*. 1989;99(suppl):S68–S72.

Meyers B, Tune LE, Coyle JT. Clinical response and serum neuroleptic levels in childhood schizophrenia. *Am J Psychiatry*. 1980;137:1459–1460.

Michelson D, Allen AJ, Busner J, et al. Once-daily atomoxetine treatment for children and adolescents with attention deficit hyperactivity disorder: a randomized, placebo-controlled study. *Am J Psychiatry*. 2002;159(11):1896–1901.

Michelson D, Faries D, Wernicke J, et al. Atomoxetine in the treatment of children and adolescents with attention-deficit/hyperactivity disorder: a randomized, placebo-controlled, dose-response study. *Pediatrics*. 2001;108(5):E83.

Michelson D, Read HA, Ruff DD, et al. CYP2D6 and clinical response to atomoxetine in children and adolescents with ADHD. *J Am Acad Child Adolesc Psychiatry*. 2007;46(2):242–251.

Millard H, McLaren J, Coffey B. Lurasidone treatment in a child with autism spectrum disorder with irritability and aggression. *J Child Adolesc Psychopharmacol*. 2014;6:354–356.

Miller WR, Tonigan JS. Assessing drinkers' motivation for change: the Stages of Change and Treatment Eagerness Scale (SOCRATES). *Psychol Addict Behav*. 1996;10:81–89.

Miranda R, Ray L, Blanchard A, et al. Effects of naltrexone on adolescent alcohol cue reactivity and sensitivity: an initial randomized trial. *Addict Biol*. 2014;19(5):941–954.

Mitchell AJ, Delaffon V, Vancampfort D, et al. Guideline concordant monitoring of metabolic risk in people treated with antipsychotic medication: systematic review and meta-analysis of screening practices. *Psychol Med*. 2012;42(1):125–147.

Mitsunaga MM, Garrett A, Howe M, et al. Increased subgenual cingulate cortex volume in pediatric bipolar disorder associated with mood stabilizer exposure. *J Child Adolesc Psychopharmacol*. 2011;21(2):149–155.

MMDLN. Newsletter update: antipsychotic medication use in medicaid children and adolescents: a study of 16 state programs. *The Medicaid Medical Directors' Learning Network Newsletter*. Spring. 2011. http://chsr.rutgers.edu/MMDLNAPKIDS/mmdlnnews1.pdf. Accessed March 2, 2013.

Modabbernia A, Heidari P, Soleimani R, et al. Melatonin for prevention of metabolic side-effects of olanzapine in patients with first-episode schizophrenia: randomized double-blind placebo-controlled study. *J Psych Res.* 2014;53:133–140.

Mohammadi MR, Hafezi P, Galeiha A, et al. Buspirone versus methylphenidate in the treatment of children with attention-deficit/hyperactivity disorder: randomized double blind study. *Acta Med Iran.* 2012;50(11):723–728.

Mojtabai R, Olfson M. National trends in psychotropic medication polypharmacy in office-based psychiatry. *Arch Gen Psychiatry.* 2010;67(1):26.

Molitch M, Eccles AK. The effect of benzedrine sulfate on the intelligence scores of children. *Am J Psychiatry.* 1937;94:587–590.

Molitch M, Poliakoff S. The effect of benzedrine sulfate on enuresis. *Arch Pediatr.* 1937;54:499–501.

Molitch M, Sullivan JP. The effect of benzedrine sulfate on children taking the New Stanford Achievement Test. *Am J Orthopsychiatry.* 1937;7:519–522.

Moolchan ET, Robinson ML, Ernst M, et al. Safety and efficacy of the nicotine patch and gum for the treatment of adolescent tobacco addiction. *Pediatrics.* 2005;115(4):e407–e414.

Morrato EH, Nicol GE, Maahs D, et al. Metabolic screening in children receiving antipsychotic drug treatment. *Arch Pediatr Adolesc Med.* 2010;164(4):344–351.

Morselli PL, Bianchetti G, Dugas M. Therapeutic drug monitoring of psychotropic drugs in children. *Pediatr Pharmacol.* 1983;3:149–156.

Mozes T, Toren P, Chernauzan N, et al. Clozapine treatment in very early onset schizophrenia. *J Am Acad Child Adolesc Psychiatry.* 1994;33:65–70.

Mrakotsky C, Masek B, Biederman J, et al. Prospective open-label pilot trial of mirtazapine in children and adolescents with social phobia. *J Anxiety Disord.* 2008;22(1):88–97.

MTA Cooperative Group. A 14-month randomized clinical trial of treatment strategies for attention-deficit/hyperactivity disorder. *Arch Gen Psychiatry.* 1999a;56:1073–1086.

MTA Cooperative Group. Moderators and mediators of treatment response for children with attention-deficit/hyperactivity disorder. *Arch Gen Psychiatry.* 1999b;56:1088–1096.

Muramoto ML, Leischow SJ, Sherrill D, et al. Randomized, double-blind, placebo-controlled trial of 2 dosages of sustained-release bupropion for adolescent smoking cessation. *Arch Pediatr Adolesc Med.* 2007;161(11):1068–1074.

Musten LM, Firestone P, Pisterman S, et al. Effects of methylphenidate on preschool children with ADHD: cognitive and behavioral functions. *J Am Acad Child Adolesc Psychiatry.* 1997;36:1407–1415.

Mutlu C, Demirci AC, Yalcin O, et al. One-year follow-up of heroin-dependent adolescents treated with buprenorphine/naloxone for the first time in a substance treatment unit. *J Subst Abuse Treat.* 2016;67:1–8.

Myers WC, Carrera F III. Carbamazepine-induced mania with hypersexuality in a 9-year-old boy. *Am J Psychiatry.* 1989;146:400.

Nasrallah HA, White T, Nasrallah AT. Lower mortality in geriatric patients receiving risperidone and olanzapine versus haloperidol: a preliminary analysis of retrospective data. *Am J Geriatr Psychiatry.* 2004;12(4):437–439.

National Institute of Mental Health/National Institutes of Health Consensus Development Panel. Mood disorders: pharmacologic prevention of recurrences. *Am J Psychiatry.* 1985;142:469–476.

National Public Radio. Psychiatrists shift focus to drugs, not talk therapy [Internet]. October 22, 2012. http://www.npr.org/2012/10/22/163409863/psychiatrists-shift-focus-to-drugs-not-talk-therapy. Cited October 22, 2017.

Nemeth G, Laszlovszky I, Czobor P, et al. Cariprazine versus risperidone monotherapy for treatment of predominant negative symptoms in patients with schizophrenia: a randomized, double-blind, controlled trial. *Lancet.* 2017;389:1103–1113.

Neppe VM, Ward NG. The evaluation and management of neuroleptic-induced acute extrapyramidal syndromes. In: Neppe VM, ed. *Innovative Psychopharmacology.* New York, NY: Raven Press; 1989:152–176.

Newcomer JW. Metabolic considerations in the use of antipsychotic medications: a review of recent evidence. *J Clin Psychiatry.* 2007;68(suppl 1):20–27.

Newcorn JH, Spencer TJ, Biederman J, et al. Atomoxetine treatment in children and adolescents with attention-deficit/hyperactivity disorder and comorbid oppositional defiant disorder. *J Am Acad Child Adolesc Psychiatry.* 2005;44(3):240–248.

Newcorn JH, Sutton VK, Weiss MD, et al. Clinical responses to atomoxetine in attention-deficit/hyperactivity disorder: the Integrated Data Exploratory Analysis (IDEA) study. *J Am Acad Child Adolesc Psychiatry.* 2009;48(5):511–518.

Newton JEO, Cannon DJ, Couch L, et al. Effects of repeated drug holidays on serum haloperidol concentration, psychiatric symptoms, and movement disorders in schizophrenic patients. *J Clin Psychiatry.* 1989;50:132–135.

New York State Department of Health. *Safe, Effective and Therapeutically Equivalent Prescription Drugs.* 7th ed. Albany, NY: New York State Department of Health Office of Health Systems Management; 1988.

Ng QX. A systematic review of the use of bupropion for attention-deficit/hyperactivity disorder in children and adolescents. *J Child Adolesc Psychopharmacol.* 2017;27(2):112–116.

Niederhofer H, Huber M. Bupropion may support psychosocial treatment of Nicotine⊠dependent adolescents: preliminary results. *Pharmacotherapy.* 2004;24(11):1524–1528.

Niederhofer H, Staffen W. Comparison of disulfiram and placebo in treatment of alcohol dependence of adolescents. *Drug Alcohol Rev.* 2003a;22(3):295–297.

Niederhofer H, Staffen W. Acamprosate and its efficacy in treating alcohol dependent adolescents. *Eur Child Adolesc Psychiatry.* 2003b;12(3):144–148.

Nobile M, Bellotti B, Marino C, et al. An open trial of paroxetine in the treatment of children and adolescents diagnosed with dysthymia. *J Child Adolesc Psychopharmacol.* 2000;10:103–109.

Noyes R. Beta-adrenergic blockers. In: Last CG, Hersen M, eds. *Handbook of Anxiety Disorders.* New York, NY: Pergamon Press; 1988:445–459.

Nulman I, Koren G, Rovet J, et al. Neurodevelopment of children following prenatal exposure to venlafaxine, selective serotonin reuptake inhibitors, or untreated maternal depression. *Am J Psychiatry.* 2012;169(11):1165–1174.

Nurcombe B. Malpractice. In: Lewis M, ed. *Child and Adolescent Psychiatry: A Comprehensive Textbook.* Baltimore, MD: Williams & Wilkins; 1991:1127–1139.

Nurcombe B, Partlett DF. *Child Mental Health and the Law.* New York, NY: Free Press; 1994:220–272.

Olfson M, Blanco C, Liu L, et al. National trends in the outpatient treatment of children and adolescents with antipsychotic drugs. *Arch Gen Psychiatry.* 2006;63(6):679.

Olfson M, Blanco C, Wang S, et al. National trends in mental health care of children, adolescents, and adults by office-based physicians. *JAMA Psychiatry.* 2014;71(1):81.

Olfson M, Marcus SC, Druss BG. Effects of Food and Drug Administration warnings on antidepressant use in a national sample. *Arch Gen Psychiatry.* 2008;65(1):94–101.

Olvera RL, Pliszka SR, Luh J, et al. An open trial of venlafaxine in the treatment of attention-deficit/hyperactivity disorder in children and adolescents. *J Child Adolesc Psychopharmacol.* 1996;6:241–250.

Orsagh-Yentis DK, Wink LK, Stigler KA, et al. Buspirone for bruxism in a child with pervasive developmental disorder-not otherwise specified. *J Child Adolesc Psychopharmacol.* 2011;21(6):643–645.

Otasowie J, Castells X, Ehimare UP, et al. Tricyclic antidepressants for attention deficit hyperactivity disorder (ADHD) in children and adolescents. *Cochrane Database Syst Rev.* 2014;(9):CD006997.

Owens JA, Rosen CL, Mindell JA, et al. Use of pharmacotherapy for insomnia in child psychiatry practice: a national survey. *Sleep Med.* 2010;11(7):692–700.

Owley T, Walton L, Salt J, et al. An open-label trial of escitalopram in pervasive developmental disorders. *J Am Acad Child Adolesc Psychiatry.* 2005;44(4):343–348.

Oxford English Dictionary. 2nd ed. Oxford, England: Oxford University Press; 1989.

Pandina G, Bossie C, Youssef E, et al. Risperidone improves behavioral symptoms in children with autism in a randomized, double-blind, placebo-controlled trial. *J Autism Dev Disord.* 2007;37:367–373.

Papatheodorou G, Kutcher SP, Katic M, et al. The efficacy and safety of divalproex sodium in the treatment of acute mania in adolescents and young adults: an open clinical trial. *J Clin Psychopharmacol.* 1995;15:110–116.

Pappadopulos E, Woolston S, Chait A, et al. Pharmacotherapy of aggression in children and adolescents: efficacy and effect size. *J Can Acad Child Adolesc Psychiatry.* 2006;15(1):27–39.

Pappagallo M, Silva R. The effect of atypical antipsychotic agents on prolactin levels in children and adolescents. *J Child Adolesc Psychopharmacol.* 2004;14:359–371.

Pare CMB, Kline N, Hallstrom C, et al. Will amitriptyline prevent the "cheese" reaction of monoamine oxidase inhibitors? *Lancet.* 1982;2:183–186.

Parellada E, Velligan D, Emsley R, et al. Long-acting injectable antipsychotics in first-episode schizophrenia. *Schizophr Res Treatment.* 2012;2012:318535.

Parellada M, Boada L, Fraguas D, et al. Trait and state attributes of insight in first episodes of early-onset schizophrenia and other psychoses: a 2-year longitudinal study. *Schizophr Bull.* 2011;37:38–51.

Pataki CS, Carlson GA, Kelly KL, et al. Side effects of methylphenidate and desipramine alone and in combination in children. *J Am Acad Child Adolesc Psychiatry.* 1993;32:1065–1072.

Patel A, Malek N, Haq F, et al. Hirsutism in a female adolescent induced by long-acting injectable risperidone: a case report. *Prim Care Companion CNS Disord.* 2013;15:PCC.12101454.

Patel N, Delbello M, Bryan H, et al. Open-label lithium for the treatment of adolescents with bipolar depression. *J Am Acad Child Adolesc Psychiatry.* 2006;45(3):289–297.

Patrick KS, Mueller RA, Gualtieri CT, et al. Pharmacokinetics and actions of methylphenidate. In: Meltzer HY, ed. *Psychopharmacology: The Third Generation of Progress.* New York, NY: Raven Press; 1987:1387–1395.

Pavuluri MN, Henry DB, Carbray JA, et al. Divalproex sodium for pediatric mixed mania: a 6-month prospective trial. *Bipolar Disord.* 2005;7(3):266–273.

Pavuluri MN, Henry DB, Carbray JA, et al. A one-year open-label trial of risperidone augmentation in lithium nonresponder youth with preschool-onset bipolar disorder. *J Child Adolesc Psychopharmacol.* 2006;16(3):336–350.

Pavuluri MN, Henry DB, Devineni B, et al. Child Mania Rating Scale (CMRS): development, reliability and validity. *J Am Acad Child Adolesc Psychiatry.* 2006;45:550–560.

Pavuluri MN, Henry DB, Findling RL, et al. Double-blind randomized trial of risperidone versus divalproex in pediatric bipolar disorder. *Bipolar Disord.* 2010a;12(6):593–605.

Pavuluri MN, Henry DB, Moss M, et al. Effectiveness of lamotrigine in maintaining symptom control in pediatric bipolar disorder. *J Child Adolesc Psychopharm.* 2009;19(1):75–82.

Pavuluri MN, Passarotti AM, Mohammed T, et al. Enhanced working and verbal memory after lamotrigine treatment in pediatric bipolar disorder. *Bipolar Disord.* 2010b;12(2):213–220.

PDR.net. *FDA Drug Safety Communication Information for Healthcare Professionals: Suicidal Behavior and Ideation and Antiepileptic Drugs.* 2008.

PDR.net. *Drug Information: Drug Summary.* PDR.net; 2012.

Pearson DA, Lane DM, Santos CW, et al. Effects of methylphenidate treatment in children with mental retardation and ADHD: individual variation in medication response. *J Am Acad Child Adolesc Psychiatry.* 2004a;43:686–698.

Pearson DA, Santos CW, Casat CD, et al. Treatment effects of methylphenidate on cognitive functioning in children with mental retardation and ADHD. *J Am Acad Child Adolesc Psychiatry.* 2004b;43:677–685.

Pearson DA, Santos CW, Roache JD, et al. Treatment effects of methylphenidate on behavioral adjustment in children with mental retardation and ADHD. *J Am Acad Child Adolesc Psychiatry.* 2003;42:209–216.

Pelham WE, Bender ME, Caddell J, et al. Methylphenidate and children with attention deficit disorder. *Arch Gen Psychiatry.* 1985;42:948–952.

Pelham WE, Greenslade KE, Vodde-Hamilton M, et al. Relative efficacy of longacting stimulants on children with attention deficit-hyperactivity disorder: a comparison of standard methylphenidate, sustained-release methylphenidate, sustained-release dextroamphetamine, and pemoline. *Pediatrics.* 1990;86:226–237.

Pelham WE, Sturges J, Hoza JA, et al. Sustained release and standard methylphenidate effects on cognitive and social behavior in children with attention deficit disorder. *Pediatrics.* 1987;80:491–501.

Pennsylvania Department of Human Services. *Department of Human Services' Recommendations Regarding Appropriate Use and Monitoring of Psychotropic Medications. .* Harrisburg, PA: Department of Human Services; 2015. http://dhs.pa.gov/cs/groups/webcontent/documents/webcopy/c_190843.pdf. Accessed July 16, 2018.

Perepletchikova F, Nathanson D, Axelrod S, et al. Randomized clinical trial of dialectical behavior therapy for preadolescent children with disruptive mood dysregulation disorder: feasibility and outcomes. *J Am Acad Child Psychiatry.* 2017;56(10):832–840.

Perkins D, Gu H, Boteva K, et al. Relationship between duration of untreated psychosis and outcome in first-episode schizophrenia: a critical review and meta-analysis. *Am J Psychiatry.* 2005;162:1785–1804.

Perry R, Campbell M, Adams P, et al. Long-term efficacy of haloperidol in autistic children: continuous versus discontinuous drug administration. *J Am Acad Child Adolesc Psychiatry.* 1989;28:87–92.

Perry R, Campbell M, Green WH, et al. Neuroleptic-related dyskinesias in autistic children: a prospective study. *Psychopharmacol Bull.* 1985;21:140–143.

Pesikoff RB, Davis PC. Treatment of pavor nocturnus and somnambulism in children. *Am J Psychiatry.* 1971;128:778–781.

Peterson CE, Amaral S, Frosch E. Lithium-induced nephrotic syndrome in a prepubertal boy. *J Child Adolesc Psychopharmacol.* 2008;18(2):210–213.

Petti TA, Fish B, Shapiro T, et al. Effects of chlordiazepoxide in disturbed children: a pilot study. *J Clin Psychopharmacol.* 1982;2:270–273.

Peuskens J, Pani L, Detraux J, et al. The effects of novel and newly approved antipsychotics on serum prolactin levels: a comprehensive review. *CNS Drugs.* 2014;28(5):421–453.

Pfeffer CR, Jiang H, Domeshek LJ. Buspirone treatment of psychiatrically hospitalized children with symptoms of anxiety and moderately severe aggression. *J Child Adolesc Psychopharmacol.* 1997;7:145–155.

Pfefferbaum G, Overall JE, Boren HA, et al. Alprazolam in the treatment of anticipatory and acute situational anxiety in children with cancer. *J Am Acad Child Adolesc Psychiatry.* 1987;26: 532–535.

Phan H, Casavant M, Crockett S, et al. Serotonin syndrome following a single 50 mg dose of sertraline in a child. *Clin Toxicol.* 2008;46(9):845–849.

Physicians' Desk Reference (PDR). 44th ed. Oradell, NJ: Medical Economics; 1990.

Physicians' Desk Reference (PDR). 49th ed. Oradell, NJ: Medical Economics; 1995.

Physicians' Desk Reference (PDR). 54th ed. Oradell, NJ: Medical Economics; 2000.

Physician's Desk Reference (PDR). 57th ed. Montvale, NJ: Thomson PDR; 2004.

Physician's Desk Reference (PDR). 58th ed. Montvale, NJ: Thomson PDR; 2005.

Physicians' Desk Reference (PDR). 59th ed. Montvale, NJ: Thomson PDR; 2006.

Piacentini J, Bennett S, Compton SN, et al. 24- and 36-week outcomes for the Child/Adolescent Anxiety Multimodal Study (CAMS). *J Am Acad Child Adolesc Psychiatry.* 2014;53(3):297–310.

Piontek CM, Wisner KL. Appropriate clinical management of women taking valproate. *J Clin Psychiatry.* 2000;61:161–163.

Platt JE, Campbell M, Green WH, et al. Cognitive effect of lithium carbonate and haloperidol in treatment resistant aggressive children. *Arch Gen Psychiatry.* 1984;41:657–662.

Pleak RR, Birmaher B, Gavrilescu A, et al. Mania and neuropsychiatric excitation following carbamazepine. *J Am Acad Child Adolesc Psychiatry.* 1988;27:500–503.

Pliszka S, Bernet W, Bukstein O, et al. Practice parameter for the assessment and treatment of children and adolescents with attention-deficit/hyperactivity disorder. *J Am Acad Child Adolesc Psychiatry.* 2007;46(7):894–921.

Pliszka SR. Tricyclic antidepressants in the treatment of children with attention deficit disorder. *J Am Acad Child Adolesc Psychiatry.* 1987;26:127–132.

Pliszka SR, Browne RG, Olvera RL, et al. A double-blind, placebo-controlled study of Adderall and methylphenidate in the treatment of attention-deficit/hyperactivity disorder. *J Am Acad Child Adolesc Psychiatry.* 2000;39:619–626.

Pliszka SR, Crismon ML, Hughes CW, et al. The Texas children's medication algorithm project: revision of the algorithm for pharmacotherapy of attention-deficit/hyperactivity disorder. *J Am Acad Child Adolesc Psychiatry.* 2006;45(6):642–657.

Pliszka SR, Greenhill LL, Crismon ML, et al. The Texas Children's Medication Algorithm Project: report of the Texas Consensus Conference Panel on Medication Treatment of Childhood Attention-Deficit/Hyperactivity Disorder: part I, attention-deficit/hyperactivity disorder. *J Am Acad Child Adolesc Psychiatry.* 2000a;39:908–919.

Pliszka SR, Greenhill LL, Crismon ML, et al. The Texas Children's Medication Algorithm Project: report of the Texas Consensus Conference Panel on Medication Treatment of Childhood Attention-Deficit/Hyperactivity Disorder: part II, tactics. *J Am Acad Child Adolesc Psychiatry.* 2000b;39:920–927.

Pool D, Bloom W, Mielke DH, et al. A controlled evaluation of loxitane in seventy-five adolescent schizophrenic patients. *Curr Ther Res Clin Exp.* 1976;19:99–104.

Pope S, Zaara S. Efficacy of long acting injectable antipsychotics in adolescents. *J Child Adolesc Psychopharmacol.* 2016;26:391–394.

Popper C. Medical unknown and ethical consent: prescribing psychotropic medications for children in the face of uncertainty. In: Popper C, ed. *Psychiatric Pharmacosciences of Children and Adolescents.* Washington, DC: American Psychiatric Press; 1987a.

Popper C, ed. *Psychiatric Pharmacosciences of Children and Adolescents.* Washington, DC: American Psychiatric Press; 1987b.

Popper CW. Combining methylphenidate and clonidine: pharmacologic questions and news reports about sudden death. *J Child Adolesc Psychopharmacol.* 1995;5:157–166.

Popper CW, Zimnitzky B. Sudden death putatively related to desipramine treatment in youth: a fifth case and a review of speculative mechanisms. *J Child Adolesc Psychopharmacol.* 1995;5:283–300.

Potenza MN, Holmes JP, Kanes SJ, et al. Olanzapine treatment of children, adolescents, and adults with pervasive developmental disorders: an open-label pilot study. *J Clin Psychopharmacol.* 1999;19:37–44.

Potter WZ, Calil HM, Sutfin TA, et al. Active metabolites of imipramine and desipramine in man. *Clin Pharmacol Ther.* 1982;31:393–401.

Poussaint AF, Ditman KS. A controlled study of imipramine (Tofranil) in the treatment of childhood enuresis. *J Pediatr.* 1965;67:283–290.

Prakash A, Lobo E, Kratochvil CJ, et al. An open-label safety and pharmacokinetics study of duloxetine in pediatric patients with major depression. *J Child Adolesc Psychopharmacol*. 2012;22:48–55.

Preskorn SH, Bupp SJ, Weller EB, et al. Plasma levels of imipramine and metabolites in 68 hospitalized children. *J Am Acad Child Adolesc Psychiatry*. 1989a;28:373–375.

Preskorn SH, Jerkovich GS, Beber JH, et al. Therapeutic drug monitoring of tricyclic antidepressants: a standard of care issue. *Psychopharmacol Bull*. 1989b;25:281–284.

Preskorn SH, Weller EB, Hughes CW, et al. Depression in prepubertal children: dexamethasone nonsuppression predicts differential response to imipramine vs. placebo. *Psychopharmacol Bull*. 1987;23:128–133.

Preskorn SH, Weller EB, Jerkovich G, et al. Depression in children: concentration dependent CNS toxicity of tricyclic antidepressants. *Psychopharmacol Bull*. 1988;24:275–279.

Prien RF. Methods and models for placebo use in pharmacotherapeutic trials. *Psychopharmacol Bull*. 1988;24:4–8.

Prince JB, Wilens TE, Biederman J, et al. A controlled study of nortriptyline in children and adolescents with attention deficit hyperactivity disorder. *J Child Adolesc Psychopharmacol*. 2000;10:193–204.

Psychopharmacology Bulletin. Special issue: *Pharmacotherapy of Children*. Rockville, MD: US Department of Health, Education, and Welfare; 1973. Publication No (HSM) 73–9002.

Puente RM. The use of carbamazepine in the treatment of behavioural disorders in children. In: Birkmayer W, ed. *Epileptic Seizures-Behaviour-Pain*. Bern, Germany: Hans Huber Publishers; 1976:243–252.

Puig-Antich J. Major depression and conduct disorder in prepuberty. *J Am Acad Child Adolesc Psychiatry*. 1982;21:118–128.

Puig-Antich J. Affective disorders in children and adolescents: diagnostic validity and psychobiology. In: Meltzer HY, ed. *Psychopharmacology: The Third Generation of Progress*. New York, NY: Raven Press; 1987:843–859.

Puig-Antich J, Perel JM, Lupatkin W, et al. Imipramine in prepubertal major depressive disorders. *Arch Gen Psychiatry*. 1987;44:81–89.

Puri B. Progressive structural brain changes in schizophrenia. *Expert Rev Neurother*. 2010;10:33–42.

Quiason H, Ward D, Kitchen T. Buspirone for aggression [letter]. *J Am Acad Child Adolesc Psychiatry*. 1991;30:1026.

Quinn PO, Rapoport JL. One-year follow-up of hyperactive boys treated with imipramine or methylphenidate. *Am J Psychiatry*. 1975;132:241–245.

Quintana H, Birmaher B, Stedge D, et al. Use of methylphenidate in the treatment of children with autistic disorder. *J Autism Dev Disord*. 1995;25:283–294.

Rall TW. Hypnotics and sedatives; ethanol. In: Gilman AG, Rall TW, Nies AS, et al, eds. *Goodman and Gilman's The Pharmacological Basis of Therapeutics*. 8th ed. New York, NY: Pergamon Press; 1990:345–382.

Rapoport J, Kasoff L, Ahn K, et al. Strong treatment response and high maintenance rates of clozapine in childhood-onset schizophrenia. *J Child Adolesc Psychopharmacol*. 2016;26:428–435.

Rapoport JL, Buchsbaum MS, Weingartner H, et al. Dextroamphetamine: its cognitive and behavioral effects in normal and hyperactive boys and normal men. *Arch Gen Psychiatry*. 1980a;37:933–943.

Rapoport JL, Buchsbaum MS, Zahn TP, et al. Dextroamphetamine: cognitive and behavioral effects in normal prepubertal boys. *Science*. 1978a;199:560–563.

Rapoport JL, Mikkelsen EJ. Antidepressants. In: Werry JS, ed. *Pediatric Psychopharmacology: The Use of Behavior Modifying Drugs in Children*. New York, NY: Brunner/Mazel; 1978b:208–233.

Rapoport JL, Mikkelsen EJ, Werry JS. Antimanic, antianxiety, hallucinogenic and miscellaneous drugs. In: Werry JS, ed. *Pediatric Psychopharmacology: The Use of Behavior Modifying Drugs in Children*. New York, NY: Brunner/Mazel; 1978c:316–355.

Rapoport JL, Mikkelsen EJ, Zavadil A, et al. Childhood enuresis: psychopathology, plasma tricyclic concentration and antienuretic effect. *Arch Gen Psychiatry*. 1980b;37:1146–1152.

Rapoport JL, Quinn PO, Bradbard G, et al. Imipramine and methylphenidate treatment of hyperactive boys. *Arch Gen Psychiatry*. 1974;30:789–798.

Rapport MD, Carlson GA, Kelly KL, et al. Methylphenidate and desipramine in hospitalized children: I, separate and combined effects on cognitive function. *J Am Acad Child Adolesc Psychiatry*. 1993;32:333–342.

Rapport MD, Denney C, DuPaul GJ, et al. Attention deficit disorder and methylphenidate: normalization rates, clinical effectiveness, and response prediction in 76 children. *J Am Acad Child Adolesc Psychiatry*. 1994;33:882–893.

Raskind MA, Peskind ER, Hoff DJ, et al. A parallel group placebo controlled study of prazosin for trauma nightmares and sleep disturbance in combat veterans with post-traumatic stress disorder. *Biol Psychiatry*. 2007;61:928–934.

Rasmussen D, Marck B, Boldt B, et al. Suppression of hypothalamic pro-opiomelanocortin (POMC) gene expression by daily melatonin supplementation in aging rats. *J Pineal Res*. 2003;34(2):127–133.

Rating scales and assessment instruments for use in pediatric psychopharmacology research. *Psychopharmacol Bull*. 1985;21:713–1124.

Realmuto G. Neurobiological assessment. In: Klykylo W, Kay J, eds. *Clinical Child Psychiatry*. 3rd ed. Chichester, England: John Wiley & Sons; 2012.

Realmuto GM, August GJ, Garfinkel BD. Clinical effect of buspirone in autistic children. *J Clin Psychopharmacol*. 1989;9:122–125.

Realmuto GM, Erickson WD, Yellin AM, et al. Clinical comparison of thiothixene and thioridazine in schizophrenic adolescents. *Am J Psychiatry*. 1984;141:440–442.

Redden L, DelBello M, Wagner KD, et al. Long-term safety of divalproex sodium extended-release in children and adolescents with bipolar I disorder. *J Child Adolesc Psychopharmacol*. 2009;19(1):83–89.

Reisberg B, Gershon S. Side effects associated with lithium therapy. *Arch Gen Psychiatry*. 1979;36:879–887.

Reiss AL, O'Donnell DJ. Carbamazepine-induced mania in two children: case report. *J Clin Psychiatry*. 1984;45:272–274.

Reite ML, Nagel KE, Ruddy JR. *Concise Guide to Evaluation and Management of Sleep Disorders*. Washington, DC: American Psychiatric Press; 1990.

Remschmidt H. The psychotropic effect of carbamazepine in non-epileptic patients, with particular reference to problems posed by clinical studies in children with behavioural disorders. In: Birkmayer W, ed. *Epileptic Seizures-Behaviour-Pain*. Bern, Germany: Hans Huber Publishers; 1976:253–258.

Remschmidt H, Schulz E, Martin PDM. An open trial of clozapine in thirty-six adolescents with schizophrenia. *J Child Adolesc Psychopharmacol*. 1994;4:31–41.

The Research Units on Pediatric Psychopharmacology Anxiety Study Group. The pediatric anxiety rating scale (PARS): development and psychometric properties. *J Am Acad Child Adolesc Psychiatry*. 2002;41(9):1061–1069.

Rexulti [package insert]. Tokyo, Japan: Otsuka Pharmaceutical Co, Ltd; 2017.

Richardson MA, Haugland G, Craig TJ. Neuroleptic use, parkinsonian symptoms, tardive dyskinesia and associated factors in child and adolescent psychiatric patients. *Am J Psychiatry*. 1991;148:1322–1328.

Riddle MA, ed. Pediatric psychopharmacology I [entire issue]. *Child Adolesc Psychiatr Clin N Am*. 1995a;4:1–260.

Riddle MA, ed. Pediatric psychopharmacology II [entire issue]. *Child Adolesc Psychiatr Clin N Am*. 1995b;4:261–520.

Riddle MA, Geller B, Ryan N. Another sudden death in a child treated with desipramine. *J Am Acad Child Adolesc Psychiatry*. 1993;32:792–797.

Riddle MA, Geller B, Ryan ND. The safety of desipramine: reply [letter]. *J Am Acad Child Adolesc Psychiatry*. 1994;33:589–590.

Riddle MA, Hardin MT, Cho SC, et al. Desipramine treatment of boys with attention-deficit hyperactivity disorder and tics: preliminary clinical experiences. *J Am Acad Child Adolesc Psychiatry*. 1988;27:811–814.

Riddle MA, Hardin MT, King R, et al. Fluoxetine treatment of children and adolescents with Tourette's and obsessive compulsive disorders: preliminary clinical experience. *J Am Acad Child Adolesc Psychiatry*. 1990;29:45–48.

Riddle MA, King RA, Hardin MT, et al. Behavioral side effects of fluoxetine in children and adolescents. *J Child Adolesc Psychopharmacol*. 1990/1991;1:193–198.

Riddle MA, Nelson JC, Kleinman CS, et al. Sudden death in children receiving norpramin: a review of three reported cases and commentary. *J Am Acad Child Adolesc Psychiatry*. 1991;30:104–108.

Riddle MA, Reeve EA, Yaryura-Tobias JA, et al. Fluvoxamine for children and adolescents with obsessive-compulsive disorder: a randomized, controlled, multicenter trial. *J Am Acad Child Adolesc Psychiatry*. 2001;40(2):222–229.

Riddle MA, Scahill L, King RA, et al. Double-blind, crossover trial of fluoxetine and placebo in children and adolescents with obsessive-compulsive disorder. *J Am Acad Child Adolesc Psychiatry*. 1992;31:1062–1069.

Rifkin A, Karajgi B, Dicker R, et al. Lithium treatment of conduct disorders in adolescents. *Am J Psychiatry*. 1997;154:554–555.

Rifkin A, Quitkin F, Klein DF. Akinesia: a poorly recognized drug-induced extrapyramidal behavior disorder. *Arch Gen Psychiatry*. 1975;32:672–674.

Riggs PD, Leon SL, Mikulich SK, et al. An open trial of bupropion for ADHD in adolescents with substance use disorders and conduct disorder. *J Am Acad Child Adolesc Psychiatry*. 1998;37:1271–1278.

Risperdal [package insert]. Titusville, NJ: Janssen Pharmaceuticals, Inc; 2010.

Risperdal for consistency change to: [package insert]. Titusville, NJ: Janssen L.P; 2007.

Rivera-Calimlim L, Griesbach PH, Perlmutter R. Plasma chlorpromazine concentrations in children with behavioral disorders and mental illness. *Clin Pharmacol Ther.* 1979;26:114–121.

Rivera-Calimlim L, Nasrallah H, Strauss J, et al. Clinical response and plasma levels: effect of dose, dosage schedules, and drug interactions on plasma chlorpromazine levels. *Am J Psychiatry.* 1976;133:646–652.

Rizzo R, Eddy CM, Cali P, et al. Metabolic effects of aripiprazole and pimozide in children with Tourette syndrome. *Pediatr Neurol.* 2012;47:419–422.

Robb AS, Cueva JE, Sporn J, et al. Sertraline treatment of children and adolescents with posttraumatic stress disorder: a double-blind placebo-controlled trial. *J Child Adolesc Psychopharmacol.* 2010;20(6):463–471.

Robinson AA, Malow BA. Gabapentin shows promise in treating refractory insomnia in children. *J Child Neurol.* 2013;28(12):1618–1621.

Roessner V, Schoenefeld K, Buse J, et al. Pharmacological treatment of tic disorders and Tourette syndrome. *Neuropharmacology.* 2012;68:143–149.

Romo-Nava F, Alvarez-Icaza G, Fresán-Orellana A, et al. Melatonin attenuates antipsychotic metabolic effects: an eight-week randomized, double-blind, parallel-group, placebo-controlled clinical trial. *Bipolar Disord.* 2014;16(4):410–421.

Rosenbaum JF, Fava M, Hoog SL, et al. Selective serotonin reuptake inhibitor discontinuation syndrome: a randomized clinical trial. *Biol Psychiatry.* 1998;44:77–87.

Rosenberg DR, Davanzo PA, Gershon S. *Pharmacotherapy for Child and Adolescent Psychiatric Disorders.* 2nd ed. New York, NY: Marcel Dekker, Inc; 2002.

Rosenberg DR, Holttum J, Gershon S. *Textbook of Pharmacotherapy for Child and Adolescent Psychiatric Disorders.* New York, NY: Brunner/Mazel; 1994.

Rosenberg DR, Johnson K, Sahl R. Evolving mania in an adolescent treated with low-dose fluoxetine. *J Child Adolesc Psychopharmacol.* 1992;2:299–306.

Rosenberg DR, Stewart CM, Fitzgerald KD, et al. Paroxetine open-label treatment of pediatric outpatients with obsessive-compulsive disorder. *J Am Acad Child Adolesc Psychiatry.* 1999;38:1180–1185.

Ross DC, Piggott LR. Clonazepam for OCD [letter]. *J Am Acad Child Adolesc Psychiatry.* 1993;32:470–471.

Rosse RB, Giese AA, Deutsch SI, et al. *Laboratory Diagnostic Testing in Psychiatry.* Washington, DC: American Psychiatric Press; 1989.

Rossenu S, Cleton A, Talluri K, et al. Evaluation of the pharmacokinetics of an extended-release formulation of paliperidone with an immediate-release formulation of risperidone. *Clin Pharm Ther.* 2007;81(suppl 1):S62.

Rossenu SAC, Rusch S, Janssens S, et al. Extended-release formulation of paliperidone shows dose proportional pharmacokinetics. Presented at: the American Association of Pharmaceutical Sciences Annual Meeting and Exposition; October 29–November 2, 2006; San Antonio, TX; 2006. Poster number: T3123.

Rubinstein ML, Benowitz NL, Auerback GM, et al. A randomized trial of nicotine nasal spray in adolescent smokers. *Pediatrics.* 2008;122(3):e595–e600.

Rudorfer MV, Potter WZ. Pharmacokinetics of antidepressants. In: Meltzer HY, ed. *Psychopharmacology: The Third Generation of Progress.* New York, NY: Raven Press; 1987:1353–1363.

Russell JL, Spiller HA, Chounthirath T, et al. Pediatric ingestion of vilazodone compared to other selective serotonin reuptake inhibitor medications. *Clin Toxicol.* 2017;55(5):352–356.

Russo RM, Gururaj VJ, Allen JE. The effectiveness of diphenhydramine HCl in pediatric sleep disorders. *J Clin Pharmacol.* 1976;4:284–288.

Ryan ND. Heterocyclic antidepressants in children and adolescents. *J Child Adolesc Psychopharmacol.* 1990;1:21–31.

Ryan ND, Meyer V, Dachille S, et al. Lithium antidepressant augmentation in TCA-refractory depression in adolescents. *J Am Acad Child Adolesc Psychiatry.* 1988a;27:371–376.

Ryan ND, Puig-Antich J, Cooper T, et al. Imipramine in adolescent major depression: plasma level and clinical response. *Acta Psychiatr Scand.* 1986;73:275–288.

Ryan ND, Puig-Antich J, Rabinovich H, et al. MAOIs in adolescent major depression unresponsive to tricyclic antidepressants. *J Am Acad Child Adolesc Psychiatry.* 1988b;27:755–758.

Rynn M, Siqueland L, Rickels K. Placebo-controlled trial of sertraline in the treatment of children with generalized anxiety disorder. *Am J Psychiatry.* 2001;158:2008–2014.

Rynn M, Wagner KD, Donnelly C, et al. Long-term sertraline treatment of children and adolescents with major depressive disorder. *J Child Adolesc Psychopharmacol.* 2006;16(1–2):103–116.

Rynn MA, Walkup JT, Compton SN, et al. Child/adolescent anxiety multimodal study: evaluating safety. *J Am Acad Child Adolesc Psychiatry.* 2015;54(3):180–190.

Sabuncuoglu O, Ekinci O, Berkem M. Fluoxetine-induced sleep bruxism in an adolescent treated with buspirone: a case report. *Spec Care Dentist.* 2009;29(5):215–217.

Sadock B. *Synopsis of Psychiatry.* 10th ed. New-York, NY: Wolters Kluwer; 2007.

Safer D, Allen RP, Barr E. Depression of growth in hyperactive children on stimulant drugs. *N Engl J Med.* 1972;287:217–220.

Safer DJ, Krager M. A survey of medication treatment for hyperactive/inattentive students. *JAMA.* 1988;260:2256–2258.

Safer DJ, Zito JM. Treatment-emergent adverse events from selective serotonin reuptake inhibitors by age group: children versus adolescents. *J Child Adolesc Psychopharmacol.* 2006;16(1–2):159–169.

Saito E, Correll CU, Gallelli K, et al. A prospective study of hyperprolactinemia in children and adolescents treated with atypical antipsychotic agents. *J Child Adolesc Psychopharmacol.* 2004;14:350–358.

Sakarcan A, Thomas DB, O'Reilly KP, et al. Lithium-induced nephrotic syndrome in a young pediatric patient. *Pediatr Nephrol.* 2002;17(4):290–292.

Sakkas P, Davis JM, Han J, et al. Pharmacotherapy of NMS. *Psychiatr Ann.* 1991;21:157–164.

Salazar DE, Frackiewicz EJ, Dockens R. Pharmacokinetics and tolerability of buspirone during oral administration to children and adolescents with anxiety disorder and normal healthy adults. *J Clin Pharmacol.* 2001;41:1351–1358.

Sallee FR, DeVane CL, Ferrell RE. Fluoxetine-related death in a child with cytochrome P-450 2D6 genetic deficiency. *J Child Adolesc Psychopharmacol.* 2000a;10:27–34.

Sallee FR, Kurlan R, Goetz CG, et al. Ziprasidone treatment of children and adolescents with Tourette's syndrome: a pilot study. *J Am Acad Child Adolesc Psychiatry.* 2000b;39(3):292–299.

Sallee FR, Nesbitt L, Jackson C, et al. Relative efficacy of haloperidol and pimozide in children and adolescents with Tourette's disorder. *Am J Psychiatry.* 1997;154:1057–1062.

Sallee FR, Sethuraman G, Rock CM. Effects of pimozide on cognition in children with Tourette syndrome: interaction with comorbid attention deficit hyperactivity disorder. *Acta Psychiatr Scand.* 1994;90(1):4–9.

Salzman C. Benzodiazepine dependency: summary of the APA task force on benzodiazepines. *Psychopharmacol Bull.* 1990;26:61–62.

Saphris [package insert]. Parsippany, NJ: Allergan; 2017.

Saraf KR, Klein DF, Gittelman-Klein R, et al. Imipramine side effects in children. *Psychopharmacologia (Berlin).* 1974;37:265–274.

Saul RC. Nortriptyline in attention deficit disorder. *Clin Neuropharmacol.* 1985;8:382–384.

Scahill L, Chappell PB, Kim YS, et al. Guanfacine in the treatment of children with tic disorders and ADHD: a placebo-controlled study [Abstract, 40th Annual NCDEU meeting]. *J Child Adolesc Psychopharmacol.* 2000;10:250.

Scahill L, Chappell PB, Kim YS, et al. A placebo-controlled study of guanfacine in the treatment of children with tic disorders and attention deficit hyperactivity disorder. *Am J Psychiatry.* 2001;158(7):1067–1074.

Scahill L, McCracken J, Mcdougle CJ, et al. Methodological issues in designing a multisite trial of risperidone in children and adolescents with autism. *J Child Adolesc Psychopharmacol.* 2001;11:377–388.

Scahill L, Riddle MA, McSwiggin-Hardin M, et al. Children's Yale-Brown obsessive compulsive scale: reliability and validity. *J Am Acad Child Adolesc Psychiatry.* 1997;36(6):844–852.

Scharko AM, Schumacher J. Prolonged QTc interval in a 14-year-old girl with escitalopram overdose. *J Child Adolesc Psychopharmacol.* 2008;18(3):297–298.

Scherphof CS, van den Eijnden RJ, Engels RC, et al. Short-term efficacy of nicotine replacement therapy for smoking cessation in adolescents: a randomized controlled trial. *J Subst Abuse Treat.* 2014a;46(2):120–127.

Scherphof CS, van den Eijnden RJ, Engels RC, et al. Long-term efficacy of nicotine replacement therapy for smoking cessation in adolescents: a randomized controlled trial. *Drug Alcohol Depend.* 2014b;140:217–220.

Schmid I, Burcu M, Zito JM. Medicaid prior authorization policies for pediatric use of antipsychotic medications. *JAMA.* 2015(313):966–968.

Schmidt MH, Trott G-E, Blanz B, et al. Clozapine medication in adolescents. In: Stefania CN, Rabavilas AD, Soldatos CR, eds. *Psychiatry: A World Perspective.* Vol 1. Proceedings of the Eighth World Congress of Psychiatry. Amsterdam, The Netherlands: Excerpta Medica; 1990:1100–1104.

Schooler N, Gharabawi G, Bossie C, et al. A virtual comparison of paliperidone ER and oral risperidone in patients with schizophrenia. Presented at: the 45th Annual Meeting of the American College of Neuropharmacology; December 3–7, 2006; Hollywood, FL; 2006.

Schooler NR, Kane JM. Research diagnoses for tardive dyskinesia. *Arch Gen Psychiatry.* 1982;38:486–487.

Schou M. Lithium: elimination rate, dosage, control, poisoning, goiter, mode of action. *Acta Psychiatr Scand.* 1969;207(suppl):49–59.

Schroeder JS, Mullin AV, Elliott GR, et al. Cardiovascular effects of desipramine in children. *J Am Acad Child Adolesc Psychiatry.* 1989;28:376–379.

Schumann A, Ewigman B. Can metformin undo weight gain induced by antipsychotics? *J Fam Pract.* 2008;57(8):526–530.

Schwarz A. Thousands of toddlers are medicated for ADHD, report finds, raising worries. *New York Times (New York Ed.).* 2014:A11.

Scott LL. Iloperidone: in schizophrenia. *CNS Drugs.* 2009;23(10):867–880.

Sethy RR, Sinha VK. Effect of lithium on thyroid function in adolescents with mood disorder. *Asian J Psychiatr.* 2016;24:41–45.

Shamseddeen W, Clarke G, Keller MB, et al. Adjunctive sleep medications and depression outcome in the treatment of serotonin-selective reuptake inhibitor resistant depression in adolescents study. *J Child Adolesc Psychopharmacol.* 2012;22(1):29–36.

Shapiro AK, Shapiro E. Do stimulants provoke, cause, or exacerbate tics and Tourette syndrome? *Compr Psychiatry.* 1981;22:265–273.

Shapiro AK, Shapiro E. Controlled study of pimozide vs. placebo in Tourette's syndrome. *J Am Acad Child Psychiatry.* 1984;23:161–173.

Shapiro AK, Shapiro E. Tic disorders. In: Kaplan HI, Sadock BJ, eds. *Comprehensive Textbook of Psychiatry.* 5th ed. Baltimore, MD: Williams & Wilkins; 1989:1865–1878.

Shapiro AK, Shapiro E, Eisenkraft GJ. Treatment of Gilles de la Tourette syndrome with pimozide. *Am J Psychiatry.* 1983;140:1183–1186.

Shapiro M, Reid A, Olsen B. Topiramate, zonisamide and weight loss in children and adolescents prescribed psychiatric medications: a medical record review. *Int J Psychiatry Med.* 2016;51(1):56–68.

Sharko AM. Selective serotonin reuptake inhibitor-induced sexual dysfunction in adolescents: a review. *J Am Acad Child Adolesc Psychiatry.* 2004;43:1071–1079.

Shaw P, Sporn A, Gogtay N, et al. Childhood-onset schizophrenia: a double-blind, randomized clozapine-olanzapine comparison. *Arch Gen Psychiatry.* 2006;63:721–730.

Shea S, Turgay A, Carroll A, et al. Risperidone in the treatment of disruptive behavioral symptoms in children with autistic and other pervasive developmental disorders. *Pediatrics.* 2004;114(5):634–641.

Sheitman BB, Bird PM, Binz W, et al. Olanzapine-induced elevation of plasma triglyceride levels. *Am J Psychiatry.* 1999;156:1471–1472.

Shin L, Bregman H, Breeze J, et al. Metformin for weight control in pediatric patients on atypical antipsychotic medication. *J Child Adolesc Psychopharmacol.* 2009;3:275–279.

Shirazi E, Alaghband-Rad J. An open trial of citalopram in children and adolescents with depression. *J Child Adolesc Psychopharmacol.* 2005;15:233–239.

Shojaei AH, Rong-Kun C, Pennick M. Guanfacine extended release tablets as treatment for attention-deficit/hyperactivity disorder: formulation characteristics. Poster presented at: USPMH Congress; November 16, 2006; New Orleans, LA.

Sholevar EH, Baron DA, Hardie TL. Treatment of childhood-onset schizophrenia with olanzapine. *J Child Adolesc Psychopharmacol.* 2000;10:69–78.

Shon SH, Joo Y, Lee JS, et al., Lamotrigine treatment of adolescents with unipolar and bipolar depression: a retrospective chart review. *J Child Adolesc Psychopharmacol.* 2014;24(5):285–287.

Siefen G, Remschmidt H. Behandlungsergebnisse mit clozapin bei schizophrenen jugendlichen [Clozapine in the treatment of adolescents with schizophrenia: treatment outcome]. *Zeitschrift fur Kinder-und-Jugendpsychiatrie.* 1986;14:245–257.

Siegel M, Beresford CA, Bunker M, et al. Preliminary investigation of lithium for mood disorder symptoms in children and adolescents with autism spectrum disorder. *J Child Adolesc Psychopharmacol.* 2014;24(7):399–402.

Sikich L, Frazier JA, McClellan J, et al. Double-blind comparison of first- and second-generation antipsychotics in early-onset schizophrenia and schizoaffective disorder: findings from the Treatment of Early-Onset Schizophrenia Spectrum Disorders (TEOSS) study. *Am J Psychiatry.* 2008;165(11):1420–1431.

Silva RR. May-June 2012 update: psychopharmacology news and views. *J Child Adolesc Psychopharmacol.* 2012;22(3):249.

Silva RR, Muniz R, Pestreich L, et al. Efficacy and duration of effect of extended-release dexmethylphenidate versus placebo in schoolchildren with attention-deficit/hyperactivity disorder. *J Child Adolesc Psychopharmacol.* 2006;16:239–251.

Silva RR, Munoz DM, Alpert M. Carbamazepine use in children and adolescents with features of attention-deficit hyperactivity disorder: a meta-analysis. *J Am Acad Child Adolesc Psychiatry.* 1996;35:352–358.

Simeon JG, Carrey NJ, Wiggins DM, et al. Risperidone effects in treatment-resistant adolescents: preliminary case reports. *J Child Adolesc Psychopharmacol.* 1995;5:69–79.

Simeon JG, Dinicola VF, Ferguson HB, et al. Adolescent depression: a placebo-controlled fluoxetine treatment study and follow-up. *Prog Neuropsychopharmacol Biol Psychiatry.* 1990;14:791–795.

Simeon JG, Ferguson HB. Recent developments in the use of antidepressant and anxiolytic medications. *Psychiatr Clin N Am.* 1985;8:893–907.

Simeon JG, Ferguson HB. Alprazolam effects in children with anxiety disorders. *Can J Psychiatry.* 1987;32:570–574.

Simeon JG, Ferguson HB, Fleet JVW. Bupropion effects in attention deficit and conduct disorder. *Can J Psychiatry.* 1986;31:581–585.

Simeon JG, Ferguson HB, Knott V, et al. Clinical, cognitive, and neurophysiological effects of alprazolam in children and adolescents with overanxious and avoidant disorders. *J Am Acad Child Adolesc Psychiatry.* 1992;31:29–33.

Simeon JG, Knott VJ, DuBois C, et al. Buspirone therapy of mixed anxiety disorders in childhood and adolescence: a pilot study. *J Child Adolesc Psychopharmacol.* 1994;4:159–170.

Simon GE, Savarino J, Operskalski B, et al. Suicidal risk during antidepressant treatment. *Am J Psychiatry.* 2006;163:41–47.

Singer HS. Treatment of tics and Tourette syndrome. *Curr Treat Options Neurol.* 2010;12(6):539–561.

Singh AB, Bousman CA, Ng CH, et al. High impact child abuse may predict risk of elevated suicidality during antidepressant initiation. *Aust N Z J Psychiatry.* 2013;47(12):1191–1195.

Singh D, Akingbola A, Ross-Ascuitto N, et al. Electrocardiac effects associated with lithium toxicity in children: an illustrative case and review of the pathophysiology. *Cardiol Young.* 2016;26:221–229.

Singh S, Loke YK, Spangler JG, et al. Risk of serious adverse cardiovascular events associated with varenicline: a systematic review and meta-analysis. *Can Med Assoc J.* 2011;183(12):1359–1366.

Skapinakis P, Caldwell D, Hollingsworth W, et al. A systematic review of the clinical effectiveness and cost-effectiveness of pharmacological and psychological interventions for the management of obsessive-compulsive disorder in children/adolescents and adults. *Health Technol Assess.* 2016;20(43):13–92.

Skarphedinsson G, Weidle B, Thomsen PH, et al. Continued cognitive-behavior therapy versus sertraline for children and adolescents with obsessive-compulsive disorder that were non-responders to cognitive-behavior therapy: a randomized controlled trial. *Eur Child Adolesc Psychiatry.* 2015;24(5):591–602.

Sleator EK. Diagnosis. In: Sleator EK, Pelham WE Jr, eds. *Attention Deficit Disorder: Dialogues in Pediatric Management.* Vol 1, No 3. Norwalk, CT: Appleton-Century-Crofts; 1986:11–42.

Sleator EK, von Neumann A, Sprague RL. Hyperactive children: a continuous long-term placebo-controlled follow-up. *JAMA.* 1974;229:316–317.

Small JG, Milstein V, Marhenke JD, et al. Treatment outcome with clozapine in tardive dyskinesis, neuroleptic sensitivity, and treatment resistant psychosis. *J Clin Psychiatry.* 1987;48:263–267.

Smathers SA, Wilson JG, Nigro MA. Topiramate effectiveness in Prader-Willi syndrome. *Pediatr Neurol.* 2003;28(2):130–133.

Smith TA, House RF Jr, Croghan IT, et al. Nicotine patch therapy in adolescent smokers. *Pediatrics.* 1996;98(4, Pt 1):659–667.

Smith TC, Wollman H. History and principles of anaesthesiology. In: Gilman AF, Goodman LS, Rall TW, et al, eds. *Goodman and Gilman's The Pharmacological Basis of Therapeutics.* 7th ed. New York, NY: Macmillan; 1985:260–275.

Snyder R, Turgay A, Aman M, et al; and the Risperidone Conduct Study Group. Effects of risperidone on conduct and disruptive behavior disorders in children with subaverage IQs. *J Am Acad Child Adolesc Psychiatry.* 2002;41:1026–1036.

Sokol MS, Campbell M. Novel psychoactive agents in the treatment of developmental disorders. In: Aman MG, Singh NN, eds. *Psychopharmacology of the Developmental Disabilities.* New York, NY: Springer-Verlag; 1988:147–167.

Sondheimer AN, Klykylo WM. The Ethics Committees of the American Academy of Child and Adolescent Psychiatry and the American Psychiatric Association: history, process, education, and advocacy. *Child Adolesc Psychiatr Clin N Am.* 2008;17(1):225–236.

Sorgi P, Ratey JJ, Knoedler DW, et al. Rating aggression in the clinical setting: a retrospective adaptation of the Overt Aggression Scale: preliminary results. *J Neuropsychiatry Clin Neurosci.* 1991;3:S52–S56.

Soutullo CA, Casuto LS, Keck PE Jr. Gabapentin in the treatment of adolescent mania: a case report. *J Child Adolesc Psychopharmacol*. 1998;8(1):81–85.

Soutullo CA, Diez-Suarez A, Figueroa-Quintana A. Adjunctive lamotrigine treatment for adolescents with bipolar disorder: retrospective report of five cases. *J Child Adolesc Psychopharmacol*. 2006;16(3):357–364.

Spencer EK, Kafantaris V, Padron-Gayol MV, et al. Haloperidol in schizophrenic children: early findings from a study in progress. *Psychopharmacol Bull*. 1992;28:183–186.

Spencer T, Biederman J, Kerman K, et al. Desipramine treatment of children with attention-deficit hyperactivity disorder and tic disorder or Tourette's syndrome. *J Am Acad Child Adolesc Psychiatry*. 1993a;32:354–360.

Spencer T, Biederman J, Steingard R, et al. Bupropion exacerbates tics in children with attention-deficit hyperactivity disorder and Tourette's syndrome. *J Am Acad Child Adolesc Psychiatry*. 1993b;32:211–214.

Spencer T, Biederman J, Wilens T, et al. Nortriptyline treatment of children with attention-deficit hyperactivity disorder and tic disorder or Tourette's syndrome. *J Am Acad Child Adolesc Psychiatry*. 1993c;32:201–210.

Spitzer RL, Endicott J, Robins E. Research diagnostic criteria. *Arch Gen Psychiatry*. 1978;35:773–782.

Sporn AL, Vermani A, Greenstein DK, et al. Clozapine treatment of childhood-onset schizophrenia: evaluation of effectiveness, adverse effects, and long-term outcome. *J Am Acad Child Adolesc Psychiatry*. 2007;46:1349–1356.

Sprague RL, Sleator EK. Methylphenidate in hyperkinetic children: differences in dose effects on learning and social behavior. *Science*. 1977;198:1274–1276.

Stahl SM. *Essential Psychopharmacology: Neuroscientific Basis and Practical Applications*. 2nd ed. Cambridge, England: Cambridge; 2000.

Staller JA. Intramuscular ziprasidone in youth: a retrospective chart review. *J Child Adolesc Psychopharmacol*. 2004;14:590–592.

Staller JA, Kunwar A, Simionescu M. Oxcarbazepine in the treatment of child psychiatric disorders: a retrospective review. *J Child Adolesc Psychopharmacol*. 2005;15:964–969.

Stanley B. An integration of ethical and clinical considerations in the use of placebos. *Psychopharmacol Bull*. 1988;24:18–20.

Starr HL, Kemner J. Multicenter, randomized, open-label study of OROS methylphenidate versus atomoxetine: treatment outcomes in African-American children with ADHD. *J Natl Med Assoc*. 2005;97(10 suppl):11S–16S.

Steiner H, Petersen ML, Saxena K, et al. Divalproex sodium for treatment of conduct disorder: a randomized controlled clinical trial. *J Clin Psychiatry*. 2003;64:1183–1191.

Steingard R, Biederman J, Spencer T, et al. Comparison of clonidine response in the treatment of attention-deficit hyperactivity disorder with and without comorbid tic disorders. *J Am Acad Child Adolesc Psychiatry*. 1993;32:350–353.

Steingard R, Khan A, Gonzales A, et al. Neuroleptic malignant syndrome: review of experience with children and adolescents. *J Child Adolesc Psychopharmacol*. 1992;2:183–198.

Stevens J, Prince J, Prager L, et al. Psychotic disorders in children and adolescents: a primer on contemporary evaluation and management. *Prim Care Companion CNS Disord*. 2014;16. doi:10.4088/PCC.13f01514.

Stigler K, Erickson C, Mullet J, et al. Paliperidone for irritability in autistic disorder [letters to the editor]. *J Child Adolesc Psychopharmacol*. 2010;20(1):75–78.

Stoddard FJ, Luthra R, Sorrentina EA, et al. A randomized controlled trial of sertraline to prevent posttraumatic stress disorder in burned children. *J Child Adolesc Psychopharmacol*. 2011;21(5):469–477.

Strawn JR, Prakash A, Zhang Q, et al. A randomized, placebo-controlled study of duloxetine for the treatment of children and adolescents with generalized anxiety disorder. *J Am Acad Child Adolesc Psychiatry*. 2015;54(4):283–293.

Strayhorn JM, Rapp N, Donina W, et al. Randomized trial of methylphenidate for an autistic child. *J Am Acad Child Adolesc Psychiatry*. 1988;27:244–247.

Strober M, Freeman R, Rigali J. The pharmacotherapy of depressive illness in adolescents: I, an open label trial of imipramine. *Psychopharmacol Bull*. 1990;26:80–84.

Strober M, Freeman R, Rigali J, et al. The pharmacotherapy of depressive illness in adolescents: II, effects of lithium augmentation in nonresponders to imipramine. *J Am Acad Child Adolesc Psychiatry*. 1992;31:16–20.

Stuhec, M, Munda B, Svab V, et al. Comparative efficacy and acceptability of atomoxetine, lisdexamfetamine, bupropion and methylphenidate in treatment of attention deficit hyperactivity disorder in children and adolescents: a meta-analysis with focus on bupropion. *J Affect Disord.* 2015;178:149–159.

Sudden death in children treated with a tricyclic antidepressant. *Med Lett.* 1990;32:53.

Sussman N. The potential benefits of serotonin receptor-specific agents. *J Clin Psychiatry.* 1994a;55(suppl 1):45–51.

Sussman N. The uses of buspirone in psychiatry. *J Clin Psychiatry Monograph.* 1994b;12:3–19.

Sussman N, Ginsberg D. Valproate and risk of polycystic ovary syndrome. *Prim Psychiatry.* 1998;5:42–48.

Sverd J. Methylphenidate treatment for children with attention deficit hyperactivity disorder and tic disorder: inadvisable or indispensable? In: Greenhill LL, Osman BB, eds. *Ritalin: Theory and Practice.* 2nd ed. Larchmont, NY: Mary Ann Liebert, Inc; 2000:301–319.

Swanson J, Greenhill L, Pelham W, et al. Initiating Concerta (OROS methylphenidate HCl) qd in children with attention-deficit hyperactivity disorder. *J Clin Res.* 2000;3:59–76.

Swanson JM, Connor DF, Cantwell D. Combining methylphenidate and clonidine: ill-advised/ and negative rebuttal (debate forum). *J Am Acad Child Adolesc Psychiatry.* 1999;38: 614–622.

Swanson JM, Flockhart D, Udrea D, et al. Clonidine in the treatment of ADHD: questions about safety and efficacy [letter]. *J Child Adolesc Psychopharmacol.* 1995;5:301–304.

Swanson JM, Lerner M, Cantwell D. Blood levels and tolerance to stimulants in ADDH children. *Clin Neuropharmacol.* 1986;9(suppl 4):523–525.

Swanson JM, Lerner MA, Gupta S, et al. Development of a new once-a-day formulation of meth-ylphenidate for the treatment of ADHD. *Arch Gen Psychiatry.* 2003;60:204–211.

Swanson JM, Wigal S, Greenhill LL, et al. Analog classroom assessment of Adderall in children with ADHD. *J Am Acad Child Adolesc Psychiatry.* 1998;37:519–526.

Szigethy E, Wiznitzer M, Branicky LA, et al. Risperidone-induced hepatotoxicity in children and adolescents? A chart review study. *J Child Adolesc Psychopharmacol.* 1999;9:93–98.

Tauscher-Wisniewski S, Nilsson M, Caldwell C, et al. Meta-analysis of aggression and/or hostility-related events in children and adolescents treated with fluoxetine compared with placebo. *J Child Adolesc Psychopharmacol.* 2007;17(5):713–718.

Taylor E, Schachar R, Thorley G, et al. Which boys respond to stimulant medication? A controlled trial of methylphenidate in boys with disruptive behavior. *Psychol Med.* 1987;17:121–143.

Teicher MH, Baldessarini RJ. Developmental pharmacodynamics. In: Popper C, ed. *Psychiatric Pharmacosciences of Children and Adolescents.* Washington, DC: American Psychiatric Press; 1987:45–80.

Teitelbaum M. Oxcarbazepine in bipolar disorder [letter]. *J Am Acad Child Adolesc Psychiatry.* 2001;40:993–994.

Texas Department of Family and Protective Services. *Psychotropic Medication Utilization Param-eters for Children and Youth in Foster Care.* 5th ed. Austin, TX: University of Texas at Austin College of Pharmacy; 2016.

Thase ME, Kupfer DJ, Frank E, et al. Treatment of imipramine-resistant recurrent depression: II, an open clinical trial of lithium augmentation. *J Clin Psychiatry.* 1989;50:413–417.

Thompson PM, Vidal C, Giedd JN, et al. Mapping adolescent brain change reveals a dynamic wave of accelerated gray matter loss in very early-onset schizophrenia. *Proc Natl Acad Sci U S A.* 2001;98(20):11650–11655.

Thomsen PH. Child and adolescent obsessive-compulsive disorder treated with citalopram: findings from an open trial of 23 cases. *J Child Adolesc Psychopharmacol.* 1997;7:157–166.

Tierney E, Joshi PT, Llinas JF, et al. Sertraline for major depression in children and adolescents: preliminary clinical experience. *J Child Adolesc Psychopharmacol.* 1995;5:13–27.

Tiihonen J, Haukka J, Taylor M, et al. A nationwide cohort study of oral and depot antipsychotics after first hospitalization for schizophrenia. *Am J Psychiatry.* 2011;168:603–609.

Tourian L, LeBoeuf A, Breton J, et al. Treatment options for the cardinal symptoms of disruptive mood dysregulation disorder. *J Can Acad Child Adolesc Psychiatry.* 2015;24(1):41–54.

Trivedi H, Chang K. *Psychopharmacology, an Issue of Child and Adolescent Psychiatric Clinics of North America.* Vol 21-4. Philadelphia, PA: WB Saunders; 2012.

Tsapakis EM, Soldani F, Tondo L, et al. Efficacy of antidepressants in juvenile depression: meta-analysis. *Br J Psychiatry.* 2008;193:10–17.

Tschoner A, Engl J, Laimer M, et al. Metabolic side effects of antipsychotic medication. *Int J Clin Pract.* 2007;61:1356–1370.

Uchida M, Spencer AE, Kenworth T, et al. A pilot study: cardiac parameters in children receiving new-generation antidepressants. *J Clin Psychopharmacol.* 2017;37(3):359–362.

United States Pharmacopeial Dispensing Information (USPDI). *Drug Information for the Health Care Professional*. Rockville, MD: United States Pharmacopeial Convention; 1990.

United States Pharmacopeial Dispensing Information (USPDI). Thompson Healthcare, eds. *Drug Information for the Health Care Professional*. 25th ed. Vol 1. Greenwood Village, CO: Thomson MICROMEDEX; 2005.

Upadhyahya HP, Brady KT, Wang W. Bupropion SR in adolescents with comorbid ADHD and nicotine dependence: a pilot study. *J Am Acad Child Adolesc Psychiatry*. 2004;43(2):199–205.

Usala T, Clavenna A, Zuddas A, et al. Randomised controlled trials of selective serotonin reuptake inhibitors in treating depression in children and adolescents: a systematic review and meta-analysis. *Eur Neuropsychopharmacol*. 2008;18(1):62–73.

US Food and Drug Administration. FDA statement regarding the anti-depressant paxil for pediatric population. *FDA Talk Paper*. 2003.

Van Putten T, Marder SR. Behavioral toxicity of antipsychotic drugs. *J Clin Psychiatry*. 1987;48(suppl 9):13–19.

Van Putten T, May PRA, Marder SR. Akathisia with haloperidol and thiothixene. *Arch Gen Psychiatry*. 1984;41:1036–1039.

Varley CK, McClellan J. Case study: two additional sudden deaths with tricyclic antidepressants. *J Am Acad Child Adolesc Psychiatry*. 1997;36:390–394.

Veatch RM. *The Patient-Physician Relation: The Patient As Partner, Part 2*. Bloomington, IN: Indiana University Press; 1991.

Venkataraman S, Naylor MW, King CA. Mania associated with fluoxetine treatment in adolescents. *J Am Acad Child Adolesc Psychiatry*. 1992;31:276–281.

Verdoux H, Tournier M, Bégaud B. Antipsychotic prescribing trends: a review of pharmaco-epidemiological studies. *Acta Psychiatr Scand*. 2010;121(1):4.

Vermeir M, Boom S, Naessens I, et al. Absorption, metabolism and excretion of a single oral dose of 14C-paliperidone 1 mg in healthy subjects. *Eur Neuropsychopharmacol*. 2005;30:S191–S192.

Veselinovic T, Paulzen M, Gründer G. Cariprazine, a new, orally active dopamine D2/3 receptor partial agonist for the treatment of schizophrenia, bipolar mania and depression. *Expert Rev Neurother*. 2013;13(11):1141–1159.

Vetro A, Szentistvanyi I, Pallag L, et al. Therapeutic experience with lithium in childhood aggressivity. *Pharmacopsychiatry*. 1985;14:121–127.

Villeneuve A. The rabbit syndrome: a peculiar extrapyramidal reaction. *Can Psychiatr Assoc J*. 1972;17:69–72.

Vincent J, Varley CK, Leger P. Effects of methylphenidate on early adolescent growth. *Am J Psychiatry*. 1990;147:501–502.

Vitiello B, Behar D, Malone R, et al. Pharmacokinetics of lithium carbonate in children. *J Clin Psychopharmacol*. 1988;8:355–359.

Vitiello B, Emslie G, Clarke G, et al. Long-term outcome of adolescent depression initially resistant to selective serotonin reuptake inhibitor treatment: a follow-up study of the TORDIA sample. *J Clin Psychiatry*. 2011;72(3):388–396.

Volavka J. The effects of clozapine on aggression and substance abuse in schizophrenic patients. *J Clin Psychiatry*. 1999;60(suppl 12):43–46.

Volkers AC, Heerdink ER, van Dijk L. Antidepressant use and off-label prescribing in children and adolescents in Dutch general practice (2001–2005). *Pharmacoepidemiol Drug Saf*. 2007;16(9):1054–1062.

Vraylar [package insert]. Parsippany, NJ: Actavis Pharma, Inc; 2015.

Vyvanse [package insert]. Wayne, PA: Shire US Inc; 2007.

Wade A, McConnachie A, Crawford G, et al. Nightly treatment of primary insomnia with prolonged release melatonin for 6 months: a randomized placebo controlled trial on age and endogenous melatonin as predictors of efficacy and safety. *BMC Med*. 2010;8(51):1–18.

Wagner K, Ambrosini P, Rynn M, et al. Sertraline pediatric depression study group. Efficacy of sertraline in the treatment of children and adolescents with major depressive disorder: two randomized controlled trials. *JAMA*. 2003;290:1033–1041.

Wagner K, Jonas J, Findling R, et al. A double-blind, randomized, placebo-controlled trial of escitalopram in the treatment of pediatric depression. *J Am Acad Child Adolesc Psychiatry*. 2006;45:280–288.

Wagner KD, Ambrosinie P, Rynn M, et al. Efficacy of sertraline in the treatment of children and adolescents with major depressive disorder two randomized controlled trials. *JAMA*. 2003;290:1033–1041.

Wagner KD, Arsarnow JR, Vitiello B, et al. Out of the black box: treatment of resistant depression in adolescents and the antidepressant controversy. *J Child Adolesc Psychopharmacol*. 2012;22(1):5–10.

Wagner KD, Berard R, Stein MB, et al. A multicenter, randomized, double-blind, placebo-controlled trial of paroxetine in children and adolescents with social anxiety disorder. *Arch Gen Psychiatry.* 2004a;61:1153–1162.

Wagner KD, Kowatch RA, Emslie GJ, et al. A double-blind, randomized, placebo-controlled trial of oxcarbazepine in the treatment of bipolar disorder in children and adolescents. *Am J Psychiatry.* 2006;163(7):1179–1186.

Wagner KD, Redden L, Kowatch R, et al. A double-blind, randomized, placebo-controlled trial of divalproex extended-release in the treatment of bipolar disorder in children and adolescents. *J Am Acad Child Adolesc Psychiatry.* 2009;48(5):519–532.

Wagner KD, Robb AS, Findling RL, et al. A randomized placebo-controlled trial of citalopram for the treatment of major depression in children and adolescents. *Am J Psychiatry.* 2004b;161(6):1079–1083.

Wagner KD, Weller E, Carlson G, et al. An open-label trial of divalproex in children and adolescents with bipolar disorder. *J Am Acad Child Adolesc Psychiatry.* 2002;41(10):1224–1230.

Waizer J, Hoffman SP, Polizos P, et al. Outpatient treatment of hyperactive school children with imipramine. *Am J Psychiatry.* 1974;131:587–591.

Walkup J, Cottingham E. Antipsychotic-induced weight gain and metformin. *J Am Acad Child Adolesc Psychiatry.* 2017;56(10):808–810.

Walkup JT, Albano AM, Piacentini J, et al. Cognitive behavioral therapy, sertraline, or a combination in childhood anxiety. *N Engl J Med.* 2008;359:2753–2766.

Walkup JT, Labellarte MJ, Riddle MA, et al. Fluvoxamine for the treatment of anxiety disorders in children and adolescents. *N Engl J Med.* 2001;344:1279–1285.

Walsh BT, ed. *Child Psychopharmacology.* Washington, DC: American Psychiatric Press; 1998.

Walsh BT, Giardina EG, Sloan RP, et al. Effects of desipramine on autonomic control of the heart. *J Am Acad Child Adolesc Psychiatry.* 1994;33:191–197.

Walsh BT, Greenhill LL, Giardina EG, et al. Effects of desipramine on autonomic input to the heart. *J Am Acad Child Adolesc Psychiatry.* 1999;38:1186–1192.

Wang H, Woo Y, Bahk W. The role of melatonin and melatonin agonists in counteracting antipsychotic-induced metabolic side effects: a systematic review. *Int Clin Psychopharmacol.* 2016;31(6):301–306.

Wang HD, Dunnavant FD, Jarman T, et al. Effects of antipsychotic drugs on neurogenesis in the forebrain of adult rat. *Neuropsychopharmacology.* 2004;29(7):1230–1238.

Warden D, Subramaniam GA, Carmody T, et al. Predictors of attrition with buprenorphine/naloxone treatment in opioid dependent youth. *Addict Behav.* 2012;37(9):1046–1053.

Ware JC, Pittard JT. Increased deep sleep after trazodone use: a double-blind placebo-controlled study in healthy young adults. *J Clin Psychiatry.* 1990;51:18–22.

Waxmonsky J, Pelham W, Gnagy E, et al. The efficacy and tolerability of methylphenidate and behavior modification in children with attention-deficit/hyperactivity disorder and severe mood dysregulation. *J Child Adolesc Psychopharmacol.* 2008;18(6):573–588.

Wechsler D. *Manual for the Wechsler Intelligence Scale for Children—Revised.* San Antonio, TX: The Psychological Corporation; 1974.

Wehmeier PM, Schacht A, Dittmann RW, et al. Minor differences in ADHD-related difficulties between boys and girls treated with atomoxetine for attention-deficit/hyperactivity disorder. *Atten Defic Hyperact Disord.* 2010;2(2):73–85.

Wehmeier PM, Schacht A, Dittmann RW, et al. Effect of atomoxetine on quality of life and family burden: results from a randomized, placebo-controlled, double-blind study in children and adolescents with ADHD and comorbid oppositional defiant or conduct disorder. *Qual Life Res.* 2011;20(5):691–702.

Wehmeier PM, Schacht A, Escobar R, et al. Differences between children and adolescents in treatment response to atomoxetine and the correlation between health-related quality of life and attention deficit/hyperactivity disorder core symptoms: meta-analysis of five atomoxetine trials. *Child Adolesc Psychiatry Ment Health.* 2010;4:30.

Wei YJ, Liu X, Rao N, et al. Physical health outcomes in preschoolers with prior authorization for antipsychotics. *J Child Adolesc Psychopharmacol.* 2017;27(9):833–839.

Weiden PJ. Switching antipsychotics as a treatment strategy for antipsychotic-induced weight gain and dyslipidemia. *J Clin Psychiatry.* 2007;68(suppl 4):34–39.

Weihs KL, Murphy W, Abbas R, et al. Desvenlafaxine versus placebo in a fluoxetine-referenced study of children and adolescents with major depressive disorder. *J Child Adolesc Psychopharmacol.* 2018;28(1):36–46.

Weiner JM, Jaffe SL. Historical overview of childhood and adolescent psychopharmacology. In: Weiner JM, ed. *Diagnosis and Psychopharmacology of Childhood and Adolescent Disorders.* New York, NY: John Wiley; 1985:3–50.

Weiner N. Norepinephrine, epinephrine, and the sympathomimetic amines. In: Gilman AG, Goodman LS, Gilman A, eds. *Goodman and Gilman's The pharmacological Basis of Therapeutics.* 6th ed. New York, NY: Macmillan; 1980:138–175.

Weiss G, Hechtman LT. *Hyperactive Children Grown Up: Empirical Findings and Theoretical Considerations.* New York, NY: Guilford Press; 1986.

Weiss G, Kruger E, Danielson U, et al. Effect of long-term treatment of hyperactive children with methylphenidate. *Can Med Assoc J.* 1975;112:159–165.

Weiss M, Tannock R, Kratochvil C, et al. A randomized, placebo-controlled study of once-daily atomoxetine in the school setting in children with ADHD. *J Am Acad Child Adolesc Psychiatry.* 2005;44(7):647–655.

Weiss M, Wasdell M, Bomben M, et al. Sleep hygiene and melatonin treatment for children and adolescents with ADHD and initial insomnia. *J Am Acad Child Adolesc Psychiatry.* 2006;45(5):512–519.

Weizman A, Weitz R, Szekely GA, et al. Combination of neuroleptic and stimulant treatment in attention deficit disorder with hyperactivity. *J Am Acad Child Psychiatry.* 1984;23:295–298.

Weller EB, Weller RA, Fristed MA. Lithium dosage guide for prepubertal children: a preliminary report. *J Am Acad Child Psychiatry.* 1986;25:92–95.

Weller EB, Weller RA, Preskorn SH, et al. Steady-state plasma imipramine levels in prepubertal depressed children. *Am J Psychiatry.* 1982;139:506–508.

Wender PH. Attention deficit hyperactivity disorder. In: Howells JG, ed. *Modern Perspectives in Clinical Psychiatry.* New York, NY: Brunner/Mazel; 1988:149–169.

Wernicke JF. The side effect profile and safety of fluoxetine. *J Clin Psychiatry.* 1985;46:59–67.

Werry J, Aman M. Methylphenidate and haloperidol in children: effects on attention, memory, and activity. *Arch Gen Psychiatry.* 1975;32:790–795.

Werry J, Aman MG, Diamond E. Imipramine and methylphenidate in hyperactive children. *J Child Psychol Psychiatry.* 1980;21:27–35.

Werry J, Weiss G, Douglas V, et al. Studies on the hyperactive child III: the effects of chlorpromazine upon behavior and learning ability. *J Am Acad Child Psychiatry.* 1966;5:292–312.

Werry JS, ed. *Pediatric Psychopharmacology: The Use of Behavior Modifying Drugs in Children.* New York, NY: Brunner/Mazel; 1978.

Werry JS. The safety of desipramine [letter]. *J Am Acad Child Adolesc Psychiatry.* 1994;33:588–589.

Werry JS, Aman MG, eds. *Practitioner's Guide to Psychoactive Drugs for Children and Adolescents.* 2nd ed. New York, NY: Plenum Medical Book; 1999.

West A, Weinstein S, Peters A, et al. Child- and family-focused cognitive-behavioral therapy for pediatric bipolar disorder: a randomized clinical trial. *J Am Acad Child Adolesc Psychiatry.* 2014;53(11):1168–1178.

West L, Brunssen S, Waldrop J. Review of the evidence for treatment of children with autism with selective serotonin reuptake inhibitors. *J Spec Pediatr Nurs.* 2009;14:183–191.

Whalen CK, Henker B, Swanson JM, et al. Natural social behaviors in hyperactive children: dose effects of methylphenidate. *J Consult Clin Psychol.* 1987;55:187–193.

White L, Tursky B, Schwartz GE, eds. *Placebo: Theory, Research, and Mechanisms.* New York, NY: Guilford Press; 1985.

Wigal S, Swanson JM, Feifel D, et al. A double-blind, placebo-controlled trial of dexmethylphenidate hydrochloride and *d, l-threo-*methylphenidate hydrochloride in children with attention-deficit/hyperactivity disorder. *J Am Acad Child Adolesc Psychiatry.* 2004;43:1406–1414.

Wigal SB, McGough JJ, McCracken JT, et al. A laboratory school comparison of mixed amphetamine salts extended release (Adderall XR) and atomoxetine (Strattera) in school-aged children with attention deficit/hyperactivity disorder. *J Atten Disord.* 2005;9(1):275–289.

Wijemanne S, Wu LJ, Jankovic J. Long-term efficacy and safety of fluphenazine in patients with Tourette syndrome. *Mov Disord.* 2014;29:126–130.

Wilens T, McBurnett K, Stein M, et al. ADHD treatment with once-daily OROS methylphenidate: final results from a long-term open-label study. *J Am Acad Child Adolesc Psychiatry.* 2005;44:1015–1023.

Wilens TE, Biederman J, Baldessarini RJ, et al. Developmental changes in serum concentrations of desipramine and 2-hydroxydesipramine during treatment with desipramine. *J Am Acad Child Adolesc Psychiatry.* 1992;31:691–698.

Wilens TE, Biederman J, Baldessarini RJ, et al. Electrocardiographic effects of desipramine and 2-hydroxydesipramine in children, adolescents, and adults treated with desipramine. *J Am Acad Child Adolesc Psychiatry.* 1993a;32:798–804.

Wilens TE, Biederman J, Geist DE, et al. Nortriptyline in the treatment of ADHD: a chart review of 58 cases. *J Am Acad Child Adolesc Psychiatry.* 1993b;32:343–349.

Wilens TE, Biederman J, March JS, et al. Absence of cardiovascular adverse effects of sertraline in children and adolescents. *J Am Acad Child Adolesc Psychiatry.* 1999;38:573–577.

Wilens TE, Biederman J, Spencer T. Clonidine for sleep disturbances associated with attention-deficit hyperactivity disorder. *J Am Acad Child Adolesc Psychiatry.* 1994;33:424–426.

Wilens TE, Spencer TJ. Combining methylphenidate and clonidine: a clinically sound medication option/ and affirmative rebuttal [Debate Forum]. *J Am Acad Child Adolesc Psychiatry.* 1999;38:614–622.

Wilens TE, Spencer TJ. The stimulants revisited. *Child Adolesc Psychiatr Clin N Am.* 2000;9:573–603.

Williams D, Mehl R, Yudofsky S, et al. The effect of propranolol on uncontrolled rage outbursts in children and adolescents with organic brain dysfunction. *J Am Acad Child Adolesc Psychiatry.* 1982;21(2):129–135.

Winsberg BG, Kupietz SS, Sverd J, et al. Methylphenidate oral dose plasma concentrations and behavioral response in children. *Psychopharmacology.* 1982;76:329–332.

Wisniewski A. New treatment option in resistant schizophrenia in adolescence. *Eur Psychiatry.* 2012;60:5239.

Wolf DV, Wagner KD. Tardive dyskinesia, tardive dystonia, and tardive Tourette's syndrome in children and adolescents. *J Child Adolesc Psychopharmacol.* 1993;3:175–198.

Wolraich ML, Bard DE, Neas B, et al. The psychometric properties of the Vanderbilt attention-deficit hyperactivity disorder diagnostic teacher rating scale in a community population. *J Dev Behav Pediatr.* 2013;34(2):83–93. doi:10.1097/DBP.0b013e31827d55c3.

Woody GE, Poole SA, Subramaniam G, et al. Extended vs short-term buprenorphine-naloxone for treatment of opioid-addicted youth: a randomized trial. *JAMA.* 2008;300(17):2003–2011. Erratum in: *JAMA.* 2009;301(8):830.

Woolston J. Case study: carbamazepine treatment of juvenile-onset bipolar disorder. *J Am Acad Child Adolesc Psychiatry.* 1999;38:335–338.

Wozniak J, Mick E, Waxmonsky J, et al. Comparison of open-label 8-week trials of olanzapine monotherapy and topiramate augmentation of olanzapine for the treatment of pediatric bipolar disorder. *J Child Adolesc Psychopharmacol.* 2009;19(5):539–545.

Wright B, Sims D, Smart S, et al. Melatonin versus placebo in children with autism spectrum conditions and severe sleep problems not amenable to behaviour management strategies: a randomized controlled crossover trial. *J Autism Dev Disord.* 2011;41(2):175–184.

Wu RR, Zhao J-P, Jin H, et al. Lifestyle intervention and metformin for treatment of antipsychotic-induced weight gain: a randomized controlled trial. *JAMA.* 2008;299:185–193.

Wudarsky M, Nicolson R, Hamburger SD, et al. Elevated prolactin in pediatric patients on typical and atypical antipsychotics. *J Child Adolesc Psychopharmacol.* 1999;9:239–245.

Wysowski DK, Barash D. Adverse behavioral reactions attributed to triazolam in the Food and Drug Administration's spontaneous reporting system. *Arch Intern Med.* 1991;151:2003–2008.

Yepes LE, Balka EB, Winsberg BG, et al. Amitriptyline and methylphenidate treatment of behaviorally disordered children. *J Child Psychol Psychiatry.* 1977;18:39–52.

Zametkin A, Rapoport JL, Murphy DL, et al. Treatment of hyperactive children with monoamine oxidase inhibitors: I, clinical efficacy. *Arch Gen Psychiatry.* 1985;42:962–966.

Zametkin AJ, Rapoport JL. Noradrenergic hypothesis of attention deficit disorder with hyperactivity: a critical review. In: Meltzer HY, ed. *Psychopharmacology: The Third Generation of Progress.* New York, NY: Raven Press; 1987:837–842.

Zito JM, Safer DJ, Sai D, et al. Psychotropic medication patterns among youth in foster care. *Pediatrics.* 2008;121(1):157.

Zonfrillo MR, Penn JV, Leonard HL. Pediatric psychotropic polypharmacy. *Psychiatry (Edgmont).* 2005;2(8):14.

Zrull JP, Westman JC, Arthur B, et al. A comparison of chlordiazepoxide, d-amphetamine, and placebo in the treatment of the hyperkinetic syndrome in children. *Am J Psychiatry.* 1963;120:590–591.

Zrull JP, Westman JC, Arthur B, et al. A comparison of diazepam, d-amphetamine, and placebo in the treatment of the hyperkinetic syndrome in children. *Am J Psychiatry.* 1964;121:388–389.

Zubieta JK, Alessi NE. Acute and chronic administration of trazodone in the treatment of disruptive behavior disorders in children. *J Clin Psychopharmacol.* 1992;12:346–351.

Zubieta JK, Bueller JA, Jackson LR, et al. Placebo effects mediated by endogenous opioid activity on μ-opioid receptors. *J Neurosci.* 2005;25(34):7754–7762.

Zuckerman ML, Vaughan BL, Whitney J, et al. Tolerability of selective serotonin reuptake inhibitors in thirty-nine children under age seven: a retrospective chart review. *J Child Adolesc Psychopharmacol.* 2007;17(2):165–174.

Zwier KJ, Rao U. Buspirone use in an adolescent with social phobia and mixed personality disorder (cluster A type). *J Am Acad Child Adolesc Psychiatry.* 1994;33:1007–1011.

Zyprexa [package insert]. Indianapolis, IN: Lilly USA, LLC; 2011.

Index